# Nursing
# Procedures
# & Protocols

# Nursing
# Procedures
# & Protocols

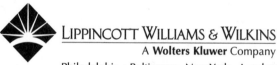

LIPPINCOTT WILLIAMS & WILKINS
A **Wolters Kluwer** Company

Philadelphia • Baltimore • New York • London
Buenos Aires • Hong Kong • Sydney • Tokyo

**STAFF**

**Publisher**
Judith A. Schilling McCann, RN, MSN

**Editorial Director**
William J. Kelly

**Clinical Director**
Joan M. Robinson, RN, MSN

**Senior Art Director**
Arlene Putterman

**Clinical Project Managers**
Denise D. Hayes, RN, CRNP, CCRN, MSN; Beverly Ann Tscheschlog, RN, BS

**Senior Editor**
Ann E. Houska

**Editors**
Rita Doyle, Nancy Priff, Jenifer F. Walker

**Digital Composition Services**
Diane Paluba (manager), Joyce Rossi Biletz (senior desktop assistant), Donna S. Morris (project manager)

**Cover Illustration**
Kris Magyarits

**Manufacturing**
Patricia K. Dorshaw (senior manager), Beth Janae Orr (book production coordinator)

**Editorial Assistants**
Danielle J. Barsky, Carol Caputo, Beverly Lane, Linda Ruhf

**Librarian**
Catherine M. Heslin

**Indexer**
Barbara Hodgson

P&P- D N O S A J J M A M

05 04 03  10 9 8 7 6 5 4 3 2 1

**Library of Congress Cataloging-in-Publication Data**
Nursing procedures & protocols.
    p. ; cm.
Includes index.
    1. Nursing care plans—Handbooks, manuals, etc.
    [DNLM: 1. Nursing Care. 2. Nursing Assessment. WY 100 N9737 2003]
I. Title: Nursing procedures and protocols. II. Lippincott Williams & Wilkins.
    RT49.N88 2003
    610.73—dc21
ISBN 1-58255-237-1 (pbk. : alk. paper)        2002156113

# Contents

# Contributors and consultants

**Elizabeth Archer, RN, EdD(C)**
Assistant Professor
Baptist College of Health Sciences
Memphis

**Susan D. Bell, RN, MS, CNRN, CNP**
Neurosurgery Nurse Practitioner
Ohio State University Medical Center
Columbus

**Nancy L. Bocchino, MSN, CRNP**
Geriatric Nurse Practitioner
Graduate Hospital
Philadelphia

**Mary Bouchaud, RN, MSN, CNS, CRRN**
Faculty
Thomas Jefferson University
College of Health Professions
Philadelphia

**Cheryl Brady, RN, MSN**
Adjunct Faculty
Youngstown Ohio State University

**Barbara Shelton Broome, MSN, PhD**
Chair, Community Mental Health
University of South Alabama, College of
    Nursing
Mobile

**Carol Calianno, RN, MSN, CWOCN**
Wound, Ostomy, Continence Nurse
    Specialist
Abramson's Center for Jewish Life
North Wales, Pa.

**Louise Diehl-Opinger, RN, MSN, APRN, BC,**
    **CCRN, CLNC**
Pokave-Mascarenhas Cardiology
Phillipsburg, N.J.

**Laurie Donaghy, RN**
Emergency Department Charge Nurse
Nazareth Hospital
Philadelphia

**Shelba Durston, RN, MSN, CCRN**
Adjunct Faculty
San Joaquin Delta College
Stockton, Calif.

**Maryann Foley, RN, BSN**
Independent Consultant
Flourtown, Pa.

**Athena A. Foreman, RN, MSN**
Nursing Coordinator
Stanly Community College
Albemarle, N.C.

**Ellie Z. Franges, MSN, CNRN**
Director of Neuroscience Services
Sacred Heart Hospital
Allentown, Pa.

**Mary F. Gerard, RN, BSN, CCRN**
Staff Nurse, Critical Care
Phoenix Health Care
Englewood Cliffs, N.J.

**Patricia Greer, RN**
Instructor, Practical Nursing
Tennessee Technology Center
Paris, Tenn.

**Elaine L. Gross, RN, MSN**
Assistant Professor
Temple University
Philadelphia

**Sandy Hamilton, RN, BSN, MEd, CRNI**
Regional Coordinator of Pharmacy
    Nursing Services
Kindred Pharmacy Services
Las Vegas

**Nancy Haynes, RN, MN, CCRN**
Assistant Professor
Saint Luke's College
Kansas City, Mo.

**Shelton M. Hisley, RNC, WHNP, PhD**
Assistant Professor, School of Nursing
University of North Carolina at
  Wilmington

**Gary R. Jones, MSN, ARNP**
ARNP Coordinator
Mercy Disease Management Program and
  Heart Failure Program
Mercy Health Center
Fort Scott, Kan.

**JoAnne Konick-McMahan, RN, MSN, CCRN**
Inglis Foundation
School of Nursing
University of Pennsylvania
Philadelphia

**Patricia A. Lange-Otsuka, MSN, EdD,**
  **APRN, BC**
Associate Professor of Nursing
Hawaii Pacific University
Kaneohe

**Linda Laskowski-Jones, RN, MS, CCRN,**
  **CEN, CS**
Director, Trauma, Emergency and
  Aeromedical Services
Christiana Hospital
Newark, Del.

**Anita Lockhart, RN,C, MSN**
Independent Consultant
Wynnewood, Pa.

**Lynda A. Mackin, RN, MS, ANP, CN, CNS**
Assistant Clinical Professor
University of California
San Francisco

**Jennifer McWha, RN, MSN**
Vocational Nursing Instructor
Delmar College
Corpus Christi, Tex.

**Donna Marie Mohr, RN, BSN**
Clinical Coordinator of Outpatient
  Neuroscience Services
Sacred Heart Hospital
Allentown, Pa.

**Maureen A. Seckel, RN, MSN, APN, CCRN**
Medical and Pulmonary Clinical Nurse
  Specialist
Christiana Care Health System
Newark, Del.

**Amy Shay, RN, MS, CCRN, CS**
Pulmonary Clinical Nurse Specialist
Miami Valley Hospital
Dayton, Ohio

**Concha Carrollo Sitter, MS, APN, FNP, CGRN**
GI Nurse Practitioner
Sterling Rock Falls Clinic
Sterling, Ill.

**Mary A. Stahl, RN, MSN, APRN, BC, CCRN**
Clinical Nurse Specialist
St. Luke's Hospital
Kansas City, Mo.

**Linda Wood, RN, MSN**
Director of Practical Nursing
Massanutten Technical Center
Harrisonburg, Va.

**Karen Zulkowski, RN, DNSC, CWS**
Assistant Professor, College of Nursing
Montana State University
Bozeman

# Foreword

In this era of increased scrutiny regarding patient safety and the drive toward standardizing patient care to control spiraling health care costs, nurses need and want reliable, research-based protocols and procedures. *Nursing Procedures & Protocols* provides both in a single quick-access, easy-to-use book.

The protocols and procedures in *Nursing Procedures & Protocols* are designed to help nurses react quickly and correctly to a wide range of clinical situations — an essential benefit in today's environment where smaller staffs mean fewer colleagues to turn to for expert advice.

This authoritative book presents scores of peer-reviewed clinical protocols, which are the frameworks for managing disorders, and hundreds of associated procedures, which are detailed, step-by-step processes. Each of the 12 chapters gives you the associated protocols and procedures for a particular topic area: fundamentals, infection control, medication administration, intravascular therapy, cardiovascular care, pulmonary care, neurologic care, gastrointestinal care, renal and urologic care, musculoskeletal care, skin care, and endocrine and hematologic care. For example, in chapter 6, you'll find, in the Protocols section, the complete protocol for managing a patient requiring ventilatory assistance, along with a list of the procedures related to that protocol: arterial puncture for blood gas analysis, endotracheal intubation, endotracheal tube care, end-tidal carbon dioxide monitoring, I.V. bolus injection, manual ventilation, mechanical ventilation, mixed venous oxygen saturation monitoring, oxygen administration, peripheral I.V. line maintenance, prone positioning, pulse and ear oximetry, tracheal cuff-pressure measurement, tracheal suction, tracheostomy care, total parenteral nutrition, and venipuncture. To complete the protocol, if you need to double-check the procedure for performing arterial puncture for blood gas analysis, you'll turn to the alphabetized Procedures section of the chapter, where each procedure is given in its entirety. In some cases, a particular procedure associated with a protocol in one chapter will be detailed in another chapter; this is because protocol topics are fluid and overlap in some areas.

To make *Nursing Procedures & Protocols* an easy-to-use reference, the contributors and editors use a consistent, logical format for all protocols and procedures. Thus, once you take a few moments to look at the book, you'll always know exactly where to go for the specific information you need. Plus, each protocol and procedure includes references and supporting documentation that assures the credibility of the nursing care described.

The text also provides more than 300 illustrations, checklists, tables, and flowcharts to augment and further clarify the protocols and procedures. *Nurs-*

*ing Procedures & Protocols* also uses logos to draw your eye to some important recurring themes:

▶ The *Evidence base* logo signals key information based on current research results.

▶ The *Troubleshooting* logo accompanies ready-access information on diagnosing and correcting equipment problems.

▶ The *Alert!* logo draws your attention to potential dangers — in some cases, life-threatening dangers — and tells you how to avoid them.

Given the current demand for efficient, cost-effective, standardized care, we all need reliable guidance in the form of well-researched, clearly written nursing protocols and procedures. *Nursing Procedures & Protocols* meets these needs — as you'll see when you flip through it and, more important, when you use it in your daily practice.

**Michelle L. Dumpe, RN, MS, PhD**
Director of Research, Education, and
    Quality Management
Division of Nursing
Cleveland Clinic Foundation

# 1

# Fundamentals

**F**OR MOST PEOPLE, HOSPITALIZATION IS ONE OF THE MOST DIFFICULT TIMES IN THEIR LIFE. Being in the hospital involves illness and causes disrupted daily routine, loss of privacy, and loss of control over life events. In addition to being the direct caregiver, the nurse may need to provide for the patient and his family, offering teaching, counseling, coordination of services, development of community support systems, and assistance in coping with health-related lifestyle changes. In many facilities, staff nurses, primary nurses, clinical nurse specialists, and advanced practitioners provide some or all of these vital services.

This chapter covers the fundamentals of nursing: physical assessment and preoperative and postoperative care. Besides providing a review of nursing fundamentals, this chapter also covers procedures such as passive range-of-motion exercises, use of restraints, care of the dying patient, spiritual care, and postmortem care.

This chapter also covers nursing protocols such as managing the dying patient, managing the patient at risk for falls, and managing the patient who needs physical restraint.

# Protocols

## Managing the dying patient

### Purpose
To provide for the physical, spiritual, and psychosocial well-being of the dying patient and his family, to ensure patient and family dignity, and to encourage their control over care and treatment decisions

### Collaborative level
Interdependent

### Expected patient outcomes
▶ The patient in the end-stage of life will maintain his dignity and will receive maximum physical, psychological, and spiritual comfort.
▶ The patient's family and significant others will be able to assist in the physical and psychological care of their loved one and will be given emotional support during the grief process.

### Definition of terms
▶ *Hospice care:* A health care system that incorporates the concept of palliative care and is designed to support the physical, psychosocial, and spiritual needs of the patient and his family at the end of life. This type of care affirms the idea that the patient and his family deserve to be completely in-

formed about the patient's medical condition and all treatment alternatives.
▶ *Bereavement counseling:* Support services provided for surviving family members and significant others who are going through the grief process as they try to cope with their loss.

### Indications
Treatment
▶ Physical pain and discomfort
▶ Patient and family grief
▶ Loss of dignity

Prevention
▶ Advance Directive to ensure proper communication of the patient's care and treatment choices to the health care team
▶ Chaplain services or other spiritual support
▶ Family counseling to assist both the patient and family through the grief process

### Assessment guidance
Signs and symptoms
▶ Pain and discomfort
▶ Expressions of anger toward caregivers
▶ Difficulty expressing emotions
▶ Cheyne-Stokes respirations (shortly before death)

## Diagnostic studies
▶ Only if requested, to diagnose a treatable source of pain such as new tumor growth.

## Nursing interventions
▶ Help the patient and his family go through the five stages of the grief process: shock and denial, anger, bargaining, depression, and acceptance.
▶ Provide pain relief and comfort measures and discuss inadequate pain relief with the doctor.
▶ Antidepressants and anticonvulsants may also be used to help alleviate pain.
▶ Anticipate and promptly treat adverse effects of pain medications.
▶ Prevent skin breakdown by using turning regimens and pressure-reducing mattresses, by frequently inspecting the patient's skin, and by keeping the skin clean and dry.
▶ Use passive range-of-motion (ROM) exercises to optimize circulation and prevent painful muscle contractures.
▶ Explore respiratory-assistive options with the patient, his family, or both to help minimize the discomfort in a patient having difficulty breathing.
▶ Be familiar with the patient's and his family's cultural beliefs about death and dying.
▶ Ensure that the Advance Directive still meets the patient's and his family's wishes.
▶ Inform the patient's family about support groups and other services to help them through the grief process.
▶ Provide postmortem care, according to hospital policy.
▶ Allow time for the patient's family to be alone with their loved one after death.

## Patient teaching
▶ Provide grief support for the patient and his family, encouraging them to discuss their feelings openly with each other.
▶ Provide assistance when needed in making end-of-life care decisions.
▶ Provide information regarding support groups and bereavement counseling.
▶ Be knowledgeable of the patient's cultural beliefs about death and dying.
▶ Inform his family about passive ROM exercises, if appropriate.

## Precautions
▶ Ensure that everyone on the health care team is familiar with the patient's Advance Directive.
▶ Occasionally, the health care team may need help coping with the care of a dying patient. Provide support group sessions for the team members, as needed, so they can give their patient the best care and support.

## Contraindications
The patient's Advance Directive should be reviewed to determine contraindications to treatment.

## Documentation
▶ Document that an Advance Directive exists in the patient's chart.
▶ Document postmortem care properly, according to hospital policy.
▶ Document all care given to patient and family before and during hospitalization, and all postmortem care.

## Related procedures
▶ Alignment and pressure-reducing devices
▶ Care of the dying patient
▶ Clinitron therapy bed
▶ Passive range-of-motion exercises
▶ Physical assessment
▶ Postmortem care
▶ Spiritual care

### REFERENCES
Abrahm, J.L. "Management of Pain and Spinal Cord Compression in Patients with Advanced Cancer," *Annals of Internal Medicine* 13(1):37-46, July 1999.

Block, S.D. "Assessing and Managing Depression in the Terminally Ill Patient," *Annals of Internal Medicine* 132(3):209-18, February 2000.

Easley, M.K., and Elliott, S. "Managing Pain at the End of Life," *Nursing Clinics of North America* 36(4):779-94, December 2001.

Kessler, D. *The Needs of the Dying: A Guide for Bringing Hope, Comfort and Love to Life's Final Chapter.* New York: Harper Collins, 2000.

Whitecar, P.S., et al. "Managing Pain in the Dying Patient," *American Family Physician* 61(3):755-64, February 2000.

# Managing the immobile patient

## Purpose
To prevent multisystem complications caused by immobility and to provide timely assessments and interventions when signs of complications arise; to provide for the psychosocial well-being of the patient and family

## Collaborative level
Interdependent

## Expected patient outcomes
▶ The patient will be free from multisystem complications resulting from immobility. These systems include cardiopulmonary, cardiovascular, musculoskeletal, integumentary, gastrointestinal (GI), and genitourinary (GU).
▶ The patient and his family will develop appropriate coping mechanisms to adapt to temporary or permanent loss of mobility.

## Definition of terms
▶ *Immobility:* The temporary or permanent state in which a patient can't move, or has difficulty moving in the environment, to complete tasks. Immobility may result from prolonged bedrest caused by illness, chronic disease or disability states, old age, obesity, or recovery periods after surgery. It's important to note that physical complications from immobility can occur within 48 hours of immobilization.

## Indications
### Treatment
▶ Pulmonary effects, such as increased congestion, shallow breathing
▶ Cardiovascular effects, such as hypotension, leg edema, thrombophlebitis
▶ Breakdown in skin integrity such as pressure ulcers
▶ Muscle weakness, joint stiffness
▶ Nutritional and fluid imbalances
▶ Bowel incontinence or constipation
▶ Urinary incontinence or retention
▶ Psychosocial needs such as recreational activities
▶ Educational needs of the patient and his family

### Prevention
▶ Pneumonia
▶ Falls from hypotensive reactions
▶ Deep vein thrombosis (DVT)
▶ Skin breakdown
▶ Muscle atrophy and joint contractures
▶ Negative nitrogen balance
▶ Bowel impaction, ileus
▶ Renal calculi and renal infection

## Assessment guidance
### Signs and symptoms
▶ Ineffective breathing patterns
▶ Ineffective airway clearance
▶ Vertigo
▶ Leg pain (especially in lower leg or calf)
▶ Decreased skin sensation in any area
▶ Joint pain
▶ Muscle aches or difficulty with ROM
▶ Poor appetite
▶ Abdominal pain
▶ Nausea and vomiting
▶ Pain or burning with urination
▶ Flank pain
▶ Adventitious lung sounds (crackles, rhonchi, wheezes)
▶ Elevated temperature
▶ Increase in sputum production
▶ Change in sputum color, consistency, odor
▶ Orthostatic hypotension
▶ Lower leg or thigh edema, tightness
▶ Calf redness, warmth
▶ Decreased pedal pulses
▶ Skin redness or breaks in skin integrity
▶ Improper alignment of body
▶ Decreased ROM or new pain with movement
▶ Decreased bowel sounds
▶ Abdominal tenderness
▶ Change in pattern of urine output
▶ Increased urinary sediment
▶ Changes in input and output patterns

### Diagnostic studies
#### Laboratory tests
▶ Sputum culture
▶ Urinalysis and urine cultures
▶ Creatinine level
▶ White blood cell (WBC) count
▶ Electrolytes (especially calcium level)

#### Imaging tests
▶ Flat plate abdomen
▶ Bone films
▶ Venogram
▶ Doppler studies

*Other*
▶ Pulmonary function tests
▶ Electrocardiogram (ECG)

## Nursing interventions
▶ Change the patient's position every 2 hours, ensuring that his body weight is evenly distributed and body alignment is normal.
▶ Inspect the skin over pressure points, especially over bony prominences, with each position change.
▶ Keep bed linens dry and free from wrinkles.
▶ Provide regular toileting to prevent incontinence.
▶ Use rotating beds and other specialized mattresses for patients who are most at risk for complications.
▶ Avoid the use of donut-shaped cushions. These only create further compression surrounding the initial problem site.
▶ If pressure ulcer occurs, intervene immediately to prevent further breakdown. For example, a stage 1 or 2 ulcer can be treated with a hydrocolloid dressing to prevent advancement to a stage 3 ulcer.
▶ Encourage regular use of incentive spirometers every hour while awake.
▶ Encourage the patient to lie on his side, unless contraindicated.
▶ Auscultate lung fields and report variances.
▶ Explain to the patient and his family the need for ongoing exercise and physical therapy to limit the degree of deconditioning.
▶ Use isotonic (dynamic) and isometric (static) exercise routines as part of the patient's daily therapy schedule. If a joint is inflamed, use isometric exercise.
▶ Encourage the patient to follow a well-balanced diet and maintain adequate fluid intake. Ensure that a dietitian is monitoring the patient.
▶ Monitor electrolyte values.
▶ Advise the use of support hose or sequential compression devices to prevent clot formation and ensure circulatory health.
▶ Assess bowel sounds each shift. Provide stool softeners and laxatives for constipation. If needed, assess patient digitally for fecal impaction.
▶ Monitor and report signs of urinary retention.
▶ Encourage the patient to participate in individual and group activities.

▶ Play therapy is ideal for hospitalized children. Encourage crafts, reading, or other activities, depending on the patient's interests and hobbies.
▶ Always involve the patient and his family in the care plan. Give positive reinforcement for every small gain.

## Patient teaching
▶ Teach the patient and his family proper body mechanics for moving or repositioning the patient.
▶ Teach caregivers the signs and symptoms of complications related to immobility and how to deal with them.
▶ Give the patient and his family important information regarding community resources, support groups, home health agencies, and meal delivery services.
▶ Provide all available written educational materials to help reinforce verbal education.

## Precautions
▶ For the paralyzed patient, always ensure proper alignment of all extremities to prevent complications. Avoid pressure over areas where nerves run superficially over bony prominences, and avoid pressure over the brachial plexus.

## Contraindications
The doctor should specify the contraindications, according to the patient's condition. For example, if a patient develops DVT, ROM exercises to the affected extremity may be contraindicated.

## Documentation
▶ All measures to prevent complications of immobility on the nursing care plans and flow sheets
▶ All systemic complications caused by the patient being immobilized, including appropriate assessments and interventions taken as well as patient response to treatment
▶ Teaching sessions with the patient and his family, noting if further reinforcement is needed

## Related procedures
▶ Alignment and pressure-reducing devices
▶ Clinitron therapy bed
▶ Passive range-of-motion exercises
▶ Physical assessment

▶ Postoperative care
▶ Rotation beds
▶ Sequential compression therapy
▶ Spiritual care

## REFERENCES

"Immobility," *Core Curriculum for Ortho-paedic Nurses,* 4th ed. Pitman, N.J.: National Association of Orthopaedic Nurses, 2001.

Markey, D.W., and Brown, R.J. "An Interdisciplinary Approach to Addressing Patient Activity and Mobility in the Medical-Surgical Patient," *Journal of Nursing Care Quality* 16(4):1-12, July 2002.

Melland, H.I., et al. "Clinical Evaluation of an Automated Turning Bed," *Orthopaedic Nursing* 18(4):65-70, July-August 1999.

# Managing the patient at risk for falling

## Purpose
To prevent patient injury by providing a safe physical environment and by instituting nursing measures that minimize the patient's risk of falls

## Collaborative level
Interdependent

## Expected patient outcomes
▶ The patient at risk for falling will be protected from injury through astute nursing assessments and safety interventions.
▶ The patient and his family will be well-informed about home safety issues.

## Definition of terms
▶ *Fall:* A sudden, unanticipated change in the body's center of gravity that may cause injury.
▶ *Falls risk assessment:* A nursing assessment tool that categorizes patients as having a low, moderate, or high risk for falls. Indicators include history of chronic disease, such as diabetes and osteoporosis; altered elimination patterns; sensory impairments; medications, such as steroids, tranquilizers, narcotics, antidepressants, and antihypertensive; and altered cognitive functioning.

## Indications
### Treatment
▶ Need for a fall safety care plan individualized for each patient
▶ Injuries resulting from falls, such as fractures, sprains, and strains

### Prevention
▶ Injuries resulting from falls, such as fractures, sprains, and strains
▶ Pain
▶ Neurovascular impairment
▶ Infection
▶ Complications from immobility, such as pneumonia, DVT, pulmonary embolus, pressure ulcers, ileus, urinary tract infections, and muscle atrophy and contractures
▶ Loss of independence
▶ Loss of self-esteem
▶ Depression and anxiety
▶ Death

## Assessment guidance
### Signs and symptoms
▶ Previous falls
▶ Immobilization or prolonged period of immobilization
▶ Increased age
▶ Poor appetite
▶ Fatigue, weakness, or lethargy
▶ Continence problems
▶ Depression and anxiety
▶ Unsteady gait
▶ Diminished mental capacity or confusion
▶ Sensory, visual, and perceptual impairments
▶ History of chronic disease
▶ Malnutrition
▶ Dehydration (dry or poor skin turgor, dry mucosal membranes, sunken eyes)
▶ Alteration in elimination
▶ Use of steroids, tranquilizers, antidepressants
▶ Noncompliance

### Diagnostic studies
*Laboratory tests*
▶ Complete blood count (CBC)
▶ Urinalysis for occult blood
▶ Cardiac enzymes

*Imaging tests*
▶ X-ray
▶ Magnetic resonance imaging (MRI)
▶ Computed tomography (CT)
▶ Bone scan

## Nursing interventions

▶ Assess the patient's falls risk on admission with a thorough nursing history.
▶ Implement an individualized falls assessment and safety plan for the patient to minimize the risk of injury.
▶ Reevaluate the patient's falls risk every shift, every day, or at other set intervals established by the health care facility.
▶ Place beds in low positions with brakes locked.
▶ Place call signal and personal items within the patient's reach.
▶ Maintain a clutter-free room, ensuring all pathways and doorways are obstacle free.
▶ Keep floors dry; wipe up all spills.
▶ Turn on the bathroom light or night-light during the evening and night shifts.
▶ Give the patient nonskid footwear.
▶ Position side rails up, down, or halfway up, according to hospital guidelines and the patient's circumstances.
▶ Assess the patient's response to all medications and report any deviations from expected outcomes.
▶ Implement an exercise regimen to improve and maintain the patient's strength and endurance, as appropriate.
▶ Suggest that a geriatric nurse practitioner be consulted to provide guidance in developing the patient's care plan.
▶ Assess and provide for regular elimination patterns, to avoid incontinence.
▶ Assess patient for restraint-free safety and positioning devices, and implement, as needed.
▶ Communicate the patient's falls risk level to the multidisciplinary team.
▶ Place signs at the head of the bed to alert the patient's family and all staff of his higher risk for falls.
▶ Place a color-coded armband on the patient that identifies him as at risk for falling.
▶ Ensure prompt responses to the call signal.
▶ Enlist the support of the patient's family to sit with him.
▶ Institute the restraint policy only when all interventions have been unsuccessful and the patient is determined to be a risk to himself.

## Patient teaching

▶ Teach the patient and his family about the facility's Fall Safety program.
▶ Instruct the patient about the possible risks and complications of a fall.
▶ Instruct the patient to use the call signal if he needs assistance.
▶ Teach the patient and his family about wheelchair safety (for example, locking brakes).
▶ Train the patient in the use of assistive devices, if indicated.
▶ Teach the patient and his family how to maintain a safe home environment and provide written materials when available. Have an occupational therapist make a home visit, if possible, to make recommendations for a safe environment.
▶ Instruct the patient on proper footwear and shoe fit to prevent foot problems and falls.

## Precautions

▶ Increased risk for falls as patient's confusion increases.

## Documentation

▶ Make sure an initial Falls Risk Assessment is documented in the nursing history and physical.
▶ Start the standard care plan for falls prevention, or expand on the standard plan to individualize it to the patient at higher risk for falls.
▶ If a patient falls, whether he's injured or not, the progress notes should contain:
  – objective account of a witnessed fall or how a patient was found if the fall wasn't witnessed
  – patient activity at the time of the fall
  – location of the fall
  – symptoms reported by the patient before falling
  – documentation of injuries or patient complaints
  – doctor notification and follow-up documentation
  – notification of the patient's family, if indicated
  – use of assistive devices or restraints at the time of the fall
  – modifications of interventions instituted as a result of the fall.
▶ Document all patient and family teaching.

## Related procedures

▶ Alignment and pressure-reducing devices
▶ Passive ROM exercises
▶ Physical assessment
▶ Postoperative care

▶ Seizure precautions
▶ Sequential compression therapy

## REFERENCES
Parker, R. "Assessing the Risk of Falls among Older Inpatients," *Professional Nurse* 15(8): 511-14, May 2000.

Richmond, T.S., et al. "Characteristics and Outcomes of Serious Traumatic Injury in Older Adults," *Journal of the American Geriatric Society* 50(2):215-22, February 2002.

Vassallo, M., et al. "Characteristics of Single Fallers and Recurrent Fallers among Hospital In-patients," *Gerontology* 48(3): 147-50, May-June 2002.

# Managing the patient who needs physical restraint

## Purpose
To provide restraint-free care, patient safety, and patient comfort and well-being when physical restraints are used

## Collaborative level
Interdependent

## Expected patient outcomes
▶ The patient will have restraint-free care.
▶ The patient will have restraints applied only after alternative interventions to restraints have been evaluated and have failed to:
 –preserve indwelling lines and tubes
 –prevent injury to the patient or to others.

## Definition of terms
▶ *Restraint:* The direct application of physical force to a patient, with or without the patient's permission, to restrict his freedom of movement. The physical force may be human, mechanical devices, or a combination thereof. Restraints should be used only in situations when it's essential to protect patients from harming themselves, other patients, or staff. Health care providers need to be aware of the associated risks of using restraints.
▶ *Medical immobilization:* Customary safety devices required to limit a patient's movement for the purpose of performing medical, surgical, or diagnostic procedures, which are based on standard practice for the procedure.

▶ *Adaptive devices:* Devices providing postural support, protection, and comfort to patients with neurologic, orthopedic, or muscular impairment.
▶ *Forensic restraints:* restraints used for security purposes by law enforcement agencies and officers. This exception doesn't apply to restraints used in the clinical care of such patients.
▶ *Soft restraints:* Restraints that feel soft and are usually made of cloth. Examples are limb, vest, lap, and mitt restraints.
▶ *Hard restraints:* Restraints in the form of limb cuffs that are made of leather or hard synthetic material. They may have locks and keys.
▶ *Seclusion:* The involuntary confinement of a person in a locked room.
▶ *Behavioral health care restraint and seclusion standards:* The behavioral health care standards for restraint and seclusion apply to any use of restraint and seclusion for behavioral health care reasons. Restraint or seclusion for a behavioral health care disorder is different from restraint to promote medical or surgical healing.
▶ *Behavioral health care settings:* Facilities where restraint or seclusion is used, such as free-standing psychiatric hospitals, psychiatric units in general hospitals, and residential treatment centers.
▶ *Nonbehavioral health care settings:* Nonbehavioral health care facilities in which restraint or seclusion is used for behavioral health care reasons, such as acute care hospitals and emergency departments. These patients are usually restrained to kept from harming themselves or others because of hostile, aggressive behavior.
▶ *Restraint or seclusion for behavioral health care reasons:* Restraint used primarily to protect the patient against injury to self or others because of an emotional or behavioral disorder.
▶ *Restraint for medical or surgical reasons:* Restraint standards for medical or surgical purposes apply when the primary reason for use directly supports medical healing.
▶ *Chemical restraint:* A drug used to control behavior or to restrict a patient's freedom of movement that isn't part of the standard treatment for the patient's medical or psychiatric condition. Psychoactive drugs given as needed aren't considered chemical restraints.

## Indications
### Treatment
▶ Noncompliance with treatment
▶ Risk of falling
▶ Wandering
▶ Hostile, aggressive behavior

### Prevention
▶ Injury and death from potentially harmful patient actions

## Assessment guidance
### Signs and symptoms
▶ Change in mental status
▶ Impaired judgment
▶ Pulling on indwelling lines and tubes
▶ Lack of safety awareness
▶ Unable to follow caregiver safety instructions
▶ Attempting to get up without assistance in presence of an unsteady gait
▶ Unsafe wandering
▶ Combative behavior
▶ Hostile, aggressive behavior

### Diagnostic studies
*Laboratory tests*
▶ WBC count
▶ Blood cultures

*Imaging tests*
▶ MRI
▶ CT scan

*Other*
▶ Blood urea nitrogen (BUN) and creatinine
▶ Thyroid-stimulating hormone
▶ Blood toxicology
▶ ECG

## Nursing interventions
### Decision-making and restraint order requirements
▶ Notify the doctor of any significant change in the patient's condition so a medical workup and treatment can be started.
▶ Base your assessment of the patient's individual needs on his behaviors and on the fact that a cognitively impaired patient may not be able to verbally express his needs. In these patients, ascertain patient needs by what the patient does because behavior may be the method of communication the patient finds easiest to use. For example, a patient unsafely trying to get out of bed may be communicating his need to go to the toilet.
▶ As an alternative to restraint, try other ways to meet the patient's needs. If alternative measures have been evaluated and have failed to meet the patient's safety needs, restrain the patient and get a doctor's time-limited order according to institution policy.

### Restraint for medical or surgical reasons
▶ Obtain a time-limited order, which must contain date and time of order, type of restraint, maximum length of time restraint may be used, behaviors that present a danger to the patient or others requiring the use of restraint, and behaviors that must be exhibited by the patient in order for the restraint to be discontinued.
▶ Renew the order 24 hours after the initial restraint application and then every calendar day thereafter that the patient continues to be restrained. The patient must be evaluated daily in person by a doctor.

### Restraint for behavioral health care reasons
▶ The patient must be evaluated by a doctor within 1 hour of restraint application and every 24 hours thereafter for continued restraint.
▶ After nursing assessment of the continued need for restraint, get a time-limited order renewal by telephone:
 – every 4 hours for adults
 – every 2 hours for children ages 9 to 18
 – every 1 hour for children younger than age 9.
▶ A time-limited restraint order must contain: Date and time, type of restraint, maximum length of time restraint may be used, behaviors that present a danger to the patient or others requiring the use of restraint, and behaviors that must be exhibited by the patient in order for the restraint to be discontinued.
▶ A patient behaving hostilely or aggressively may be given a drug as a restraint, to calm him or to protect him or others from harm. A doctor or other licensed independent practitioner must see and evaluate this patient within 1 hour of starting the drug.

### Restraint application
▶ Teach staff alternatives to restraints, how to apply and remove restraints, and how to

monitor restrained patients. (Instruction for behavioral health care facility staff is more comprehensive than that for staff in nonbehavioral health care facilities without a psychiatric unit.)
▶ Perform a baseline assessment of distal pulses and assess skin integrity before applying restraints.
▶ Secure restraints to a stationary frame, never to side rails, removable head boards or footboards, or any moving parts, to allow for quick release.

### Care of the restrained patient
▶ Visually observe the patient for safety, agitation, or mental status changes, proper restraint placement, and accessibility of the call signal at frequency defined in institutional policy for those restrained for medical or surgical reasons.
▶ Patients restrained for behavioral health care reasons should be observed every 15 minutes.
▶ Remove restraints every 2 hours, and then follow these steps:
  – Check distal pulses.
  – Check skin integrity under the restraint.
  – Perform ROM exercises.
  – Change the patient's position.
  – Offer fluids, if appropriate.
  – Help the patient with meals and hygiene.
  – Offer the bedpan or a urinal or help the patient to the bathroom.
▶ Reassess the treatment plan, the continued need for restraints, and alternatives to restraints if the patient has been restrained for more than 72 hours continuously or has been restrained more than four separate times in 7 days, before reapplication. Remove restraints if appropriate or consider using less-restrictive restraints.
▶ Walk with the patient at least every 4 hours, depending on the patient's condition.

## Patient teaching
▶ Explain to the patient why he's being restrained, including specific behaviors exhibited by the patient.
▶ Explain that restraints will be used only until an effective alternative is in place.
▶ Explain to the patient's family that if they can sit with him, restraints may not be necessary.

## Precautions
▶ Incontinence
▶ Contractures
▶ Muscle wasting and deconditioning
▶ Pressure ulcers
▶ Injury
▶ Emotional or psychological distress
▶ Loss of dignity
▶ Strangulation or asphyxiation (in frail, restless patients who become trapped between the side rail and the mattress)
▶ Increased agitation
▶ Possible risk of compromised respiratory status (with vest restraints)

## Contraindications
▶ Severely agitated patients who fight the restraint
▶ Some patients at risk for seizures

## Documentation
▶ Doctor notification of significant change in condition and doctor response
▶ Assessment of patient behavior before application of restraints
▶ Behavior that triggered restraint use and reason for restraint use (clinical justification required if restraints used)
▶ Alternatives to restraints tried before restraint applied
▶ Type of restraint chosen as the least-restrictive device according to individual needs
▶ Care of the patient while restrained, including when the care occurred (restraint care flow sheets required at many facilities to fulfill documentation requirements)
▶ Reassessment of the treatment plan
▶ Patient and family instruction and response to the instruction
▶ Patient response to the use of restraint for behavioral health care reasons
▶ Rationale for renewal of telephone order in patient restrained for behavioral health care reasons
▶ Specimens obtained and sent to the laboratory
▶ Diagnostic study results

## Related procedures
▶ Alternatives to physical restraint
▶ Arterial puncture for blood gas analysis
▶ Electrocardiography
▶ Passive range-of-motion exercises
▶ Physical assessment
▶ Pulse oximetry

❯ Restraint application
❯ Urine/sputum collection

## REFERENCES
Capezuti, E., et al. "Individualized Assessment and Intervention in Bilateral Side Rail Use," *Geriatric Nursing* 19(6):322-30, November-December 1998.

## ORGANIZATIONS
Food and Drug Administration: *www.fda.gov*
Joint Commission for Accreditation of Healthcare Organizations Standards: *www.jcaho.org*
The Centers for Medicare and Medicaid Services: *www.cms.hhs.gov*

# Managing the patient having a surgical procedure

## Purpose
To teach about and provide care and treatment to ensure the surgical patient a positive outcome

## Collaborative level
Interdependent

## Expected patient outcomes
❯ The patient and his family will be informed and prepared both physically and psychologically for the surgical procedure.
❯ Safety and comfort measures will be provided throughout the preoperative, intraoperative, and postoperative phases of the surgical procedure.
❯ The patient will recover from the procedure free from systemic complications.

## Definition of terms
❯ *Preoperative:* The phase that begins with the patient's decision to have surgery and ends with transfer of the patient into the care of the operating room staff
❯ *Intraoperative:* The phase that begins with transfer of the patient into the surgical suite and ends with his transfer to the recovery room
❯ *Postoperative:* The phase that begins with transfer of the patient to the recovery room and ends with his return to preoperative functioning

## Indications
### Treatment
#### Preoperative
❯ Verification of procedure
❯ Verification of informed consent
❯ Vital signs
❯ Assessment of skin condition
❯ Assessment of mobility
❯ Verification of allergies
❯ Assessment of body systems, noting abnormalities and injuries
❯ Documentation of previous surgeries
❯ Documentation and intervention for sensory impairments
❯ Neurovascular assessment
❯ Review of diagnostic studies and deviations
❯ Presence of implants and prostheses
❯ Substance abuse screening
❯ Begin discharge planning
❯ Verification of nothing-by-mouth status, if indicated
❯ Administration of preoperative medication, if ordered

#### Intraoperative
❯ Collaboration with other members of the surgical team, including anesthesia, to physiologically monitor and assure continuity of care
❯ Proper positioning to assure good skin integrity
❯ Provision of warmth
❯ Provision of thermal regulation, if indicated
❯ Maintenance of patient dignity and respect
❯ Creation and maintenance of a sterile field
❯ Performing sponge, sharps, and instrument counts
❯ Documenting all aspects of intraoperative patient care
❯ Recording all implants, as indicated

#### Postoperative
❯ Initiating an individualized nursing care plan
❯ Collaboration with other members of the multidisciplinary team for care activities
❯ Provision of safety and comfort
❯ Provision of pain relief
❯ Prevention of potential multisystem problems, including musculoskeletal, neurologic, infection, cardiopulmonary, integumentary, GI, fluid balance, and GU

▶ Initiation of a discharge plan that includes family members, social services, if indicated, and community resources
▶ Provision of psychological and spiritual support, if indicated

### Prevention
▶ Pneumonia
▶ Excessive pain
▶ DVT
▶ Muscle contractures
▶ Paresthesia
▶ Infection
▶ Ileus
▶ Pressure ulcers
▶ Depression
▶ Loss of dignity and self-respect
▶ Death

## Assessment guidance
### Signs and symptoms
▶ Anxiety about the procedure or discharge plans
▶ Postoperatively, patient complaints of neurovascular compromise, muscle or joint stiffness, abdominal pains, urinary dysfunction, respiratory difficulty, loss of skin sensation, and generalized or localized pain
▶ Numbness, tingling of extremities
▶ Muscle or joint pain, or both, with range of motion
▶ Abdominal tenderness
▶ Diminished or absent bowel sounds
▶ Fever
▶ Blood in the urine
▶ Adventitious lung sounds
▶ Skin redness or breakdown
▶ Expressions of fear, anger, crying, or withdrawal from staff or family
▶ Inadequate pain relief

### Diagnostic studies
#### Laboratory tests
*Preoperative*
▶ CBC
▶ Prothrombin time
*Postoperative*
▶ Laboratory studies, as ordered, for patient diagnosis and procedure

#### Imaging tests
*Preoperative*
▶ Chest X-ray
▶ MRI
▶ CT scan

*Postoperative*
▶ Imaging tests, as ordered, for patient diagnosis and procedure

## Nursing interventions
▶ Interpret assessment data preoperatively and postoperatively.
▶ Identify actual and potential patient problems; and develop a nursing care plan specific to the patient and the surgical procedure.
▶ Assess the patient's psychosocial health, including his perception of surgery, coping mechanisms, cognitive level, religious and cultural practices, and availability of family support systems.
▶ Monitor the patient for changes in physical status as well as behavioral changes (for example, level of consciousness).
▶ Give I.V. fluids and blood products.
▶ Provide adequate and consistent pain relief to keep the patient comfortable and able to participate in his daily treatment regimen.
▶ Use multidisciplinary clinical pathways to streamline care and to help reduce the length of stay.

## Patient teaching
▶ Provide educational materials or information about preoperative classes available at your hospital.
▶ Postoperatively, reinforce deep-breathing exercises and use of the incentive spirometer.
▶ Tell the patient and his family the reasons for specific therapeutic devices such as sequential compression boots.
▶ Encourage the patient to perform bed exercises approved by his doctor and taught by physical therapy.
▶ If he's able, encourage the patient to change his position every 2 hours while in bed. Provide assistance, if needed.
▶ Tell the patient to alert the staff if abdominal pain, nausea, or vomiting occurs.
▶ Teach the patient who can tolerate a regular diet the importance of good nutrition for proper wound healing.
▶ Teach alternative methods of pain control, such as deep breathing, imagery, or meditation.
▶ Encourage the patient to request pain medication at the first instance of discomfort. Tell him that delaying pain relief only

adds to his anxiety, which can increase pain.

▶ Involve the patient's family in discharge planning.

▶ Encourage as much independence with self-care as possible.

▶ Be available to answer questions and address concerns, whether physical or emotional.

▶ Provide a list of community resources and support groups to assist the patient and his family in their return to wellness.

## Precautions

▶ Ensure that informed consent has been obtained and is in the patient's chart.

▶ Determine whether the patient has an Advance Directive and, if so, place it in the chart.

## Documentation

▶ Document all assessment data with progress notes, flow sheets, and operating room checklists.

▶ Record appropriately on all "pain control" flow sheets, such as patient-controlled analgesia and epidural analgesia forms.

▶ Maintain an updated care plan that shows daily progress, educational needs, and multidisciplinary involvement in interventions to promote health.

▶ Document all system complications with appropriate nursing assessments, interventions, and evaluations of responses.

▶ Maintain an individual patient- and family-teaching record that notes teaching sessions, demonstrations, return demonstrations by the patient and his family, and areas that need further reinforcement or follow-up with home care.

## Related procedures

▶ Alignment and pressure-reducing devices
▶ Epidural analgesia
▶ Hand washing
▶ Hyperthermia and hypothermia blanket
▶ Indwelling catheter insertion
▶ Passive range-of-motion exercises
▶ Physical assessment
▶ Preoperative care
▶ Postoperative care
▶ Preoperative skin preparation
▶ Rotation beds
▶ Sequential compression therapy
▶ Spiritual care
▶ Standard precautions
▶ Surgical wound care

### REFERENCES

Armstrong, D., and Bortz, P. "An Integrative Review of Pressure Relief in Surgical Patients," *AORN* 73(3):645-48, 650-53, 656-57, March 2001.

Good, M., et al. "Relaxation and Music Reduce Pain after Gynecologic Surgery," *Pain Management* 3(2):61-70, June 2002.

Todaro, T., and Schott-Baer, D. "Plan Faster, Healthier Recovery after Orthopedic Surgery," 31(1):24-26, January 2000.

# Procedures

# Alignment and pressure-reducing devices

Various devices can be used to maintain correct body positioning and help prevent complications that often arise when a patient must be on prolonged bed rest. These devices include boots to protect the heels and help prevent skin breakdown and foot-drop; abduction pillows to help prevent internal hip rotation after femoral fracture, hip fracture, or surgery; trochanter rolls to help prevent external hip rotation; and hand rolls to help prevent hand contractures.

Several of these devices—boots, trochanter rolls, and hand rolls—are especially useful when caring for patients who

## Common preventive devices

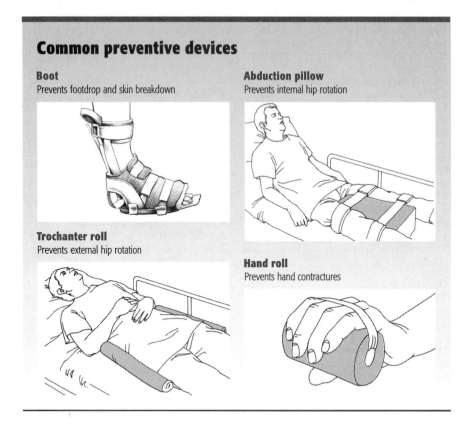

**Boot**
Prevents footdrop and skin breakdown

**Abduction pillow**
Prevents internal hip rotation

**Trochanter roll**
Prevents external hip rotation

**Hand roll**
Prevents hand contractures

have a loss of sensation, mobility, or consciousness.

### Equipment

Protective boots ● abduction pillow ● trochanter roll ● hand roll (See *Common preventive devices*.)

*Protective boots* are made of soft material that cradles the heel to prevent pressure on the heel. Other models are made of aluminum frames with fleece lining and a toe extension that protects the toes and prevents hip adduction. High-topped sneakers may be used to help prevent footdrop, but they don't prevent external hip rotation or heel pressure.

The *abduction pillow* is a wedge-shaped piece of sponge rubber with lateral indentations for the patient's thighs. Its straps wrap around the thighs to maintain correct positioning. A properly shaped bed pillow may temporarily substitute for the commercial abduction pillow, but it's difficult

to apply and fails to maintain the correct lateral alignment.

The commercial *trochanter roll* is made of sponge rubber, but you can also improvise one from a rolled blanket or sheet, or use a pillow. The *hand roll,* available in hard and soft materials, is held in place by fixed or adjustable straps. It can be improvised from a rolled washcloth secured with roller gauze and adhesive tape.

### Preparation of equipment

If you're using a device that's available in different sizes, select the appropriate size for the patient.

### Implementation

Explain the purpose and steps of the procedure to the patient.

#### Applying a boot

▶ Open the slit on the superior surface of the boot. Then place the patient's foot in the boot and fasten the ankle and foot

straps. If the patient is positioned laterally, you may apply the boot only to the bottom foot and support the flexed top foot with a pillow.
▶ If appropriate, insert the other heel in the second boot.
▶ Position the patient's legs in proper alignment to prevent strain on hip ligaments and pressure on bony prominences.

### Applying an abduction pillow
▶ Position the patient supine and place the pillow between the patient's legs. Slide it toward the groin so that it touches the legs all along their lengths.
▶ Place the upper part of both legs in the pillow's lateral indentations and secure the straps to prevent the pillow from slipping.

### Applying a trochanter roll
▶ Position one roll along the outside of the thigh, from the iliac crest to mid-thigh. Then place another roll along the other thigh. Make sure neither roll extends as far as the knee to avoid peroneal nerve compression and palsy, which can lead to foot-drop.
▶ If you've fashioned trochanter rolls from a rolled up sheet or blanket, leave several inches unrolled and tuck this under the patient's thigh to hold the device in place and maintain the patient's position.

### Applying a hand roll
▶ Place one roll in the patient's hand to maintain the neutral position. Then secure the strap, if present, or apply roller gauze and secure with hypoallergenic or adhesive tape.
▶ Place another roll in the other hand.

### Special considerations
▶ Remember that the use of assistive devices doesn't preclude regularly scheduled patient positioning, range-of-motion exercises, and skin care.

### Home care
▶ Explain the use of appropriate devices to the patient and caregiver.
▶ Demonstrate how to use each device, emphasizing proper alignment of extremities, and have the patient or caregiver give a return demonstration so you can check for proper technique.
▶ Emphasize measures needed to prevent pressure ulcers.

### Complications
Contractures and pressure ulcers may occur with the use of a hand roll and possibly with other assistive devices. To avoid these problems, remove a soft hand roll every 4 hours (every 2 hours if the patient has hand spasticity); remove a hard hand roll every 2 hours.

### Documentation
▶ Record the use of these devices in the patient's chart and the nursing plan of care, and indicate assessment for complications. Reevaluate your patient care goals as needed.

### REFERENCES
"Clinical Update: An Ounce of Prevention," *Nursing98* 28(4):30-31, April 1998.
IPRO. "A Quality Improvement Study: Impact Results of a Statewide Effort to Improve Pressure Ulcer Prevention in New York State." *IPRO HCQIP Publication No. 99-05,* April 1999.
Stimler, C. "A Pressure Ulcer Toolbox for Facilitating Hospital-wide Quality," *Advances in Wound Care* 11(3):13, May-June 1998.
The Joanna Briggs Institute of Evidence Based Nursing, *Best Practice: Pressure Sores— Part 1: Prevention of Pressure Related Damage* 1(1), 1997.

# Care of the dying patient

A patient needs intensive physical and emotional support as he approaches death. Signs of impending death include reduced respiratory rate and depth, decreased or absent blood pressure, weak or erratic pulse rate, lowered skin temperature, decreased level of consciousness (LOC), diminished sensorium and neuromuscular control, diaphoresis, pallor, cyanosis, and mottling.

Emotional support for the dying patient and his family most commonly means reassurance and the nurse's physical presence to help ease fear and loneliness. More intense emotional support is important at much earlier stages, especially for patients with long-term progressive illnesses who can work through the stages of dying. (See *Five stages of dying,* page 16.)

Respect the patient's wishes about extraordinary means of supporting life.

# Five stages of dying

According to Elisabeth Kübler-Ross, author of *On Death and Dying*, the dying patient may progress through five psychological stages in preparation for death. Although each patient experiences these stages differently, and not necessarily in this order, understanding the stages will help you meet the patient's needs.

### Denial
When the patient first learns that his illness is terminal, he may refuse to accept the diagnosis. He may experience physical symptoms similar to those of a stress reaction – shock, fainting, pallor, sweating, tachycardia, and nausea and other GI disorders. During this stage, be honest with the patient but not blunt or callous. Maintain communication with him so he can discuss his feelings when he accepts the reality of death. Don't force the patient to confront this reality.

### Anger
When the patient stops denying his impending death, he may show deep resentment toward those who will live on after he dies – to you, to the facility staff, and to his own family. Although you may instinctively draw back from the patient or even resent this behavior, remember that he's dying and has a right to be angry. After you accept the patient's anger, help him find different ways to express it and help his family understand it.

### Bargaining
Although the patient acknowledges his impending death, he may secretly try to bargain with God or fate for more time. If he does confide in you, don't urge him to keep his promises.

### Depression
In this stage, the patient may first have regrets about his past and then grieve about his current condition. He may withdraw from his friends, his family, his doctor, and you. He may suffer from anorexia, increased fatigue, or self-neglect. You may find him sitting alone, in tears. Accept the patient's sorrow and if he talks to you, listen. Provide comfort by touch, as appropriate. Resist the temptation to make optimistic remarks or cheerful small talk.

### Acceptance
In this last stage, the patient accepts the inevitability and imminence of his death – without emotion. The patient may simply desire the quiet company of a family member or friend. If, for some reason, a family member or friend can't be present, stay with the patient to satisfy his final need. Remember, though, that many patients die before reaching this stage.

---

▶ The ordinary Power of Attorney doesn't give another person the legal right to make decisions about medical care for the patient. Only a Durable Medical Power of Attorney authorizes another person to make such decisions for a patient when the patient is unable to communicate his wishes.

The patient may have signed a living will. This document, legally binding in most states, declares the patient's desire for a death unimpeded by the artificial support of defibrillators, ventilators, life-sustaining drugs, auxiliary hearts, and so on. If the patient has signed such a document, the nurse must respect his wishes and communicate the doctor's "no code" order to all staff members.

## Equipment
Bed linens ● gowns ● gloves ● water-filled basin ● soap ● washcloth ● towels ● lotion ● linen-saver pads ● petroleum jelly ● suction equipment, as necessary ● optional: indwelling urinary catheter

## Implementation
Assemble equipment at the patient's bedside, as needed.

### Meeting physical needs
▶ Take vital signs often and observe for pallor, diaphoresis, and decreased LOC.
▶ Reposition the patient in bed at least every 2 hours because sensation, reflexes, and mobility diminish first in the legs and gradually in the arms. Make sure the bed

sheets cover him loosely to reduce discomfort caused by pressure on arms and legs.
▶ When the patient's vision and hearing start to fail, turn his head toward the light and speak to him from near the head of the bed. Because hearing may be acute despite loss of consciousness, avoid whispering or speaking inappropriately about the patient in his presence.
▶ Change the bed linens and the patient's gown as needed. Provide skin care during gown changes and adjust the room temperature for patient comfort, if necessary.
▶ Observe for incontinence or anuria, which is a result of diminished neuromuscular control or decreased renal function. If necessary, obtain an order to catheterize the patient or place linen-saver pads beneath the patient's buttocks. Put on gloves and provide perineal care with soap, a washcloth, and towels to prevent irritation.
▶ With suction equipment, suction the patient's mouth and upper airway to remove secretions. Elevate the head of the bed to decrease respiratory resistance. As the patient's condition deteriorates, he may breathe mostly through his mouth.
▶ Offer fluids frequently and lubricate the patient's lips and mouth with petroleum jelly to counteract dryness.
▶ If the comatose patient's eyes are open, provide eye care to prevent corneal ulceration. Such ulceration can cause blindness and prevent the use of these tissues for transplantation should the patient die.
▶ Provide ordered pain medication as needed. Keep in mind that, as circulation diminishes, medications given I.M. will be poorly absorbed. Medications should be given I.V., if possible, for optimum results.

### Meeting emotional needs
▶ Fully explain all care and treatments to the patient even if he's unconscious because he may still be able to hear. Answer any questions as candidly as possible without sounding callous.
▶ Allow the patient to express his feelings, which may range from anger to loneliness. Take time to talk with the patient. Sit near the head of the bed and avoid looking rushed or unconcerned.
▶ Notify family members, if they're absent, when the patient wishes to see them. Let the patient and his family discuss death at their own pace.

---

## Understanding organ and tissue donation

A federal regulation enacted in 1998 requires that facilities report all deaths to the regional organ procurement organization. This regulation was enacted so that no potential donor is missed. The regulation ensures that the family of every potential donor will understand the option to donate. According to the American Medical Association, about 25 kinds of organs and tissues are being transplanted. Donor organ requirements vary, but the typical donor must be age 60 or younger and free from transmissible disease. Tissue donations are less restrictive, and some tissue banks will accept skin from donors up to age 75.

Collection of most organs, such as the heart, liver, kidney, or pancreas, requires that the patient be pronounced brain dead and kept physically alive until the organs are harvested. Tissue, such as eyes, skin, bone, and heart valves, may be taken after death. Contact your regional organ procurement organization for specific organ donation criteria or to identify a potential donor. If you don't know the regional organ procurement organization in your area, call the United Network for Organ Sharing at (804) 330-8500.

---

▶ Offer to contact a member of the clergy or social services department, if appropriate.

### Special considerations
▶ If the patient has signed a living will, the doctor will write a "no code" order on his progress notes and order sheets. Know your state's policy regarding the living will. If it's legal, transfer the "no code" order to the patient's chart or Kardex and, at the end of your shift, inform the incoming staff of this order.
▶ At an appropriate time, ask the family whether they have considered organ and tissue donation. Check the patient's records to determine whether he completed an organ donor card. (See *Understanding organ and tissue donation*.)
▶ If family members remain with the patient, show them the location of bathrooms, lounges, and cafeterias. Explain the patient's needs, treatments, and plan of care to them. If appropriate, offer to teach

them specific skills so they can take part in nursing care. Emphasize that their efforts are important and effective. As the patient's death approaches, give them emotional support.

### Documentation
▶ Record changes in the patient's vital signs, intake and output, and LOC.
▶ Note the times of cardiac arrest and the end of respiration and notify the doctor when these occur.

#### REFERENCES
Harvey, J. "Debunking Myths about Post-mortem Care," *Nursing2001* 31(7):44-45, July 2001.
Jenkins, C., and Bruers, E. "Assessment and Management of Medically Ill Patients Who Refuse Life-Prolonging Treatment: Two Case Reports and Proposed Guidelines," *Journal of Palliative Care* 14(1):18-24, 1998.
Quill, T., and Boyd, I. "Responding to Intractable Terminal Suffering: The Role of Terminal Sedation and Voluntary Refusal of Food and Fluids," *Annals of Internal Medicine* 132(5):408-13, March 2000.

## Clinitron therapy bed

Originally designed for managing burns, the Clinitron therapy bed is now used for patients with various debilities. The bed promotes comfort and healing by allowing harmless contact between its surface and grafted sites.

The bed is actually a large tub that supports the patient on a thick layer of silicone-coated microspheres of lime glass. (See *A look at the Clinitron therapy bed.*) A monofilament polyester filter sheet covers the microsphere-filled tub. Warmed air, propelled by a blower beneath the bed, passes through it. The resulting fluidlike surface reduces pressure on the skin to avoid obstructing capillary blood flow, thereby helping to prevent pressure ulcers and promote wound healing. The bed's air temperature can be adjusted to help control hypothermia and hyperthermia.

The Clinitron therapy bed is contraindicated for patients with an unstable spine. It may also be contraindicated for the patient unable to mobilize and expel pulmonary

### A look at the Clinitron therapy bed

The Clinitron therapy bed is a large tub filled with microspheres suspended by air pressure that gives the patient fluidlike support. The bed provides the advantages of flotation without the disadvantages of instability, patient positioning difficulties, and immobility.

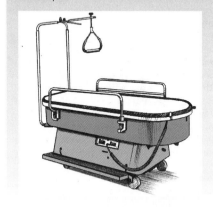

secretions because the lack of back support impairs productive coughing. Operation of the Clinitron therapy bed is complex and requires special training.

### Equipment
Clinitron therapy bed with microspheres (about 1,650 lb [750 kg]) ● filter sheet ● six aluminum rails (for restraining and sealing filter sheet) ● flat sheet ● elastic cord

#### Preparation of equipment
Normally, a manufacturer's representative or a trained staff member prepares the bed for use. If you must help with the preparation, make sure the microspheres reach to within ½" (1.3 cm) of the top of the tank. Then position the filter sheet on the bed with its printed side facing up. Match the holes in the sheet to the holes in the edge of the bed's frame. Place the aluminum rails on the frame, with the studs in the proper holes. Depress the rails firmly, and secure them by tightening the knurled knobs to seal the filter sheet. Place a flat sheet over the filter sheet and secure it

with the elastic cord. Turn on the air current to activate the microspheres and to ensure that the bed is working properly; then turn it off.

## Implementation
▶ Explain and, if possible, demonstrate the operation of the Clinitron therapy bed. Tell the patient the reason for its use and that he'll feel as though he's floating.
▶ With the help of three or more coworkers, transfer the patient to the bed using a lift sheet.
▶ Turn on the air pressure to activate the bed.
▶ Adjust the air temperature as necessary. Because the bed usually operates within 10° to 12° F (5.5° to 6.7° C) of ambient air temperature, set the room temperature to 75° F (24° C). If microsphere temperature reaches 105° F (40.6° C), the bed automatically shuts off. It restarts automatically after 30 minutes.

## Special considerations
▶ Monitor fluid and electrolyte status because the Clinitron therapy bed increases evaporative water loss. Because of this drying effect, always cover a mesh graft for the first 2 to 8 days. If the patient has excessive upper respiratory tract dryness, use a humidifier and mask . Encourage coughing and deep breathing. After prolonged use of a Clinitron bed, watch for hypocalcemia and hypophosphatemia.
▶ To position a bedpan, roll the patient away from you, place the bedpan on the flat sheet, and push it into the microspheres. Then reposition the patient. To remove the bedpan, hold it steady and roll the patient away from you. Turn off the air pressure and remove the bedpan. Then turn the air on and reposition the patient.
▶ Don't wear a watch when handling the microspheres because they can damage the mechanism. Don't secure the filter sheet with pins or clamps, which may puncture the sheet and release microspheres. Take care not to puncture the bed when giving injections. Repair any holes or tears with iron-on patching tape. Sieve the microspheres monthly or between patients to remove any clumped microspheres. Handle them carefully to avoid spills; spilled microspheres may cause falls. Treat a soiled filter sheet and clumped microspheres as contaminated items; handle according to policy. Change the filter sheet and operate the unit unoccupied for 24 hours between patients.
▶ Assess the patient's skin and reposition him every 2 hours. Specialty beds don't end the need for frequent assessment and position changes.

## Documentation
▶ Record the duration of therapy and the patient's response to it.
▶ Document the condition of the patient's skin, pressure ulcers, and other wounds.
▶ Record the patient's position change schedule.

### REFERENCES
Jastremski, C.A. "Pressure Relief Bedding To Prevent Pressure Ulcer Development in Critical Care," *Journal of Critical Care* 17(2):122-25, June 2002.
Sae-Sia, W., and Wipke-Tevis, D. "Pressure Ulcer Prevention and Treatment Practices in Inpatient Rehabilitation Facilities," *Rehabilitation Nursing* 27(5):192-98, September-October 2002.

# Passive range-of-motion exercises

Used to move the patient's joints through as full a range of motion as possible, passive ROM exercises improve or maintain joint mobility and help prevent contractures. Performed by a nurse, a physical therapist, or a caregiver of the patient's choosing, these exercises are indicated for the patient with temporary or permanent loss of mobility, sensation, or consciousness. Performed properly, passive ROM exercises require recognition of the patient's limits of motion and support of all joints during movement.

Passive ROM exercises are contraindicated in patients with septic joints, acute thrombophlebitis, severe arthritic joint inflammation, or recent trauma with possible hidden fractures or internal injuries.

## Implementation
▶ Determine the joints that need ROM exercises and consult the doctor or physical

## Glossary of joint movements

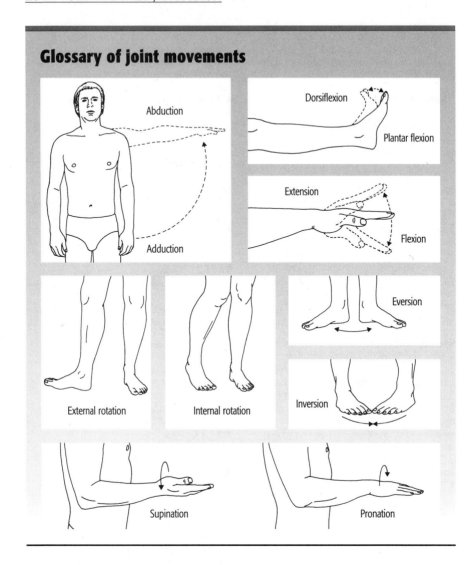

therapist about limitations or precautions for specific exercises. The exercises below treat all joints, but they don't have to be performed in the order given or all at once. You can schedule them over the course of a day, whenever the patient is in the most convenient position. Remember to perform all exercises slowly, gently, and to the end of the normal ROM or to the point of pain but no further. (See *Glossary of joint movements*.)

▶ Before you begin, raise the bed to a comfortable working height.

### Exercising the neck
▶ Support the patient's head with your hands and extend the neck, flex the chin to the chest, and tilt the head laterally toward each shoulder.
▶ Rotate the head from right to left.

### Exercising the shoulders
▶ Support the patient's arm in an extended, neutral position; then extend the forearm and flex it back. Abduct the arm outward from the side of the body and adduct it back to the side.

Rotate the shoulder so that the arm crosses the midline and bend the elbow so that the hand touches the opposite shoulder, then touches the mattress of the bed for complete internal rotation.

Return the shoulder to a neutral position and, with elbow bent, push the arm backward so that the back of the hand touches the mattress for complete external rotation.

### Exercising the elbow
Place the patient's arm at his side with his palm facing up.

Flex and extend the arm at the elbow.

### Exercising the forearm
Stabilize the patient's elbow and then twist the hand to bring the palm up (supination).

Twist it back again to bring the palm down (pronation).

### Exercising the wrist
Stabilize the forearm and flex and extend the wrist. Then rock the hand sideways for lateral flexion and rotate the hand in a circular motion.

### Exercising the fingers and thumb
Extend the patient's fingers and then flex the hand into a fist; repeat extension and flexion of each joint of each finger and thumb separately.

Spread two adjoining fingers apart (abduction) and then bring them together (adduction).

Oppose each fingertip to the thumb and rotate the thumb and each finger in a circle.

### Exercising the hip and knee
Fully extend the patient's leg and then bend the hip and knee toward the chest, allowing full joint flexion.

Next, move the straight leg sideways, out and away from the other leg (abduction), and then back, over, and across it (adduction).

Rotate the straight leg internally toward the midline, then externally away from the midline.

### Exercising the ankle
Bend the patient's foot so that the toes push upward (dorsiflexion) and then bend the foot so that the toes push downward (plantar flexion).

Rotate the ankle in a circular motion.

Invert the ankle so that the sole of the foot faces the midline and evert the ankle so that the sole faces away from the midline.

### Exercising the toes
Flex the patient's toes toward the sole and then extend them back toward the top of the foot.

Spread two adjoining toes apart (abduction) and bring them together (adduction).

## Special considerations
Because joints begin to stiffen within 24 hours of disuse, start passive ROM exercises as soon as possible and perform them at least once a shift, particularly while bathing or turning the patient. Use proper body mechanics and repeat each exercise at least three times.

Patients who experience prolonged bed rest or limited activity without profound weakness can also be taught to perform ROM exercises on their own (called active ROM), or they may benefit from isometric exercises. (See *Learning about isometric exercises,* page 22.)

If the disabled patient requires long-term rehabilitation after discharge, consult with a physical therapist and teach a family member or caregiver to perform passive ROM exercises.

## Documentation
Record which joints were exercised, the presence of edema or pressure areas, any pain resulting from the exercises, any limitation of ROM, and the patient's tolerance of the exercises.

### REFERENCES
Goldsmith, J.R., et al: "The Effects of Range-of-Motion Therapy on the Plantar Pressures of Patients with Diabetes Mellitus." *Journal of the American Podiatric Medical Association* 92(9):483-90, October 2002.

Kozier, B., et al. *Fundamentals of Nursing,* 6th ed. Englewood Cliffs, N.J.: Prentice Hall, 2000.

# Learning about isometric exercises

The patient can strengthen and increase muscle tone by contracting muscles against resistance (from other muscles or from a stationary object, such as a bed or a wall) without joint movement. These exercises require only a comfortable position, either standing, sitting, or lying down, and proper body alignment. For each exercise, instruct the patient to hold each contraction for 2 to 5 seconds and to repeat it three to four times daily, below peak contraction level for the first week and at peak level thereafter.

### Neck rotators

The patient places the heel of his hand above one ear. Then he pushes his head toward the hand as forcefully as possible, without moving his head, neck, or arm. He repeats the exercise on the other side.

### Neck flexors

The patient places both palms on his forehead. Without moving his neck, he pushes his head forward while resisting with his palms.

### Neck extensors

The patient clasps his fingers behind his head, then pushes his head against the clasped hands without moving his neck.

### Shoulder elevators

Holding his right arm straight down at his side, the patient grasps his right wrist with his left hand. He then tries to shrug his right shoulder but prevents it from moving by holding his arm in place. He repeats this exercise, alternating arms.

### Shoulder, chest, and scapular musculature

The patient places his right fist in his left palm and raises both arms to shoulder height. He pushes his fist into his palm as forcefully as possible without moving either arm. Then with his arms in the same position, he clasps his fingers and tries to pull his hands apart. He repeats the pattern, beginning with his left fist in his right palm.

### Elbow flexors and extensors

With his right elbow bent 90 degrees and his right palm facing upward, the patient places his left fist against his right palm. He tries to bend his right elbow further while resisting with his left fist. He repeats the pattern, bending his left elbow.

### Abdomen

The patient assumes a sitting position and bends slightly forward with his hands in front of the middle of his thighs. He tries to bend further forward, resisting by pressing his palms against his thighs.

Alternatively, in the supine position, he clasps his hands behind his head. Then he raises his shoulders about 1" (2.5 cm), holding this position for a few seconds.

### Back extensors

In a sitting position, the patient bends forward and places his hands under his buttocks. He tries to stand up, resisting with both hands.

### Hip abductors

While standing, the patient squeezes his inner thighs together as tightly as possible. Placing a pillow between the knees supplies resistance and increases the effectiveness of this exercise.

### Hip extensors

The patient squeezes his buttocks together as tightly as possible.

### Knee extensors

The patient straightens his knee fully. Then he vigorously tightens the muscle above the knee so that it moves the kneecap upward. He repeats this exercise, alternating legs.

### Ankle flexors and extensors

The patient pulls his toes upward, holding briefly. Then he pushes them down as far as possible, again holding briefly.

# Physical assessment

Nurses perform a complete physical assessment when the patient is admitted to the facility and partial reassessments as the patient's condition warrants. A complete assessment includes a thorough health history and physical examination. The health history includes the chief complaint, a history of the current illness, general medical and surgical histories, a family history, a social history, and a review of systems. Typically, the physical examination follows a methodical, head-to-toe format. Patient preparation includes providing a clear explanation of the examination, as well as proper positioning and draping before and during the examination. During this procedure, the nurse must make every effort to recognize and respect the patient's feelings (particularly embarrassment and anxiety), as well as to provide comfort measures and follow appropriate safety precautions.

## Equipment

Scale with height measurement bar • urine specimen container and laboratory request form • sphygmomanometer • watch with second hand stethoscope • thermometer • gown (for patient) • examining table (with stirrups if necessary) • gloves • drapes (sheet, bath blanket, or towel, as needed) • adhesive tape • spotlight or gooseneck lamp • flashlight • laryngeal mirror • tongue blades • percussion (reflex) hammer • otoscope • tuning fork • ear specula • tape measure • visual acuity chart • ophthalmoscope • test tubes of hot and cold water • containers of odorous materials (such as coffee or chocolate) • substances for taste assessment (sugar, salt, vinegar) • coin, pin, and cotton • paper clip • fecal occult blood test kit • linen-saver pad • water-soluble lubricant • facial tissues • cotton-tipped applicators • nursing assessment form

## Preparation of equipment

Adjust the température in the examining room and close the doors to prevent drafts. Cover the examining table with a clean sheet or disposable paper. Then assemble the appropriate equipment for the examination.

## Implementation

Review the patient's health history to obtain subjective data about the patient and insight into problem areas and subtle physical changes. Investigate the patient's chief complaint. (See *Exploring a patient's symptoms,* page 24.)

▶ Obtain biographical data, including the patient's name, address, telephone number, contact person, sex, age and birth date, birthplace, Social Security number, marital status, education, religion, occupation, race, nationality, and cultural background, as well as the names of persons living with the patient.

▶ Ask about health and illness patterns, the reason for seeking health care, current and past health status, family health status, and condition of body systems.

▶ Ask about health promotion and protection patterns, including health beliefs, personal habits, sleep and wake cycles, exercise, recreation, nutrition, stress level and coping skills, socioeconomic status, environmental health conditions, and occupational health hazards.

▶ Explore the patient's role and relationship patterns, including self-concept, cultural and religious influences, family roles and relationships, sexuality and reproductive patterns, social support systems, and any other psychosocial considerations.

▶ Explain the physical examination and answer questions. (See *Performing a head-to-toe assessment,* pages 25 to 34.)

▶ Instruct the patient to void if possible. You may need to collect a urine specimen. Emptying the bladder increases patient comfort during the examination.

▶ Help the patient undress, and provide a gown. Then measure and record height, weight, and vital signs.

▶ Assist the patient onto the examination table. Requirements for positioning and draping vary with the body system and region being assessed. To examine the head, neck, and anterior and posterior thorax, have the patient sit on the edge of the examination table or the bed. For the ab-

## Exploring a patient's symptoms

A clear understanding of the patient's symptoms is essential to a complete physical assessment. One method of gaining that understanding involves using the mnemonic device PQRST as a guide.

### Provocative or palliative

What causes the symptom? What makes it better or worse?

▶ What were you doing when you first noticed it?
▶ What seems to trigger it? Stress? Position? Certain activities? An argument? (For a sign such as an eye discharge: What seems to cause it or make it worse? For a psychological symptom such as depression: Does the depression occur after specific events?)
▶ What relieves the symptom? Changing diet? Changing position? Taking medication? Being active?
▶ What makes the symptom worse?

### Quality or quantity

How does the symptom feel, look, or sound? How much of it are you experiencing now?

▶ How would you describe the symptom — how it feels, looks, or sounds?
▶ How much are you experiencing now? Is it so much that it prevents you from performing any activities? Is it more or less than you experienced at any other time?

### Region or radiation

Where is the symptom located? Does it spread?
▶ Where does the symptom occur?

▶ In the case of pain, does it travel down your back or arms, up your neck, or down your legs?

### Severity

How does the symptom rate on a scale of 1 to 10, with 10 being the most severe?
▶ How bad is the symptom at its worst? Does it force you to lie, sit, or slow?
▶ Does the symptom seem to be getting better, worse, or staying about the same?

### Timing

When did the symptom begin? Did it occur suddenly or gradually? How often does it occur?
▶ On what date and time did the symptom first occur?
▶ How did the symptom start? Suddenly? Gradually?
▶ How often do you experience the symptom? Hourly? Daily? Weekly? Monthly?
▶ When do you usually experience the symptom? During the day? At night? In the early morning? Does it awaken you? Does it occur before, during, or after meals? Does it occur seasonally?
▶ How long does an episode of the symptom last?

---

domen and cardiovascular system, place the patient in a supine position and stand to his right. For a female patient, place a towel over her breasts and upper thorax during abdominal assessment. Pull the sheet down as far as her symphysis pubis, but no farther.
▶ Perform a physical examination.

### Documentation

▶ Document significant normal and abnormal findings in an organized manner according to body systems.

### REFERENCES

Bickley, L. *Bates' Guide to Physical Examination and Health History Taking,* 7th ed. Philadelphia: Lippincott Williams & Wilkins, 1999.
JCAHO. "Standards: Frequently Asked Questions: Hospital." *www.jcaho.org/standard/ faq/hos.html.* Posted March 26, 2001.
Kozier, B., et al. *Fundamentals of Nursing,* 6th ed. Englewood Cliffs, N.J.: Prentice Hall, 2000.
Perry, A., and Potter, P. *Clinical Nursing Skills and Techniques,* 4th ed. St. Louis: Mosby–Year Book, Inc., 1998.

*(Text continues on page 35.)*

# Performing a head-to-toe assessment

This table provides guidelines for a systematic head-to-toe assessment. It groups assessment techniques by body region and nurse-patient positioning to make the assessment as efficient as possible and to avoid tiring the patient. Each entry describes assessment techniques for each body system or region and the *normal findings* for adults.

| Technique | Normal findings | Special considerations |
|---|---|---|
| *Head and neck* | | |
| Inspect the patient's head. Note hair color, texture, and distribution. Palpate from the forehead to the posterior triangle of the neck for the posterior cervical lymph nodes. | Symmetrical, rounded normocephalic head positioned at midline and erect with no lumps or ridges | ▶ This technique can detect asymmetry, size changes, enlarged lymph nodes, and tenderness.<br>▶ Wear gloves for palpation if the patient has scalp lesions.<br>▶ Inspect and gently palpate the fontanels and sutures in an infant. |
| Palpate in front of and behind the ears, under the chin, and in the anterior triangle for the anterior cervical lymph nodes. | Nonpalpable lymph nodes or small, round, soft, mobile, nontender lymph nodes | ▶ This technique can detect enlarged lymph nodes.<br>▶ Palpable lymph nodes may be normal in a patient under age 12. |
| Palpate the left and then the right carotid artery. | Bilateral equality in pulse amplitude and rhythm | ▶ This technique evaluates circulation through the carotid pulse. |
| Auscultate the carotid arteries. | No bruit on auscultation | ▶ Auscultation in this area can detect a bruit, a sign of turbulent blood flow. |
| Palpate the trachea. | Straight, midline trachea | ▶ This technique evaluates trachea position. |
| Palpate the suprasternal notch. | Palpable pulsations with an even rhythm | ▶ Palpation in this area allows evaluation of aortic arch pulsations. |
| Palpate the supraclavicular area. | Nonpalpable lymph nodes | ▶ This technique can detect enlarged lymph nodes. |
| Palpate the thyroid gland and auscultate for bruits. | Thin, mobile thyroid isthmus; nonpalpable thyroid lobes | ▶ Palpation detects thyroid enlargement, tenderness, or nodules. |
| Have the patient touch his chin to his chest and to each shoulder, each ear to the corresponding shoulder, then tip his head back as far as possible. | Symmetrical strength and movement of neck muscles | ▶ These maneuvers evaluate range of motion (ROM) in the neck. |
| Place your hands on the patient's shoulders while he shrugs them against resistance. Then place your hand on the patient's left cheek, then the right, and have the patient push against it. | Symmetrical strength and movement of neck muscles | ▶ This procedure checks cranial nerve XI (accessory nerve) functioning and trapezius and sternocleidomastoid muscle strength. |

*(continued)*

# Performing a head-to-toe assessment *(continued)*

| Technique | Normal findings | Special considerations |
|---|---|---|
| ***Head and neck*** *(continued)* | | |
| Have the patient smile, frown, wrinkle the forehead, and puff out the cheeks. | Symmetrical smile, frown, and forehead wrinkles; equal puffing out of the cheeks | ▸ This maneuver evaluates the motor portion of cranial nerve VII (facial nerve). |
| Occlude one nostril externally with your finger while the patient breathes through the other. Repeat on the other nostril. | Patent nostrils | ▸ This technique checks the patency of the nasal passages. |
| Inspect the internal nostrils using a nasal speculum or an ophthalmoscope handle with a nasal attachment. | Moist, pink to red nasal mucosa without deviated septum, lesions, or polyps | ▸ This technique can detect edema, inflammation, and excessive drainage.<br>▸ Use only a flashlight to inspect an infant's or toddler's nostrils; a nasal speculum is too sharp. |
| Palpate the nose. | No bumps, lesions, edema, or tenderness | ▸ This technique assesses for structural abnormalities in the nose.<br>▸ An infant's nose usually is slightly flattened. |
| Palpate and percuss the frontal and maxillary sinuses. If palpation and percussion elicit tenderness, assess further by transilluminating the sinuses. | No tenderness on palpation or percussion | ▸ These techniques are used to elicit tenderness, which may indicate sinus congestion or infection.<br>▸ In a child under age 8, frontal sinuses commonly are too small to assess. |
| Palpate the temporomandibular joints as the patient opens and closes the jaws. | Smooth joint movement without pain; correct approximation | ▸ This action assesses the temporomandibular joints and the motor portion of cranial nerve V (trigeminal nerve). |
| Inspect the oral mucosa, gingivae, teeth, and salivary gland openings, using a tongue blade and a penlight. | Pink, moist, smooth oral mucosa without lesions or inflammation; pink, moist slightly irregular gingivae without sponginess or edema; 32 teeth with correct occlusion | ▸ This technique evaluates the condition of several oral structures.<br>▸ A child may have up to 20 temporary (baby) teeth.<br>▸ Slight gingival swelling may be normal during pregnancy. |
| Observe the tongue and the hard and soft palates. | Pink, slightly rough tongue with a midline depression; pink to light red palates with symmetrical lines | ▸ Observation provides information about the patient's hydration status and the condition of these oral structures. |
| Ask the patient to stick out his tongue. | Midline tongue without tremors | ▸ This procedure tests cranial nerve XII (hypoglossal nerve). |
| Ask the patient to say "Ahh" while sticking out his tongue. Inspect the visible oral structures. | Symmetrical rise in soft palate and uvula during phonation; pink, midline, cone-shaped uvula; +1 tonsils (both tonsils behind the pillars) | ▸ Phonation ("Ahh'") checks portions of cranial nerves IX and X (glossopharyngeal and vagus nerves). Lowering the tongue aids viewing. |

# Performing a head-to-toe assessment *(continued)*

| Technique | Normal findings | Special considerations |
| --- | --- | --- |
| **Head and neck** *(continued)* | | |
| Test the gag reflex using a tongue blade. | Gagging | ▶ Gagging during this procedure indicates that cranial nerves IX and X are intact. |
| Place the tongue blade at the side of the tongue while the patient pushes it to the left and right with the tongue. | Symmetrical ability to push tongue blade to left and right | ▶ This action tests cranial nerve XII. |
| Test the sense of smell using a test tube of coffee, chocolate, or another familiar substance. | Correct identification of smells in both nostrils | ▶ This action tests cranial nerve I (olfactory nerve).<br>▶ Make sure the patient keeps both eyes closed during the test. |
| **Eyes and ears** | | |
| Perform a visual acuity test using the standard Snellen eye chart or another visual acuity chart, with the patient wearing corrective lenses if needed. | 20/20 vision | ▶ This test assesses the patient's distance vision (central vision) and evaluates cranial nerve II (optic nerve). |
| Ask the patient to identify the pattern in a specially prepared page of color dots or plates. | Correct identification of pattern | ▶ This test assesses the patient's color perception. |
| Test the six cardinal positions of gaze. | Bilaterally equal eye movement without nystagmus | ▶ This test evaluates the function of each of the six extraocular muscles and tests cranial nerves III, IV, and VI (oculomotor, trochlear, and abducens nerves). |
| Inspect the external structures of the eyeball (eyelids, eyelashes, and lacrimal apparatus). | Bright, clear, symmetrical eyes free of nystagmus; eyelids close completely; no lesions, scaling, or inflammation | ▶ This inspection allows detection of such problems as ptosis, ectropion (outward-turning eyelids), entropion (inward-turning eyelids), and styes. |
| Inspect the conjunctiva and sclera. | Pink palpebral conjunctiva and clear bulbar conjunctiva without swelling, drainage, or hyperemic blood vessels; white, clear sclera | ▶ Inspection detects conjunctivitis and the scleral color changes that may occur with systemic disorders. |
| Inspect the cornea, iris, and anterior chamber by shining a penlight tangentially across the eye. | Clear, transparent cornea and anterior chamber; illumination of total iris | ▶ This technique assesses anterior chamber depth and the condition of the cornea and iris.<br>▶ An elderly patient may exhibit a thin, grayish ring in the cornea (called arcus senilis). |
| Examine the pupils for equality of size, shape, reaction to light, and accommodation. | Pupils equal, round, reactive to light and accommodation (PERRLA), directly and consensually | ▶ Testing the pupillary response to light and accommodation assesses cranial nerves III, IV, and VI. |

*(continued)*

# Performing a head-to-toe assessment *(continued)*

| Technique | Normal findings | Special considerations |
| --- | --- | --- |
| **Eyes and ears** *(continued)* | | |
| Observe the red reflex using an ophthalmoscope. | Sharp, distinct orange-red glow | ▶ Presence of the red reflex indicates that the cornea, anterior chamber, and lens are free from opacity and clouding. |
| Inspect the ear. Perform an otoscopic examination if indicated. | Nearly vertically positioned ears that line up with the eye, match the facial color, are similarly shaped, and are in proportion to the face; no drainage, nodules, or lesions | ▶ A dark-skinned patient may have darker orange or brown cerumen (earwax); a fair-skinned patient typically will have yellow cerumen. |
| Palpate the ear and mastoid process. | No pain, swelling, nodules, or lesions | ▶ This assessment technique can detect inflammation or infection. It may also uncover other abnormalities, such as nodules or lesions. |
| Perform the whispered voice test or the watch-tick test on one ear at a time. | Whispered voice heard at a distance of 1' to 2' (30 to 61 cm); watch-tick heard at a distance of 5" (13 cm) | ▶ This test provides a gross assessment of cranial nerve VIII (acoustic nerve). |
| Perform Weber's test using a 512 or 1024 hertz (Hz) tuning fork. | Tuning fork vibrations heard equally in both ears or in the middle of the head | ▶ This test differentiates conductive from sensorineural hearing loss. <br> ▶ The sound is heard best in the ear with a conductive loss. |
| Perform the Rinne test using a 512 or 1024 Hz tuning fork. | Tuning fork vibrations heard in front of the ear for as long as they are heard on the mastoid process | ▶ This test helps differentiate conductive from sensorineural hearing loss. |
| **Posterior thorax** | | |
| Observe the skin, bones, and muscles of the spine, shoulder blades, and back as well as symmetry of expansion and accessory muscle use. | Even skin tone; symmetrical placement of all structures; bilaterally equal shoulder height; symmetrical expansion with inhalation; no accessory muscle use | ▶ Observation provides information about lung expansion and accessory muscle use during respiration. It may also detect a deformity that can alter ventilation such as scoliosis. |
| Assess the anteroposterior and lateral diameters of the thorax. | Lateral diameter up to twice the anteroposterior diameter (2:1) | ▶ This assessment may detect abnormalities such as an increased anteroposterior diameter (barrel chest may be as low as 1:1). <br> ▶ Normal anteroposterior diameters vary with age. <br> ▶ Measure an infant's chest circumference at the nipple line. |

# Performing a head-to-toe assessment *(continued)*

| Technique | Normal findings | Special considerations |
|---|---|---|
| *Posterior thorax* (continued) | | |
| Palpate down the spine. | Properly aligned spinous processes without lesions or tenderness; firm, symmetrical, evenly spaced muscles | ▸ This technique detects pain in the spine and paraspinous muscles. It also evaluates the muscles' consistency. |
| Palpate over the posterior thorax. | Smooth surface; no lesions, lumps, or pain | ▸ This technique helps detect musculoskeletal inflammation. |
| Assess respiratory excursion. | Symmetrical expansion and contraction of the thorax | ▸ This technique checks for equal expansion of the lungs. |
| Palpate for tactile fremitus as the patient repeats the word "ninety-nine." | Equally intense vibrations of both sides of the chest | ▸ Palpation provides information about the content of the lungs; vibrations increase over consolidated or fluid-filled areas and decrease over gas-filled areas. |
| Percuss over the posterior and lateral lung fields. | Resonant percussion note over the lungs that changes to a dull note at the diaphragm | ▸ This technique helps identify the density and location of the lungs, diaphragm, and other anatomic structures.<br>▸ Percussion may produce hyperresonant sounds in a patient with chronic obstructive pulmonary disease or an elderly patient because of hyperinflation of lung tissue. |
| Percuss for diaphragmatic excursion on each side of the posterior thorax. | Excursion from 1¼″ to 2¼″ (3 to 6 cm) | ▸ This technique evaluates diaphragm movement during respiration. |
| Auscultate the lungs through the posterior thorax as the patient breathes slowly and deeply through the mouth. Also auscultate lateral areas. | Bronchovesicular sounds (soft, breezy sounds) between the scapulae; vesicular sounds (soft, swishy sounds about two notes lower than bronchovesicular sounds) in the lung periphery | ▸ Lung auscultation helps detect abnormal fluid or mucus accumulation as well as obstructed passages.<br>▸ Auscultate a child's lungs before performing other assessment techniques that may cause crying, which increases the respiratory rate and interferes with clear auscultation.<br>▸ A child's breath sounds are normally harsher or more bronchial than an adult's. |
| *Anterior thorax* | | |
| Observe the skin, bones, and muscles of the anterior thoracic structures as well as symmetry of expansion and accessory muscle use during respiration. | Even skin tone; symmetrical placement of all structures; symmetrical costal angle of less than 90 degrees; symmetrical expansion with inhalation; no accessory muscle use | ▸ Observation provides information about lung expansion and accessory muscle use. It may also detect a deformity that can prevent full lung expansion, such as pigeon chest. |
| Inspect the anterior thorax for lifts, heaves, or thrusts. Also check for the apical impulse. | No lifts, heaves, or thrusts; apical impulse not usually visible | ▸ Apical impulse may be visible in a thin or young patient. |

*(continued)*

# Performing a head-to-toe assessment *(continued)*

| Technique | Normal findings | Special considerations |
|---|---|---|
| *Anterior thorax (continued)* | | |
| Palpate over the anterior thorax. | Smooth surface; no lesions, lumps, or pain | ▸ This technique helps detect musculoskeletal inflammation. |
| Assess respiratory excursion. | Symmetrical expansion and contraction of the thorax | ▸ This technique checks for equal expansion of the lungs. |
| Palpate for tactile fremitus as the patient repeats the word "ninety-nine." | Equally intense vibrations of both sides of the chest, with more vibrations in the upper chest than in the lower chest | ▸ Palpation provides information about the content of the lungs. |
| Percuss over the anterior thorax. | Resonant percussion note over lung fields that changes to a dull note over ribs and other bones | ▸ This technique helps identify the density and location of the lungs, diaphragm, and other anatomic structures.<br>▸ Percussion is unreliable in an infant because of the infant's small chest size.<br>▸ Percussion may produce hyperresonant sounds in an elderly patient because of hyperinflation of lung tissue. |
| Auscultate the lungs through the anterior thorax as the patient breathes slowly and deeply through the mouth. Also auscultate lateral areas. | Bronchovesicular sounds (soft, breezy sounds) between the scapulae; vesicular sounds (soft, swishy sounds about two notes lower than bronchovesicular sounds) in the lung periphery | ▸ Lung auscultation helps detect abnormal fluid or mucus accumulation.<br>▸ Auscultate a child's lungs before performing other assessment techniques that may cause crying.<br>▸ Breath sounds are normally harsher or more bronchial in a child. |
| Inspect the breasts and axillae with the patient's hands resting at the sides of the body, placed on the hips, and raised above the head. | Symmetrical, convex, similar-looking breasts with soft, smooth skin and bilaterally similar venous patterns; symmetrical axillae with varying amounts of hair, but no lesions; nipples at same level on chest and of same color | ▸ This technique evaluates the general condition of the breasts and axillae and detects such abnormalities as retraction, dimpling, and flattening.<br>▸ Expect to see enlarged breasts with darkened nipples and areolae and purplish linear streaks if the patient is pregnant. |
| Palpate the axillae with the patient's arms resting against the side of the body. | Nonpalpable nodes | ▸ This technique detects nodular enlargements and other abnormalities. |
| Palpate the breasts and nipples with patient lying supine. | Smooth, relatively elastic tissue without masses, cracks, fissures, areas of induration (hardness), or discharge | ▸ This technique evaluates the consistency and elasticity of the breasts and nipples and may detect nipple discharge.<br>▸ The premenstrual patient may exhibit breast tenderness, nodularity, and fullness.<br>▸ A pregnant patient may discharge colostrum from the nipple and may exhibit nodular breasts with prominent venous patterns. |

# Performing a head-to-toe assessment *(continued)*

| Technique | Normal findings | Special considerations |
|---|---|---|
| ***Anterior thorax*** *(continued)* | | |
| Inspect the neck for jugular vein distention with the patient lying supine at a 45-degree angle. | No visible pulsations | ▸ This technique assesses right-sided heart pressure. |
| Palpate the precordium for the apical impulse. | Apical impulse present in the apical area (fifth intercostal space at the midclavicular line) | ▸ This action evaluates the size and location of the left ventricle. |
| Auscultate the aortic, pulmonic, tricuspid, and mitral areas for heart sounds. | $S_1$ and $S_2$ heart sounds with a regular rhythm and an age–appropriate rate | ▸ Auscultation over the precordium evaluates the heart rate and rhythm and can detect other abnormal heart sounds.<br>▸ A child or a pregnant woman in the third trimester may have functional (innocent) heart murmurs. |
| ***Abdomen*** | | |
| Observe the abdominal contour. | Symmetrical flat or rounded contour | ▸ This technique determines whether the abdomen is distended or scaphoid.<br>▸ An infant or a toddler will have a rounded abdomen. |
| Inspect the abdomen for skin characteristics, symmetry, contour, peristalsis, and pulsations. | Symmetrical contour with no lesions, striae, rash, or visible peristaltic waves | ▸ Inspection can detect an incisional or umbilical hernia, or an abnormality caused by bowel obstruction. |
| Auscultate all four quadrants of the abdomen. | Normal bowel sounds in all four quadrants; no bruits | ▸ Abdominal auscultation can detect abnormal bowel sounds. |
| Percuss from below the right breast to the inguinal area down the right midclavicular line. | Dull percussion note over the liver; tympanic note over the rest of the abdomen | ▸ Percussion in this area helps evaluate the size of the liver. |
| Percuss from below the left breast to the inguinal area down the left midclavicular line. | Tympanic percussion note | ▸ Percussion that elicits a dull note in this area can detect an enlarged spleen. |
| Palpate all four abdominal quadrants. | Nontender organs without masses | ▸ Palpation provides information about the location, size, and condition of the underlying structures. |
| Palpate for the kidneys on each side of the abdomen. | Nonpalpable kidneys or solid, firm, smooth kidneys (if palpable) | ▸ This technique evaluates the general condition of the kidneys. |
| Palpate the liver at the right costal border. | Nonpalpable liver or smooth, firm, nontender liver with a rounded, regular edge (if palpable) | ▸ This technique evaluates the general condition of the liver. |

*(continued)*

# Performing a head-to-toe assessment *(continued)*

| Technique | Normal findings | Special considerations |
|---|---|---|
| ***Abdomen** (continued)* | | |
| Palpate for the spleen at the left costal border. | Nonpalpable spleen | ▶ This procedure detects splenomegaly (spleen enlargement). |
| Palpate the femoral pulses in the groin. | Strong, regular pulse | ▶ Palpation assesses vascular patency. |
| ***Arms*** | | |
| Observe the skin and muscle mass of the arms and hands. | Uniform color and texture with no lesions; elastic turgor; bilaterally equal muscle mass | ▶ The skin provides information about hydration and circulation. Muscle mass provides information about injuries and neuromuscular disease. |
| Ask the patient to extend the arms forward and then rapidly turn the palms up and down. | Steady hands with no tremor or pronator drift | ▶ This maneuver tests proprioception and cerebellar function. |
| Place your hands on the patient's upturned forearms while the patient pushes up against resistance. Then place your hands under the forearms while the patient pushes down. | Symmetrical strength and ability to push up and down against resistance | ▶ This procedure checks the muscle strength of the arms. |
| Inspect and palpate the fingers, wrists, and elbow joints. | Smooth, freely movable joints with no swelling | ▶ An elderly patient may exhibit osteoarthritic changes. |
| Palpate the patient's hands to assess skin temperature. | Warm, moist skin with bilaterally even temperature | ▶ Skin temperature assessment provides data about circulation to the area. |
| Palpate the radial and brachial pulses. | Bilaterally equal rate and rhythm | ▶ Palpation of pulses helps evaluate peripheral vascular status. |
| Inspect the color, shape, and condition of the patient's fingernails, and test for capillary refill. | Pink nail beds with smooth, rounded nails; brisk capillary refill; no clubbing | ▶ Nail assessment provides data about the integumentary, cardiovascular, and respiratory systems. |
| Place two fingers in each of the patient's palms while the patient squeezes your fingers. | Bilaterally equal hand strength | ▶ This maneuver tests muscle strength in the hands. |
| ***Legs*** | | |
| Inspect the legs and feet for color, lesions, varicosities, hair growth, nail growth, edema, and muscle mass. | Even skin color; symmetrical hair and nail growth; no lesions, varicosities, or edema; bilaterally equal muscle mass | ▶ Inspection assesses adequate circulatory function. |
| Test for pitting edema in the pretibial area. | No pitting edema | ▶ This test assesses for excess interstitial fluid. |

# Performing a head-to-toe assessment *(continued)*

| Technique | Normal findings | Special considerations |
|---|---|---|
| **Legs** *(continued)* | | |
| Palpate for pulses and skin temperature in the posterior tibial, dorsalis pedis, and popliteal areas. | Bilaterally even pulse rate, rhythm, and skin temperature | ▶ Palpation of pulses and temperature in these areas evaluates the patient's peripheral vascular status. |
| Perform the straight leg test on one leg at a time. | Painless leg lifting | ▶ This test checks for vertebral disk problems. |
| Palpate for crepitus as the patient abducts and adducts the hip. Repeat on the opposite leg. | No crepitus; full ROM without pain | ▶ Perform Ortolani's maneuver on an infant to assess hip abduction and adduction. |
| Ask the patient to raise his thigh against the resistance of your hands. Repeat this procedure on the opposite thigh. | Each thigh lifts easily against resistance | ▶ This maneuver tests the motor strength of the upper legs. |
| Ask the patient to push outward against the resistance of your hands. | Each leg pushes easily against resistance | ▶ This maneuver tests the motor strength of the lower legs. |
| Ask the patient to pull backward against the resistance of your hands. | Each leg pulls easily against resistance | ▶ This maneuver tests the motor strength of the lower legs. |
| **Nervous system** | | |
| Lightly touch the ophthalmic, maxillary, and mandibular areas on each side of the patient's face with a cotton-tipped applicator and a pin. | Correct identification of sensation and location | ▶ This test evaluates the function of cranial nerve V (trigeminal nerve). |
| Touch the dorsal and palmar surfaces of the arms, hands, and fingers with a cotton-tipped applicator and a pin. | Correct identification of sensation and location | ▶ This test evaluates the function of the ulnar, radial, and medial nerves. |
| Touch several nerve distribution areas on the legs, feet, and toes with a cotton-tipped applicator and a pin. | Correct identification of sensation and location | ▶ This test evaluates the function of the dermatome areas randomly. |
| Place your fingers above the patient's wrist and tap them with a reflex hammer. Repeat on the other arm. | Normal reflex reaction | ▶ This procedure elicits the brachioradialis deep tendon reflex (DTR). |
| Place your fingers over the antecubital fossa and tap them with a reflex hammer. Repeat on the other arm. | Normal reflex reaction | ▶ This procedure elicits the biceps DTR. |

*(continued)*

# Performing a head-to-toe assessment *(continued)*

| Technique | Normal findings | Special considerations |
|---|---|---|
| ***Nervous system*** *(continued)* | | |
| Place your fingers over the triceps tendon area and tap them with a reflex hammer. Repeat on the other arm. | Normal reflex reaction | ▶ This procedure elicits the triceps DTR. |
| Tap just below the patella with a reflex hammer. Repeat this procedure on the opposite patella. | Normal reflex reaction | ▶ This procedure elicits the patellar DTR. |
| Tap over the Achilles tendon area with a reflex hammer. Repeat this procedure on the opposite ankle. | Normal reflex reaction | ▶ This procedure elicits the Achilles DTR. |
| Stroke the sole of the patient's foot with the end of the reflex hammer handle. | Plantar reflex | ▶ This procedure elicits plantar flexion of all toes.<br>▶ Expect Babinski's sign in children age 2 and under. |
| Ask the patient to demonstrate dorsiflexion by bending both feet upward against resistance. | Both feet lift easily against resistance | ▶ This procedure tests foot strength and ROM. |
| Ask the patient to demonstrate plantar flexion by bending both feet downward against resistance. | Both feet push down easily against resistance | ▶ This procedure tests foot strength and ROM. |
| Inspect the feet and toes for lesions and lumps. | No lesions or lumps | ▶ Condition of the feet and toes helps evaluate peripheral vascular status. |
| Using your finger, trace a one-digit number in the palm of the patient's hand. | Correct identification of traced number | ▶ This procedure evaluates the patient's tactile discrimination through graphesthesia. |
| Place a familiar object, such as a key or a coin, in the patient's hand. | Correct identification of object | ▶ This procedure evaluates the patient's tactile discrimination. |
| Observe the patient while he walks with a regular gait, on the toes, on the heels, and heel-to-toe. | Steady gait, good balance, and no signs of muscle weakness or pain in any style of walking | ▶ This technique evaluates the cerebellum and motor system and checks for vertebral disk problems. |
| Inspect the scapulae, spine, back, and hips as the patient bends forward, backward, and from side to side. | Full ROM, easy flexibility, and no signs of scoliosis or varicosities | ▶ Inspection evaluates the patient's ROM and detects musculoskeletal abnormalities such as scoliosis. |
| Perform the Romberg test. Ask the patient to stand straight with both eyes closed and both arms extended, with hands palms up. | Steady stance with minimal weaving | ▶ This test checks cerebellar functioning and evaluates balance and coordination. |

# Postmortem care

After the patient dies, care includes preparing him for family viewing, arranging transportation to the morgue or funeral home, and determining the disposition of the patient's belongings. In addition, postmortem care entails comforting and supporting the patient's family and friends and providing for their privacy.

Postmortem care usually begins after a doctor certifies the patient's death. If the patient died violently or under suspicious circumstances, postmortem care may be postponed until the medical examiner completes an autopsy.

## Equipment

Gauze or soft string ties ● gloves ● chin straps ● ABD pads ● cotton balls ● plastic shroud or body wrap ● three identification tags ● adhesive bandages to cover wounds or punctures ● plastic bag for patient's belongings ● water-filled basin ● soap ● towels ● washcloths ● stretcher

A commercial morgue pack usually contains gauze or string ties, chin straps, a shroud, and identification tags.

## Implementation

▶ Document any auxiliary equipment, such as a mechanical ventilator, still present. Put on gloves.
▶ Place the body in the supine position, arms at sides and head on a pillow. Elevate the head of the bed 30 degrees to prevent discoloration from blood settling in the face.
▶ If the patient wore dentures and your facility's policy permits, gently insert them, then close the mouth. Close the eyes by gently pressing on the lids with your fingertips. If they don't stay closed, place moist cotton balls on the eyelids for a few minutes, and then try again to close them. Place a folded towel under the chin to keep the jaw closed, if necessary.
▶ Remove all indwelling urinary catheters, tubes, and tape, and apply adhesive bandages to puncture sites. Replace soiled dressings.
▶ Collect all the patient's valuables to prevent loss. If you're unable to remove a ring, cover it with gauze, tape it in place, and tie the gauze to the wrist to prevent slippage and subsequent loss.

▶ Clean the body thoroughly, using soap, a basin, and washcloths. Place one or more ABD pads between the buttocks to absorb rectal discharge or drainage.
▶ Cover the body up to the chin with a clean sheet.
▶ Offer comfort and emotional support to the family and intimate friends. Ask if they wish to see the patient. If they do, allow them to do so in private. Ask if they would prefer to leave the patient's jewelry on the body.
▶ After the family leaves, remove the towel from under the chin of the deceased patient. Pad the chin, and wrap chin straps under the chin and tie them loosely on top of the head. Then, pad the wrists and ankles to prevent bruises and tie them together with gauze or soft string ties.
▶ Fill out the three identification tags. Each tag should include the deceased patient's name, room and bed numbers, date and time of death, and doctor's name. Tie one tag to the deceased patient's hand or foot, but don't remove his identification bracelet to ensure correct identification.
▶ Place the shroud or body wrap on the morgue stretcher and, after obtaining assistance, transfer the body to the stretcher. Wrap the body and tie the shroud or wrap with the string provided. Attach another identification tag and cover the shroud or wrap with a clean sheet. If a shroud or wrap isn't available, dress the deceased patient in a clean gown and cover the body with a sheet.
▶ Place the deceased patient's personal belongings, including valuables, in a bag and attach the third identification tag to it.
▶ If the patient died of an infectious disease, label the body according to your facility's policy.
▶ Close the doors of adjoining rooms if possible. Then take the body to the morgue. Use corridors that aren't crowded and, if possible, use a service elevator.

## Special considerations

▶ Give the deceased patient's personal belongings to his family or bring them to the morgue. If you give the family jewelry or money, make sure a coworker is present as a witness. Obtain the signature of an adult family member to verify receipt of valuables or to state their preference that jewelry remain on the patient.

▶ Offer emotional support to the deceased patient's family and friends, and to the patient's facility roommate, if appropriate.

## Documentation

▶ Document that postmortem care was provided.

▶ Although the extent of documentation varies among facilities, always record the disposition of the patient's possessions, especially jewelry and money.

▶ Note the date and time the patient was transported to the morgue.

### REFERENCES

Harvey, J. "Debunking Myths about Postmortem Care," *Nursing2001* 31(7):44-45, July 2001.

Jenkins, C., and Bruers, E. "Assessment and Management of Medically Ill Patients Who Refuse Life-Prolonging Treatment: Two Case Reports and Proposed Guidelines," *Journal of Palliative Care* 14(1):18-24, 1998.

Quill, T., and Boyd, I. "Responding to Intractable Terminal Suffering: The Role of Terminal Sedation and Voluntary Refusal of Food and Fluids," *Annals of Internal Medicine* 132(5):408-13, March 2000.

# Postoperative care

Postoperative care begins when the patient arrives in the postanesthesia care unit (PACU) and continues as he moves on to the short procedure unit, medical-surgical unit, or critical care area. Postoperative care aims to minimize postoperative complications by early detection and prompt treatment. After anesthesia, a patient may experience pain, inadequate oxygenation, or adverse physiologic effects of sudden movement.

Recovery from general anesthesia takes longer than induction because the anesthetic is retained in fat and muscle. Fat has a meager blood supply; thus, it releases the anesthetic slowly, providing enough anesthesia to maintain adequate blood and brain levels during surgery. The patient's recovery time varies with his amount of body fat, his overall condition, his premedication regimen, and the type, dosage, and duration of anesthesia.

## Equipment

Thermometer ● watch with second hand ● stethoscope ● sphygmomanometer ● postoperative flowchart or other documentation tool

## Implementation

▶ Assemble the equipment at the patient's bedside.

▶ Obtain the patient's record from the PACU nurse. This should include a summary of operative procedures and pertinent findings; type of anesthesia; vital signs (preoperative, intraoperative and postoperative); medical history; medication history, including preoperative, intraoperative, and postoperative medications; fluid therapy, including estimated blood loss, type and number of drains, amount of drainage, catheters, and characteristics of drainage; and notes on the condition of the surgical wound. If the patient had vascular surgery, for example, knowing the location and duration of blood vessel clamping can prevent postoperative complications.

▶ Transfer the patient from the PACU stretcher to the bed, and position him properly. Get a coworker to help if necessary. When moving the patient, keep transfer movements smooth to minimize pain and postoperative complications and avoid back strain among team members. Use a transfer board to facilitate transfer.

▶ If the patient has had orthopedic surgery, always get a coworker to help transfer him. Ask the coworker to move only the affected extremity.

▶ If the patient is in skeletal traction, you may receive special orders for moving him. If you must move him, have a coworker move the weights as you and another coworker move the patient.

▶ Make the patient comfortable and raise the bed's side rails to ensure his safety.

▶ Assess the patient's LOC, skin color, and mucous membranes.

▶ Monitor the patient's respiratory status by assessing his airway. Note breathing rate and depth, and auscultate for breath sounds. Administer oxygen and initiate pulse oximetry to monitor oxygen saturation, if ordered.

▶ Monitor the patient's pulse rate. It should be strong and easily palpable. The heart rate should be within 20% of the preoperative heart rate.

▶ Compare postoperative blood pressure to preoperative blood pressure. It should be within 20% of the preoperative level unless the patient suffered a hypotensive episode during surgery.

▶ Assess the patient's temperature because anesthesia lowers body temperature. Body temperature should be at least 95° F (35° C). If it's lower, apply blankets to warm the patient.

▶ Assess the patient's infusion sites for redness, pain, swelling, or drainage. This would indicate infiltration and would require discontinuing the I.V. and restarting at another site.

▶ Assess surgical wound dressings; they should be clean and dry. If they're soiled, assess the characteristics of the drainage and outline the soiled area. Note the date and time of assessment on the dressing. Assess the soiled area frequently; if it enlarges, reinforce the dressing and alert the doctor.

▶ Note the presence and condition of any drains and tubes. Note the color, type, odor, and amount of drainage. Make sure all drains are properly connected and free of kinks and obstructions.

▶ If the patient has had vascular or orthopedic surgery, assess the appropriate extremity—or all extremities, depending on the surgical procedure. Assess color, temperature, sensation, movement, and presence and quality of pulses, and notify the doctor of any abnormalities.

▶ As the patient recovers from anesthesia, monitor his respiratory and cardiovascular status closely. Be alert for signs of airway obstruction and hypoventilation caused by laryngospasm, or for sedation, which can lead to hypoxemia. Cardiovascular complications, such as arrhythmias and hypotension, may result from the anesthetic agent or the operative procedure.

▶ Encourage coughing and deep-breathing exercises. Don't encourage them if the patient has just had nasal, ophthalmic, or neurologic surgery, to avoid increasing intracranial pressure.

▶ Give postoperative medications, such as antibiotics, analgesics, antiemetics, or reversal agents, as appropriate.

▶ Remove all fluids from the patient's bedside until he's alert enough to eat and drink. Before giving him liquids, assess his gag reflex to prevent aspiration. To do this, lightly touch the back of his throat with a cotton swab. The patient will gag if the reflex has returned. Do this test quickly to prevent a vagal reaction.

▶ Monitor the patient's input and output.

▶ Assess for presence of bowel sounds, especially after abdominal surgery, and passage of flatus before patient can be allowed food.

## Special considerations

▶ Fear, pain, anxiety, hypothermia, confusion, and immobility can upset the patient and jeopardize his safety and postoperative status. Offer emotional support to the patient and his family. Keep in mind that the patient who has lost a body part or who has been diagnosed with an incurable disease will need ongoing emotional support. Refer him and his family for counseling, as needed.

▶ As the patient recovers from general anesthesia, reflexes appear in reverse order to that in which they disappeared. Hearing recovers first, so avoid holding inappropriate conversations.

▶ The patient under general anesthesia can't protect his own airway because of muscle relaxation. As he recovers, his cough and gag reflexes reappear. If he can lift his head without assistance, he's usually able to breathe on his own.

▶ If the patient received spinal anesthesia, he will need to remain supine with the bed adjusted to between 0 degrees and 20 degrees for at least 6 hours to reduce the risk of spinal headache from leakage of cerebrospinal fluid. The patient won't be able to move his legs, so be sure to reassure him that sensation and mobility will return.

▶ If the patient has had epidural anesthesia for postoperative pain control, monitor his respiratory status closely. Respiratory arrest may result from paralysis of the diaphragm by the anesthetic. He may also suffer nausea, vomiting, or pruritus.

▶ If the patient will be using a patient-controlled anesthesia (PCA) unit, make sure he understands how to use it. Caution him to activate it only when he has pain, not when he feels sleepy or is pain-free. Review your facility's criteria for PCA use.

## Complications

Postoperative complications may include arrhythmias, hypotension, hypovolemia, septicemia, septic shock, atelectasis, pneumonia, thrombophlebitis, pulmonary embolism, urine retention, wound infection, wound dehiscence, evisceration, abdominal distention, paralytic ileus, constipation, altered body image, and postoperative psychosis.

## Documentation

▸ Document vital signs on the appropriate flowchart.

▸ Record the condition of dressings and drains and the characteristics of drainage.

▸ Document all interventions taken to alleviate pain and anxiety and the patient's responses to them.

▸ Document any complications and interventions taken.

### REFERENCES

American Association for Respiratory Care. "Directed Cough," *Respiratory Care* 38(5): 495-99, May 1993. [Reviewed 2000.]

Leinonen, T., and Leino-Kilpi, H. "Research in Peri-operative Nursing Care," *Journal of Clinical Nursing* 8(2):123-38, March 1999.

# Preoperative care

Preoperative care begins when surgery is first planned and ends with the administration of anesthesia. This phase of care includes a preoperative interview and assessment to collect baseline subjective and objective data from the patient and his family; diagnostic tests, such as urinalysis, ECG, and chest radiography; preoperative teaching; securing informed consent from the patient; and physical preparation.

## Equipment

Thermometer ● sphygmomanometer ● stethoscope ● watch with second hand ● weight scale ● tape measure

### Preparation of equipment

Assemble all equipment needed at the patient's bedside or in the admission area.

## Implementation

▸ If the patient is having same-day surgery, make sure he knows ahead of time not to eat or drink anything for 8 hours before surgery. Confirm with him what time he's scheduled to arrive at the facility, and tell him to leave all jewelry and valuables at home. Also make sure the patient has arranged for someone to accompany him home after surgery.

▸ Obtain a health history and assess the patient's knowledge, perceptions, and expectations about his surgery. Ask about previous medical and surgical interventions. Also determine the patient's psychosocial needs; ask about occupational well-being, financial matters, support systems, mental status, and cultural beliefs. Use your facility's preoperative surgical assessment database, if available, to gather this information. Obtain a drug history. Ask about current prescription and over-the-counter medications and about known allergies to foods, drugs, and latex.

▸ Measure the patient's height, weight, and vital signs.

▸ Identify risk factors that may interfere with a positive expected outcome. Be sure to consider age, general health, medications, mobility, nutritional status, fluid and electrolyte disturbances, and lifestyle. Also consider the primary disorder's duration, location, and nature, and the extent of the surgical procedure.

▸ Explain preoperative procedures to the patient. Include typical events that he can expect. Discuss equipment that may be used postoperatively, such as nasogastric tubes and I.V. equipment. Explain the typical incision, dressings, and staples or sutures that will be used. Preoperative teaching can help reduce postoperative anxiety and pain, increase patient compliance, hasten recovery, and decrease length of stay.

▸ Talk the patient through the sequence of events from operating room to PACU back to patient's room. Some patients may be transferred from the PACU to an intensive care unit or surgical care unit. Your patient may also benefit from a tour of the areas he'll see during the perioperative events.

▸ Tell the patient that when he goes to the operating room, he may have to wait a short time in the holding area. Explain that the doctors and nurses will wear surgical dress, and even though they'll be observing him closely, they'll refrain from talking to him very much. Explain that minimal conversation will help the preoperative medication take effect.

▸ When discussing transfer procedures and techniques, describe sensations that the patient will experience. Tell him that he'll be taken to the operating room on a stretcher and transferred from the stretcher to the operating room table. For his own safety, he'll be held securely to the table with soft restraints. The operating room nurses will check his vital signs frequently.

▶ Warn the patient that the operating room may feel cool. Electrodes may be put on his chest to monitor his heart rate during surgery. Describe the drowsy floating sensation he'll feel as the anesthetic takes effect. Tell him it's important that he relax at this time.

▶ Tell the patient about exercises that he may be expected to perform after surgery, such as deep-breathing, coughing (while splinting the incision if necessary), extremity exercises, and movement and ambulation to minimize respiratory and circulatory complications. If the patient will undergo ophthalmic or neurologic surgery, he won't be asked to cough because coughing increases intracranial pressure.

▶ On the day of surgery, important interventions include giving morning care, verifying that the patient has signed an informed consent form (see *Obtaining informed consent*), giving preoperative medications, completing the preoperative checklist and chart, and supporting the patient and his family.

▶ Other immediate preoperative interventions may include preparing the GI tract (restricting food and fluids for about 8 hours before surgery) to reduce vomiting and the risk of aspiration, cleaning the lower GI tract of fecal material by enemas before abdominal or GI surgery, and giving antibiotics for 2 or 3 days preoperatively to prevent contamination of the peritoneal cavity by GI bacteria.

▶ Just before the patient is moved to the surgical area, make sure he is wearing a hospital gown, has his identification band in place, and has his vital signs recorded. Check to see that hairpins, nail polish, and jewelry have been removed. Note whether dentures, contact lenses, or prosthetic devices have been removed or left in place.

## Special considerations

▶ Preoperative medications must be given on time to enhance the effect of ordered anesthesia. The patient should take nothing by mouth preoperatively. Don't give oral medications unless ordered. Be sure to raise the bed's side rails immediately after giving preoperative medications.

## Obtaining informed consent

Informed consent means that the patient has agreed to a procedure after receiving a full explanation of the procedure, its risks and complications, and the risk if the procedure isn't performed at this time. Although obtaining informed consent is the doctor's responsibility, the nurse is responsible for verifying that this step has been taken.

You may be asked to witness the patient's signature. However, if you didn't hear the doctor's explanation to the patient, you must sign that you are witnessing the patient's signature only.

Consent forms must be signed before the patient receives preoperative medication because forms signed after sedatives are given are legally invalid. Adults and emancipated minors can sign their own consent forms. Consent forms of children or of adults with impaired mental status must be signed by a parent or guardian.

▶ If family members or others are present, direct them to the appropriate waiting area and offer support as needed.

## Documentation

▶ Complete the preoperative checklist used by your facility.

▶ Record all nursing care measures and preoperative medications, results of diagnostic tests, and the time the patient is transferred to the surgical area.

▶ The chart and the surgical checklist must accompany the patient to surgery.

## REFERENCES

Centers for Disease Control and Prevention. "Guideline for Prevention of Surgical Site Infection, 1999," *www.guideline.gov.*

Matiti, M., and Sharman, J. "Dignity: A Study of Pre-operative Patients," *Nursing Standards* 14(13-15):32-35, December 1999.

Shuldham, C. "Pre-operative Education: A Review of the Research Design," *International Journal of Nursing Studies* 36:179-87, April 1999.

Shuldham, C. "A Review of the Impact of Pre-operative Education in Recovery from Surgery," *International Journal of Nursing Studies* 36:171-77, April 1999.

# Preoperative skin preparation

Proper preparation of the patient's skin for surgery renders it as free as possible from microorganisms, thereby reducing the risk of infection at the incision site. It doesn't duplicate or replace the full sterile preparation that immediately precedes surgery. Rather, it may involve a bath, shower, or local scrub with an antiseptic detergent solution, followed by hair removal. (See *Removing hair for surgery*.)

The Association of Operating Room Nurses recommends that hair not be removed from the area surrounding the operative site unless it's thick enough to interfere with surgery because hair removal may increase the risk of infection. Each facility has a hair removal policy.

The area of preparation always exceeds that of the expected incision to minimize the number of microorganisms in the areas adjacent to the proposed incision and to allow surgical draping of the patient without contamination.

## Equipment

Antiseptic soap solution • warm tap water • bath blanket • two clean basins • linen-saver pad • adjustable light • sterile razor with sharp new blade, if needed • scissors • liquid soap • optional: 4″ × 4″ gauze pads, cotton-tipped applicators, acetone or nail polish remover, orangewood stick, trash bag, towel, and gloves

### Preparation of equipment
Use warm tap water because heat reduces the skin's surface tension and facilitates removal of soil and hair. Dilute the antiseptic soap solution with warm tap water in one basin for washing, and pour plain warm water into the second basin for rinsing.

## Implementation

▶ Check the doctor's order and explain the procedure to the patient, including the reason for the extensive preparations, to avoid causing undue anxiety. Provide privacy, wash your hands thoroughly, and put on gloves.
▶ Place the patient in a comfortable position, drape him with the bath blanket, and expose the preparation area. For most surgeries, this area extends 12″ (30.5 cm) in each direction from the expected incision

site. However, to ensure privacy and avoid chilling the patient, expose only one small area at a time while performing skin preparation.
▶ Position a linen-saver pad beneath the patient to catch spills and avoid linen changes. Adjust the light to illuminate the preparation area.
▶ Assess skin condition in the preparation area and report any rash, abrasion, or laceration to the doctor before beginning the procedure. Any break in the skin increases the risk of infection and could cause cancellation of planned surgery.
▶ Have the patient remove all jewelry in or near the operative site.
▶ Begin removing hair from the preparation area by clipping any long hairs with scissors. If ordered, shave all remaining hair within the area to remove microorganisms. Perform the procedure as near to the time of surgery as possible so that microorganisms will have minimal time to proliferate. Use only a sterilized or sterile disposable razor with a sharp new blade to avoid the risk of infection from a contaminated razor.
▶ Use a gauze pad to spread liquid soap over the shave site.
▶ Pull the skin taut in the direction opposite the direction of hair growth because this makes the hair rise and facilitates shaving.
▶ Holding the razor at a 45-degree angle, shave with short strokes in the direction of hair growth to avoid skin irritation and achieve a smooth clean shave.
▶ If possible, avoid lifting the razor from the skin and placing it down again to minimize the risk of lacerations. Also, avoid applying pressure because this can cause abrasions, particularly over bony prominences.
▶ Rinse the razor frequently and reapply liquid soap to the skin, as needed, to keep the area moist.
▶ Change the rinse water, if necessary. Then rinse the soap solution and loose hair from the preparation area and inspect the skin. Immediately notify the doctor of any new nicks, lacerations, or abrasions, and file a report if your facility requires it.
▶ Proceed with a 10-minute scrub to ensure a clean preparation area. Wash the area with a gauze pad dipped in the antiseptic soap solution. Using a circular motion, start at the expected incision site and

# Removing hair for surgery

### Shoulder and upper arm

On operative side, remove hair from fingertips to hairline and center chest to center spine, extending to iliac crest and including the axilla.

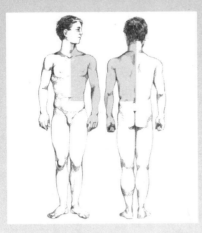

### Chest

Remove hair from chin to iliac crests and side to midline of back on operative side (2″ [5 cm] beyond midline of back for thoracotomy). Include axilla and entire arm to elbow on operative side.

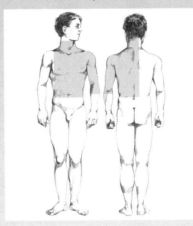

### Forearm, elbow, and hand

On operative side, remove hair from fingertips to shoulder. Include the axilla unless surgery is for hand. Trim and clean fingernails.

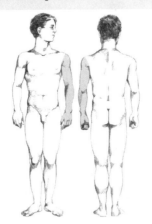

### Abdomen

Remove hair from 3″ (7.6 cm) above nipples to upper thighs, including pubic area.

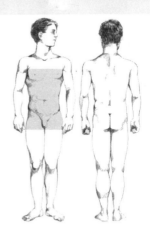

*(continued)*

work outward toward the periphery of the area to avoid recontaminating the clean area. Apply light friction while washing to improve the antiseptic effect of the solution. Replace the gauze pad as necessary.

◗ Carefully clean skin folds and crevices because they harbor greater numbers of mi-

# Removing hair for surgery *(continued)*

### Thigh

On operative side, remove hair from toes to 3" (7.6 cm) above umbilicus and from midline front to midline back, including pubis. Clean and trim toenails.

### Lower abdomen

Remove hair from 2" (5 cm) above umbilicus to midthigh, including pubic area; for femoral ligation, to midline of thigh in back; and for hernioplasty and embolectomy, to costal margin and down to knee.

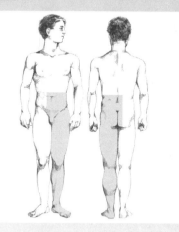

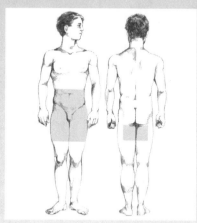

### Ankle and foot

On operative side, remove hair from toes to 3" above the knee. Clean and trim toenails.

### Spine

Remove all hair from the axillae and back, including the shoulders and neck to the hairline, down to both knees.

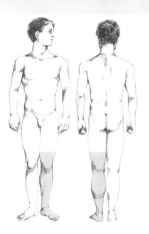

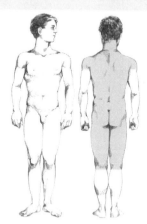

croorganisms. Scrub the perineal area last, if it's part of the preparation area, for the same reason. Pull loose skin taut. If necessary, use cotton-tipped applicators to clean the umbilicus and an orangewood stick to clean under nails. Remove any nail polish with acetone or nail polish remover because the anesthetist uses nail bed color to

# Removing hair for surgery *(continued)*

### Knees and lower leg
On operative side, remove hair from toes to groin. Clean and trim toenails.

### Perineum
Remove hair from pubis, perineum, and perianal area and from the waist to at least 3″ below the groin in front and at least 3″ below the buttocks in back.

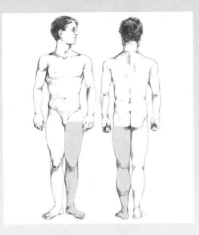

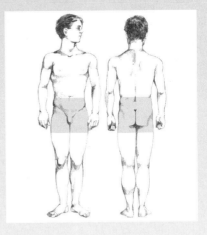

### Hip
On operative side, remove hair from toes to nipples and at least 3″ beyond midline back and front, including the pubis. Clean and trim toenails.

### Flank
On operative side, remove hair from nipples to pubis, 3″ beyond midline in back and 2″ past abdominal midline. Include pubic area and, on affected side, upper thigh and axilla.

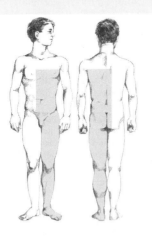

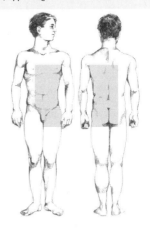

determine adequate oxygenation and may place a probe on the nail to measure oxygen saturation.

▶ Dry the area with a clean towel and remove the linen-saver pad.
▶ Give the patient any special instructions for care of the prepared area and remind

him to keep the area clean for surgery. Make sure the patient is comfortable.
▶ Properly dispose of solutions and the trash bag, and clean or dispose of soiled equipment and supplies according to your facility's policy.

### Special considerations
▶ Avoid shaving facial or neck hair on women and children unless ordered. Never shave eyebrows because this disrupts normal hair growth and the new growth may prove unsightly. Scalp shaving is usually performed in the operating room, but if you're required to prepare the patient's scalp, put all hair in a plastic or paper bag and store it with the patient's possessions.
▶ If the patient won't hold still for shaving, remove hair with a depilatory cream. Although this method produces clean, intact skin without risking lacerations or abrasions, it can cause skin irritation or rash, especially in the groin area. If possible, cut long hairs with scissors before applying the cream because removal of remaining hair then requires less cream. Then use a glove to apply the cream in a layer ½″ (1.3 cm) thick. After about 10 minutes, remove the cream with moist gauze pads. Next, wash the area with antiseptic soap solution, rinse, and pat dry.

### Complications
Rashes, nicks, lacerations, and abrasions are the most common complications of skin preparation. They also increase the risk of postoperative infection.

### Documentation
▶ Record the date, time, and area of preparation; skin condition before and after preparation; any complications; and the patient's tolerance.
▶ If your facility requires it, complete an incident report if the patient suffers nicks, lacerations, or abrasions during skin preparation.

### REFERENCES
Craven, R., and Hirnle, C.J. *Fundamentals of Nursing: Human Health and Function,* 4th ed. Philadelphia: Lippincott Williams & Wilkins, 2002.

Simmons, M. "Pre-operative Skin Preparation," *Professional Nurse* 13(7):446-47, April 1998.

# Restraint application

Restraints are used only when other less restrictive measures have been ineffective in protecting the patient and others from harm. Various soft restraints limit movement to prevent the confused, disoriented, or combative patient from injuring himself or others. Vest and belt restraints, which are used to prevent falls from a bed or a chair, permit full movement of arms and legs. Limb restraints, which are used to prevent removal of supportive equipment, such as I.V. lines, indwelling catheters, and nasogastric tubes, allow only slight limb motion. Like limb restraints, mitts prevent removal of supportive equipment, keep the patient from scratching rashes or sores, and prevent the combative patient from injuring himself or others. Body restraints, which are used to control the combative or hysterical patient, immobilize all or most of the body.

When soft restraints aren't sufficient and sedation is dangerous or ineffective, leather restraints can be used. Depending on the patient's behavior, leather restraints may be applied to all limbs (four-point restraints) or to one arm and one leg (two-point restraints). The duration of such restraint is governed by state law and by facility policy.

Restraints must be used cautiously in seizure-prone patients because they increase the risk of fracture and trauma. Restraints can cause skin irritation and restrict blood flow, so they shouldn't be applied directly over wounds or I.V. catheters. Vest restraints should be used with caution in patients who have heart failure or respiratory disorders. Such restraints can tighten with movement, further limiting circulation and respiratory function.

Any measure used to restrict a patient's movements, such as a lap tray, geriatric chair, bedside table, or side rails in considered a restraint.

### Equipment
For soft restraints: Restraint (such as a vest, limb, mitt, belt, or body as needed) ● gauze pads, if needed

For leather restraints: Two wrist and two ankle leather restraints ● four straps ● key ● large gauze pads to cushion each extremity

## Preparation of equipment

Before entering the patient's room, make sure the restraints are the correct size, using the patient's build and weight as a guide. If you use leather restraints, make sure that the straps are unlocked and the key fits the locks.

◆ **ALERT!** For children, typically too small for standard restraints, use a child restraint. (See *Types of child restraints,* page 46.)

## Implementation

▶ Obtain a doctor's order for the restraint. Keep in mind that the doctor's order must be time limited: 4 hours for adults, 2 hours for children and adolescents ages 9 to 17, and 1 hour for children younger than age 9. The original order may only be renewed for a total of 24 hours. After the original order expires, the doctor must see and evaluate the patient before a new order can be written.

▶ If necessary, obtain adequate assistance to restrain the patient before entering his room. Enlist the aid of several coworkers and organize their effort, giving each person a specific task; for example, one person explains the procedure to the patient and applies the restraints while the others immobilize the patient's arms and legs.

▶ Tell the patient what you're about to do and describe the restraints to him. Assure him that they're being used to protect him from injury rather than to punish him.

### Applying a vest restraint

▶ Assist the patient to a sitting position, if his condition permits. Then slip the vest over his gown. Crisscross the cloth flaps at the front, placing the V-shaped opening at the patient's throat. Be sure there is clothing between the skin and vest to decrease chance of skin irritation and breakdown. Never crisscross the flaps in the back because this may cause the patient to choke if he tries to squirm out of the vest.

▶ Pass the tab on one flap through the slot on the opposite flap. Then adjust the vest for the patient's comfort. You should be able to slip your fist between the vest and the patient. Avoid wrapping the vest too tightly because it may restrict respiration.

▶ Tie all restraints securely to the frame of the bed, chair, or wheelchair and out of the patient's reach. Use a bow or a knot that can be released quickly and easily in an emergency. (See *Knots for securing soft restraints,* page 47.) Never tie a regular knot to secure the straps. Leave 1″ to 2″ (2.5 to 5 cm) of slack in the straps to allow room for movement.

◆ **ALERT!** Never tie a restraint to a side rail of the bed because this will tighten the vest and restrict respirations when the side rails are lowered.

▶ After applying the vest, check the patient's respiratory rate and breath sounds regularly. Be alert for signs of respiratory distress. Also, make sure the vest hasn't tightened with the patient's movement. Loosen the vest at least every 2 hours for at least 20 minutes so the patient can stretch, turn, and breathe deeply.

### Applying a limb restraint

▶ Wrap the patient's wrist or ankle with gauze pads to reduce friction between the patient's skin and the restraint, helping to prevent irritation and skin breakdown. Then wrap the restraint around the gauze pads.

▶ Pass the strap on the narrow end of the restraint through the slot in the broad end and adjust for a snug fit. Or fasten the buckle or Velcro cuffs to fit the restraint. You should be able to slip one or two fingers between the restraint and the patient's skin. Avoid applying the restraint too tightly because it may impair circulation distal to the restraint.

▶ Tie the restraint, as above.

▶ After applying limb restraints, be alert for signs of impaired circulation in the extremity distal to the restraint. If the skin appears blue or feels cold, or if the patient complains of a tingling sensation or numbness, loosen the restraint. Perform ROM exercises every 2 hours when restraints are removed to stimulate circulation and prevent contractures and resultant loss of mobility.

### Applying a mitt restraint

▶ Wash and dry the patient's hands.

▶ Roll up a washcloth or gauze pad and place it in the patient's palm. Have him form a loose fist, if possible; then pull the mitt over it and secure the closure.

▶ To restrict the patient's arm movement, attach the strap to the mitt and tie it securely, using a bow or a knot that can be released quickly and easily in an emergency.

# Types of child restraints

You may need to restrain an infant or a child to prevent injury or to facilitate examination, diagnostic tests, or treatment. If so, take the following steps:

▶ Provide a simple explanation, reassurance, and constant observation to minimize the child's fear.
▶ Explain the restraint to the parents and enlist their help.
▶ Reassure them that it won't hurt the child.

▶ Make sure restraint ties or safety pins are secured outside the child's reach to prevent injury.
▶ When using a mummy restraint, secure the infant's arms in proper alignment with the body to avoid dislocation and other injuries.

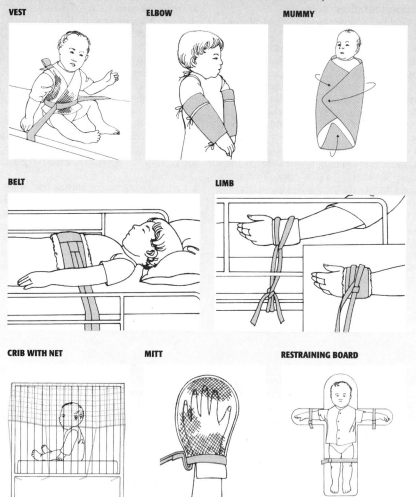

VEST   ELBOW   MUMMY

BELT   LIMB

CRIB WITH NET   MITT   RESTRAINING BOARD

▶ When using mitts made of transparent mesh, check hand movement and skin color frequently to assess circulation. Remove the mitts at least every 2 hours for at least 20 minutes to stimulate circulation, and perform passive ROM exercises to prevent contractures.

### Applying a belt restraint
▶ Center the flannel pad of the belt on the bed. Then wrap the short strap of the belt around the bed frame and fasten it under the bed.
▶ Position the patient on the pad. Then have him roll slightly to one side while you guide the long strap around his waist and through the slot in the pad.
▶ Wrap the long strap around the bed frame and fasten it under the bed.
▶ After applying the belt, slip your hand between the patient and the belt to ensure a secure but comfortable fit. A loose belt can be raised to chest level; a tight one can cause abdominal discomfort.

### Applying a body (Posey net) restraint
▶ Place the restraint flat on the bed, with arm and wrist cuffs facing down and the "V" at the head of the bed.
▶ Place the patient in the prone position on top of the restraint.
▶ Lift the "V" over the patient's head. Thread the chest belt through one of the loops in the "V" to ensure a snug fit.
▶ Secure the straps around the patient's chest, thighs, and legs, then turn the patient on his back.
▶ Secure the straps to the bed frame to anchor the restraint. Then secure the straps around the patient's arms and wrists.

### Applying leather restraints
▶ Position the patient supine on the bed, with each arm and leg securely held down to minimize combative behavior and to prevent injury to the patient and others. Immobilize the patient's arms and legs at the joints — knee, ankle, shoulder, and wrist — to minimize his movement without exerting excessive force.
▶ Apply pads to the patient's wrists and ankles to reduce friction between his skin and the leather, preventing skin irritation and breakdown.
▶ Wrap the restraint around the gauze pads. Then insert the metal loop through the hole that gives the best fit. Apply the restraints securely but not too tightly. You should be able to slip one or two fingers between the restraint and the patient's skin. A tight restraint can compromise circulation; a loose one can slip off or move up

## Knots for securing soft restraints

When securing soft restraints, use knots that can be released quickly and easily, such as those shown below. Remember, never secure restraints to the bed's side rails.

**MAGNUS HITCH**

**CLOVE HITCH**

**LOOPCLOVE HITCH**

**REVERSE CLOVE HITCH**

the patient's arm or leg, causing skin irritation and breakdown.
▶ Thread the strap through the metal loop on the restraint, close the metal loop, and secure the strap to the bed frame, out of the patient's reach.
▶ Lock the restraint by pushing in the button on the side of the metal loop, and tug it gently to make sure it's secure. Once the restraint is secure, a coworker can release the arm or leg. Flex the patient's arm or leg slightly before locking the strap to allow room for movement and to prevent frozen joints and dislocations.
▶ Place the key in a readily accessible location that all staff are of aware in case of emergency.
▶ After applying leather restraints, observe the patient regularly to give emotional support and to reassess the need for continued use of the restraint. Check his pulse rate and vital signs at least every 2 hours. Remove or loosen the restraints one at a time, every 2 hours, and perform passive ROM exercises, if possible. Watch for signs of impaired peripheral circulation such as cool, cyanotic skin. To unlock the restraint, insert the key into the metal loop, opposite

the locking button. This releases the lock, and the metal loop can be opened.

### Special considerations

▶ Some facilities may require that a consent form be signed by the family indicating that they agree to the application of restraints, if they're absolutely necessary.

▶ When the patient is at high risk for aspiration, restrain him on his side. Never secure all four restraints to one side of the bed because the patient may fall out of bed.

▶ When loosening restraints, have a coworker on hand to assist in restraining the patient, if necessary.

▶ After assessing the patient's behavior and condition, you may decide to use a two-point restraint, which should restrain one arm and the opposite leg, for example, the right arm and the left leg. Never restrain the arm and leg on the same side because the patient may fall out of bed.

▶ Don't apply a limb restraint above an I.V. site because the constriction may occlude the infusion or cause infiltration into surrounding tissue.

▶ Never secure restraints to the side rails because someone might inadvertently lower the rail before noticing the attached restraint. This may jerk the patient's limb or body, causing him discomfort and trauma. Never secure restraints to the fixed frame of the bed if the patient's position is to be changed.

▶ Don't restrain a patient in the prone position. This position limits his field of vision, intensifies feelings of helplessness and vulnerability, and impairs respiration, especially if the patient has been sedated.

▶ Because the restrained patient has limited mobility, his nutrition, elimination, and positioning become your responsibility. To prevent pressure ulcers, reposition the patient regularly and massage and pad bony prominences and other vulnerable areas.

▶ Continually monitor, assess, and evaluate the condition of the restrained patient. Document restraint use hourly on a Restraint Flow Sheet. Release the restraints every 2 hours; assess the patient's pulse and skin condition, and perform ROM exercises.

### Complications

Excessively tight limb restraints can reduce peripheral circulation; tight vest restraints can impair respiration. Apply restraints carefully and check them regularly.

Skin breakdown can also occur under limb and vest restraints. To prevent this, pad the patient's wrists and ankles, loosen or remove the restraints at least every 2 hours, and provide regular skin care.

Long periods of immobility can predispose the patient to pneumonia, urine retention, constipation, and sensory deprivation. Reposition the patient and attend to his elimination requirements as needed.

Some patients resist restraints by biting, kicking, scratching, or head butting, in the course of which they may injure themselves or others.

### Documentation

▶ Record the behavior that necessitated restraints; what measures or interventions were used or attempted, and their results, before restraints were applied; when the restraints were applied and removed, and the type of restraints used.

▶ Document the patient's behavior during release of restraints. Record any ROM exercises and skin care provided. Also document how the patient's elimination and nutritional needs are being met.

▶ Record vital signs, skin condition, respiratory status, peripheral circulation, and mental status.

**REFERENCES**

"JCAHO Revises Restraints Standards," *Contemporary Long Term Care* 23(8):9, August 2000.

Lusis, S. "Update on Restraint Use in Acute Care Settings," *Plastic Surgical Nursing* 20(3):145, Fall 2000.

McConnell, E.A. "Applying a Wrist Restraint," *Nursing2000* 30(9):22, September 2000.

McConnell, E.A. "Applying a Vest Restraint," *Nursing2000* 30(10):22, September 2000.

Rogers, P.D., and Bocchino, N.L. "Restraint-free Care: Is It Possible?" *AJN* 99(1):26-33, October 1999.

Schiff, L. "JCAHO and HFCA Now Agree on Restraint Standards," *RN* 64(1):14, January 2001.

# Rotation beds

Because of their constant motion, rotation beds, such as the Roto Rest or Roto Rest Kinetic Treatment Table, promote postural drainage, kidney drainage, and peristalsis and help prevent the complications of immobility while maintaining spinal alignment. The bed rotates from side to side in a cradlelike motion, achieving a maximum elevation of 62 degrees and full side-to-side turning approximately every 4½ minutes.

Because the bed holds the patient motionless, it's especially helpful for patients with spinal cord injury, multiple trauma, stroke, multiple sclerosis, coma, severe burns, hypostatic pneumonia, and atelectasis or other unilateral lung involvement causing poor ventilation and perfusion.

Rotation beds, such as the Roto Rest bed, can accommodate cervical traction devices and tongs. One type of Roto Rest bed has an access hatch underneath for the perineal area; another type has access hatches for the perineal, cervical, and thoracic areas. Both have arm and leg hatches that fold down to allow ROM exercises. Other features include variable angles of rotation, a fan, access for X-rays, and supports and clips for chest tubes, catheters, and drains. Racks beneath the bed hold X-ray plates in place for chest and spinal films. (See *Understanding the Roto Rest bed,* page 50.)

Rotation beds are contraindicated for the patient who has severe claustrophobia or who has an unstable cervical fracture without neurologic deficit and the complications of immobility. Patient transfer and positioning on the bed should be performed by at least two persons to ensure the patient's safety.

The instructions given below apply to the Roto Rest bed.

## Equipment

Rotation bed with appropriate accessories • pillowcases or linen-saver pads • flat sheet or padding

### Preparation of equipment

When using the Roto Rest bed, carefully inspect the bed and run it through a complete cycle in both automatic and manual modes to ensure that it's working properly. If you're using the Mark I model, check the tightness of the set screws at the head of the bed.

To prepare the bed for the patient, remove the counterbalance weights from the keel and place them in the base frame's storage area. Release the connecting arm by pulling down on the cam handle and depressing the lower side of the footboard. Next, lock the table in the horizontal position and place all side supports in the extreme lateral position by loosening the cam handles on the underside of the table. Slide the supports off the bed. Note that all supports and packs are labeled RIGHT or LEFT on the bottom to facilitate reassembly.

Remove the knee packs by depressing the snap button and rotating and pulling the packs from the tube. Then remove the abductor packs (the Mark III model has only one) by depressing and sliding them toward the head of the bed. Next, loosen the foot and knee assemblies by lifting the cam handle at its base and slide them to the foot of the bed. Finally, loosen the shoulder clamp assembly and knobs; swing the shoulder clamps to the vertical position and retighten them.

If you're using the Mark I model, remove the cervical, thoracic, and perineal packs. Cover them with pillowcases or linen-saver pads, smooth all wrinkles, and replace the packs. If you're using the Mark III model, remove the perineal pack, cover the pack, and replace it. Cover the upper half of the bed, which is a solid unit, with padding or a sheet. Install new disposable foam cushions for the patient's head, shoulders, and feet.

## Implementation

▶ If possible, show the patient the bed before use. Explain and demonstrate its operation and reassure the patient that the bed will hold him securely.

▶ Before positioning the patient on the bed, make sure it's turned off. Then place and lock the bed in horizontal position, out of gear. Latch all hatches and lock the wheels.

▶ Obtain assistance and transfer the patient. Move him gently to the center of the bed to prevent contact with the pillar posts and to ensure proper balance during bed operation. Smooth the pillowcase or linen-saver pad beneath his hips. Then place any tubes through the appropriate notches in the hatches and ensure that any traction weights hang freely.

▶ Insert the thoracic side supports in their posts. Adjust the patient's longitudinal po-

## Understanding the Roto Rest bed

Driven by a silent motor, this bed turns the immobilized patient slowly and continuously, more than 300 times daily. The motion provides constant passive exercise and peristaltic stimulation without depriving the patient of sleep or risking further injury. The bed is radiolucent, permitting X-rays to be taken through it without moving the patient. It also has a built-in cooling fan and allows access for surgery on multiple-trauma patients without disrupting spinal alignment or traction.

The bed's hatches provide access to various parts of the patient's body. Arm hatches permit full range of motion and have holes for chest tubes. Leg hatches allow full hip extension. The perineal hatch provides access for bowel and bladder care, the thoracic hatch for chest auscultation and lumbar puncture, and the cervical hatch for wound care, bathing, and shampooing.

**TOP VIEW**

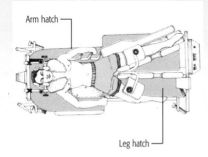

Arm hatch

Leg hatch

**BACK VIEW**

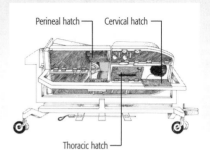

Perineal hatch — Cervical hatch

Thoracic hatch

---

sition to allow a 1″ (2.5 cm) space between the axillae and the supports, thereby avoiding pressure on the axillary blood vessels and the brachial plexus. Push the supports against his chest and lock the cam arms securely to provide support and ensure patient safety.

▶ Place the disposable supports under his legs to remove pressure from his heels and prevent pressure ulcers.

▶ Install and adjust the foot supports so that the patient's feet lie in the normal anatomic position, thereby helping to prevent footdrop. The foot supports should be in position for only 2 hours of every shift to prevent excessive pressure on the soles and toes.

▶ Place the abductor packs in the appropriate supports, allowing a 6″ (15.2 cm) space between the packs and the patient's groin. Tighten the knobs on the bed's underside at the base of the support tubes.

▶ Install the leg side supports snugly against the patient's hips and tighten the cam arms. Position the knee assemblies

slightly above his knees and tighten the cam arms. Then place your hand on the patient's knee and move the knee pack until it rests lightly on the top of your hand. Repeat for the other knee.

▶ Loosen the retaining rings on the crossbar and slide the head and shoulder assembly laterally. The retaining rings maintain correct lateral position of the shoulder clamp assembly and head support pack.

▶ Carefully lower the head and shoulder assembly into place and slide it to touch the patient's head.

▶ Place your hand on the patient's shoulder and move the shoulder pack until it touches your hand. Tighten it in place. Repeat for the other shoulder. The 1″ clearance between the shoulders and the packs prevents excess pressure, which can lead to pressure ulcers.

▶ Place the head pack close to, but not touching, the patient's ears or tongs.

▶ Tighten the head and shoulder assembly securely so it won't lift off the bed. Position

the restraining rings next to the shoulder assembly bracket and tighten them.
▶ Place the patient's arms on the disposable supports. Install the side arm supports and secure the safety straps, placing one across the shoulder assembly and the other over the thoracic supports. If necessary, cover the patient with a flat sheet.

### Balancing the bed
▶ Place one hand on the footboard to prevent the bed from turning rapidly if it's unbalanced. Then remove the locking pin. If the bed rotates to one side, reposition the patient in its center; if it tilts to the right, gently turn it slightly to the left and slide the packs on the right side toward the patient; if it tilts to the left, reverse the process. If a large imbalance exists, you may have to adjust the packs on both sides.
▶ After the patient is centered, gently turn the bed to the 62-degree position.
▶ Measure the space between the patient's chest, hip, and thighs and the inside of the packs. If this space exceeds ½″ (1.3 cm) for the Mark III model or 1″ for the Mark I, return the bed to the horizontal position, lock it in place, and slide the packs inward on both sides. If the space appears too tight, proceed as above but slide both packs outward. Excessively loose packs cause the patient to slide from side to side during turning, possibly resulting in unnecessary movement at fracture sites, skin irritation from shearing force, and bed imbalance. Overly tight packs can place pressure on the patient during turning.
▶ After adjusting the packs, check the bed; balance it, and make any necessary adjustments.
▶ If you're using the Mark III model bed and the patient weighs more than 160 lb (72.6 kg), the bed may become top-heavy. To correct this, place counterbalance weights in the appropriate slots in the keel of the bed. Add one weight for every 20 lb (9.1 kg) over 160 lb, but remember that placement of weights doesn't replace correct patient positioning.
▶ If you're using the Mark I model, it may be necessary to add weights for the patient weighing less than 160 lb. Place one weight for each 20 lb less than 160 lb in the proper bracket at the foot of the bed.

### Initiating automatic bed rotation
▶ Ensure that all packs are securely in place. Then hold the footboard firmly and remove the locking pin to start the bed's motor. The bed will continue to rotate until the pin is reinserted.
▶ Raise the connecting arm cam handle until the connecting assembly snaps into place, locking the bed into automatic rotation.
▶ Remain with the patient for at least three complete turns from side to side to evaluate his comfort and safety. Observe his response and offer him emotional support.

## Special considerations
▶ If the patient develops cardiac arrest while on the bed, perform cardiopulmonary resuscitation after taking the bed out of gear, locking it in the horizontal position, removing the side arm support and the thoracic pack, lifting the shoulder assembly, and dropping the arm pack. Doing all these steps takes only 5 to 10 seconds. You won't need a cardiac board because of the bed's firm surface.
▶ If the electricity fails, lock the bed in the horizontal or lateral position and rotate it manually every 30 minutes to prevent pressure ulcers. If cervical traction causes the patient to slide upward, place the bed in reverse Trendelenburg's position; if extremity traction causes the patient to migrate toward the foot of the bed, use Trendelenburg's position.
▶ Lock the bed in the extreme lateral position for access to the back of the head, thorax, and buttocks through the appropriate hatches. Clean the mattress and nondisposable packs during patient care and rinse them thoroughly to remove all soap residue. When replacing the packs and hatches, take care not to pinch the patient's skin between the packs. This can cause pain and tissue necrosis.
▶ Expect increased drainage from any pressure ulcers for the first few days the patient is on the bed because the motion helps debride necrotic tissue and improves local circulation.
▶ Perform or schedule daily ROM exercises because the bed allows full access to all extremities without disturbing spinal alignment. Drop the arm hatch for shoulder rotation, remove the thoracic packs for shoulder abduction, and drop the leg hatch and

remove leg and knee packs for hip rotation and full leg motion.

▶ For female patients, tape an indwelling urinary catheter to the thigh before bringing it through the perineal hatch. For the male patient with spinal cord lesions, tape the catheter to the abdomen and then to the thigh to facilitate gravity drainage. Hang the drainage bag on the clips provided and make sure it doesn't become caught between the bed frames during rotation.

▶ If the patient has a tracheal or endotracheal tube and is on mechanical ventilation, attach the tube support bracket between the cervical pack and the arm packs. Tape the connecting T tubing to the support and run it beside the patient's head and off the center of the table to help prevent reflux of condensation.

▶ For a patient with pulmonary congestion or pneumonia, suction secretions more often during the first 12 to 24 hours on the bed because the motion will increase drainage. A vibrator is available for use under the thoracic hatch of the Mark I to help mobilize pulmonary secretions more quickly.

## Complications

Some patients may develop motion sickness because they can't tolerate the continuous oscillation of this bed. May also increase the patient's agitation.

## Documentation

▶ Record changes in the patient's condition and his response to therapy in your progress notes.

▶ Note turning times and ongoing care on the flowchart.

### REFERENCES

Davis, K. Jr., et al. "The Acute Effects of Body Position Strategies and Respiratory Therapy in Paralyzed Patients with Acute Lung Injury," *Critical Care* 5(2):81-87, 2001.

Staudinger, T., et al. "Comparison of Prone Positioning and Continuous Rotation of Patients with Adult Respiratory Distress Syndrome: Results of a Pilot Study," *Critical Care Medicine* 29(1):51-56, January 2001.

# Sequential compression therapy

Safe, effective, and noninvasive, sequential compression therapy helps prevent DVT in surgical patients. This therapy massages the legs in a wavelike, milking motion that promotes blood flow and deters thrombosis.

Typically, sequential compression therapy complements other preventive measures, such as antiembolism stockings and anticoagulant medications. Although patients at low risk for DVT may require only antiembolism stockings, those at moderate to high risk may require both antiembolism stockings and sequential compression therapy. These preventive measures are continued for as long as the patient remains at risk.

Both antiembolism stockings and sequential compression sleeves are commonly used preoperatively and postoperatively because blood clots tend to form during surgery. About 20% of blood clots form in the femoral vein. Sequential compression therapy counteracts blood stasis and coagulation changes—two of the three major factors that promote DVT. It reduces stasis by increasing peak blood flow velocity, helping to empty the femoral vein's valve cusps of pooled or static blood. Also, the compressions cause an anticlotting effect by increasing fibrinolytic activity, which stimulates the release of a plasminogen activator.

## Equipment

Measuring tape and sizing chart for the brand of sleeves you're using ● pair of compression sleeves in correct size ● connecting tubing ● compression controller

## Implementation

▶ Explain the procedure to the patient to increase cooperation.

### Determining proper sleeve size

▶ Before applying the compression sleeve, determine the proper size of sleeve that you need. Begin by washing your hands.

▶ Then measure the circumference of the upper thigh while the patient rests in bed. Do this by placing the measuring tape under the thigh at the gluteal furrow (as shown top of next page).

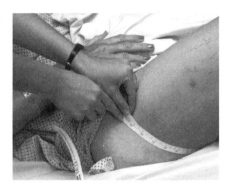

▶ Hold the tape snugly, but not tightly, around the patient's leg. Note the exact circumference.

▶ Find the patient's thigh measurement on the sizing chart and locate the corresponding size of the compression sleeve.

▶ Remove the compression sleeves from the package and unfold them.

▶ Lay the unfolded sleeves on a flat surface with the cotton lining facing up (as shown below).

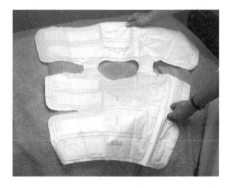

▶ Notice the markings on the lining denoting the ankle and the area behind the knee at the popliteal pulse point. Use these markings to position the sleeve at the appropriate landmarks.

## Applying the sleeves

▶ Place the patient's leg on the sleeve lining. Position the back of the knee over the popliteal opening.

▶ Make sure that the back of the ankle is over the ankle marking.

▶ Starting at the side opposite the clear plastic tubing, wrap the sleeve snugly around the patient's leg.

▶ Fasten the sleeve securely with the Velcro fasteners. For the best fit, first secure the ankle and calf sections and then the thigh.

▶ The sleeve should fit snugly but not tightly. Check the fit by inserting two fingers between the sleeve and the patient's leg at the knee opening. Loosen or tighten the sleeve by readjusting the Velcro fastener.

▶ Using the same procedure, apply the second sleeve (as shown below).

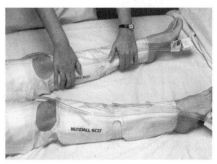

## Operating the system

▶ Connect each sleeve to the tubing leading to the controller. Both sleeves must be connected to the compression controller for the system to operate. Line up the blue arrows on the sleeve connector with the arrows on the tubing connectors and push the ends together firmly. Listen for a click, signaling a firm connection. Make sure that the tubing isn't kinked.

▶ Plug the compression controller into the proper wall outlet. Turn on the power.

▶ The controller automatically sets the compression sleeve pressure at 45 mm Hg, which is the midpoint of the normal range (35 to 55 mm Hg).

▶ Observe the patient to see how well he tolerates the therapy and the controller as the system completes its first cycle. With the instrument, each cycle lasts 71 seconds — 11 seconds of compression and 60 seconds of decompression.

▶ Check the AUDIBLE ALARM key. The green light should be lit, indicating that the alarm is working.

▶ The compression sleeves should function continuously (24 hours daily) until the patient is fully ambulatory. Check the sleeves at least once each shift to ensure proper fit and inflation.

### Removing the sleeves

▶ You may remove the sleeves when the patient is walking, bathing, or leaving the room for tests or other procedures. Reapply them immediately after any of these activities. To disconnect the sleeves from the tubing, press the latches on each side of the connectors and pull the connectors apart.

▶ Store the tubing and compression controller according to facility protocol. This equipment isn't disposable.

## Special considerations

▶ The compression controller also has a mechanism to help cool the patient.

▶ If you're applying only one sleeve — for example, if the patient has a cast — leave the unused sleeve folded in the plastic bag. Cut a small hole in the bag's sealed bottom edge and pull the sleeve connector (the part that holds the connecting tubing) through the hole. Then you can join both sleeves to the compression controller.

▶ If a malfunction triggers the instrument's alarm, you'll hear beeping. The system shuts off whenever the alarm is activated.

▶ To respond to the alarm, remove the operator's card from the slot on the top of the compression controller.

▶ Follow the instructions printed on the card next to the matching code.

## Complications

▶ Acute DVT (or DVT diagnosed within the past 6 months)

▶ Severe arteriosclerosis or any other ischemic vascular disease

▶ Massive edema of the legs resulting from pulmonary edema or heart failure

▶ Any local condition that the compression sleeves would aggravate, such as dermatitis, vein ligation, gangrene, and recent skin grafting. A patient with a pronounced leg deformity also would be unlikely to benefit from the compression sleeves.

## Documentation

▶ Document the procedure, the patient's response to and understanding of the procedure, and the status of the alarm and cooling settings.

### REFERENCES

Robertson, K.A., et al. "Patient Compliance and Satisfaction with Mechanical Devices for Preventing Deep Venous Thrombosis After Joint Replacement," *Journal of the Southern Orthopaedic Association* 9(3):182-86, Fall 2000.

Segers, P., et al. "Excessive Pressure in Multi-chambered Cuffs Used for Sequential Compression Therapy," *Physical Therapy* 82(10):1000-08, October 2002.

# Spiritual care

Religious beliefs can profoundly influence a patient's recovery rate, attitude toward treatment, and overall response to hospitalization. In certain religious groups, beliefs can preclude diagnostic tests and therapeutic treatments, require dietary restrictions, and prohibit organ donation and artificial prolongation of life.

Consequently, effective patient care requires recognition of and respect for the patient's religious beliefs. Recognizing his beliefs and need for spiritual care may require close attention to his nonverbal cues or to seemingly casual remarks that express his spiritual concerns. Respecting his beliefs may require setting aside your own beliefs to help the patient follow his. Providing spiritual care may require contacting an appropriate member of the clergy in the facility or community, gathering equipment needed to help the patient perform rites and administer sacraments, and preparing him for a pastoral visit.

## Equipment

Clean towels (one or two) • teaspoon or 1-oz (30-ml) medicine cup (for baptism) • container of water (for emergency baptism)

Some facilities, particularly those with a religious affiliation, provide baptismal trays. The clergy member may bring holy water, holy oil, or other religious articles to minister to the patient.

### Preparation of equipment

For baptism, cover a small table with a clean towel. Fold a second towel and place it on the table, along with the teaspoon or medicine cup. For communion and anointing, cover the bedside stand with a clean towel.

## Implementation

▶ Check the patient's admission record to determine his religious affiliation. Remember that some patients may claim no religious beliefs. However, even an agnostic may wish to speak with a clergy member, so watch and listen carefully for subtle expressions of this desire.

▶ Evaluate the patient's behavior for signs of loneliness, anxiety, or fear—emotions that may signal his need for spiritual counsel. Also consider whether the patient is facing a health crisis, which may occur with chronic illness and before childbirth, surgery, or impending death. Remember that a patient may feel acutely distressed because of his inability to participate in religious observances. Help such a patient verbalize his beliefs to relieve stress. Listen to him and let him express his concerns, but carefully refrain from imposing your beliefs on him to avoid conflict and further stress. If the patient requests, arrange a visit by an appropriate member of the clergy. Consult this clergy member if you need more information about the patient's beliefs.

▶ If your patient faces the possibility of abortion, amputation, transfusion, or other medical procedures with important religious implications, try to discover his spiritual attitude. Also, try to determine your patient's attitude toward the importance of laying on of hands, confession, communion, observance of holy days (such as the Sabbath), and restrictions in diet or physical appearance. Helping the patient continue his normal religious practices during hospitalization can help reduce stress.

▶ If the patient is pregnant, find out her beliefs concerning infant baptism and circumcision, and comply with them after delivery. If a neonate is in critical condition, call an appropriate clergy member immediately. To perform an emergency baptism, the minister or priest pours a small amount of holy water into a teaspoon or a medicine cup and sprinkles a few drops of water over the infant's head while saying, "(Name of child), I baptize you in the name of the Father, the Son, and the Holy Spirit. Amen." In an extreme emergency, you can perform a Roman Catholic baptism, using a container of any available water. If you do so, be sure to notify the priest because this sacrament must be given only once.

▶ If a Jewish woman delivers a male infant prematurely or by cesarean birth, ask her whether she plans to observe the rite of circumcision, or a bris, a significant ceremony performed on the 8th day after birth. (Because a patient who delivers a healthy, full-term baby vaginally is usually discharged quickly, this ceremony is normally performed outside the facility.) For a bris, ensure privacy and, if requested, sterilize the instruments.

▶ If the patient requests communion, prepare him for it before the clergy member arrives. First, place him in Fowler's or semi-Fowler's position if his condition permits. Otherwise, allow him to remain supine. Tuck a clean towel under his chin and straighten the bed linens.

▶ If a terminally ill patient requests the Sacrament of the Sick (Last Rites) or special treatment of his body after death, call an appropriate clergy member. For the Roman Catholic patient, call a Roman Catholic priest to administer the sacrament, even if the patient is unresponsive or comatose. To prepare the patient for this sacrament, uncover his arms and fold back the top linens to expose his feet. After the clergy member anoints the patient's forehead, eyes, nose, mouth, hands, and feet, straighten and retuck the bed linens.

## Special considerations

▶ Handle the patient's religious articles carefully to avoid damage or loss.

▶ Become familiar with religious resources in your facility. Some facilities employ one or more clergy members who counsel patients and staff and link patients to other pastoral resources.

▶ If the patient tries to convert you to his personal beliefs, tell him that you respect his beliefs but are content with your own. Likewise, avoid attempts to convert the patient to your personal beliefs.

## Documentation

▶ Complete a baptismal form and attach it to the patient's record; send a copy of the form to the appropriate clergy member.

▶ Record the rites of circumcision and last rites in your notes. Also, record last rites in red on the Kardex so it won't be repeated unnecessarily.

### REFERENCES

Govier, I. "Spiritual Care in Nursing: A Systematic Approach," *Nursing Standard* 14(17):32-36, January 12-18, 2000.

# 2

# Infection control

**D**ESPITE OUR INCREASED UNDERSTANDING OF INFECTIOUS DISEASES AND THE ADVENT OF programs to survey, prevent, identify, and control them, more than 2 million nosocomial infections develop each year. They raise health care costs by about $4.5 billion, lengthen hospital stays, and lead directly or indirectly to about 25,000 patient deaths annually.

Not all nosocomial infections can be prevented. Immunodeficient patients and those receiving immunosuppressive therapy, for example, may succumb to nosocomial infections despite all precautions. However, studies have shown that about one-third of all nosocomial infections could be prevented every year by faithful adherence to infection control principles. This chapter contains detailed instructions for using these principles effectively.

# Protocols

## Managing the patient at risk for or experiencing myelosuppression

### Purpose
To minimize the susceptibility to infection in the neutropenic or immunocompromised patient (those with leukemia or other cancers, acquired immunodeficiency syndrome [AIDS], severe burns or other extensive skin conditions, and those receiving radiation, chemotherapy, and antimetabolic therapy are highly susceptible to infection)

### Collaborative level
Interdependent

### Expected patient outcomes
▶ The patient who has neutropenia or is immunocompromised will remain free from infection.

### Definition of terms
▶ *Myelosuppression:* Suppression of the bone marrow, which makes blood cells and platelets, reducing white blood cell (WBC), red blood cell, and platelet counts, resulting in leukopenia, anemia, and thrombocytopenia, respectively.
▶ *Neutropenia:* Abnormal lowering of neutrophils, a type of WBC that fights infection. Neutropenia isn't a disease; rather, it's a sign caused by many diseases, such as

cancer and AIDS. If severe, it can result in blood, lung, kidney, and skin infections.

### Indications
Treatment
▶ Underlying conditions resulting in myelosuppression or neutropenia

Prevention
▶ Infections
▶ Complications caused by infections

### Assessment guidance
Signs and symptoms
▶ High fever
▶ Thrombocytopenia
▶ Weakness
▶ Pallor
▶ Chills
▶ Malaise and fatigue
▶ Tachycardia, palpitations, dyspnea, bleeding, opportunistic infections with disease progression

Diagnostic studies
*Laboratory tests*
▶ Complete blood count with differential
▶ Blood, sputum, urine, and wound cultures
▶ Bone marrow aspirate, biopsy
▶ Lumbar puncture
▶ Pathology stains
▶ Cytogenetic analysis
▶ Chromosome analysis of peripheral blood or bone marrow

### Nursing interventions
▶ Comfort the patient.
▶ Monitor vital signs at appropriate intervals.
▶ Maintain a patent I.V. access line.
▶ Provide antibiotic, antifungal, and antiviral drugs, as needed.
▶ Administer whole blood and blood products, as ordered.
▶ Continually assess nutrition and hydration, which are critical to the immune system.

### Patient teaching
▶ Teach the patient and his family of the risks of blood product transfusion.
▶ Teach the patient and his family how to help reduce the risk of infection in the home, community, or both.
▶ Advise the patient and his family that fresh fruit, live flowers, and plants may be reservoirs for bacterial growth and may colonize in the immunocompromised patient or on the hands of caregivers.
▶ Teach the patient and his family about proper hand-washing techniques.
▶ Teach about coughing and deep-breathing exercises.

### Precautions
▶ Ensure that informed consent is obtained before blood transfusions.
▶ Properly identify the patient and blood products before transfusion to make sure the correct blood product is given to the correct patient.
▶ Monitor the patient for signs and symptoms of a transfusion reaction.
▶ Proper hand washing is vital in the care of the myelosuppressed patient.
▶ Ensure that the patient is in a private room.
▶ Don't allow fresh fruit, flowers, or plants in the room, because they're reservoirs for bacterial growth.
▶ Limit visitors to avoid exposure to other persons with infections.
▶ Inspect mouth, skin, and mucous membranes (especially the anal area) as frequently as ordered.
▶ Ensure strict aseptic technique with dressing changes or procedures.

### Contraindications
Contraindications vary depending on the patient's history.

### Documentation
▶ Document the date and time of reaction.
▶ Record the type and amount of blood product received.
▶ Record nursing assessments, including frequent vital signs.
▶ Document subjective symptoms reported by the patient.
▶ Note laboratory specimens sent.
▶ Record nursing interventions and patient response to treatment.
▶ Document patient teaching.
▶ Document doctor notification and interventions.

### Related procedures
▶ Airborne precautions
▶ Blood culture
▶ Contact precautions
▶ Droplet precautions
▶ Hand washing
▶ Latex allergy precautions
▶ Neutropenic precautions
▶ Standard precautions
▶ Swab specimens
▶ Use of isolation equipment

**REFERENCES**
*Atlas of Pathophysiology.* Springhouse, Pa.: Springhouse Corp., 2002.
Association of Professionals in Infection Control. *Infection Control and Applied Epidemiology: Principles and Practices.* St. Louis: Mosby–Year Book, Inc., 1996.
Young, J. "Transfusion Reaction," *Nursing 2000* 30(12):33, December 2000.

**ORGANIZATIONS**
Centers for Disease Control and Prevention: *www.cdc.gov*

# Managing the patient at risk for or experiencing sepsis

### Purpose
To minimize the number of risk factors predisposing a patient to an infectious process; and to appropriately manage and treat the patient with sepsis

### Collaborative level
Interdependent

## Expected patient outcomes
▶ The patient will show no signs of sepsis.
▶ The patient with sepsis will undergo early intervention and management of sepsis to restore optimal health.

## Definition of terms
▶ *Infection:* Invasion and multiplication of microorganisms in or on body tissue that have the potential of causing disease. Infections usually result in an immune response.
▶ *Sepsis:* Pathologic state resulting from microorganisms and their byproducts in the bloodstream; an overwhelming inflammatory and coagulation response can rapidly lead to organ dysfunction and death.
▶ *Shock:* Circulatory dysfunction in which oxygen delivery to tissues and organs is compromised; if untreated, multiple organ failure or death can result.
▶ *Septic shock:* Shock caused by infectious process with gram-positive or gram-negative bacteria, viruses, fungi, parasites, rickettsiae, yeast, protozoa, or mycobacteria.

## Indications
Treatment
▶ Patient with sepsis
▶ Patient with septic shock

Prevention
▶ Respiratory failure
▶ Multiorgan failure
▶ Disseminated intravascular coagulation
▶ Death

## Assessment guidance
Signs and symptoms
*Sepsis*
▶ Fever
▶ Edema from local vasodilatation
▶ Pain or loss of function of a specific body part as a direct result of edema and pain
▶ Increasing malaise
▶ Poor skin integrity
▶ Altered nutrition

*Septic shock*
▶ Tachycardia with bounding pulse
▶ Restlessness
▶ Irritability
▶ Hypotension
▶ Tachypnea with shallow respirations
▶ Decreased urinary output

▶ Warm, dry skin (as opposed to cool, clammy skin with other types of shock)
▶ Weak, rapid pulse

*Irreversible stage*
▶ Absent reflexes, rapidly falling blood pressure, Cheyne-Stokes respirations, anuria

## Diagnostic studies
*Laboratory tests*
▶ Blood, urine, and sputum cultures (Gram, acid-fast, and silver stains)
▶ Complete blood count
▶ Coagulation studies
▶ White blood cell count
▶ Erythrocyte sedimentation rate
▶ Blood urea nitrogen and creatinine levels
▶ Glucose level
▶ Protein level
▶ Cardiac enzyme and protein levels
▶ Arterial blood gas analysis

*Imaging tests*
▶ Chest X-ray
▶ Echocardiogram

## Nursing interventions
Diagnostic procedures
▶ Monitor hemodynamic status.
▶ Monitor electrocardiography results.

Preventing sepsis
▶ Maintain good skin integrity.
▶ Ensure that patient is receiving proper nutrition and proteins; malnutrition has been linked directly to the incidence of nosocomial infections.
▶ Incorporate proper hand washing before and after all patient care or contact.
▶ Maintain adequate hydration.
▶ Use pulmonary toileting, if necessary (for example, chest physiotherapy).
▶ Administer antibiotic therapy, as prescribed.

Treating patients with septic shock
▶ Manage the underlying cause.
▶ Provide continuous cardiac monitoring.
▶ Maintain a patent airway.
▶ Maintain a patent I.V. access line.
▶ Give antibiotics.
▶ Monitor hemodynamic status.
▶ Maintain Swan-Ganz catheter and arterial line.

▶ Monitor oxygen saturation.
▶ Maintain hyperalimentation.

### Patient teaching
▶ Inform the patient's family of the importance of proper hand washing.
▶ Give the patient and his family the rationale for any precautions being taken with the patient.
▶ Teach the patient at risk for sepsis or who has recovered from a septic episode and his family about the importance of good hygiene in promoting normal host defenses.
▶ Teach the patient and his family about the need for proper nutrition and a balanced diet for an effective immune system.
▶ Teach the patient and his family about the need for adequate protein, which helps produce antibodies.

### Precautions
▶ Use friction when washing your hands; scrub between the webs of the fingers and under the nails because improper hand washing is the primary reason for spread of infection.
▶ Always wash your hands before and after patient contact and before putting on gloves.

### Documentation
▶ Document all initial signs and symptoms exhibited, in the case of septic shock.
▶ Record all nursing assessments and interventions in chronological order.
▶ Record the patient's response to all interventions.
▶ Record all doctor interventions.

### Related procedures
▶ Airborne precautions
▶ Blood culture
▶ Contact precautions
▶ Droplet precautions
▶ Hand washing
▶ Latex allergy precautions
▶ Neutropenic precautions
▶ Standard precautions
▶ Swab specimens
▶ Use of isolation equipment

### REFERENCES
Astiz, M.E., and Rachow, E.C. "Septic Shock," *Lancet* 351(9114):1501-05, May 1998.

*Atlas of Pathophysiology.* Springhouse, Pa.: Springhouse Corp., 2002.
Levi, M., and Ten Cate, H. "Disseminated Intravascular Coagulation," *New England Journal of Medicine* 341(8):586-92, December 1999.
Wheeler, A.P., and Bernard, G.R. "Treating Patients with Severe Sepsis," *New England Journal of Medicine* 340(3):207-14, January 1999.

### ORGANIZATIONS
Centers for Disease Control and Prevention: *www.cdc.gov*

# Managing the patient at risk for latex allergy response

### Purpose
To minimize the risk of allergic or hypersensitivity reactions in patients with actual or potential latex sensitivity

### Collaborative level
Interdependent

### Expected patient outcomes
▶ The patient will be maintained in a latex-free environment.
▶ The patient will avoid hypersensitivity and anaphylactic reactions.
▶ The patient and his family will be educated about environmental latex hazards, preventive measures, and the rationale for precautions.

### Definition of terms
▶ *Latex:* Milky sap derived from a rubber tree; contains proteins that may act as allergens.
▶ *Latex-free environment:* An environment in which equipment, supplies, and pharmaceutical products have been removed or altered.
▶ *Anaphylaxis:* An acute, hypersensitivity reaction that usually occurs within minutes after reexposure to an antigen; severe reactions cause vascular collapse, respiratory distress, shock, and sometimes death.

### Indications
Treatment
▶ Hypersensitivity reactions
▶ Anaphylactic reactions

## Prevention
▶ Bronchospasm
▶ Circulating shock

## Assessment guidance
### Signs and symptoms
*Irritant contact dermatitis (nonallergic, non–life-threatening)*
▶ Acute: redness, burning, itching
▶ Chronic: dry, thickened skin; cracking, sores, bumps

*Allergic contact dermatitis (non–life-threatening)*
▶ Acute: small, clustered bumps, itching, redness, pain
▶ Chronic: dry, thickened skin; cracking, sores, bumps

*Urticaria (immediate hypersensitivity; life-threatening)*
▶ Hives, watery eyes, running nose, swelling, difficulty breathing, dizziness, abdominal cramps, rapid heart rate, low blood pressure, anaphylactic shock

### Diagnostic studies
No single diagnostic test can identify anaphylaxis.

## Nursing interventions
▶ Have emergency medications readily available on the code cart for potential latex reactions.
▶ For patient experiencing anaphylaxis, immediately give epinephrine to cause vasoconstriction and reverse bronchoconstriction.
▶ Have oxygen therapy available as well as an emergency respiratory box for potential tracheostomy or endotracheal intubation and mechanical ventilation.
▶ Maintain a patent I.V. access line.
▶ Always wash your hands before entering a latex-free environment to eliminate transference of latex proteins into the patient's environment.
▶ When a latex substitute isn't available, use a barrier, such as Webril or gauze, between the product and the patient's skin.
▶ Evaluate the patient's response to treatment.
▶ Ask questions about latex sensitivity when taking the patient history. For example, ask about history of multiple medical or surgical procedures; history of nondrug

anaphylactic reactions; and history of sensitivity to bananas, kiwi, passion fruit, avocado, chestnuts, or pineapple. Populations at risk for latex sensitivity include health care and rubber industry workers and patients with spina bifida and congenital urinary anomalies as well as those with a known history of natural rubber sensitivity.
▶ Place latex allergy bracelets on patients who are sensitive.
▶ Alert staff of latex-sensitive patient by using appropriate signs on doors of patient rooms and procedure rooms.
▶ Always use nonlatex gloves and substitute latex-free products whenever possible.
▶ Use stopcocks for drug injection in I.V. lines and tape over any latex ports.
▶ Wrap blood pressure tubing with gauze to avoid contact with patient's skin.
▶ Use gauze under latex tourniquets, or use Velcro tourniquets.
▶ Avoid the use of multidose medication vials.
▶ Notify Pharmacy and Central Supply of the need for latex-free supplies for this patient.

## Patient teaching
▶ Give the patient and his family the rationale for precautions.
▶ Teach the patient and his family how to assess home environmental hazards.
▶ Encourage the patient to obtain a medical identification bracelet or other form of identification that indicates a latex allergy.
▶ Advise the patient to carry a latex-free EpiPen.
▶ Encourage the patient to take a supply of latex-free examination gloves with him to all doctor visits.
▶ Suggest that the patient include an allergist as part of his medical team.
▶ Give the patient and his family written educational materials.

## Precautions
▶ Place a latex allergy bracelet on all patients sensitive to latex.
▶ Alert staff of a patient's latex sensitivity with appropriate signs on the patient's room and procedure rooms the patient may be in.
▶ Wash your hands thoroughly before entering a patient's room to ensure removal of latex proteins from the surrounding environment.

## Documentation
▶ Document date and time of reaction.
▶ Record subjective symptoms reported.
▶ Document objective signs assessed by nursing staff.
▶ Document specimens obtained.
▶ Record doctor notification and interventions.

## Related procedures
▶ Airborne precautions
▶ Blood culture
▶ Contact precautions
▶ Droplet precautions
▶ Hand washing
▶ Latex allergy precautions
▶ Neutropenic precautions
▶ Standard precautions
▶ Swab specimens
▶ Use of isolation equipment

## REFERENCES
*Atlas of Pathophysiology.* Springhouse, Pa.: Springhouse Corp., 2002.

Buhr, V. "Screening Patients for Latex Allergies," *Journal of the American Academy of Nurse Practitioners* 12(9):380-83, September 2000.

Gehring, L.L., and Ring, P. "Latex Allergy: Creating a Safe Environment," *Dermatology Nursing* 12(3):197-201, June 2000.

Thurlow, K.L. "Latex Allergies: Management and Clinical Responsibility," *Home Healthcare Nurse* 19(6):369-75, June 2001.

# Managing reportable diseases

## Purpose
To provide the patient in a health care facility or in the community with appropriate assessments, effective treatments, ongoing evaluation, and education about contagious disease prevention. Reporting is increasingly essential because of population movement, international travel and food commerce, deforestation and urbanization, and antimicrobial resistance.

The most commonly reported diseases include hepatitis, measles, salmonellosis, shigellosis, syphilis, and gonorrhea.

## Collaborative level
Interdependent

## Expected patient outcomes
▶ The patient in a health care facility or in the community will receive quality care and education through:
  – surveillance of disease processes
  – control of disease outbreaks
  – education and prevention of future disease outbreaks.

## Definition of terms
▶ *Epidemiology:* The study of both the distribution and determinants of disease processes in human populations; enables effective planning and evaluation of interventions and prevention measures.
▶ *Surveillance:* Systematic method of collecting data regarding the determinants and distribution of disease or other events; consolidation and analysis of the data are followed by dissemination to those who are dedicated to outcome improvement.
▶ *Communicable disease:* Diseases and conditions that warrant reporting because of the potential risk to the immediate or general populations; it's important to note that some diseases, such as anthrax and tetanus, although designated as reportable, aren't considered communicable.

## Indications
Treatment
▶ Contagious diseases that must be reported to health officials

Prevention
▶ Spread of disease or escalation of a specific condition

## Assessment guidance
Signs and symptoms
▶ Signs and symptoms will be specific to the disease or condition.

Diagnostic studies
▶ Diagnostic studies will be specific to the disease or condition.

## Nursing interventions
▶ Designated personnel, such as an infection control practitioner or laboratory worker, must report all reportable commu-

nicable and designated noncommunicable diseases to the local health department.
▶ For in-house patients, institute appropriate precautions, as needed; for example, standard, contact, droplet, or airborne precautions.
▶ Teach the patient and his family about the specific condition; explain why the precautions are imperative.

## Patient teaching
▶ Teach the patient and his family about the specific disease or condition.
▶ Tell the patient and his family why specific precautions are warranted for certain conditions.
▶ Provide educational materials at patient discharge.

## Precautions
▶ Precautions will be specific to the disease or condition.

## Documentation
▶ Doctors are required by law to report all cases of communicable and certain designated noncommunicable diseases to their local health departments. Written report forms provided by local health departments are generally available from the facility's Infection Control office.

▶ Logs should be kept by each health care facility of all diseases reported to local health departments.

## Related procedures
▶ Airborne precautions
▶ Blood culture
▶ Contact precautions
▶ Droplet precautions
▶ Hand washing
▶ Latex allergy precautions
▶ Neutropenic precautions
▶ Standard precautions
▶ Swab specimens
▶ Use of isolation equipment

## REFERENCES
Heymann, D.L., and Rodier, G.R. "Global Surveillance of Communicable Diseases," *Emerging Infectious Diseases* 4(3):362-65. Geneva, Switzerland: The World Health Organization, July-September 1998.
*Infection Control and Applied Epidemiology: Principles and Practices.* Association for Professionals in Infection Control. St. Louis: Mosby–Year Book, Inc., 1996.

## ORGANIZATIONS
Centers for Disease Control and Prevention: *www.cdc.gov*

# Procedures

# Airborne precautions

Airborne precautions, used in addition to standard precautions, prevent the spread of infectious diseases transmitted by airborne pathogens that are breathed, sneezed, or coughed into the environment. (See *Diseases requiring airborne precautions,* page 64.) This precaution category includes the former categories of acid-fast bacillus isolation and respiratory isolation.

Effective airborne precautions require a negative-pressure room with the door kept closed to maintain the proper air pressure balance between the isolation room and the adjoining hallway or corridor. An anteroom is preferred. The negative air pressure must be monitored, and the air is either vented directly to the outside of the building or filtered through high-efficiency particulate air (HEPA) filtration before recirculation.

All persons who enter the room must wear respiratory protection, provided by a

## Diseases requiring airborne precautions

| Disease | Precautionary period |
|---------|---------------------|
| Chickenpox (varicella) | Until lesions are crusted and no new lesions appear |
| Herpes zoster (disseminated) | Duration of illness |
| Herpes zoster (localized in immunocompromised patient) | Duration of illness |
| Measles (rubeola) | Duration of illness |
| Tuberculosis (pulmonary or laryngeal, confirmed or suspected) | Depends on clinical response; patient must be on effective therapy, be improving clinically (decreased cough and fever and improved findings on chest radiograph), and have three consecutive negative sputum smears collected on different days, or tuberculosis must be ruled out |

disposable N95 or HEPA respirator or a reusable HEPA or powered air-purifying respirator (PAPR). Whatever type of respirator is used, ensure proper fit to the face each time it's worn. If the patient must leave the room for an essential procedure, he should wear a surgical mask to cover his nose and mouth while out of the room.

### Equipment
Disposable N95 or HEPA respirator or reusable HEPA or PAPR • surgical masks • isolation door card • other personal protective equipment

Gather any additional supplies for patient care, such as a thermometer, stethoscope, and blood pressure cuff.

### Preparation of equipment
Keep all airborne precaution supplies outside the patient's room in a cart or anteroom.

### Implementation
▶ Situate the patient in a negative-pressure room with the door closed. If possible, the room should have an anteroom. The negative pressure should be monitored. If necessary, two patients with the same infection may share a room. Explain isolation precautions to the patient and his family.
▶ Keep the patient's door (and the anteroom door) closed at all times, to maintain the negative pressure and contain the airborne pathogens. Put the airborne precautions sign on the door to notify anyone entering the room.
▶ Pick up your respirator and put it on according to the manufacturer's directions. Adjust the straps for a firm but comfortable fit. Check the fit. (See *Respirator seal check.*)
▶ Instruct the patient to cover his nose and mouth with a facial tissue while coughing or sneezing.
▶ Tape an impervious bag to the patient's bedside so he can dispose of facial tissues correctly.
▶ Make sure that all visitors wear respiratory protection while in the patient's room.
▶ Limit the patient's movement from the room. If he must leave the room for essential procedures, make sure he wears a surgical mask over his nose and mouth. Notify the receiving department or area of the patient's isolation precautions so that the precautions will be maintained and the patient can be returned to the room promptly.

### Special considerations
Before leaving the room, remove gloves (if worn) and wash your hands. Remove your respirator outside the patient's room after closing the door.

Depending on the type of respirator and recommendations from the manufacturer,

## Respirator seal check

Before using a respirator, always check the respirator seal. To do this, place both hands over the respirator and exhale. If air leaks around your nose, adjust the nosepiece. If air leaks at the respirator's edges, adjust the straps along the side of your head. Recheck respirator fit after this adjustment.

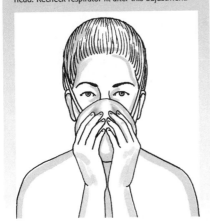

follow your facility's policy and either discard your respirator or store it until the next use. If your respirator is to be stored until the next use, store it in a dry, well-ventilated place (not a plastic bag) to prevent microbial growth. Nondisposable respirators must be cleaned according to the manufacturer's recommendations.

### Documentation

Record the need for airborne precautions on the nursing plan of care and as required by your facility. Document initiation and maintenance of the precautions, the patient's tolerance of the procedure, and any patient or family teaching. Also document the date airborne precautions were discontinued.

### REFERENCES

Garner, J.S. "Hospital Infection Control Practices Advisory Committee Guideline for Isolation Precautions in Hospitals," *Infection Control and Hospital Epidemiology* 17(1):53-80, January 1996.

# Blood culture

Normally bacteria-free, blood is susceptible to infection through infusion lines, as well as from thrombophlebitis, infected shunts, and bacterial endocarditis caused by prosthetic heart valve replacements. Bacteria may also invade the vascular system from local tissue infections through the lymphatic system and the thoracic duct.

Blood cultures are performed to detect bacterial invasion (bacteremia) and the systemic spread of such an infection (septicemia) through the bloodstream. In this procedure, a laboratory technician, doctor, or nurse collects a venous blood sample by venipuncture at the patient's bedside and then transfers it into two bottles, one containing an anaerobic medium and the other an aerobic medium. The bottles are incubated, encouraging any organisms that are present in the sample to grow in the media. Blood cultures identify 67% of pathogens within 24 hours and up to 90% within 72 hours.

Although some authorities consider the timing of culture collections debatable and possibly irrelevant, others advocate drawing three blood samples at least 1 hour apart. The first of these should be collected at the earliest sign of suspected bacteremia or septicemia. To check for suspected bacterial endocarditis, collect three or four samples at 5- to 30-minute intervals before starting antibiotic therapy.

### Equipment

Tourniquet, gloves, alcohol or povidone-iodine pads ● 10-ml syringe for an adult ● 6-ml syringe for a child ● three or four 20G 1" needles ● two or three blood culture bottles (50-ml bottles for adults, 20-ml bottles for infants and children) with sodium polyethanol sulfonate added (one aerobic bottle containing a suitable medium, such as Trypticase soy broth with 10% carbon dioxide atmosphere; one anaerobic bottle with prereduced medium; and, possibly, one hyperosmotic bottle with 10% sucrose medium) ● laboratory request form ● 2" × 2" gauze pads ● small adhesive bandages ● labels

### Preparation of equipment
Check the expiration dates on the culture bottles and replace outdated bottles.

### Implementation
▶ Tell the patient that you need to collect a series of blood samples to check for infection. Explain the procedure to ease his anxiety and promote cooperation. Explain that the procedure usually requires three blood samples collected at different times.
▶ Wash your hands and put on gloves.
▶ Tie a tourniquet 2″ (5 cm) proximal to the area chosen.
▶ Clean the venipuncture site with an alcohol or a povidone-iodine pad. Don't wipe off the povidone-iodine with alcohol because alcohol cancels the effect of povidone-iodine. Start at the site and work outward in a circular motion. Wait 30 to 60 seconds for the skin to dry.
▶ Perform a venipuncture, drawing 10 ml of blood from an adult.
▶ Remove the tourniquet. Apply pressure to the venipuncture site using a 2″ × 2″ dressing. Then cover the site with a small adhesive bandage.

> ◆ **ALERT!** Draw only 2 to 6 ml of blood from a child.

▶ Wipe the diaphragm tops of the culture bottles with a povidone-iodine pad, and change the needle on the syringe used to draw the blood.
▶ Inject 5 ml of blood into each 50-ml bottle or 2 ml into each 20-ml pediatric culture bottle. (Bottle size may vary according to the facility's protocol, but the sample dilution should always be 1:10.)
▶ Label the culture bottles with the patient's name and room number, doctor's name, and date and time of collection. Indicate the suspected diagnosis and the patient's temperature and note on the laboratory request form any recent antibiotic therapy. Send the samples to the laboratory immediately.
▶ Discard syringes, needles, and gloves in the appropriate containers.

### Special considerations
▶ Obtain each set of cultures from a different site.
▶ Avoid using existing blood lines for cultures unless the sample is drawn when the line is inserted or catheter sepsis is suspected.

### Complications
The most common complication of venipuncture is formation of a hematoma.

If a hematoma develops, apply warm soaks to the site.

### Documentation
Record the date and time of blood sample collection, name of the test, amount of blood collected, number of bottles used, patient's temperature, and adverse reactions to the procedure.

### REFERENCES
Calfee, D.P., and Farr, B.M. "Comparison of Four Antiseptic Preparations for Skin in the Prevention of Contamination of Percutaneously Drawn Blood Cultures: A Randomized Trial," *Journal of Clinical Microbiology* 40(5):1660-65, May 2002.
Penwarden, L.M., and Montgomery, P.G. "Developing a Protocol for Obtaining Blood Cultures from Central Venous Catheters and Peripheral Sites," *Clinical Journal of Oncology Nursing* 6(5):268-70, September-October 2002.

# Contact precautions

Contact precautions prevent the spread of infectious diseases transmitted by contact with body substances containing the infectious agent or items contaminated with the body substances containing the infectious agent. Contact precautions apply to patients who are infected or colonized (presence of microorganism without clinical signs or symptoms of infection) with epidemiologically important organisms that can be transmitted by direct or indirect contact. (See *Diseases requiring contact precautions.*)

Effective contact precautions require a single room and the use of gloves and gowns by anyone having contact with the patient, the patient's support equipment, or items soiled with body substances containing the infectious agent. Thorough hand washing and proper handling and disposal of articles contaminated by the body substance containing the infectious agent are also essential.

### Equipment
Gloves ● gowns or aprons ● masks, if necessary ● isolation door card ● plastic bags

Gather any additional supplies, such as a thermometer, stethoscope, and blood pressure cuff.

# Diseases requiring contact precautions

| Disease | Precautionary period |
| --- | --- |
| Infection or colonization with multidrug-resistant bacteria | Until off antibiotics and culture negative |
| *Clostridium difficile* enteric infection | Duration of illness |
| *Escherichia coli* disease, in diapered or incontinent patient | Duration of illness |
| Shigellosis, in diapered or incontinent patient | Duration of illness |
| Hepatitis A, in diapered or incontinent patient | Duration of illness |
| Rotavirus infection, in diapered or incontinent patient | Duration of illness |
| Respiratory syncytial virus infection, in infants and young children | Duration of illness |
| Parainfluenza virus infection, in diapered or incontinent patient | Duration of illness |
| Enteroviral infection, in diapered or incontinent patient | Duration of illness |
| Scabies | Until 24 hours after initiation of effective therapy |
| Diphtheria (cutaneous) | Duration of illness |
| Herpes simplex virus infection (neonatal or mucocutaneous) | Duration of illness |
| Impetigo | Until 24 hours after initiation of effective therapy |
| Major abscesses, cellulitis, or pressure ulcers | Until 24 hours after initiation of effective therapy |
| Pediculosis (lice) | Until 24 hours after initiation of effective therapy |
| Rubella, congenital syndrome | Place infant on precautions during any admission until age 1, unless nasopharyngeal and urine cultures are negative for virus after age 3 months |
| Staphylococcal furunculosis in infants and young children | Duration of illness |
| Acute viral (acute hemorrhagic) conjunctivitis | Duration of illness |
| Viral hemorrhagic infections (Ebola, Lassa, Marburg) | Duration of illness |
| Zoster (chickenpox, disseminated zoster, or localized zoster in immunodeficient patient) | Until all lesions are crusted, requires airborne precautions |
| Acquired immunodeficiency syndrome | Until white blood cell count reaches 1,000 µl or more, or according to facility guidelines |
| Agranulocytosis | Until remission |

*(continued)*

## Diseases requiring contact precautions *(continued)*

| Disease | Precautionary period |
|---------|---------------------|
| Burns, extensive noninfected | Until skin surface heals substantially |
| Dermatitis, noninfected vesicular, bullous, or eczematous disease (when severe and extensive) | Until skin surface heals substantially |
| Immunosuppressive therapy | Until patient's immunity is adequate |
| Lymphomas and leukemia, especially late stages of Hodgkin's disease or acute leukemia | Until clinical improvement is substantial |

### Preparation of equipment

Keep all contact precaution supplies outside the patient's room in a cart or anteroom.

### Implementation

▶ Situate the patient in a single room with private toilet facilities and an anteroom if possible. If necessary, two patients with the same infection may share a room. Explain isolation procedures to the patient and his family.
▶ Place a contact precautions card on the door to notify anyone entering the room.
▶ Wash your hands before entering and after leaving the patient's room and after removing gloves.
▶ Place any laboratory specimens in impervious, labeled containers, and send them to the laboratory at once. Attach requisition slips to the outside of the container.
▶ Instruct visitors to wear gloves and a gown while visiting the patient and to wash their hands after removing the gown and gloves.
▶ Place all items that have come in contact with the patient in a single impervious bag, and arrange for their disposal or disinfection and sterilization.
▶ Limit the patient's movement from the room. If the patient must be moved, cover any draining wounds with clean dressings. Notify the receiving department or area of the patient's isolation precautions so that the precautions will be maintained and the patient can be returned to the room promptly.

### Special considerations

▶ Cleaning and disinfection of equipment between patients is essential.
▶ Try to dedicate certain reusable equipment (thermometer, stethoscope, blood pressure cuff) for the patient in contact precautions to reduce the risk of transmitting infection to other patients.
▶ Remember to change gloves during patient care as indicated by the procedure or task. Wash your hands after removing gloves and before putting on new gloves.

### Documentation

▶ Record the need for contact precautions on the nursing care plan and as required by your facility.
▶ Document initiation and maintenance of the precautions, the patient's tolerance of the procedure, and any patient or family teaching.
▶ Document the date contact precautions were discontinued.

### REFERENCES

Garner, J.S. "Hospital Infection Control Practices Advisory Committee Guidelines for Isolation Precautions in Hospitals," *Infection Control and Hospital Epidemiology* 17(1):53-80, January 1996.

## Droplet precautions

Droplet precautions prevent the spread of infectious diseases (including some diseases formerly included in respiratory isolation) that are transmitted when nasal or oral secretions from the infected patient

# Diseases requiring droplet precautions

| Disease | Precautionary period |
|---|---|
| Invasive *Haemophilus influenzae* type b disease, including meningitis, pneumonia, and sepsis | Until 24 hours after initiation of effective therapy |
| Invasive *Neisseria meningitidis* disease, including meningitis, pneumonia, epiglottiditis, and sepsis | Until 24 hours after initiation of effective therapy |
| Diphtheria (pharyngeal) | Until off antibiotics and two cultures taken at least 24 hours apart are negative |
| *Mycoplasma pneumoniae* infection | Duration of illness |
| Pertussis | Until 5 days after initiation of effective therapy |
| Pneumonic plague | Until 72 hours after initiation of effective therapy |
| Streptococcal pharyngitis, pneumonia, or scarlet fever in infants and young children | Until 24 hours after initiation of effective therapy |
| Adenovirus infection in infants and young children | Duration of illness |
| Influenza | Duration of illness |
| Mumps | For 9 days after onset of swelling |
| Human parvovirus B19 | Duration of hospitalization when chronic disease occurs in an immunodeficient patient; 7 days for patients with transient aplastic crisis or red-cell crisis |
| Rubella (German measles) | Until 7 days after onset of rash |

come in contact with the mucous membranes of the susceptible host. The droplets of moisture, which arise from coughing or sneezing, are heavy and generally fall to the ground within 3′ (0.9 m); the organisms that the droplets contain don't become airborne or suspended in the air. (See *Diseases requiring droplet precautions*.)

Effective droplet precautions require a single room (not necessarily a negative-pressure room), and the door doesn't need to be closed. Persons having direct contact with and those who will be within 3′ of the patient should wear a surgical mask covering the nose and mouth.

When handling infants or young children who require droplet precautions, you may also need to wear gloves and a gown to prevent soiling of clothing with nasal and oral secretions.

## Equipment

Masks, gowns, and gloves, if necessary ● plastic bags ● droplet precautions door card

Gather any additional supplies needed for routine patient care, such as a thermometer, stethoscope, and blood pressure cuff.

### Preparation of equipment

Keep all droplet precaution supplies outside the patient's room in a cart or anteroom.

## Implementation

▶ Place the patient in a single room with private toilet facilities and an anteroom, if possible. If necessary, two patients with the same infection may share a room. Explain isolation procedures to the patient and his family.

▶ Put a droplet precautions card on the door to notify anyone entering the room.
▶ Wash your hands before entering and after leaving the room and during patient care, as indicated.
▶ Pick up your mask by the top strings, adjust it around your nose and mouth, and tie the strings for a comfortable fit. If the mask has a flexible metal nose strip, adjust it to fit firmly but comfortably.
▶ Instruct the patient to cover his nose and mouth with a facial tissue while coughing or sneezing.
▶ Tape a plastic bag to the patient's bedside so that he can dispose of facial tissues correctly.
▶ Make sure all visitors wear masks and, if necessary, gowns and gloves when they're within 3' (0.9 m) of the patient.
▶ If the patient must leave the room for essential procedures, make sure he wears a surgical mask over his nose and mouth. Notify the receiving department or area of the patient's isolation precautions so that the precautions will be maintained and the patient can be returned to the room promptly.

### Special considerations
▶ Before removing your mask, remove your gloves (if worn) and wash your hands.
▶ Untie the strings and dispose of the mask, handling it only by the strings.

### Documentation
▶ Record the need for droplet precautions on the nursing plan of care and as required by your facility.
▶ Document initiation and maintenance of the precautions, the patient's tolerance of the procedure, and any patient or family teaching. Also document the date droplet precautions were discontinued.

### REFERENCES
Garner, J.S. "Hospital Infection Control Practices Advisory Committee Guidelines for Isolation Precautions in Hospitals," *Infection Control and Hospital Epidemiology* 17(1):53-80, January 1996.
Hughes, J.M. "Guideline for Handwashing and Hospital Environmental Control, 1985," *MMWR* 37(24), June 1988. *www.cdc. gov/ncidod/hip/guide/handwash.htm.*

# Hand washing

The hands are the conduits for almost every transfer of potential pathogens from one patient to another, from a contaminated object to the patient, or from a staff member to the patient. Thus, hand washing is the single most important procedure for preventing infection. To protect patients from nosocomial infections, hand washing must be performed routinely and thoroughly. In effect, clean and healthy hands with intact skin, short fingernails, and no rings minimize the risk of contamination. Artificial nails may serve as a reservoir for microorganisms, and microorganisms are more difficult to remove from rough or chapped hands.

### Equipment
Soap or detergent (from a dispenser) ● warm running water ● paper towels ● optional: antiseptic cleaning agent, fingernail brush, disposable sponge brush or plastic cuticle stick

### Implementation
▶ Remove rings as your facility's policy dictates because they harbor dirt and skin microorganisms. Remove your watch or wear it well above the wrist. Note: Artificial fingernails and nail polish must be kept in good repair to minimize their potential to harbor microorganisms; refer to your facility's policy pertaining to nail polish and artificial nails.
▶ Wet your hands and wrists with warm water and apply soap from a dispenser. Don't use bar soap because it allows cross-contamination. Hold your hands below elbow level to prevent water from running up your arms and back down, thus contaminating clean areas. (See *Proper hand-washing technique.*)
▶ Work up a generous lather by rubbing your hands together vigorously for about 10 seconds. Soap and warm water reduce surface tension and this, aided by friction, loosens surface microorganisms, which wash away in the lather.
▶ Pay special attention to the area under fingernails and around cuticles and to the thumbs, knuckles, and sides of the fingers and hands because microorganisms thrive in these protected or overlooked areas. If you don't remove your wedding band,

move it up and down your finger to clean beneath it.

▶ Avoid splashing water on yourself or the floor because microorganisms spread more easily on wet surfaces and because slippery floors are dangerous.

▶ Avoid touching the sink or faucets because they're considered contaminated.

▶ Rinse hands and wrists well because running water flushes suds, soil, soap or detergent, and microorganisms away.

▶ Pat hands and wrists dry with a paper towel. Avoid rubbing, which can cause abrasion and chapping.

▶ If the sink isn't equipped with knee or foot controls, turn off faucets by gripping them with a dry paper towel to avoid recontaminating your hands.

### Special considerations

▶ Before participating in any sterile procedure or whenever your hands are grossly contaminated, wash your forearms also, and clean under the fingernails and in and around the cuticles with a fingernail brush, disposable sponge brush, or plastic cuticle stick. Use these softer implements because brushes, metal files, or other hard objects may injure your skin and, if reused, may be a source of contamination.

▶ Follow your facility's policy concerning when to wash with soap and when to use an antiseptic cleaning agent. Typically, you'll wash with soap before coming on duty; before and after direct or indirect patient contact; before and after performing any bodily functions, such as blowing your nose or using the bathroom; before preparing or serving food; before preparing or administering medications; after removing gloves or other personal protective equipment; and after completing your shift.

▶ Use an antiseptic cleaning agent before performing invasive procedures, wound care, and dressing changes and after contamination. Antiseptics are also recommended for hand washing in isolation rooms and neonate and special care nurseries as well as before caring for any highly susceptible patient.

▶ If your hands aren't visibly soiled, an alcohol-based hand rub can be used for routine decontamination.

▶ Wash your hands before and after performing patient care or procedures or having contact with contaminated objects, even though you may have worn gloves.

## Proper hand-washing technique

To minimize the spread of infection, follow these basic hand-washing instructions. With your hands angled downward under the faucet, adjust the water temperature until it's comfortably warm.

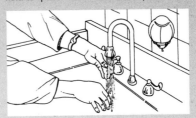

Work up a generous lather by scrubbing vigorously for 10 seconds. Make sure you clean beneath your fingernails, around your knuckles, and along the sides of your fingers and hands.

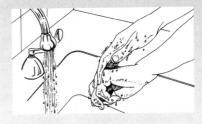

Rinse your hands completely to wash away suds and microorganisms. Pat dry with a paper towel. To prevent recontaminating your hands on the faucet handles, cover each one with a dry paper towel when turning off the water.

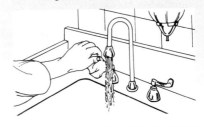

Always wash your hands after removing gloves.

### Home care

If you're providing care in the patient's home, bring your own supply of soap and disposable paper towels. If there is no running water, disinfect your hands with an antiseptic cleaning agent.

## Complications

Because frequent hand washing strips the skin of natural oils, this simple procedure can result in dryness, cracking, and irritation. However, these effects are probably more common after repeated use of antiseptic cleaning agents, especially in people with sensitive skin. To help minimize irritation, rinse your hands thoroughly, making sure they're free from any residue.

To prevent your hands from becoming dry or chapped, apply an emollient hand cream after each washing or switch to a different cleaning agent. Make sure that the hand cream or lotion you use won't cause the material in your gloves to deteriorate. If you develop dermatitis, your employee health care provider may need to evaluate you to determine whether you should continue to work until the condition resolves.

**REFERENCES**

Boyce, J.M., et al. "Guideline for Hand Hygiene in Health-Care Settings. Recommendations of the Healthcare Infection Control Practices Advisory Committee and the HICPAC/SHEA/APIC/IDSA Hand Hygiene Task Force. Society for Healthcare Epidemiology of America/Association for Professionals in Infection Control/Infectious Diseases Society of America." *MMWR* 51(RR-16):1-45, October 2002.

Earl, M.L., et al. "Improved Rates of Compliance with Hand Antisepsis Guidelines: A Three-Phase Observational Study," *AJN* 101(3):26-33, March 2001.

Garner, J.S. "Hospital Infection Control Practices Advisory Committee Guidelines for Isolation Precautions in Hospitals," *Infection Control and Hospital Epidemiology* 17(1):53-80, January 1996.

Gerberding, J.L. "Hospital-onset Infections: A Patient Safety Issue." *Annals of Internal Medicine* 15;137(8):665-70, October 2002.

## Latex allergy precautions

Latex—a natural product of the rubber tree—is used in many products in the health care field as well as other areas. With the increased use of latex in barrier protection and medical equipment, more

### Latex allergy screening

To determine if the patient has a latex sensitivity or allergy, ask the following screening questions:
▶ What is your occupation?
▶ Have you experienced an allergic reaction, local sensitivity, or itching following exposure to any latex products, such as balloons or condoms?
▶ Do you have shortness of breath or wheezing after blowing up balloons or after a dental visit?
▶ Do you have itching in or around your mouth after eating a banana?

If the patient answers "yes" to any of these questions, proceed with the following questions:
▶ Do you have a history of allergies, dermatitis, or asthma? If so, what type of reaction do you have?
▶ Do you have any congenital abnormalities? If yes, explain.
▶ Do you have any food allergies? If so, what specific allergies do you have? Describe your reaction.
▶ If you experience shortness of breath or wheezing when blowing up latex balloons, describe your reaction.
▶ Have you had any previous surgical procedures? Did you experience associated complications? If so, describe them.
▶ Have you had previous dental procedures? Did complications result? If so, describe them.
▶ Are you exposed to latex in your occupation? Do you experience a reaction to latex products at work? If so, describe your reaction.

and more nurses and patients are becoming hypersensitive to it. Certain groups of people are at an increased risk for developing latex allergy. These include people who have had or will undergo multiple surgical procedures (especially those with a history of spina bifida), health care workers (especially those in the emergency department and operating room), workers who manufacture latex and latex-containing products, and people with a genetic predisposition to latex allergy.

People who are allergic to certain cross-reactive foods, including apricots, cherries, grapes, kiwis, passion fruit, bananas, avocados, chestnuts, tomatoes, and peaches, may also be allergic to latex. Exposure to latex elicits an allergic response similar to the one elicited by the foods.

For people with latex allergy, latex becomes a hazard when the protein in latex

# Anesthesia induction and latex allergy

Latex allergy can cause symptoms in conscious and anesthetized patients.

| Causes of intraoperative reaction | Symptoms in conscious patient | Symptoms in anesthetized patient |
|---|---|---|
| ▶ Latex contact with mucous membrane <br> ▶ Latex contact with intraperitoneal serosal lining <br> ▶ Inhalation of airborne latex particles during anesthesia <br> ▶ Injection of antibiotics and anesthetic agents through latex ports | ▶ Abnormal cramping <br> ▶ Anxiety <br> ▶ Bronchoconstriction <br> ▶ Diarrhea <br> ▶ Feeling of faintness <br> ▶ Generalized pruritus <br> ▶ Itchy eyes <br> ▶ Nausea <br> ▶ Shortness of breath <br> ▶ Swelling of soft tissue (such as the hands, face, and tongue) <br> ▶ Vomiting | ▶ Bronchospasm <br> ▶ Cardiopulmonary arrest <br> ▶ Facial edema <br> ▶ Flushing <br> ▶ Hypotension <br> ▶ Laryngeal edema <br> ▶ Tachycardia <br> ▶ Urticaria <br> ▶ Wheezing |

comes in direct contact with mucous membranes or is inhaled, which happens when powdered latex surgical gloves are used. People with asthma are at greater risk for developing worsening symptoms from airborne latex.

The diagnosis of latex allergy is based on the patient's history and physical examination. Laboratory testing should be performed to confirm or eliminate the diagnosis. Skin testing can be done, but the Alastat test, Hycor assay, and Pharmacia Cap test are the only Food and Drug Administration-approved blood tests available. Some laboratories may also choose to perform an enzyme-linked immunosorbent assay.

Latex allergy can produce myriad symptoms, including generalized itching (on the hands and arms, for example); itchy, watery, or burning eyes; sneezing and coughing (hay fever-type symptoms); rash; hives; bronchial asthma, scratchy throat, or difficulty breathing; edema of the face, hands, or neck; and anaphylaxis.

To help identify people at risk for latex allergy, ask latex allergy-specific questions during the health history. (See *Latex allergy screening*.) If the patient's history reveals a latex sensitivity, the doctor assigns him to one of three categories based on the extent of his sensitization. Group 1 includes patients who have a history of anaphylaxis or a systemic reaction when exposed to a natural latex product. Group 2 patients have a clear history of an allergic reaction of a nonsystemic type. Group 3 patients don't have a previous history of latex hypersensitivity but are designated as high risk because of an associated medical condition, occupation, or cross-over allergy.

If you determine that your patient has a sensitivity to latex, make sure that he doesn't come in contact with latex because such contact could result in a life-threatening hypersensitivity reaction. Creating a latex-free environment is the only way to safeguard your patient. Many facilities now designate latex-free equipment, which is usually kept on a cart that can be moved into the patient's room.

## Equipment

Latex allergy patient identification wristband ● latex-free equipment, including room contents ● anaphylaxis kit ● optional: LATEX ALLERGY sign

### Preparation of equipment

After you've determined that the patient has a latex allergy or is sensitive to latex, arrange for him to be placed in a private room. If that isn't possible, make the room latex-free, even if the roommate hasn't been designated as hypersensitive to latex. This prevents the spread of airborne parti-

## Managing a latex allergy reaction

If you determine that the patient is having an allergic reaction to a latex product, act immediately. Make sure that you perform emergency interventions using latex-free equipment. If the latex product that caused the reaction is known, remove it and perform the following measures:

▶ If the allergic reaction develops during medication administration or a procedure, stop the medication or procedure immediately.

▶ Assess airway, breathing, and circulation.

▶ Administer 100% oxygen with continuous pulse oximetry.

▶ Start I.V. volume expanders with lactated Ringer's solution or normal saline solution.

▶ Administer epinephrine and famotidine, as ordered.

▶ If bronchospasm is evident, treat it with nebulized albuterol, as ordered.

▶ Secondary treatment for latex allergy reaction is aimed at treating the swelling and tissue reaction to the latex as well as breaking the chain of events associated with the allergic reaction. It includes:
  – diphenhydramine
  – methylprednisolone
  – famotidine

▶ Document the event and the exact cause (if known). If latex particles have entered the I.V. line, insert a new I.V. line with a new catheter, new tubing, and new infusion attachments as soon as possible.

cles from latex products used on the other patient.

### Implementation

For all patients in groups 1 and 2:

▶ Assess for possible latex allergy in all patients being admitted to the delivery room or short procedure unit or having a surgical procedure.

▶ If the patient has a confirmed latex allergy, bring a cart with latex-free supplies into his room.

▶ Document in the patient's chart (according to facility policy) that he has a latex allergy. If policy requires that the patient wear a latex allergy identification bracelet, place it on him.

▶ If the patient will be receiving anesthesia, make sure that "latex allergy" is clearly visible on the front of his chart. (See *Anesthesia induction and latex allergy,* page 73.) Notify the circulating nurse in the surgical unit, the postanesthesia care unit nurses, and any other team members that the patient has a latex allergy.

▶ If the patient must be transported to another area of the hospital, make certain that the latex-free cart accompanies him and that all health care workers who come in contact with him are wearing nonlatex gloves. The patient should wear a mask with cloth ties when leaving his room to protect him from inhaling airborne latex particles.

▶ If the patient will have an I.V. line, make sure that I.V. access is accomplished using all latex-free products. Post a latex allergy sign on the I.V. tubing to prevent access of the line using latex products.

▶ Flush I.V. tubing with 50 ml of I.V. solution because of latex ports in the I.V. tubing.

▶ Place a warning label on I.V. bags that says "Do not use latex injection ports."

▶ Use a nonlatex tourniquet. If none are available, use a latex tourniquet over clothing.

▶ Use latex-free oxygen administration equipment. Remove the elastic and tie equipment on with gauze.

▶ Wrap your stethoscope with a nonlatex product to protect the patient from latex contact.

▶ Wrap Tegaderm over the patient's finger before using pulse oximetry.

▶ Use latex-free syringes when administering medication through a syringe.

▶ Make sure an anaphylaxis kit is readily available. If the patient has an allergic reaction to latex, you must act immediately. (See *Managing a latex allergy reaction.*)

### Special considerations

▶ Remember that signs and symptoms of latex allergy usually occur within 30 minutes of anesthesia induction. However, the time of onset can range from 10 minutes to 5 hours.

▶ Don't forget that, as a health care worker, you're in a position to develop a latex hypersensitivity. If you suspect that you're sensitive to latex, contact the employee health services department concerning facility protocol for latex-sensitive employ-

ees. Use latex-free products whenever possible to help reduce your exposure to latex.
▶ Don't assume that if something doesn't look like rubber it isn't latex. Latex can be found in a wide variety of equipment, including electrocardiograph leads, oral and nasal airway tubing, tourniquets, nerve stimulation pads, temperature strips, and blood pressure cuffs.

## REFERENCES

Burt, S. "What You Need to Know about Latex Allergy," *Nursing99* 30(8):20-25, November 1999.

Centers for Disease Control and Prevention. National Institute for Occupational Safety and Health. "Latex Allergy: A Prevention Guide." Department of Health and Human Services (NIOSH) Publication No. 98-113. *www.cdc.gov/niosh/98-113.html.*

Charous, B.L. "Latex Allergy: A New and Common Problem," *American Family Physician* 57(1):42, 47, January 1998.

Reddy, S. "Latex Allergy," *American Family Physician* 57(1):93-102, January 1998.

# Neutropenic precautions

Unlike other types of precaution procedures, neutropenic precautions (also known as protective precautions and reverse isolation) guard the patient at increased risk for infection against contact with potential pathogens. These precautions are used primarily for patients with extensive noninfected burns, for those who have leukopenia or a depressed immune system, and for those who are receiving immunosuppressive treatments. (See *Conditions and treatments requiring neutropenic precautions,* page 76.)

Neutropenic precautions require a single room equipped with positive air pressure, if possible, to force suspended particles down and out of the room. The degree of precautions may range from using a single room, thorough hand-washing technique, and limitation of traffic into the room, to more extensive precautions including use of gowns, gloves, and masks by staff and visitors. The extent of neutropenic precautions may vary from facility to facility, depending on the reason for and the degree of the patient's immunosuppression.

To care for patients who have temporarily increased susceptibility, such as those who have undergone bone marrow transplantation, neutropenic precautions may also require a patient isolator unit and the use of sterile linens, gowns, gloves, and head and shoe coverings. In such cases, all other items taken into the room should be sterilized or disinfected. The patient's diet also may be modified to eliminate raw fruits and vegetables and to allow only cooked foods and, possibly, only sterile beverages.

## Equipment

Gloves, gowns, masks, shoe covers, if required ● neutropenic precautions door card

Gather any additional supplies, such as a thermometer, stethoscope, and blood pressure cuff, so you don't have to leave the isolation room unnecessarily.

### Preparation of equipment

Keep supplies in a clean enclosed cart or in an anteroom outside the room.

## Implementation

▶ After placing the patient in a single room, explain isolation precautions to the patient and his family to ease patient anxiety and promote cooperation.
▶ Place a neutropenic precautions card on the door to caution those entering the room.
▶ Wash your hands with an antiseptic agent before putting on gloves, after removing gloves, and as indicated during patient care.
▶ Wear gloves and gown according to standard precautions, unless the patient's condition warrants sterile gown, gloves, and mask.
▶ Avoid transporting the patient out of the room; if he must be moved, make sure he wears a gown and mask. Notify the receiving department or area so that the precautions will be maintained and the patient will be returned to the room promptly.
▶ Don't allow visits by anyone known to be ill or infected.

## Special considerations

▶ Don't perform invasive procedures, such as urethral catheterization, unless absolutely necessary, because these procedures risk serious infection in the patient with impaired resistance.

## Conditions and treatments requiring neutropenic precautions

| Condition and treatment | Precautionary period |
| --- | --- |
| Acquired immunodeficiency syndrome | Until white blood cell count reaches 1,000/µl or more, or according to facility guidelines |
| Agranulocytosis | Until remission |
| Burns, extensive noninfected | Until skin surface heals substantially |
| Dermatitis, noninfected vesicular, bullous, or eczematous | Until skin surface heals substantially |
| Immunosuppressive therapy | Until patient's immunity is adequate |
| Lymphomas and leukemia, especially late stages of Hodgkin's disease or acute leukemia | Until clinical improvement is substantial |

▶ Instruct the housekeeping staff to put on gowns, gloves, and masks before entering the room; no ill or infected person should enter.

▶ Make sure that the room is cleaned with new or scrupulously clean equipment. Because the patient doesn't have a contagious disease, materials leaving the room need no special precautions beyond standard precautions.

### Documentation

▶ Document the need for neutropenic precautions on the nursing plan of care and as required by your facility.

### REFERENCES

Craven, R., and Hirnle, C.J. *Fundamentals of Nursing: Human Health and Function,* 4th ed. Philadelphia: Lippincott Williams & Wilkins, 2002.

Garner, J.S. "Hospital Infection Control Practices Advisory Committee Guidelines for Isolation Precautions in Hospitals," *Infection Control and Hospital Epidemiology* 17(1):53-80, January 1996.

## Standard precautions

Standard precautions were developed by the Centers for Disease Control and Prevention (CDC) to provide the widest possible protection against the transmission of infection. CDC officials recommend that health care workers handle all blood, body fluids (including secretions, excretions, and drainage), tissues, and contact with mucous membranes and broken skin as if they contain infectious agents, regardless of the patient's diagnosis.

Standard precautions encompass much of the isolation precautions previously recommended by the CDC for patients with known or suspected blood-borne pathogens, as well as the precautions previously known as body substance isolation. They're to be used in conjunction with other transmission-based precautions, including airborne, droplet, and contact precautions.

Standard precautions recommend wearing gloves for any known or anticipated contact with blood, body fluids, tissue, mucous membrane, and nonintact skin. (See *Choosing the right glove.*) If the task or procedure being performed may result in splashing or splattering of blood or body fluids to the face, a mask and goggles or a face shield should be worn. If the task or procedure being performed may result in splashing or splattering of blood or body fluids to the body, a fluid-resistant gown or apron should be worn. Additional protective clothing, such as shoe covers, may be appropriate to protect the caregiver's feet in situations that may expose him to large

# Choosing the right glove

Health care workers may develop allergic reactions as a result of their exposure to latex gloves and other products containing natural rubber latex. Patients may also have latex sensitivity.

Take the following steps to protect yourself and the patient from allergic reactions to latex:
▶ Use nonlatex (for example, vinyl or synthetic) gloves for activities that aren't likely to involve contact with infectious materials (such as food preparation, routine cleaning, and so forth).
▶ Use appropriate barrier protection when handling infectious materials. If you choose latex gloves, use powder-free gloves with reduced protein content.
▶ After wearing and removing gloves, wash your hands with soap and dry them thoroughly.
▶ When wearing latex gloves, don't use oil-based hand creams or lotions (which can cause gloves to deteriorate) unless they have been shown to maintain glove barrier protection.
▶ Refer to the material safety data sheet for the appropriate glove to wear when handling chemicals.

▶ Learn procedures for preventing latex allergy, and learn how to recognize the following signs of latex allergy: skin rashes; hives; flushing; itching; nasal, eye, or sinus symptoms; asthma; and shock.
▶ If you have (or suspect you have) a latex sensitivity, use nonlatex gloves, avoid contact with latex gloves and other latex-containing products, and consult a doctor experienced in treating latex allergy.

## For latex allergy

If you have latex allergy, consider the following precautions:
▶ Avoid contact with latex gloves and other products that contain latex.
▶ Avoid areas where you might inhale the powder from latex gloves worn by other workers.
▶ Inform your employers and your health care providers (such as doctors, nurses, dentists, and others).
▶ Wear a medical alert bracelet.
▶ Follow your doctor's instructions for dealing with allergic reactions to latex

amounts of blood, body fluids, or both, such as care of a trauma patient in the operating room or emergency department.

Airborne precautions are initiated in situations of suspected or known infections spread by the airborne route. The causative organisms are coughed, talked, or sneezed into the air by the infected person in droplets of moisture. The moisture evaporates, leaving the microorganisms suspended in the air to be breathed in by susceptible persons who enter the shared air space. Airborne precautions recommend placing the infected patient in a negative-pressure isolation room and the wearing of respiratory protection by all persons entering the patient's room.

Droplet precautions are used to protect health care workers and visitors from mucous membrane contact with oral and nasal secretions of the infected individual.

Contact precautions use barrier precautions to interrupt the transmission of specific epidemiologically important organisms by direct or indirect contact. Each institution must establish an infection control policy that lists specific barrier precautions.

## Equipment

Gloves ● face shields or masks and goggles or glasses ● gowns or aprons ● resuscitation bag ● bags for specimens ● Environmental Protection Agency (EPA)–registered tuberculocidal disinfectant or diluted bleach solution (diluted between 1:10 and 1:100, and mixed fresh daily), or both, or EPA-registered disinfectant labeled as effective against hepatitis B virus (HBV) and human immunodeficiency virus (HIV)

## Implementation

▶ Wash your hands immediately if they become contaminated with blood or body fluids, excretions, secretions, or drainage; also, wash your hands before and after patient care and after removing gloves. Hand washing removes microorganisms from your skin.
▶ Wear gloves if you will or could come in contact with blood, specimens, tissue, body fluids, secretions or excretions, mucous membrane, broken skin, or contaminated surfaces or objects.
▶ Change your gloves and wash your hands between patient contacts to avoid cross-contamination.

▶ Wear a fluid-resistant gown or apron and face shield or a mask and glasses or goggles during procedures likely to generate splashing or splattering of blood or body fluids, such as surgery, endoscopic procedures, dialysis, assisting with intubation or manipulation of arterial lines, or any other procedure with potential for splashing or splattering of body fluids.

▶ Handle used needles and other sharp instruments carefully. Don't bend, break, reinsert them into their original sheaths, remove needles from syringes, or unnecessarily handle them. Discard them intact immediately after use into a puncture-resistant disposal box. Use tools to pick up broken glass or other sharp objects. These measures reduce the risk of accidental injury or infection.

▶ Immediately notify your employer's health care provider of all needle-stick or other sharp object injuries, mucosal splashes, or contamination of open wounds or nonintact skin with blood or body fluids to allow investigation of the incident and appropriate care and documentation.

▶ Properly label all specimens collected from patients and place them in plastic bags at the collection site. Attach requisition slips to the outside of the bag.

▶ Place all items that have come in direct contact with the patient's secretions, excretions, blood, drainage, or body fluids, such as nondisposable utensils or instruments, in a single impervious bag or container before removal from the room. Place linens and trash in single bags of sufficient thickness to contain the contents.

▶ While wearing the appropriate personal protective equipment, promptly clean all blood and body fluid spills with detergent and water, followed by an EPA-registered tuberculocidal disinfectant or diluted bleach solution (diluted between 1:10 and 1:100, and mixed daily), or both, or an EPA-registered disinfectant labeled as effective against HBV and HIV, provided that the surface hasn't been contaminated with agents or volumes of or concentrations of agents for which higher-level disinfection is recommended.

▶ Disposable food trays and dishes aren't necessary.

▶ If you have an exudative lesion, avoid all direct patient contact until the condition

has resolved and you've been cleared by the employer health care provider.

▶ If you have dermatitis or other conditions resulting in broken skin on your hands, avoid situations where you may have contact with blood and body fluids, even though gloves could be worn, until the condition has resolved and you've been cleared by the employee health provider.

## Special considerations

▶ Standard precautions, such as hand washing and appropriate use of personal protective equipment, should be routine infection control practices.

▶ Keep mouthpieces, resuscitation bags, and other ventilation devices nearby to minimize the need for emergency mouth-to-mouth resuscitation, thus reducing the risk of exposure to body fluids.

◆**ALERT!** Because you may not always know what organisms may be present in every clinical situation, you must use standard precautions for every contact with blood, body fluids, secretions, excretions, drainage, mucous membranes, and nonintact skin. Use your judgment in individual cases about whether to implement additional isolation precautions, such as airborne, droplet, or contact precautions or a combination of them. In addition, if your work requires you to be exposed to blood, you should receive the HBV vaccine series.

## Complications

Failure to follow standard precautions may lead to exposure to blood-borne diseases or other infections and to all the complications they may cause.

## Documentation

▶ Record any special needs for isolation precautions on the nursing plan of care and as required by your facility.

### REFERENCES

Garner, J.S. "Hospital Infection Control Practices Advisory Committee Guidelines for Isolation Precautions in Hospitals," *Infection Control and Hospital Epidemiology* 17(1):53-80, January 1996.

Perry, J. "The Bloodborne Pathogen Standards, 2001: What's Changed?" *Nursing Management* 32(6 part 1):25-26, June 2001.

# Swab specimens

Correct collection and handling of swab specimens helps the laboratory staff identify pathogens accurately with a minimum of contamination from normal bacterial flora. Collection normally involves sampling inflamed tissues and exudates from the throat, nasopharynx, wounds, eye, ear, or rectum with sterile swabs of cotton or other absorbent material. The type of swab used depends on the part of the body affected. For example, collection of a nasopharyngeal specimen requires a cotton-tipped swab.

After the specimen has been collected, the swab is immediately placed in a sterile tube containing a transport medium and, in the case of sampling for anaerobes, an inert gas. Swab specimens are usually collected to identify pathogens and sometimes to identify asymptomatic carriers of certain easily transmitted disease organisms.

## Equipment

*For a throat specimen*
Gloves • tongue blade • penlight • sterile cotton-tipped swab • sterile culture tube with transport medium (or commercial collection kit) • label • laboratory request form

*For a nasopharyngeal specimen*
Gloves • penlight • sterile flexible cotton-tipped swab • tongue blade • sterile culture tube with transport medium • label • laboratory request form • optional: nasal speculum

*For a wound specimen*
Sterile gloves • sterile forceps • alcohol or povidone-iodine pads • sterile cotton-tipped swabs • sterile 10-ml syringe • sterile 21G needle • sterile culture tube with transport medium (or commercial collection kit for aerobic culture) • labels • special anaerobic culture tube containing carbon dioxide or nitrogen • fresh dressings for the wound • laboratory request form • optional: rubber stopper for needle

*For an ear specimen*
Gloves • normal saline solution • two 2″ × 2″ gauze pads • sterile swabs • sterile culture tube with transport medium • label • 10-ml syringe and 22G 1″ needle (for tympanocentesis) • laboratory request form

*For an eye specimen*
Sterile gloves • sterile normal saline solution • two 2″ × 2″ gauze pads • sterile swabs • sterile wire culture loop (for corneal scraping) • sterile culture tube with transport medium • label • laboratory request form

*For a rectal specimen*
Gloves • soap and water • washcloth • sterile swab • normal saline solution or sterile broth medium • sterile culture tube with transport medium • label • laboratory request form

## Implementation

▶ Explain the procedure to the patient to ease his anxiety and ensure cooperation.

### Collecting a throat specimen

▶ Tell the patient that he may gag during the swabbing but that the procedure will probably take less than 1 minute.

▶ Instruct the patient to sit erect at the edge of the bed or in a chair, facing you. Then wash your hands and put on gloves.

▶ Ask the patient to tilt his head back. Depress his tongue with the tongue blade and illuminate his throat with the penlight to check for inflamed areas.

▶ If the patient starts to gag, withdraw the tongue blade and tell him to breathe deeply. When he's relaxed, reinsert the tongue blade but not as deeply as before.

▶ Using the sterile cotton-tipped swab, wipe the tonsillar areas from side to side, including any inflamed or purulent sites. Make sure you don't touch the tongue, cheeks, or teeth with the swab to avoid contaminating it with oral bacteria.

▶ Withdraw the swab and immediately place it in the sterile culture tube. If you're using a commercial kit, crush the ampule of culture medium at the bottom of the tube and then push the swab into the medium to keep the swab moist.

▶ Remove and discard your gloves and wash your hands.

▶ Label the specimen with the patient's name and room number, the doctor's name, and the date, time, and site of collection.

▶ On the laboratory request form, indicate whether any organism is strongly suspected, especially Corynebacterium diphtheriae (requires two swabs and special growth medium), Bordetella pertussis (requires a

## Obtaining a nasopharyngeal specimen

After you've passed the swab into the nasopharynx, quickly but gently rotate the swab to collect the specimen. Then remove the swab, taking care not to injure the nasal mucous membrane.

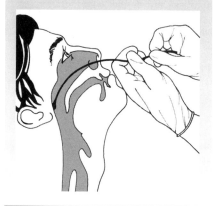

▶ While it's still in the package, bend the sterile cotton-tipped swab in a curve and then open the package without contaminating the swab.
▶ Ask the patient to tilt his head back and gently pass the swab through the more patent nostril about 3″ to 4″ (7.5 to 10 cm) into the nasopharynx, keeping the swab near the septum and floor of the nose. Rotate the swab quickly and remove it. (See *Obtaining a nasopharyngeal specimen.*)
▶ Alternatively, depress the patient's tongue with a tongue blade and pass the bent swab up behind the uvula. Rotate the swab and withdraw it.
▶ Remove the cap from the sterile culture tube, insert the swab, and break off the contaminated end. Then close the tube tightly.
▶ Remove and discard your gloves and wash your hands.
▶ Label the specimen for culture, complete a laboratory request form, and send the specimen to the laboratory immediately. If you're collecting a specimen to isolate a possible virus, check with the laboratory for the recommended collection technique.

nasopharyngeal culture and special growth medium), and Neisseria meningitidis (requires enriched selective media).
▶ Send the specimen to the laboratory immediately to prevent growth or deterioration of microbes.

### Collecting a nasopharyngeal specimen
▶ Tell the patient that he may gag or feel the urge to sneeze during the swabbing but that the procedure takes less than 1 minute.
▶ Have the patient sit erect at the edge of the bed or in a chair, facing you. Then wash your hands and put on gloves.
▶ Ask the patient to blow his nose to clear his nasal passages. Then check his nostrils for patency with a penlight.
▶ If the nostril appears narrow, use a nasal speculum to have better access to the specimen.
▶ Tell the patient to occlude one nostril first and then the other as he exhales. Listen for the more patent nostril because you'll insert the swab through it.
▶ Ask the patient to cough to bring organisms to the nasopharynx for a better specimen.

### Collecting a wound specimen
▶ Wash your hands, prepare a sterile field, and put on sterile gloves. With sterile forceps, remove the dressing to expose the wound. Dispose of the soiled dressings properly.
▶ Clean the area around the wound with an alcohol or a povidone-iodine pad to reduce the risk of contaminating the specimen with skin bacteria. Then allow the area to dry.
▶ For an aerobic culture, use a sterile cotton-tipped swab to collect as much exudate as possible, or insert the swab deeply into the wound and gently rotate it. Remove the swab from the wound and immediately place it in the aerobic culture tube. Label the tube and send it to the laboratory immediately with a completed laboratory request form. Never collect exudate from the skin and then insert the same swab into the wound; this could contaminate the wound with skin bacteria.
▶ For an anaerobic culture, insert the sterile cotton-tipped swab deeply into the wound, rotate it gently, remove it, and immediately place it in the anaerobic culture tube. (See *Anaerobic specimen collection.*)

Alternatively, insert a sterile 10-ml syringe, without a needle, into the wound and aspirate 1 to 5 ml of exudate into the syringe. Then attach the 21G needle to the syringe and immediately inject the aspirate into the anaerobic culture tube. If an anaerobic culture tube is unavailable, obtain a rubber stopper, attach the needle to the syringe, and gently push all the air out of the syringe by pressing on the plunger. Stick the needle tip into the rubber stopper, remove and discard your gloves, and send the syringe of aspirate to the laboratory immediately with a completed laboratory request form.

▶ Put on sterile gloves.
▶ Apply a new dressing to the wound.

### Collecting an ear specimen

▶ Wash your hands and put on gloves.
▶ Gently clean excess debris from the patient's ear with normal saline solution and gauze pads.
▶ Insert the sterile swab into the ear canal and rotate it gently along the walls of the canal to avoid damaging the eardrum.
▶ Withdraw the swab, being careful not to touch other surfaces to avoid contaminating the specimen.
▶ Place the swab in the sterile culture tube with transport medium.
▶ Remove and discard your gloves and wash your hands.
▶ Label the specimen for culture, complete a laboratory request form, and send the specimen to the laboratory immediately.

### Collecting a middle ear specimen

▶ Put on gloves and clean the outer ear with normal saline solution and gauze pads. Remove and discard your gloves. After the doctor punctures the eardrum with a needle and aspirates fluid into the syringe, label the container, complete a laboratory request form, and send the specimen to the laboratory immediately.

### Collecting an eye specimen

▶ Wash your hands and put on sterile gloves.
▶ Gently clean excess debris from the outside of the eye with sterile normal saline solution and gauze pads, wiping from the inner to the outer canthus.
▶ Retract the lower eyelid to expose the conjunctival sac. Gently rub the sterile

## Anaerobic specimen collection

Because most anaerobes die when exposed to oxygen, they must be transported in tubes filled with carbon dioxide or nitrogen. The anaerobic specimen collector shown here includes a rubber-stoppered tube filled with carbon dioxide, a small inner tube, and a swab attached to a plastic plunger.

Before specimen collection, the small inner tube containing the swab is held in place with the rubber stopper (as shown on the left). After collecting the specimen, quickly replace the swab in the inner tube and depress the plunger to separate the inner tube from the stopper (as shown on the right), forcing it into the larger tube and exposing the specimen to a carbon dioxide–rich environment.

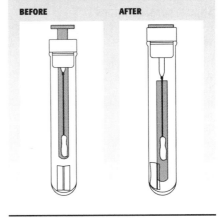

BEFORE          AFTER

swab over the conjunctiva, being careful not to touch other surfaces. Hold the swab parallel to the eye, rather than pointed directly at it, to prevent corneal irritation or trauma due to sudden movement. If a corneal scraping is required, this procedure is performed by a doctor, using a wire culture loop.

▶ Immediately place the swab or wire loop in the culture tube with transport medium.
▶ Remove and discard your gloves and wash your hands.
▶ Label the specimen for culture, complete a laboratory request form, and send the specimen to the laboratory immediately.

## Collecting a rectal specimen

▶ Wash your hands and put on gloves.
▶ Clean the area around the patient's anus using a washcloth and soap and water.
▶ Insert the sterile swab, moistened with normal saline solution or sterile broth medium, through the anus and advance it about ⅜" (1 cm) for infants or 1½" (4 cm) for adults. While withdrawing the swab, gently rotate it against the walls of the lower rectum to sample a large area of the rectal mucosa.
▶ Place the swab in a culture tube with transport medium.
▶ Remove and discard your gloves and wash your hands.
▶ Label the specimen for culture, complete a laboratory request form, and send the specimen to the laboratory immediately.

### Special considerations

▶ Note recent antibiotic therapy on the laboratory request form.

### For a wound specimen

Although you would normally clean the area around a wound to prevent contamination by normal skin flora, don't clean a perineal wound with alcohol because this could irritate sensitive tissues. Also, make sure that the antiseptic doesn't enter the wound.

### For an eye specimen

Don't use an antiseptic before culturing to avoid irritating the eye and inhibiting growth of organisms in the culture. If the patient is a child or an uncooperative adult, ask a coworker to restrain the patient's head to prevent eye trauma resulting from sudden movement.

### Documentation

Record the time, date, and site of specimen collection and any recent or current antibiotic therapy. Also, note whether the specimen has an unusual appearance or odor.

### REFERENCES

Craven, R., and Hirnle, C.J. *Fundamentals of Nursing: Human Health and Function,* 4th ed. Philadelphia: Lippincott Williams & Wilkins, 2002.
Kowalski, R.P., et al. ELVIS: A New 24-hour Culture Test for Detecting Herpes Simplex Virus from Ocular Samples," *Archives of Ophthalmology* 120(7):960-62, July 2002.

# Use of isolation equipment

Isolation procedures may be implemented to prevent the spread of infection from patient to patient, from the patient to health care workers, or from health care workers to the patient. They may also be used to reduce the risk of infection in immunocompromised patients. Essential to the success of these procedures is the selection of the proper equipment and the adequate training of those who use it.

## Equipment

Materials required for isolation typically include barrier clothing, an isolation cart or anteroom for storing equipment, and a door card announcing that isolation precautions are in effect.

*Barrier clothing*
Gowns ● gloves ● goggles ● masks
Each staff member must be trained on the proper use of these items.

*Isolation supplies*
Specially marked laundry bags (and water-soluble laundry bags, if used) ● plastic trash bags
An isolation cart may be used when the patient's room has no anteroom. It should include a work area (such as a pull-out shelf), drawers or a cabinet area for holding isolation supplies and, possibly, a pole on which to hang coats or jackets.

### Preparation of equipment

Remove the cover from the isolation cart, if necessary, and set up the work area. Check the cart or anteroom to ensure that correct and sufficient supplies are in place for the designated isolation category.

## Implementation

▶ Remove your watch, or push it well up your arm, and your rings according to facility policy. These actions help to prevent the spread of microorganisms hidden under your watch or rings.
▶ Wash your hands with an antiseptic cleaning agent to prevent the growth of microorganisms under gloves.

### Putting on isolation garb

▶ Put the gown on and wrap it around the back of your uniform. Tie the strings or fasten the snaps or pressure-sensitive tabs at the neck. Make sure your uniform is completely covered and secure the gown at the waist.

▶ Place the mask snugly over your nose and mouth. Secure ear loops around your ears or tie the strings behind your head high enough so the mask won't slip off. If the mask has a metal strip, squeeze it to fit your nose firmly but comfortably. (See *Putting on a face mask.*) If you wear eyeglasses, tuck the mask under their lower edge.

▶ Put on the gloves. Pull the gloves over the cuffs to cover the edges of the gown's sleeves.

### Removing isolation garb

▶ Remember that the outside surfaces of your barrier clothes are contaminated.

▶ While wearing gloves, untie the gown's waist strings.

▶ With your gloved left hand, remove the right glove by pulling on the cuff, turning the glove inside out as you pull. Don't touch any skin with the outside of either glove. (See *Removing contaminated gloves,* page 84.) Remove the left glove by wedging one or two fingers of your right hand inside the glove and pulling it off, turning it inside out as you remove it. Discard the gloves in a trash container that contains a plastic trash bag.

▶ Untie your mask, holding it only by the strings. Discard the mask in the trash container. If the patient has a disease spread by airborne pathogens, you may prefer to remove the mask last.

▶ Untie the neck straps of your gown. Grasp the outside of the gown at the back of the shoulders and pull the gown down over your arms, turning it inside out as you remove it to ensure containment of the pathogens.

▶ Holding the gown well away from your uniform, fold it inside out. Discard it in the specially marked laundry bags or trash container as necessary.

▶ If the sink is inside the patient's room, wash your hands and forearms with soap or antiseptic before leaving the room. Turn off the faucet using a paper towel and discard the towel in the room. Grasp the door handle with a clean paper towel to open it and discard the towel in a trash container inside the room. Close the door from the outside with your bare hand.

## Putting on a face mask

To avoid spreading airborne particles, wear a sterile or nonsterile face mask as indicated. Position the mask to cover your nose and mouth and secure it high enough to ensure stability. Tie the top strings at the back of your head above the ears. Then tie the bottom strings at the base of your neck.

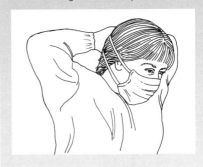

Adjust the metal nose strip if the mask has one.

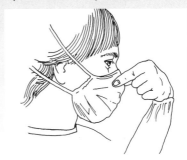

▶ If the sink is in an anteroom, wash your hands and forearms with soap or antiseptic after leaving the room.

### Special considerations

▶ Use gowns, gloves, goggles, and masks only once, and discard them in the appropriate container before leaving a contaminated area. If your mask is reusable, retain it for further use unless it's damaged or damp. Isolation garb loses its effectiveness when wet because moisture permits organisms to seep through the material. Change masks and gowns as soon as moisture is noticeable or according to the manufacturer's recommendations or your facility's policy.

# Removing contaminated gloves

Proper removal techniques are essential for preventing the spread of pathogens from gloves to your skin surface. Follow these steps carefully.

1. Using your left hand, pinch the right glove near the top. Avoid allowing the glove's outer surface to buckle inward against your wrist.

2. Pull downward, allowing the glove to turn inside out as it comes off. Keep the right glove in your left hand after removing it.

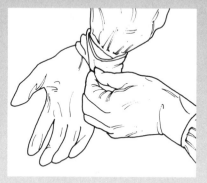
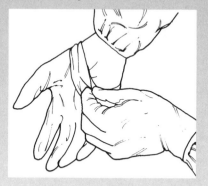

3. Next, insert the first two fingers of your ungloved right hand under the edge of the left glove. Avoid touching the glove's outer surface or folding it against your left wrist.

4. Pull downward so that the glove turns inside out as it comes off. Continue pulling until the left glove completely encloses the right one and its uncontaminated inner surface is facing out.

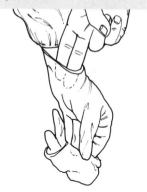
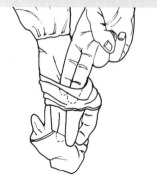

▶ At the end of your shift, restock used items for the next person. After patient transfer or discharge, return the isolation cart to the appropriate area for cleaning and restocking of supplies. An isolation room or other room prepared for isolation purposes must be thoroughly cleaned and disinfected before use by another patient.

**REFERENCES**

Craven, R., and Hirnle, C.J. *Fundamentals of Nursing: Human Health and Function,* 4th ed. Philadelphia: Lippincott Williams & Wilkins, 2002.

Garner, J.S. "Hospital Infection Control Practices Advisory Committee Guidelines for Isolation Precautions in Hospitals," *Infection Control and Hospital Epidemiology* 17(1):53-80, January 1996.

# 3

# Medication administration

**A**DMINISTERING DRUGS TO YOUR PATIENT IS ONE OF YOUR MOST CRITICAL NURSING RESPON-
sibilities. To make sure they're given safely and effectively, you'll need to be familiar
with the indications, customary dosages, and intended effects of prescribed drugs.
You'll also need to assess each patient before administering a drug, delaying or withholding it if necessary. Just as important, you'll need the skills to administer a drug capably,
minimizing your patient's anxiety and maximizing the drug's effectiveness.

Assessing a patient's response to a drug requires a thorough understanding of his condition and the drug's desired or expected effect. When assessing the patient's response to
therapy, also consider the results of laboratory tests, which can indicate a therapeutic effect, an adverse effect, or a toxic level. Monitor the patient's condition carefully; such
changes as weight gain or loss can affect the action of some drugs. Other factors, such as
the patient's age, body build, sex, and emotional state, may also affect his response to drug
therapy.

When you administer drugs, you also need to recognize and identify adverse effects,
toxic reactions, and drug allergies. Some of these effects are transient and subside as the
patient develops tolerance to the drug; others may require a change in therapy.

This chapter will help you perform these tasks by providing the information you need
to administer drugs by injection, instillation, inhalation, topical application, and the I.V.
route. You'll also learn how to add drugs to an I.V. solution, give I.V. bolus injections, and
prepare and administer chemotherapeutic drugs.

# Protocols

## Managing the patient experiencing pain

### Purpose
To relieve patient of pain and suffering interfering with his ability to achieve usual
level of activity

### Collaborative level
Interdependent

### Expected patient outcomes
▶ The patient will achieve a desired level
of comfort.
▶ The patient will participate in ongoing
treatment and rehabilitation activities.

### Indications
Treatment
▶ Acute pain
▶ Postoperative pain
▶ Chronic pain
▶ Terminal pain

Prevention
▶ Inadequate pain relief
▶ Overdose
▶ Constipation

### Assessment guidance
Signs and symptoms
*Inadequate pain relief*
▶ Complaint of continuing pain
▶ Inability to concentrate
▶ Inability to perform activities of daily
living
▶ Tachycardia
▶ Tachypnea

*Overdose*
▶ Decreased level of consciousness
▶ Bradypnea and apnea
▶ Decreased arterial $Po_2$ levels
▶ Severe lethargy
▶ Increased $Pco_2$

### Nursing interventions
▶ Notify the doctor.

▶ Make the patient as comfortable as possible and reassure him as necessary.
▶ If pain relief is inadequate, provide other means of treatment, such as diversion, biofeedback, massage, and hot or cold therapy.
▶ Check with the doctor for change in prescribed medication or in its dosage.

### Overdose
▶ Discontinue medication.
▶ Notify the doctor.
▶ Monitor vital signs as frequently as indicated by severity of respiratory depression.
▶ Administer naloxone — be prepared for withdrawal symptoms.
▶ Be prepared to assist with endotracheal intubation.

### Patient teaching
▶ Teach the patient how to assess his own pain.
▶ Make sure the patient and his family understand the symptoms of allergic reactions.
▶ Teach the patient and caregivers non–drug-related ways to reduce pain.

### Precautions
▶ Obtain thorough history, including allergies, previous reactions to narcotics, and lifestyle history, including previous or concurrent narcotic and alcohol use.

### Contraindications
Contraindications include allergy or hypersensitivity to the prescribed medication. For use of nonsteroidal anti-inflammatory drugs in the patient with previous bleeding tendencies, consult with a doctor.

### Documentation
▶ Record subjective response reported by the patient.
▶ Document length of time of patient's reported therapeutic response to medication.
▶ Record the dose of medication patient is receiving, as well as time and route, and degree of pain relief.
▶ Note objective signs recorded by the nurse.
▶ Document date, time, and type of any reactions.
▶ Document nursing interventions.
▶ Record doctor notification and intervention.

▶ Document the patient's response to treatment.
▶ Document patient teaching.

### Related procedures
▶ Admixture of drugs in a syringe
▶ Eardrops
▶ Endotracheal drugs
▶ I.M. injection
▶ I.V. bolus medication
▶ Oral drugs
▶ Endotracheal intubation
▶ Pulse and ear oximetry
▶ Mechanical ventilation
▶ Endotracheal tube care

### REFERENCES
McCaffery, M., and Pasero, C. *Pain: Clinical Manual,* 2nd ed. St. Louis: Mosby–Year Book, Inc., 1999.
*Nursing 2003 Drug Handbook.* Springhouse, Pa.: Lippincott Williams & Wilkins, 2002.
Phillips, L. *Manual of I.V. Therapeutics,* 3rd ed. Philadelphia: F.A. Davis Co., 2001.

# Managing the patient receiving epidural and intrathecal analgesia

### Purpose
To provide the patient with an analgesic level of comfort using the minimal amount of sedation

### Collaborative level
Interdependent

### Expected patient outcomes
▶ The patient will achieve desired level of comfort.
▶ The patient will participate in ongoing treatment and rehabilitation activities.

### Definition of terms
▶ *Epidural:* On or over the dura mater.
▶ *Intrathecal:* Pertaining to a structure within a sheath, surrounded by the epidural space and separated from it by the dura mater; an intrathecal injection introduces medication into the subarachnoid space (which contains cerebrospinal fluid).

## Indications
### Treatment
▶ Postsurgical patient
▶ Chronic pain when conventional treatment modalities restrict patient's mobility
▶ Cancer cells that cross the blood-brain barrier
▶ Severe spasticity in neurologically impaired patients

### Prevention
▶ Displacement of implanted catheter
▶ Local and systemic infection
▶ Respiratory depression
▶ Spinal headache

## Assessment guidance
### Signs and symptoms
*Displacement of implanted port*
▶ Inadequate pain relief
▶ Difficulty infusing epidural medication

*Narcotic overdose*
▶ Tachycardia

*Local and systemic infection*
▶ Elevated temperature
▶ Tachycardia
▶ Fever
▶ Chills
▶ General malaise

*Respiratory depression*
▶ Restlessness
▶ Anxiety
▶ Dyspnea
▶ Somnolence
▶ Tachycardia
▶ Bradypnea

*Spinal headache*
▶ Severe head pain despite narcotic administration
▶ Photophobia
▶ Tachycardia

### Diagnostic studies
*Laboratory tests*
▶ Arterial $Po_2$ levels
▶ White blood cell count

*Other*
▶ Pulse oximetry readings

## Nursing interventions
▶ Notify the doctor.
▶ Monitor vital signs every 15 minutes, or as indicated by the severity and type of reaction.
▶ Administer supplemental oxygen and medications.
▶ Make the patient as comfortable as possible and provide reassurance as necessary.

### Displacement of implanted port
▶ Gently aspirate 1 ml of fluid from the catheter to verify placement; if aspirate is blood, or blood tinged, notify the doctor; placement must be verified by the anesthesiologist.
▶ Stabilize catheter during dressing changes.

### Local and systemic infection
▶ Discontinue catheter usage.
▶ Always use preservative-free medications.
▶ Maintain sterile technique while changing dressings.

### Respiratory depression
▶ Stop the infusion.
▶ Administer naloxone and be prepared for withdrawal symptoms.
▶ Be prepared to assist with endotracheal intubation.

### Spinal headache
▶ Prepare blood patch by drawing approximately 10 ml of blood from the patient's arm and injecting the blood epidurally near the level of the original intrathecal catheter.

## Patient teaching
▶ Teach the patient's caregiver to evaluate his level of sedation.
▶ Instruct the patient on self-assessment of pain.
▶ Teach proper sterile handling of catheter site.
▶ Instruct the patient and caregiver on avoidance of catheter displacement.

## Precautions
▶ Obtain thorough history, including allergies and previous reactions to narcotics, and lifestyle history, including previous or concurrent narcotic and alcohol use.

## Contraindications

Contraindicated in patients allergic or hypersensitive to prescribed medication.

## Documentation

▶ Document adverse effects associated with site, ability to administer medication, narcotic administration, or failure to achieve therapeutic effect of medication.
▶ Record date, time, route, and dose of medication, as well as patient's degree of pain relief.
▶ Record date, time, and type of reaction.
▶ Record subjective symptoms reported by the patient.
▶ Record objective signs.
▶ Note any pertinent laboratory data.
▶ Document diagnostic study results.
▶ Record doctor notification and intervention.
▶ Document patient response to treatment.
▶ Note patient teaching.

## Related procedures

▶ I.V. bolus injection
▶ Oropharyngeal inhalers
▶ Pulse and ear oximetry
▶ Oxygen administration
▶ Endotracheal intubation
▶ Manual ventilation
▶ Mechanical ventilation
▶ Endotracheal tube care
▶ Subcutaneous injection
▶ Epidural analgesics

## REFERENCES

*Nursing 2003 Drug Handbook.* Springhouse, Pa.: Lippincott Williams & Wilkins, 2002.
Phillips, L. *Manual of I.V. Therapeutics,* 3rd ed. Philadelphia: F.A. Davis Co., 2001.

# Managing the patient receiving patient-controlled analgesia

## Purpose

To provide the patient with an analgesic level of comfort using the minimal amount of sedation

## Collaborative level

Interdependent

## Expected patient outcomes

▶ The patient will achieve desired level of comfort.
▶ The patient will participate in ongoing treatment and rehabilitation activities.

## Definition of terms

▶ *Patient-controlled analgesia* (PCA): a pain management delivery system that allows patient to self-administer I.V. narcotic pain medication by depressing a button attached to a computerized pump.

## Indications

Treatment
▶ Trauma
▶ Postsurgical condition
▶ Terminal illness

Prevention
▶ Respiratory depression
▶ Acute bronchial asthma or upper airway obstruction
▶ Renal impairment
▶ Hepatic impairment

## Assessment guidance

Signs and symptoms
*Respiratory depression*
▶ Restlessness
▶ Anxiety
▶ Dyspnea
▶ Somnolence
▶ Tachycardia
▶ Bradypnea

*Acute bronchial asthma or upper airway obstruction*
▶ Dyspnea
▶ Tachycardia
▶ Tachypnea
▶ Wheezing, stridor

*Renal impairment*
▶ Oliguria
▶ Decreased urine output

*Hepatic impairment*
▶ Nausea
▶ Vomiting
▶ Abdominal pain, tenderness
▶ Jaundice

Diagnostic studies
*Laboratory tests*
▶ Arterial $Po_2$ levels
▶ Amylase and lipase levels

*Other*
▶ Pulse oximetry

## Nursing interventions
▶ Monitor the amount of medication infused.
▶ Monitor the patient's respiratory rate.
▶ Assess the patient's degree of pain relief. If the patient reports insufficient pain relief, notify the doctor.
▶ If you suspect an overdose:
 – Assess the insertion site for signs of infiltration and catheter occlusion.
 – Discontinue PCA medication immediately.
 – Notify the doctor.
 – Monitor vital signs every 15 minutes, or as indicated by the severity and type of reaction.
 – Administer supplemental oxygen.
 – Make the patient as comfortable as possible and provide reassurance as necessary.
 – Administer epinephrine, diphenhydramine, corticosteroids, and inhaled bronchodilators.
 – Administer naloxone; be prepared for withdrawal symptoms.

## Patient teaching
▶ Instruct the patient in self-assessment of pain.
▶ Teach the proper use of PCA.
▶ Teach the patient to recognize symptoms of allergic reaction.
▶ For home care patients, teach the patient and caregivers how and when the cartridge syringe with narcotic will be changed.

## Precautions
▶ Ensure that the patient can understand and operate PCA device.
▶ Obtain thorough history, including allergies and previous reactions to narcotics, and lifestyle history, including previous or concurrent narcotic and alcohol use.

## Contraindications
PCA is contraindicated in cases of known allergy or hypersensitivity to prescribed medication.

## Documentation
▶ Record the loading dose, lockout interval, and amount the patient has received when the pump is activated.
▶ Record date, time, and type of reaction.
▶ Document subjective symptoms reported by the patient.
▶ Record objective signs observed by the nurse.
▶ Note any pertinent laboratory data.
▶ Record diagnostic study results.
▶ Note nursing interventions.
▶ Record doctor notification and intervention.
▶ Document patient response to treatment.
▶ Record all patient teaching.

## Related procedures
▶ I.V. bolus injection
▶ Oropharyngeal inhalers
▶ Pulse and ear oximetry
▶ Oxygen administration
▶ Endotracheal intubation
▶ Mechanical ventilation
▶ Endotracheal tube care
▶ Subcutaneous injection

### REFERENCES
*Nursing 2003 Drug Handbook.* Springhouse, Pa.: Lippincott Williams & Wilkins, 2002.
Phillips, L. *Manual of I.V. Therapeutics,* 3rd ed. Philadelphia: F.A. Davis Co., 2001.

### ORGANIZATIONS
American Academy of Pain Management: *www.aapainmanagement.org*
American Pain Society: *www.ampainsoc.org*

# Managing the patient undergoing chemotherapy

## Purpose
To keep the patient as comfortable as possible and able to maintain normal lifestyle while preventing complications from chemotherapeutic agents

## Collaborative level
Interdependent

## Expected patient outcomes
▶ The patient will maintain or return to normal weight.
▶ The patient will maintain or restore intact oral mucosa.
▶ The patient will maintain normal respiratory status.
▶ The patient will obtain normal serum laboratory values.
▶ The patient will remain infection-free.

## Definition of terms

▶ *Chemotherapy:* Treatment of disease with chemical agents that have a specific and toxic effect on the disease-causing microorganism.

▶ *Leukopenia:* State of low number of leukocytes in the circulating blood, which increases the patient's risk for infection.

▶ *Neutropenia:* State of low number of neutrophils in the circulating blood, which increases the patient's risk for infection.

▶ *Stomatitis:* Inflammation of the mucous membrane of the mouth.

▶ *Thrombocytopenia:* State of small number of platelets in the circulating blood, resulting in increased risk of bleeding.

## Indications

### Treatment

▶ Cancer patients, either as curative or palliative therapy

### Prevention

▶ Abnormal laboratory values (anemia, leukopenia, neutropenia, thrombocytopenia)

▶ Dehydration weight loss

▶ Infection

▶ Drug toxicity

▶ Site infiltration and extravasation

## Assessment guidance

### Signs and symptoms

▶ Abnormal laboratory values

▶ Elevated temperature

▶ Decreased intake or output

▶ Redness, warmth, or necrosis at or near catheter site

### Neutropenia and leukopenia

▶ Fever

### Thrombocytopenia

▶ Bleeding gums

▶ Petechiae

▶ Nosebleeds

▶ Bruising

▶ Hematuria

### Anemia

▶ Headache

▶ Dizziness

▶ Lightheadedness

▶ Dyspnea

▶ Fatigue

▶ Pallor

▶ Hypothermia

### Dehydration or weight loss

▶ Nausea

▶ Vomiting

▶ Diarrhea

▶ Anorexia

▶ Mouth pain

### Drug toxicity

▶ Cough

▶ Dyspnea

### Site infiltration and extravasation

▶ Pain at or near catheter insertion site

## Diagnostic studies

### Laboratory tests

▶ CBC

▶ Platelet count

▶ Hemoglobin level

▶ Blood urea nitrogen, creatinine, and alkaline phosphatase levels

▶ Arterial blood gas values

### Imaging tests

▶ Chest X-ray

▶ Echocardiogram

▶ Multiple gated acquisition (MUGA) scan

## Diagnostic procedures

▶ Pulse oximetry readings.

▶ Chest X-ray indicating heart failure

▶ Electrocardiogram displaying QRS or ST-segment changes

▶ Echocardiogram or MUGA showing decreased cardiac ejection fraction

## Nursing interventions

▶ Assess I.V. site for signs of infiltration or extravasation.

▶ Monitor laboratory values.

▶ Notify the doctor of changes in patient's physical assessment.

### Neutropenia and leukopenia

▶ Practice good hygiene and hand-washing techniques.

▶ Institute neutropenic precautions, as indicated.

▶ Maintain strict aseptic technique during procedures.

### Thrombocytopenia

▶ Institute bleeding precautions, as indicated.

## Anemia
▶ Administer Epogen and Procrit.
▶ Transfuse patient.

## Dehydration or weight loss
▶ Assess the patient for nausea, vomiting, and diarrhea.
▶ Inspect the patient's mouth.
▶ Monitor intake and output (especially if furosemide is part of drug protocol).
▶ Assess the patient's nutritional status.
▶ Weigh the patient regularly.
▶ Give an antiemetic or antidiarrheal.

## Drug toxicity
▶ Monitor patient for signs and symptoms of cardiac, pulmonary, renal, and neurologic toxicity.

## Site extravasation
▶ Stop chemotherapeutic drug infusion.
▶ Remove the catheter or needle.
▶ Administer an antidote.
▶ Apply warm compresses to the site.

## Patient teaching
▶ When teaching your patient about handling chemotherapeutic drugs, discuss appropriate safety measures. If the patient will be receiving chemotherapy at home, teach him how to dispose of contaminated equipment. Tell the patient and his family to wear gloves whenever they handle chemotherapy equipment or contaminated linens, gowns, or pajamas. Instruct them to place soiled linens in a separate washable pillowcase and to launder the pillowcase twice, with the soiled linens inside, separately from other linens.
▶ All materials used for treatment should be placed in a leakproof container and taken to a designated disposal area. The patient or his family should make arrangements with either a hospital or a private company for pickup and proper disposal of contaminated waste.
▶ Provide dietary precautions, such as foods irritating to oral membranes, if impaired; constipating foods for diarrhea; and bland foods for nausea.
▶ Instruct the patient to report fever, severe vomiting or diarrhea, or abnormal bleeding immediately.
▶ Instruct patient to report signs of drug toxicity immediately (depending on type of cancer and medication received).

## Contraindications
Contraindications vary depending on specific chemotherapeutic given but may include:
  –hypersensitivity to drug
  –preexisting severe bone marrow suppression
  –pregnancy or breast-feeding
  –chemotherapeutic drug toxicity.

## Documentation
▶ Record the date, time, and type of reaction.
▶ Document subjective symptoms, as reported by the patient.
▶ Record objective signs observed by the nurse.
▶ Note administration of medications and therapies.
▶ Record diagnostic study results.
▶ Document all nursing interventions.
▶ Record doctor notification and intervention.
▶ Document the patient's response to treatment.
▶ Document patient teaching.

## Related procedures
▶ Chemotherapeutic drug administration
▶ Chemotherapeutic drug preparation and handling
▶ Neutropenic precautions
▶ Skin medications

### REFERENCES
*Nursing 2003 Drug Handbook*. Springhouse, Pa.: Lippincott Williams & Wilkins, 2002.
Phillips, L. *Manual of I.V. Therapeutics*, 3rd ed. Philadelphia: F.A. Davis Co., 2001.

### ORGANIZATIONS
Oncolink: *www.cancer.med.upenn.edu*

# Managing medication therapy

## Purpose
To maintain or restore state of health to the patient

## Collaborative level
Interdependent

## Expected patient outcomes
▶ The patient will achieve desired therapeutic effect.
▶ The patient will verbalize relive from causative factor.
▶ The patient will demonstrate improved psychological state
▶ The patient will avoid any undesired effect of medication: pruritus, rash, shortness of breath.
▶ The patient will demonstrate vital signs indicating desired effect of medication.
▶ The patient will show laboratory values indicating desired effect of medication.

## Definition of terms
▶ *Endotracheal drugs:* Drugs that are given within the trachea.
▶ *Epidural:* On or outside the dura matter.
▶ *Intradermal injection:* An injection that is given into the corium or substance of the skin.
▶ *Intraosseous infusion:* An injection into the bone marrow because the marrow of long bones has a rich network of vessels which drain into a central venous canal, emissary veins, and ultimately into the central circulation.

## Indications
Treatment
▶ Various conditions dependent upon the desired effect of the medication

Prevention
▶ Wrong medication, dose, or route of administration
▶ Undesired effect
▶ Allergic reaction

## Assessment guidance
Signs and symptoms
▶ Will vary depending on the system affected and the disease process

## Nursing interventions
▶ Obtain drug history (including over-the-counter, herbal supplements, alcohol, and illegal drugs) from the patient, his family, or caregiver.
▶ Review the patient's medical history.
▶ Perform physical examination.
▶ Evaluate socio-economic status to determine the patient's ability to pay for medications.

▶ Assess for lifestyle factors (school, work, travel) that may interfere with taking medications at the recommended schedule.
▶ Assess cultural factors that may impact on the patient's compliance.
▶ Obtain and interpret relevant laboratory or diagnostic test results.
▶ Explore the reason for the medication.
▶ Evaluate the patient's cognitive status.
▶ Evaluate the patient's knowledge about determining the effectiveness of the drug.
▶ Evaluate age- and weight-related appropriateness of the drug.
▶ Notify the doctor of therapeutic, inadequate, or undesired effects of the medication.

## Patient teaching
▶ Teach the patient and his caregiver the proper procedure for administering a medication by the route prescribed.
▶ Discuss the effects of drug therapy and advise the patient to report new symptoms or unpredicted adverse reactions.
▶ Teach the patient about the importance of maintaining a therapeutic level of a medication.
▶ Describe the signs and symptoms of an allergic reaction.
▶ Discuss the dosing schedule of the medication prescribed.

## Precautions
▶ Observe the five rights of medication administration: right patient, right drug, right dose, right route, and right time.

## Contraindications
Contraindicated in patients with allergy or hypersensitivity to the drug.

## Documentation
▶ Document subjective data received from the patient.
▶ Document objective data recorded by the nurse.
▶ Record the date, time, and type of adverse reactions.
▶ Document any pertinent laboratory data.
▶ Record nursing interventions.
▶ Document doctor notification and his intervention.
▶ Document the patient's response to treatment.
▶ Note patient teaching.

## Related procedures
▶ Admixture of drugs in a syringe
▶ Buccal, sublingual, and translingual drugs
▶ Chemotherapeutic drug administration
▶ Chemotherapeutic drug preparation and handling
▶ Drug implants
▶ Eardrops
▶ Endotracheal drugs
▶ Epidural analgesics
▶ Eye medications
▶ Handheld oropharyngeal inhalers
▶ I.M. injection
▶ I.V. bolus injection
▶ Intradermal injection
▶ Intraosseous infusion
▶ Intrapleural drugs
▶ Nasal medications
▶ Ommaya reservoir
▶ Oral drugs
▶ Pediatric medication administration
▶ Rectal suppositories and ointments
▶ Skin medications
▶ Standard precautions
▶ Subcutaneous injection
▶ Transdermal drugs
▶ Vaginal medications
▶ Z-track injection

**REFERENCES**
Phillips, L. *Manual of I.V. Therapeutics,* 3rd ed. Philadelphia: F. A. Davis Co., 2001.
*Nursing 2003 Drug Handbook.* Springhouse, Pa.: Lippincott Williams & Wilkins, 2002.

# Procedures

## Admixture of drugs in a syringe

Combining two drugs in one syringe avoids the discomfort of two injections. Usually, drugs can be mixed in a syringe in one of four ways. They may be combined from two multidose vials (for example, regular and long-acting insulin), from one multidose vial and one ampule, from two ampules, or from a cartridge-injection system combined with either a multidose vial or an ampule.

Such combinations are contraindicated when the drugs aren't compatible and when the combined doses exceed the amount of solution that can be absorbed from a single injection site.

### Equipment
Prescribed medications ● patient's medication record and chart ● alcohol pad ● syringe and needle ● safety needle ● gauze pad ● optional: cartridge-injection system and filter needle

The type and size of the syringe and needle depend on the prescribed medications, patient's body build, and route of administration. Medications that come in prefilled cartridges require a cartridge-injection system. (See *Cartridge-injection system,* page 96.)

### Implementation
▶ Verify that the drugs to be administered agree with the patient's medication record and the doctor's orders.
▶ Calculate the dose to be given.
▶ Wash your hands.

#### Mixing drugs from two multidose vials
▶ Using an alcohol pad, wipe the rubber stopper on the first vial. This decreases the risk of contaminating the medication as you insert the needle into the vial.
▶ Pull back the syringe plunger until the volume of air drawn into the syringe equals the volume to be withdrawn from the drug vial.
▶ Without inverting the vial, insert the needle into the top of the vial, making sure that the needle's bevel tip doesn't touch the solution. Inject the air into the vial and withdraw the needle. This replaces air in

# Cartridge-injection system

A cartridge-injection system, such as Tubex or Carpuject, is a convenient, easy-to-use method of injection that facilitates accuracy and sterility. The device consists of a plastic cartridge-holder syringe and a prefilled medication cartridge with a needle attached.

The medication in the cartridge is premixed and premeasured, which saves time and helps ensure an exact dose. The medication remains sealed in the cartridge and sterile until the injection is administered to the patient.

The disadvantage of this system is that not all drugs are available in cartridge form. However, compatible drugs can be added to partially filled cartridges.

the vial, thus preventing creation of a partial vacuum on withdrawal of the drug.
❱ Repeat the steps above for the second vial. Then, after injecting the air into the second vial, invert the vial, withdraw the prescribed dose, and then withdraw the needle.
❱ Wipe the rubber stopper of the first vial again and insert the needle, taking care not to depress the plunger. Invert the vial, withdraw the prescribed dose, and then withdraw the needle.

### Mixing drugs from a multidose vial and an ampule
❱ Using an alcohol pad, clean the vial's rubber stopper.
❱ Pull back on the syringe plunger until the volume of air drawn into the syringe equals the volume to be withdrawn from the drug vial.
❱ Insert the needle into the top of the vial and inject the air. Then invert the vial and keep the needle's bevel tip below the level of the solution as you withdraw the prescribed dose. Put the sterile cover over the needle.
❱ Wrap a sterile gauze pad or an alcohol pad around the ampule's neck to protect yourself from injury in case the glass splinters. Break open the ampule, directing the force away from you.
❱ If desired, switch to the filter needle at this point to filter out any glass splinters.

❱ Insert the needle into the ampule. Be careful not to touch the outside of the ampule with the needle. Draw the correct dose into the syringe.
❱ If you switched to the filter needle, change back to a safety needle to administer the injection.

### Mixing drugs from two ampules
❱ An opened ampule doesn't contain a vacuum. To mix drugs from two ampules in a syringe, calculate the prescribed doses and open both ampules, using aseptic technique. If desired, use a filter needle to draw up the drugs. Then change to a safety needle to administer them.

## Special considerations
❱ Insert a needle through the vial's rubber stopper at a slight angle, bevel up, and exert slight lateral pressure. By using this method, you won't cut a piece of rubber out of the stopper, which can then be pushed into the vial.
❱ When mixing drugs from multidose vials, be careful not to contaminate one drug with the other. Ideally, the needle should be changed after drawing the first medication into the syringe.

◆ **ALERT!** Never combine drugs if you're unsure of their compatibility and never combine more than two drugs. Although drug incompatibility usually causes a visible reaction, such as clouding, bubbling, or precipitation, some incompatible combinations produce no visible reaction even though they alter the chemical nature and action of the drugs. Check appropriate references and consult a pharmacist when you're unsure of a specific compatibility. When in doubt, administer two separate injections.
❱ Some medications are compatible for only a brief time after being combined and should be administered within 10 minutes after mixing. After this time, environmental factors, such as temperature, exposure to light, and humidity, may alter compatibility.
❱ To reduce the risk of contamination, most facilities dispense parenteral medications in single-dose vials. Insulin is one of the few drugs still packaged in multidose vials. Be careful when mixing regular and long-acting insulin. Draw up the regular insulin first to avoid contamination by the long-acting suspension. (If a minute

amount of the regular insulin is accidentally mixed with the long-acting insulin, it won't appreciably change the effect of the long-acting insulin.) Check your facility's policy before mixing insulins.

▶ When you combine a cartridge-injection system and a multidose vial, use a separate needle and syringe to inject air into the multidose vial. This prevents contamination of the multidose vial by the cartridge-injection system.

## Documentation
▶ Record the drugs administered, injection site, and time of administration.
▶ Document adverse drug effects and other pertinent information.

### REFERENCES
Craven, R., and Hirnle, C.J. *Fundamentals of Nursing: Human Health and Function,* 4th ed. Philadelphia: Lippincott Williams & Wilkins, 2002.

Trigg, M.E., et al. "Effects of an Inadvertent Dose of Cytarabine in a Child With Fanconi's Anemia: Reducing Medication Errors," *Paediatric Drugs* 4(3):205-08, 2002.

## Buccal, sublingual, and translingual drugs

Certain drugs are given buccally, sublingually, or translingually to prevent their destruction or transformation in the stomach or small intestine. These drugs act quickly because the oral mucosa's thin epithelium and abundant vasculature allow direct absorption into the bloodstream.

Drugs given buccally include nitroglycerin and methyltestosterone; drugs given sublingually include ergotamine tartrate, isosorbide dinitrate, and nitroglycerin. Translingual drugs, which are sprayed onto the tongue, include nitrate preparations for patients with chronic angina. (See *Giving buccal and sublingual drugs.*)

### Equipment
Patient's medication record and chart ● prescribed medication ● medication cup

### Implementation
▶ Verify the order on the patient's medication record by checking it against the doctor's order on his chart.

## Giving buccal and sublingual drugs

Buccal and sublingual administration routes allow some drugs, such as nitroglycerin and methyltestosterone, to enter the bloodstream rapidly without being degraded in the GI tract. To give a drug buccally, insert it between the patient's cheek and teeth (as shown below). Ask him to close his mouth and hold the tablet against his cheek until it's absorbed.

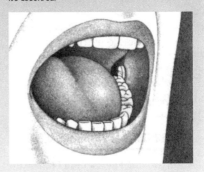

To give a drug sublingually, place it under the patient's tongue (as shown below), and ask him to leave it there until it's dissolved.

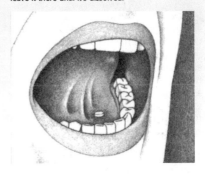

▶ Wash your hands with warm water and soap. Explain the procedure to the patient if he's never taken a drug buccally, sublingually, or translingually before.
▶ Check the label on the medication before giving it to make sure you'll be giving the prescribed medication. Verify the expiration date, of all medications.
▶ Confirm the patient's identity by asking his name and checking the name, room number, and bed number on his wristband.

### Buccal and sublingual administration

▶ For buccal administration, place the tablet in the buccal pouch, between the cheek and gum. For sublingual administration, place the tablet under the patient's tongue.

▶ Instruct the patient to keep the medication in place until it dissolves completely to ensure absorption.

▶ Caution him against chewing the tablet or touching it with his tongue to prevent accidental swallowing.

▶ Tell him not to smoke before the drug has dissolved because nicotine's vasoconstrictive effects slow absorption.

### Translingual administration

▶ To administer a translingual drug, tell the patient to hold the medication canister vertically, with the valve head at the top and the spray orifice as close to his mouth as possible.

▶ Instruct him to spray the dose onto his tongue by pressing the button firmly.

▶ Remind the patient using a translingual aerosol form that he shouldn't inhale the spray but should release it under his tongue. Also tell him to wait about 10 seconds before swallowing.

### Special considerations

▶ Don't give liquids to a patient who is receiving buccal medication because some buccal tablets can take up to 1 hour to be absorbed. Tell the patient not to rinse his mouth until the tablet has been absorbed.

▶ Tell the angina patient to wet the nitroglycerin tablet with saliva and to keep it under his tongue until it has been fully absorbed.

### Complications

Some buccal medications may irritate the mucosa. Alternate sides of the mouth for repeat doses to prevent continuous irritation of the same site. Sublingual medications — such as nitroglycerin — may cause a tingling sensation under the tongue. If the patient finds this annoying, try placing the drug in the buccal pouch instead.

### Documentation

▶ Record the medication administered, dose, date and time, and patient's reaction, if any.

**REFERENCES**
Craven, R., and Hirnle, C.J. *Fundamentals of Nursing: Human Health and Function,* 4th ed. Philadelphia: Lippincott Williams & Wilkins, 2002.
Rees, E. "The Role of Oral Transmucosal Fetanyl Citrate in the Management of Breakthrough Cancer Pain," *International Journal of Palliative Nursing* 8(6):304-08, June 2002.

# Chemotherapeutic drug administration

Administration of chemotherapeutic drugs requires skills in addition to those used when giving other drugs. For example, some drugs require special equipment or must be given through an unusual route. Others become unstable after a while, and still others must be protected from light. Finally, the drug dosage must be exact to avoid possibly fatal complications. For these reasons, only specially trained nurses and doctors should give chemotherapeutic drugs.

Chemotherapeutic drugs may be administered through a number of routes. Although the I.V. route (using peripheral or central veins) is used most commonly, these drugs may also be given orally, subcutaneously, I.M., intra-arterially, into a body cavity, through a central venous catheter, through an Ommaya reservoir into the spinal canal, or through a device implanted in a vein or subcutaneously. They may also be administered into an artery, the peritoneal cavity, or the pleural space. (See *Intraperitoneal chemotherapy: An alternative approach.*)

The administration route depends on the drug's bpharmacodynamics and the tumor's characteristics. For example, if a malignant tumor is confined to one area, the drug may be administered through a localized, or regional, method. Regional administration allows delivery of a high drug dose directly to the tumor. This is particularly advantageous because many solid tumors don't respond to drug levels that are safe for systemic administration.

Chemotherapy may be administered to a patient whose cancer is believed to have been eradicated through surgery or radiation therapy. This treatment, known as adjuvant chemotherapy, helps to ensure that

# Intraperitoneal chemotherapy: An alternative approach

Administering chemotherapeutic drugs into the peritoneal cavity has several benefits for patients with malignant ascites or ovarian cancer that has spread to the peritoneum. This technique passes drugs directly to the tumor area in the peritoneal cavity, exposing malignant cells to high concentrations of chemotherapy—up to 1,000 times the amount that could be safely given systemically. Furthermore, the semipermeable peritoneal membrane permits prolonged exposure of malignant cells to the drug.

Typically, intraperitoneal chemotherapy is performed using a peritoneal dialysis kit, but drugs can also be administered directly into the peritoneal cavity by way of a Tenckhoff catheter. This method can be performed on an outpatient basis, if necessary; it uses equipment that's readily available on most units with oncology patients.

In this technique, the chemotherapy bag is connected directly to the Tenckhoff catheter with a length of I.V. tubing, the solution is infused, and the catheter and I.V. tubing are clamped. Then the patient is asked to change positions every 10 to 15 minutes for 1 hour to move the solution around in the peritoneal cavity.

After the prescribed dwell time, the chemotherapeutic drugs are drained into an I.V. bag. The patient is encouraged to change positions to facilitate drainage. Next, the I.V. tubing and catheter are clamped, the I.V. tubing is removed, and a new intermittent infusion cap is fitted to the catheter. Finally, the catheter is flushed with a syringe of heparin flush solution.

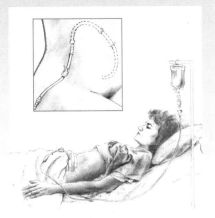

no undetectable metastasis exists. A patient may also receive chemotherapy before surgery or radiation therapy. This is called induction chemotherapy (or neoadjuvant or synchronous chemotherapy). Induction chemotherapy helps improve survival rates by shrinking a tumor before surgical excision or radiation therapy.

In general, chemotherapeutic drugs prove more effective when given in higher doses, but their adverse effects often limit the dosage. An exception to this rule is methotrexate. This drug is particularly effective against rapidly growing tumors, but it's also toxic to normal tissues that are growing and dividing rapidly. However, doctors have discovered that they can give a large dose of methotrexate to destroy cancer cells and then, before the drug has had a chance to permanently damage vital organs, give a dose of folinic acid as an antidote. The antidote stops the effects of methotrexate, thus preserving normal tissue.

## Equipment
Prescribed drug ● gloves ● aluminum foil or a brown paper bag (if the drug is photosensitive) ● normal saline solution ● syringes and needleless adapters ● infusion pump or controller ● impervious containers labeled CAUTION: BIOHAZARD.

### Preparation of equipment
Verify the drug, dosage, and administration route by checking the medication record against the doctor's order. Make sure you know the immediate and delayed adverse effects of the ordered drug. Follow administration guidelines for appropriate procedures in this chapter.

## Implementation
❯ Assess the patient's physical condition and review his medical history.
❯ Make sure you understand the drug that needs to be given and by what route and provide the necessary teaching and support to the patient and his family.

## Classifying chemotherapeutic drugs

### Irritants
▶ carmustine
▶ etoposide
▶ streptozocin

### Vesicants
▶ dacarbazine
▶ dactinomycin
▶ daunorubicin
▶ doxorubicin
▶ mechlorethamine
▶ mitomycin
▶ mitoxantrone
▶ plicamycin
▶ vinblastine
▶ vincristine

### Nonvesicants
▶ asparaginase
▶ bleomycin
▶ carboplatin
▶ cisplatin
▶ cyclophosphamide
▶ cytarabine
▶ floxuridine
▶ fluorouracil
▶ ifosfamide

▶ Determine the best site to administer the drug. When selecting the site, consider drug compatibilities, frequency of administration, and vesicant potential of the drug. (See *Classifying chemotherapeutic drugs.*) For example, if the doctor has ordered the intermittent administration of a vesicant drug, you can give it either by instilling the drug into the side port of an infusing I.V. line or by direct I.V. push. If the vesicant drug is to be infused continuously, you should administer it only through a central venous line or a vascular access device. On the other hand, nonvesicant agents (including irritants) may be given by direct I.V. push, through the side port of an infusing I.V. line, or as a continuous infusion.

Check your facility's policy before administering a vesicant. Because vein integrity decreases with time, some facilities require that vesicants be administered before other drugs. Conversely, because vesicants increase vein fragility, some facilities require that vesicants be given after other drugs.

▶ Evaluate your patient's condition, paying particular attention to the results of recent laboratory studies, specifically the complete blood count, blood urea nitrogen level, platelet count, urine creatinine level, and liver function studies.

▶ Determine whether the patient has received chemotherapy before, and note the severity of any adverse effects.

▶ Check his drug history for medications that might interact with chemotherapy. As a rule, you shouldn't mix chemotherapeutic drugs with other medications. If you have questions or concerns about giving the chemotherapeutic drug, talk with the doctor or pharmacist before you give it.

▶ Next, double-check the patient's chart for the complete chemotherapy protocol order, including the patient's name, drug's name and dosage, and route, rate, and frequency of administration. See if the drug's dosage depends on certain laboratory values. Be aware that some facilities require two nurses to read the dosage order and to check the drug and amount being administered.

▶ Check to see whether the doctor has ordered an antiemetic, fluids, a diuretic, or electrolyte supplements to be given before, during, or after chemotherapy administration.

▶ Evaluate the patient's and his family's understanding of chemotherapy and make sure the patient or a responsible family member has signed the consent form.

▶ Next, put on gloves. Keep them on through all stages of handling the drug, including preparation, priming the I.V. tubing, and administration.

▶ Before administering the drug, perform a new venipuncture proximal to the old site. Avoid giving chemotherapeutic drugs through an existing I.V. line. To identify an administration site, examine the patient's veins, starting with his hand and proceeding to his forearm.

▶ When an appropriate line is in place, infuse 10 to 20 ml of normal saline solution to test vein patency. Never test vein patency with a chemotherapeutic drug. Next, administer the drug as appropriate: nonvesicants by I.V. push or admixed in a bag of I.V. fluid; vesicants by I.V. push through a piggyback set connected to a rapidly infusing I.V. line.

▶ During I.V. administration, closely monitor the patient for signs of a hypersensitivity reaction or extravasation. Check for adequate blood return after 5 ml of the drug has been infused or according to your facility's guidelines.

▶ After infusion of the medication, infuse 20 ml of normal saline solution. Do this between administrations of different chemotherapeutic drugs and before discontinuing the I.V. line.

▶ Dispose of used needles and syringes carefully. To prevent aerosol dispersion of chemotherapeutic drugs, don't clip needles. Place them intact in an impervious container for incineration. Dispose of I.V. bags, bottles, gloves, and tubing in a properly labeled and covered trash container.

▶ Wash your hands thoroughly with soap and warm water after giving any chemotherapeutic drug, even though you have worn gloves.

### Special considerations

▶ Observe the I.V. site frequently for signs of extravasation and an allergic reaction (swelling, redness, urticaria). If you suspect extravasation, stop the infusion immediately. Leave the I.V. catheter in place and notify the doctor. A conservative method for treating extravasation involves aspirating any residual drug from the tubing and I.V. catheter, instilling an I.V. antidote, and then removing the I.V. catheter. Afterward, you may apply heat or cold to the site and elevate the affected limb. (See *Managing extravasation*.)

▶ During infusion, some drugs need protection from direct sunlight to avoid possible drug breakdown. If this is the case, cover the vial with a brown paper bag or aluminum foil.

▶ When giving vesicants, avoid sites where damage to underlying tendons or nerves may occur (veins in the antecubital fossa, near the wrist, or in the dorsal surface of the hand).

▶ If you're unable to stay with the patient during the entire infusion, use an infusion pump or controller to ensure drug delivery within the prescribed time and rate.

▶ Observe the patient at regular intervals and after treatment for adverse reactions. Monitor his vital signs throughout the infusion to assess any changes during chemotherapy administration.

▶ Maintain a list of the types and amounts of drugs the patient has received. This is especially important if he has received drugs that have a cumulative effect and that can be toxic to such organs as the heart and kidneys.

### Complications

Common adverse effects of chemotherapy are nausea and vomiting, ranging from

## Managing extravasation

Extravasation—the infiltration of a vesicant drug into the surrounding tissue—can result from a punctured vein or leakage around a venipuncture site. If vesicant drugs or fluids extravasate, severe local tissue damage may result. This may cause prolonged healing, infection, cosmetic disfigurement, and loss of function and may necessitate multiple debridements and, possibly, amputation.

Extravasation of vesicant drugs requires emergency treatment. Follow your facility's protocol. Essential steps include:

▶ Stop the I.V. flow, aspirate the remaining drug in the catheter, and remove the I.V. line, unless you need the needle to infiltrate the antidote.

▶ Estimate the amount of extravasated solution and notify the doctor.

▶ Instill the appropriate antidote according to your facility's protocol.

▶ Elevate the extremity.

▶ Record the extravasation site, patient's symptoms, estimated amount of infiltrated solution, and treatment. Include the time you notified the doctor and the doctor's name. Continue documenting the appearance of the site and associated symptoms.

▶ Ice is typically applied to all extravasated areas, with the exception of etoposide and vinca alkaloids, for 15 to 20 minutes every 4 to 6 hours for about 3 days. For etoposide and vinca alkaloids, heat is applied.

▶ If skin breakdown occurs, apply dressings as ordered.

▶ If severe tissue damage occurs, plastic surgery and physical therapy may be needed.

mild to debilitating. Another major complication is bone marrow suppression, leading to neutropenia and thrombocytopenia. Other adverse effects include intestinal irritation, stomatitis, pulmonary fibrosis, cardiotoxicity, nephrotoxicity, neurotoxicity, ototoxicity, anemia, alopecia, urticaria, radiation recall (if drugs are given with or soon after radiation therapy), anorexia, esophagitis, diarrhea, and constipation.

I.V. administration of chemotherapeutic drugs may also lead to extravasation, causing inflammation, ulceration, necrosis, and loss of vein patency.

## Documentation
▶ Record the location and description of the I.V. site before treatment or presence of blood return during bolus administration.
▶ Record the drugs and dosages administered, sequence of drug administration, needle type and size used, amount and type of flushing solution, and site condition after treatment.
▶ Document any adverse reactions, the patient's tolerance of the treatment, and topics discussed with the patient and his family.

### REFERENCES
Brown, K., et al., eds. *Chemotherapy and Biotherapy Guidelines and Recommendations for Practice.* Pittsburgh: Oncology Nursing Society, 2001.
Connor, T.H. "Permeability of Nitrile Rubber, Latex, Polyurethane Neoprene Gloves to 18 Antineoplastic Drugs," *American Journal of Health Systems* 56:2450-53, 1999.
Weinstein, S.M. *Plumer's Principles and Practice of Infusion Therapy,* 7th ed. Philadelphia: Lippincott Williams & Wilkins, 2001.

# Chemotherapeutic drug preparation and handling

When preparing chemotherapeutic drugs, take extra care, for the patient's safety and for your own. Patients who receive chemotherapeutic drugs risk teratogenic, mutagenic, and carcinogenic effects, but the people who prepare and handle the drugs are at risk as well. Although the danger from handling these drugs hasn't been fully determined, chemotherapeutic drugs can increase the handler's risk of reproductive abnormalities. These drugs also pose environmental threats, and the best method for handling them hasn't been determined.

The Occupational Safety and Health Administration (OSHA) has set certain guidelines for handling chemotherapeutic drugs. Although these guidelines are simply recommendations, adhering to them will help ensure both your safety and that of your environment.

The OSHA guidelines outline two basic requirements. The first is that all health care workers who handle chemotherapeutic drugs must be educated and trained. A key element of such training involves learning how to reduce your exposure when handling the drugs. The second requirement states that the drugs should be prepared in a class II biological safety cabinet.

■ **EVIDENCE BASE** Although little research has been done on the long-term risks at the levels of exposure encountered by unprotected health care workers, these drugs have been associated with human cancers at high (therapeutic) levels in many animal species. As a result of the research, most health care facilities developed policies, procedures, and such protocols as protective clothing, spill kits, and isolation precautions to reduce health care worker's exposure to these drugs.

## Equipment
Prescribed drug or drugs ● patient's medication record and chart ● long-sleeved gown ● latex surgical gloves ● face shield or goggles ● eyewash ● plastic absorbent pad ● alcohol pads ● sterile gauze pads ● shoe covers ● impervious container with the label CAUTION: BIOHAZARD for the disposal of any unused drug or equipment ● I.V. solution ● diluent (if necessary) ● compatibility reference source ● medication labels ● class II biological safety cabinet ● disposable towel ● hydrophobic filter or dispensing pin ● 18G needle ● syringes and needles of various sizes ● I.V. tubing with luer-lock fittings ● I.V. controller pump (if available)

Have a chemotherapeutic spill kit available. Kit includes water-resistant, nonpermeable, long-sleeved gown with cuffs and back closure, shoe covers, two pairs of gloves (for double gloving), goggles, mask, disposable dustpan, plastic scraper (for collecting broken glass), plastic-backed or absorbable towels, container of desiccant powder or granules (to absorb wet contents), two disposable sponges, puncture-proof, leakproof container labeled BIOHAZARD WASTE, container of 70% alcohol for cleaning the spill area.

## Implementation
▶ Remember to wash your hands before and after drug preparation and administration.
▶ Prepare the drugs in a class II biological safety cabinet.
▶ Wear protective garments (such as a long-sleeved gown, gloves, a face shield or gog-

gles, and shoe covers) as indicated by your facility's policy. Don't wear the garments outside the preparation area.

▶ Don't eat, drink, smoke, or apply cosmetics in the drug preparation area.

▶ Before you prepare the drug (and after you finish), clean the internal surfaces of the cabinet with 70% alcohol and a disposable towel. Discard the towel in a leakproof chemical waste container.

▶ Cover the work surface with a clean plastic absorbent pad to minimize contamination by droplets or spills. Change the pad at the end of the shift or whenever a spill occurs.

▶ Consider all the equipment used in drug preparation as well as any unused drug as hazardous waste. Dispose of them according to your facility's policy.

▶ Place all chemotherapeutic waste products in labeled, leakproof, sealable plastic bags or other appropriate impervious containers.

## Special considerations

▶ Prepare the drugs according to current product instructions, paying attention to compatibility, stability, and reconstitution technique. Label the prepared drug with the patient's name, dosage strength, and date and time of preparation.

▶ Take precautions to reduce your exposure to chemotherapeutic drugs. Systemic absorption can occur through ingestion of contaminated materials, skin contact, and inhalation. You can inhale a drug without realizing it, such as while opening a vial, clipping a needle, expelling air from a syringe, or discarding excess drug. You can also absorb a drug from handling contaminated stools or body fluids.

▶ For maximum protection, mix all chemotherapeutic drugs in an approved class II biological safety cabinet. Also, prime all I.V. bags that contain chemotherapeutic drugs under the hood. Leave the hood blower on 24 hours a day, 7 days a week.

▶ If a hood isn't available, prepare drugs in a well-ventilated work space, away from heating or cooling vents and other personnel. Vent vials with a hydrophobic filter, or use negative-pressure techniques. Also, use a needle with a hydrophobic filter to remove solution from a vial. To break an ampule, wrap a sterile gauze pad or alcohol pad around the neck of the ampule to cut the contamination risk.

▶ Make sure the biological safety cabinet is examined every 6 months or any time the cabinet is moved by a company specifically qualified to perform this work. If the cabinet passes certification, the certifying company will affix a sticker to the cabinet attesting to its approval.

▶ Use only syringes and I.V. sets that have luer-lock fittings. Label all chemotherapeutic drugs with a CHEMOTHERAPY HAZARD label.

▶ Don't clip needles, break syringes, or remove the needles from syringes. Use a gauze pad when removing syringes and needles from I.V. bags of chemotherapeutic drugs.

▶ Place used syringes and needles in a puncture-proof container, along with other sharp or breakable items.

▶ When mixing chemotherapeutic drugs, wear latex surgical gloves and a gown of low-permeability fabric with a closed front and cuffed long sleeves. When working steadily with chemotherapeutic drugs, change gloves every 30 minutes. If you spill a drug solution or puncture or tear a glove, remove the gloves at once. Wash your hands before putting on new gloves and anytime you remove your gloves.

▶ If some of the drug comes in contact with your skin, wash the involved area thoroughly with soap (not a germicidal agent) and water. If eye contact occurs, flood the eye with water or an isotonic eyewash for at least 5 minutes while holding the eyelid open. Obtain a medical evaluation as soon as possible after accidental exposure.

▶ If a major spill occurs, use a chemotherapeutic spill kit to clean the area.

▶ Discard disposable gowns and gloves in an appropriately marked, waterproof receptacle when contaminated or when you leave the work area.

▶ Don't place any food or drinks in the same refrigerator as chemotherapeutic drugs.

▶ Become familiar with drug excretion patterns and take appropriate precautions when handling a chemotherapy patient's body fluids.

▶ Give male patients a urinal with a tight-fitting lid. Wear disposable latex surgical gloves when handling body fluids. Before flushing the toilet, place a waterproof pad over the toilet bowl to avoid splashing. Wear gloves and a gown when handling linens soiled with body fluids. Place soiled linens in isolation linen bags designated for separate laundering.

▶ Women who are pregnant, trying to conceive, or breast-feeding should exercise caution when handling chemotherapeutic drugs.

### Home care

When teaching your patient about handling chemotherapeutic drugs, discuss appropriate safety measures. If the patient will be receiving chemotherapy at home, teach him how to dispose of contaminated equipment. Tell the patient and his family to wear gloves whenever handling chemotherapy equipment and contaminated linens or gowns. Instruct them to place soiled linens in a separate washable pillowcase and to launder the pillowcase twice, with the soiled linens inside, separately from other linens. When providing home care, empty waste products into the toilet close to the water to minimize splashing. Close the lid and flush two or three times.

All materials used for the treatment should be placed in a leakproof container and taken to a designated disposal area. The patient or his family should make arrangements with either a facility or a private company for pickup and proper disposal of contaminated waste.

### Complications

Chemotherapeutic drugs may be mutagenic. Chronic exposure to chemotherapeutic drugs may damage the liver or chromosomes. Direct exposure to these drugs may burn and damage the skin.

### Documentation

▶ Document each incident of exposure according to your facility's policy.

### REFERENCES

Brown, K., et al., eds. *Chemotherapy and Biotherapy Guidelines and Recommendations for Practice.* Pittsburgh: Oncology Nursing Society, 2001.

U.S. Department of Labor. Occupational Safety & Health Administration (OSHA). "Controlling Occupational Exposure to Harmful Drugs." In: TED 1-0.15A, OSHA Technical Manual. Washington, D.C.: OSHA, January 20, 1999; Section VI, chapter 2. *www.osha.gov/dts/osta_vi/otm_vi_2.htm.*

Valanis, B.G., et al. "Occupational Exposure to Antineoplastic Agents and Self-reported Infertility among Nurses and Pharmacists," *Journal of Occupational and Environmental Medicine* 39(6):574-80, June 1997.

# Drug implants

A newer method of advanced drug delivery involves implanting drugs beneath the skin — subdermally or subcutaneously — as well as targeting specific tissues with radiation implants.

With subdermal implants, flexible capsules are placed under the skin. The drug most commonly administered by this method is levonorgestrel, a synthetic hormone used for long-term contraception. Small Silastic capsules filled with the hormone are placed under the skin of the patient's upper arm, and the drug then diffuses through the capsule walls continuously.

With subcutaneous implants, drug pellets are injected into the skin's subcutaneous layer. The drug is then stored in one area of the body, called a depot. A newer treatment for prostate cancer cells calls for implants of goserelin acetate, a synthetic form of luteinizing hormone. By inhibiting pituitary gland secretion, goserelin implants reduce testosterone levels to those previously achieved only through castration. This reduction causes tumor regression and suppression of symptoms.

Radiation drug implants with a short half-life may be placed inside a body cavity, within a tumor or on its surface, or in the area from which a tumor has been removed. Implants that contain iodine-125 are used for lung and prostate tumors; gold-198, for oral and ocular tumors; and radium-226 and cesium-137, for tongue, lip, and skin therapy. These implants are usually inserted by a doctor with a nurse assisting. Some specially trained nurses may insert or inject intradermal implants. Radiation implants are usually put in place in an operating room or a radiation oncology suite.

### Equipment

*For subdermal implants*

Sterile surgical drapes ● sterile gloves ● antiseptic solution ● local anesthetic ● set of implants • needles • 5-ml syringe • #11 scalpel • #10 trocar • forceps • sutures • sterile gauze • tape

*For subcutaneous implants*
Alcohol pad • drug implant in a preloaded syringe • local anesthetic (for some patients)

*For radiation implants*
RADIATION PRECAUTION sign for the patient's door • warning labels for the patient's wristband and personal belongings • film badge or pocket dosimeter • lead-lined container • long-handled forceps • masking tape • portable lead shield • optional: tracheostomy tray

## Implementation
▶ Explain the procedure and its benefits and risks to the patient and show her a set of implants.

### Inserting subdermal implants
▶ Assist the patient into a supine position on the examination table. During the procedure, stay and provide support as necessary.
▶ After anesthetizing the upper portion of the nondominant arm, the doctor will put on sterile gloves and use a trocar to insert each capsule through a ⅛″ (2-mm) incision. After insertion, he'll remove the trocar and palpate the area. He'll then close the incision and cover it with a dry compress and sterile gauze.

The steps below describe how levonorgestrel subdermal contraceptive implants are inserted:
▶ Have the patient lie supine on the examination table and flex the elbow of her nondominant arm so that her hand is opposite her head.
▶ Swab the insertion site with antiseptic solution. The ideal insertion site is inside the upper arm about 3″ to 4″ (7.5 to 10 cm) above the elbow.
▶ Cover the arm above and below the insertion site with sterile surgical drapes.
▶ The doctor puts on sterile gloves, fills a 5-ml syringe with a local anesthetic, inserts the needle under the skin, and injects a small amount of anesthetic into several areas, in a fanlike pattern.
▶ The doctor uses the scalpel to make a small incision about ⅛″ (2 mm) through the skin.

▶ Next, he inserts the tip of the trocar through the incision at a shallow angle beneath the skin. He makes sure the trocar bevel is up so that he can place the capsules in a superficial plane. He advances the trocar slowly to the first mark near the hub of the trocar. The tip of the trocar should now be about 1½″ to 2″ (4 to 4.5 cm) from the incision site. The doctor then removes the obturator and loads the first capsule into the trocar.
▶ He gently advances the capsule with the obturator toward the tip of the trocar until he feels resistance. Next, he inserts each succeeding capsule beside the last one in a fanlike pattern. With the forefinger and middle finger of his free hand, he fixes the position of the previous capsule, advancing the trocar along the tips of his fingers. This ensures a suitable distance of about 15 degrees between capsules and keeps the trocar from puncturing the previously inserted capsules.

### Inserting subcutaneous implants
▶ Help the patient into the supine position and drape him so that his abdomen is accessible. Remove the syringe from the package and make sure you can see the drug in the chamber. Put on gloves. Then, clean a small area on the patient's upper abdominal wall with the alcohol pad.
▶ As you stretch the skin at the injection site with one hand, grip the needle with the fingers of your other hand around the barrel of the syringe. Insert the needle into subcutaneous fat at a 45-degree angle. Don't attempt to aspirate. If blood appears in the syringe, withdraw the needle and inject a new preloaded syringe and needle at another site.
▶ Next, change the direction of the needle so that it's parallel to the abdominal wall. With the barrel hub touching the patient's skin, push the needle in. Then withdraw it about ½″ (1.3 cm) to create a space for the drug. Depress the plunger. Withdraw the needle and bandage the site with sterile gauze and tape.
▶ Inspect the tip of the needle. If you can see the metal tip of the plunger, the drug has been discharged.
▶ Remove and discard your gloves.

### Inserting radiation implants
▶ To prepare for a radiation implant, place the lead-lined container and long-handled

forceps in a corner of the patient's room.
Also, place the lead shield in the back of
the room so it can be worn when providing
care. With masking tape, mark a safe line
on the floor 6′ (1.8 m) from the bed to warn
visitors of the danger of radiation exposure.
Place a RADIATION PRECAUTION sign on the
patient's door and warning labels on the
patient's wristband and personal belongings.

▶ Place an emergency tracheotomy tray in
the room if an implant will be inserted in
the patient's mouth or neck.

▶ To insert the implant, the doctor puts on
gloves, makes a small incision in the skin,
and creates a pocket in the tissue. He inserts the implant and closes the incision.
The doctor takes off the gloves and dis-
cards them. If the patient is being treated
for tonsillar cancer, he'll undergo a bronchoscopy, during which radioactive pellets
are implanted in tonsillar tissue.

▶ Your role in the implant procedure is to
explain the treatment and its goals to the
patient. Review radiation safety procedures
and visitation policies. Talk with the patient about long-term physical and emotional aspects of the therapy and discuss
home care.

## Special considerations

Special care may be necessary, depending
on the type of implant used.

### Subdermal implants

▶ Tell the patient to resume normal activities but to protect the site during the first
few days after implantation. Advise her not
to bump the insertion site and to keep the
area dry and covered with a gauze bandage
for 3 days.

▶ Tell the patient to report signs of bleeding or infection at the insertion site.

▶ Tell the patient to notify the doctor immediately if one of the implanted capsules
falls out before the skin heals over the implants. If it's a contraceptive implant, it
may no longer be effective. Advise the patient to use alternative means of contraception until she sees the doctor. If pregnancy
is suspected, the implants must be removed immediately.

### Subcutaneous implants

▶ Be aware that if an implant must be removed, a doctor will order an X-ray to locate it.

▶ Tell the patient to check the administration site for signs of infection or bleeding.

▶ Goserelin implants must be changed
every 28 days. Female patients should be
advised to use a nonhormonal form of contraception.

### Radiation implants

▶ If laboratory work is required during
treatment, a technician wearing a film
badge will obtain the specimen, affix a
RADIATION PRECAUTION label to the specimen container, and alert laboratory personnel. If urine tests are needed, ask the radiation oncology department or laboratory
technician how to transport the specimens
safely.

▶ Minimize your own exposure to radiation. Wear a personal, nontransferable film
badge or dosimeter at waist level during
your entire shift. Turn in the film badge
regularly. Pocket dosimeters measure immediate exposure.

▶ Use the principles of time, distance, and
shielding. *Time:* Plan to give care in the
shortest time possible. Less time equals
less exposure. *Distance:* Work as far away
from the radiation source as possible. Give
care from the side opposite the implant or
from a position that allows the greatest
working distance possible. Prepare the patient's meal trays outside his room. *Shielding:* Wear a portable shield, if necessary.

▶ Make sure that the patient's room is monitored daily by the radiation oncology department and that disposable items are
monitored and removed according to your
facility's policy.

▶ Keep away staff members and visitors
who are pregnant or trying to conceive or
father a child. The gonads and a developing embryo or fetus are highly susceptible
to the damaging effects of ionizing radiation.

▶ If you must take the patient out of his
room, notify the appropriate department of
the patient's status to allow time for the
necessary preparations.

▶ Collect a dislodged implant with long-
handled forceps and place it in a lead-lined
container.

▶ A patient with a permanent implant may
not be released until his radioactivity level
is less than 5 millirems/hour at a distance
of about 3′ (0.9 m).

▶ If a patient with an implant dies while
on the unit, notify the radiation oncology

staff so that a temporary implant can be properly removed and stored. If the implant was permanent, the staff will also determine which precautions should be followed after postmortem care measures.

## Complications
Complications vary, depending on the type of implant used.

### Subdermal implants
Possible adverse reactions to levonorgestrel include hyperpigmentation at the insertion site, menstrual irregularities, headache, nervousness, nausea, dizziness, adnexal enlargement, dermatitis, acne, appetite and weight changes, mastalgia, hirsutism, and alopecia. More serious reactions include breast abnormalities, mammographic changes, diabetes, elevated cholesterol or triglyceride levels, hypertension, seizures, depression, and gallbladder, heart, or kidney disease.

### Subcutaneous implants
Goserelin implants may cause anemia, lethargy, pain, dizziness, insomnia, anxiety, depression, headache, chills, fever, edema, heart failure, arrhythmias, cerebrovascular accident, hypertension, peripheral vascular disease, nausea, vomiting, diarrhea, impotence, renal insufficiency, urinary obstruction, rash, sweating, hot flashes, gout, hyperglycemia, weight increase, and breast swelling and tenderness.

### Radiation implants
Depending on the implant site and dosage, complications include implant dislodgment, tissue fibrosis, xerostomia, radiation pneumonitis, airway obstruction, muscle atrophy, sterility, vaginal dryness or stenosis, fistulas, altered bowel habits, diarrhea, hypothyroidism, infection, cystitis, myelosuppression, neurotoxicity, and secondary cancers.

## Documentation
❱ For subdermal and subcutaneous implants, document name of drug, insertion or administration site, date and time of insertion, and patient's response to the procedure. Note the date that implants should be removed and a new set inserted or the date of the next administration as appropriate.
❱ For radiation implants, document radiation precautions taken during treatment,

adverse reactions, patient and family teaching and their responses, patient's tolerance of isolation procedures and the family's compliance with procedures, and referrals to local cancer services.

## REFERENCES
Brown, D., et al. "Use of Radiation in Gynecologic and Breast Malignancies," in *Women and Cancer: A Gynecologic Oncology Nursing Perspective,* 2nd ed. Edited by G.J. Moore-Higgs, et al. Sudbury, Jones and Bartlett. 2000.
Gosselin, T.K., and Waring, J.S., "Nursing Management of Patients Receiving Brachytherapy for Gynecologic Malignancies," *Clinical Journal of Oncology Nursing,* 5(2):59-63, March-April 2001.
Velji, K. "The Experience of Women Receiving Brachytherapy for Gynecologic Cancer." *Oncology Nursing Forum* 28(4): 743-51, May 2001.

# Eardrops

Eardrops may be instilled to treat infection and inflammation, soften cerumen for later removal, produce local anesthesia, or facilitate removal of an insect trapped in the ear by immobilizing and smothering it.

Instillation of eardrops is usually contraindicated if the patient has a perforated eardrum, but it may be permitted with certain medications and adherence to sterile technique. Other conditions may also prohibit instillation of certain medications into the ear. For instance, instillation of drops containing hydrocortisone is contraindicated if the patient has herpes, another viral infection, or a fungal infection.

## Equipment
Prescribed eardrops ● patient's medication record and chart ● light source ● facial tissue or cotton-tipped applicator ● optional: cotton ball and bowl of warm water

### Preparation of equipment
Verify the order on the patient's medication record by checking it against the doctor's order.

To avoid adverse effects (such as vertigo, nausea, and pain) resulting from instillation of eardrops that are too cold, warm the medication to body temperature in the bowl of warm water or carry it in your

## Positioning the patient for eardrop instillation

Before instilling eardrops, have the patient lie on his side. Then straighten the patient's ear canal to help the medication reach the eardrum. For an adult, gently pull the auricle up and back; for an infant or a young child, gently pull down and back.

**ADULT**

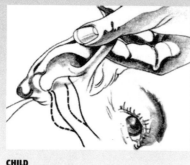

**CHILD**

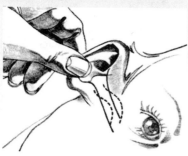

pocket for 30 minutes before administration. If necessary, test the temperature of the medication by placing a drop on your wrist. (If the medication is too hot, it may burn the patient's eardrum.)

### Implementation
❯ Wash your hands.
❯ Confirm the patient's identity by asking his name and checking the name, room number, and bed number on his wristband.
❯ Provide privacy, if possible. Explain the procedure to the patient.
❯ Have the patient lie on the side opposite the affected ear.
❯ Straighten the patient's ear canal. For an adult, pull the auricle of the ear up and

back. (See *Positioning the patient for eardrop instillation.*)
❯ For an infant or a child younger than age 3, gently pull the auricle down and back because the ear canal is straighter at this age.
❯ Using a light source, examine the ear canal for drainage. If you find any, clean the canal with the tissue or cotton-tipped applicator because drainage can reduce the medication's effectiveness.
❯ Compare the label on the eardrops with the order on the patient's medication record. Check the label again while drawing the medication into the dropper. Check the label for the final time before returning the eardrops to the shelf or drawer.
❯ To avoid damaging the ear canal with the dropper, gently support the hand holding the dropper against the patient's head. Straighten the patient's ear canal once again and instill the ordered number of drops. To avoid patient discomfort, aim the dropper so that the drops fall against the sides of the ear canal, not on the eardrum. Hold the ear canal in position until you see the medication disappear down the canal. Then release the ear.
❯ Instruct the patient to remain on his side for 5 to 10 minutes to let the medication run down into the ear canal.
❯ If ordered, tuck the cotton ball loosely into the opening of the ear canal to prevent the medication from leaking out. Be careful not to insert it too deeply into the canal because this would prevent drainage of secretions and increase pressure on the eardrum.
❯ Clean and dry the outer ear.
❯ If ordered, repeat the procedure in the other ear after 5 to 10 minutes.
❯ Assist the patient into a comfortable position.
❯ Wash your hands.

### Special considerations
❯ Remember that some conditions make the normally tender ear canal even more sensitive, so be especially gentle when performing this procedure. Wash your hands before and after caring for the patient's ear and between caring for each ear.
❯ To prevent injury to the eardrum, never insert a cotton-tipped applicator into the ear canal past the point where you can see the tip. After instilling eardrops to soften

the cerumen, irrigate the ear to facilitate its removal.

▶ If the patient has vertigo, keep the side rails of his bed up and help him during the procedure as needed. Also, move slowly and unhurriedly to avoid exacerbating his vertigo.

▶ Teach the patient to instill the eardrops correctly so that he can continue treatment at home, if necessary. Review the procedure and let the patient try it while you observe.

## Documentation

▶ Record the medication used, the ear treated, and the date, time, and number of eardrops instilled.

▶ Note any signs or symptoms the patient had during the procedure, such as drainage, redness, vertigo, nausea, and pain.

### REFERENCES

Craven, R., and Hirnle, C.J. *Fundamentals of Nursing: Human Health and Function,* 4th ed. Philadelphia: Lippincott Williams & Wilkins, 2002.

Kaplan, D.M., et al. "Intentional Ablation of Vestibular Function Using Commercially Available Topical Gentamicin-Betamethasone Eardrops in Patients with Meniere's Disease: Further Evidence for Topical Eardrop Ototoxicity," *Laryngoscope* 112(4):689-95, April 2002.

## Endotracheal drugs

When an I.V. line isn't readily available, drugs can be administered into the respiratory system through an endotracheal (ET) tube. This route allows uninterrupted resuscitation efforts and avoids such complications as coronary artery laceration, cardiac tamponade, and pneumothorax, which can occur when emergency drugs are given intracardially.

Drugs given endotracheally usually have a longer duration of action than drugs given I.V. because they're absorbed in the alveoli. For this reason, repeat doses and continuous infusions must be adjusted to prevent adverse effects. Drugs commonly given by this route include atropine, epinephrine, and lidocaine.

Endotracheal drugs are usually administered in an emergency situation by a doctor, an emergency medical technician, or a

### Administering endotracheal drugs

In an emergency, some drugs may be given through an endotracheal (ET) tube if I.V. access isn't available. They may be given using the syringe method or the adapter method.

Before injecting any drug, check for proper placement of the ET tube, using your stethoscope. Make sure that the patient is supine and that her head is level with or slightly higher than her trunk.

#### Syringe method

Remove the needle before injecting medication into the ET tube. Insert the tip of the syringe into the ET tube, and inject the drug deep into the tube.

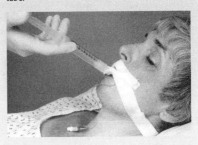

#### Adapter method

A device developed for ET drug administration provides a more closed system of drug delivery than the syringe method. A special adapter placed on the end of the ET tube allows needle insertion and drug delivery through the closed stopcock.

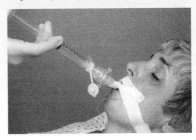

critical care nurse. Although guidelines may vary, depending on state, county, or city regulations, the basic administration method is the same. (See *Administering endotracheal drugs.*)

Endotracheal drugs may be given using the syringe method or the adapter method.

Usually used for bronchoscopy suctioning, the swivel adapter can be placed on the end of the tube and, while ventilation continues through a bag-valve device, the drug can be delivered with a needle through the closed stopcock.

## Equipment

ET tube or swivel adapter • gloves • stethoscope • handheld resuscitation bag • prescribed drug • syringe • sterile water or normal saline solution

### Preparation of equipment

Verify the order on the patient's medication record by checking it against the doctor's order. Wash your hands. Check ET tube placement by using a handheld resuscitation bag and stethoscope.

Calculate the drug dose. Adult advanced cardiac life support guidelines recommend that drugs be administered at 2 to 2½ times the recommended I.V. dose. Next, draw the drug up into a syringe. Dilute it in 10 ml of sterile water or normal saline solution. Dilution increases drug volume and contact with lung tissue.

## Implementation

▶ Put on gloves.
▶ Move the patient into the supine position and make sure his head is level with or slightly higher than his trunk.
▶ Ventilate the patient three to five times with the resuscitation bag. Then remove the bag.
▶ Remove the needle from the syringe and insert the tip of the syringe into the ET tube or the swivel adapter. Inject the drug deep into the tube.
▶ After injecting the drug, reattach the resuscitation bag and ventilate the patient briskly. This propels the drug into the lungs, oxygenates the patient, and clears the tube.
▶ Discard the syringe in an appropriate sharps container.
▶ Remove and discard your gloves.

## Special considerations

Be aware that the drug's onset of action may be quicker than it would be by I.V. administration. If the patient doesn't respond quickly, the doctor may order a repeat dose.

## Complications

Potential complications of endotracheal drug administration result from the prescribed drug, not the administration route.

## Documentation

▶ Record the date and time of drug administration, drug administered, and the patient's response.

## REFERENCES

Guidelines 2000 for Cardiopulmonary Resuscitation and Emergency Cardiovascular Care. American Heart Association, Inc., 2000.
Katz, S.H., and Falk, J.L. "Misplaced Endotracheal Tubes by Paramedics in an Urban Emergency Medical Services System," *Annals of Emergency Medicine* 37(1):32-37, January 2001.

# Epidural analgesics

In epidural analgesic administration, the doctor injects or infuses medication into the epidural space, which lies just outside the subarachnoid space where CSF flows. The drug diffuses slowly into the subarachnoid space of the spinal canal and then into the CSF, which carries it directly into the spinal area, bypassing the blood-brain barrier. In some cases, the doctor injects medication directly into the subarachnoid space. (See *Understanding intrathecal injections.*)

Epidural analgesia helps manage acute and chronic pain, including moderate to severe postoperative pain. It's especially useful in patients with cancer or degenerative joint disease. This procedure works well because opioid receptors are located along the entire spinal cord. Narcotic drugs act directly on the receptors of the dorsal horn to produce localized analgesia without motor blockade. Narcotics, such as preservative-free morphine, fentanyl, and hydromorphone are administered as a bolus dose or by continuous infusion, either alone or in combination with bupivacaine (a local anesthetic). Infusion through an epidural catheter is preferable because it allows a smaller drug dose to be given continuously.

The epidural catheter, which is inserted near the spinal cord, eliminates the risks of multiple I.M. injections, minimizes adverse cerebral and systemic effects, and eliminates the analgesic peaks and valleys that usually occur with intermittent I.M. injections. (See *Placement of a permanent epidural catheter,* page 112.)

Typically, epidural catheter insertion is performed by an anesthesiologist using aseptic technique. When the catheter has been inserted, the nurse is responsible for monitoring the infusion and assessing the patient.

Epidural analgesia is contraindicated in patients who have local or systemic infection, neurologic disease, coagulopathy, spinal arthritis or a spinal deformity, hypotension, marked hypertension, or an allergy to the prescribed medication and in those who are undergoing anticoagulant therapy.

### Equipment
Volume infusion device and epidural infusion tubing (depending on your facility's policy) • patient's medication record and chart • prescribed epidural solutions • transparent dressing • epidural tray • labels for epidural infusion line • silk tape • optional: monitoring equipment for blood pressure, pulse and apnea monitor, pulse oximeter

#### For emergency use
Oxygen • 0.4 mg of I.V. naloxone • 50 mg of I.V. ephedrine • intubation set • hand-held resuscitation bag

#### Preparation of equipment
Prepare the infusion device according to the manufacturer's instructions and your facility's policy. Obtain an epidural tray. Make sure that the pharmacy has been notified ahead of time regarding the medication order because epidural solutions require special preparation. Check the medication concentration and infusion rate against the doctor's order.

### Implementation
▶ Explain the procedure and its possible complications to the patient. Tell him that he'll feel some pain as the catheter is inserted. Answer any questions he has. Make sure that a consent form has been properly signed and witnessed.
▶ Position the patient on his side in the knee-chest position, or have him sit on the

---

## Understanding intrathecal injections

An intrathecal injection allows the doctor to inject medication into the subarachnoid space of the spinal canal. Certain drugs — such as anti-infectives or antineoplastics used to treat meningeal leukemia — are administered by this route because they can't readily penetrate the blood-brain barrier through the bloodstream. Intrathecal injection may also be used to deliver anesthetics, such as lidocaine hydrochloride, to achieve regional anesthesia (as in spinal anesthesia).

An invasive procedure performed by a doctor under sterile conditions with the nurse assisting, intrathecal injection requires the patient's informed consent. The injection site is usually between the third and fourth (or fourth and fifth) lumbar vertebrae, well below the spinal cord to avoid the risk of paralysis. This procedure may be preceded by aspiration of spinal fluid for laboratory analysis.

Contraindications to intrathecal injection include inflammation or infection at the puncture site, septicemia, and spinal deformities (especially when considered as an anesthesia route).

---

edge of the bed and lean over a bedside table.
▶ After the catheter is in place, prime the infusion device, confirm the appropriate medication and infusion rate, and then adjust the device for the correct rate.
▶ Help the anesthesiologist connect the infusion tubing to the epidural catheter. Then connect the tubing to the infusion pump.
▶ Bridge-tape all connection sites and apply an epidural infusion label to the catheter, infusion tubing, and infusion pump to prevent accidental infusion of other drugs. Then start the infusion.
▶ Tell the patient to immediately report any pain. Instruct him to use a pain scale from 0 to 10, with 0 denoting no pain and 10 denoting the worst pain imaginable. A response of 3 or less typically indicates tolerable pain. If the patient reports a higher pain score, the infusion rate may need to be increased. Call the doctor or change the rate within prescribed limits.
▶ If ordered, place the patient on an apnea monitor for the first 24 hours after beginning the infusion.

# Placement of a permanent epidural catheter

An epidural catheter is implanted beneath the patient's skin and inserted near the spinal cord at the first lumbar (L1) interspace. For temporary analgesic therapy (less than 1 week), the catheter may exit directly over the spine and be taped up the patient's back to the shoulder. For prolonged therapy, the catheter may be tunneled subcutaneously to an exit site on the patient's side or abdomen or over his shoulder.

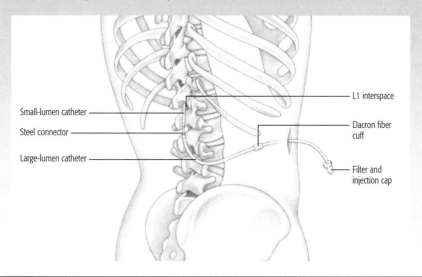

Small-lumen catheter

Steel connector

Large-lumen catheter

L1 interspace

Dacron fiber cuff

Filter and injection cap

▶ Change the dressing over the catheter's exit site every 24 to 48 hours or as needed. The dressing is usually transparent to allow inspection of drainage and commonly appears moist or slightly blood-tinged. Avoid manipulating the catheter because it usually isn't sutured in place.
▶ Change the infusion tubing every 48 hours and the solution every 24 hours, or as specified by your facility's policy.

### Removing an epidural catheter
▶ Typically, the anesthesiologist orders analgesics and removes the catheter. However, your facility's policy may allow a specially trained nurse to remove the catheter.
▶ If you feel resistance when removing the catheter, stop and call the doctor for further orders.
▶ Save the catheter. The doctor will want to examine the catheter tip to rule out any damage during removal.

## Special considerations
▶ Assess the patient's respiratory rate, oxygen saturation, and blood pressure every 2 hours for 8 hours and then every 4 hours for 8 hours during the first 24 hours after starting the infusion. Then assess the patient once per shift, depending on his condition or unless ordered otherwise. Notify the doctor if the patient's respiratory rate is less than 10 breaths/minute or if his systolic blood pressure is less than 90 mm Hg.
▶ Assess the patient's sedation level, mental status, and pain-relief status every hour initially and then every 2 to 4 hours until adequate pain control is achieved. Notify the doctor if the patient appears drowsy; experiences nausea and vomiting, refractory itching, or inability to void, which are adverse effects of certain narcotic analgesics; or complains of unrelieved pain. A change in sedation level is an early indicator of respiratory depression, which can result from narcotics use.
▶ Assess the patient's lower-extremity motor strength every 2 to 4 hours. If sensorimotor loss occurs, large motor nerve fibers have been affected and the dose may need to be decreased.
▶ Keep in mind that drugs given epidurally diffuse slowly and may cause adverse effects, including excessive sedation, up to

12 hours after the infusion has been discontinued.

▶ The patient should always have a peripheral I.V. line (either continuous infusion or saline lock) open to allow immediate administration of emergency drugs.

▶ Postdural puncture headache may result from accidental puncture of the dura during an attempted epidural insertion. This postanalgesia headache worsens with postural changes, such as standing and sitting. The headache can be treated with a "blood patch," in which the patient's own blood (about 10 ml) is withdrawn from a peripheral vein and then injected into the epidural space. When the epidural needle is withdrawn, the patient is instructed to sit up. Because the blood clots seal off the leaking area, the blood patch should relieve the patient's headache immediately. The patient need not restrict his activity after this procedure.

### Home care

Home use of epidural analgesia is possible only if the patient or a family member is willing and able to learn the care needed. The patient also must be willing and able to abstain from alcohol and street drugs because these substances potentiate opioid action.

### Complications

Complications may include infection, abscess, epidural hematoma, and catheter migration. Numbness and leg weakness may occur after the first 24 hours and are drug- and concentration-dependent. The doctor must titrate the dosage to identify the dose that provides adequate pain control without causing excessive numbness and weakness.

Other possible complications include respiratory depression, which usually occurs during the first 24 hours (treated with 0.2 to 0.4 mg of I.V. naloxone); pruritus (treated with 5 mg of I.V. nalbuphine or 25 mg of I.V. diphenhydramine); and nausea and vomiting (treated with 5 to 10 mg of I.V. prochlorperazine or 10 mg of I.V. metoclopramide).

### Documentation

▶ Record the patient's response to treatment, catheter patency, condition of dressing and insertion site, vital signs, and assessment results.

▶ Note the labeling of the epidural catheter, changing of the infusion bags, any ordered analgesics, and patient's response.

### REFERENCES

Metheny, N.M. *Fluid and Electrolyte Balance: Nursing Considerations,* 4th ed. Philadelphia: Lippincott Williams & Wilkins, 2000.

Weinstein, S.M. *Plumer's Principles and Practice of Infusion Therapy,* 7th ed. Philadelphia: Lippincott Williams & Wilkins, 2001.

# Eye medications

Eye medications — drops, ointments, and disks — serve diagnostic and therapeutic purposes. During an eye examination, eyedrops can be used to anesthetize the eye, dilate the pupil to facilitate examination, and stain the cornea to identify corneal abrasions, scars, and other anomalies. Eye medications can also be used to lubricate the eye, treat certain eye conditions (such as glaucoma and infections), protect the vision of neonates, and lubricate the eye socket for insertion of a prosthetic eye.

Understanding the ocular effects of drugs is important because certain drugs may cause eye disorders or have serious ocular effects. For example, anticholinergics are often used in eye examinations but can precipitate acute glaucoma in patients with a predisposition to the disorder.

### Equipment

Prescribed eye medication ● patient's medication record and chart ● gloves ● warm water or normal saline solution ● sterile gauze pads ● facial tissues ● optional: ocular dressing

#### Preparation of equipment

Make sure the medication is labeled for ophthalmic use. Then check the expiration date. Remember to date the container the first time you use the medication. After it's opened, an eye medication may be used for a maximum of 2 weeks to avoid contamination.

Inspect ocular solutions for cloudiness, discoloration, and precipitation but remember that some eye medications are suspensions and normally appear cloudy. Don't use any solution that appears abnormal. If the tip of an eye ointment tube has crusted, turn the tip on a sterile gauze pad to remove the crust.

# Instilling eye medications

To instill eyedrops, pull the lower lid down to expose the conjunctival sac. Have the patient look up and away and then squeeze the prescribed number of drops into the sac. Release the patient's eyelid and have him blink to distribute the medication.

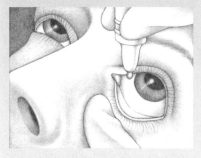

To apply an ointment, gently lay a thin strip of the medication along the conjunctival sac from the inner canthus to the outer canthus. Avoid touching the tip of the tube to the patient's eye. Then release the eyelid and have the patient roll his eye behind closed lids to distribute the medication.

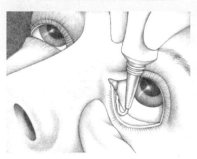

## Implementation

▶ Verify the order on the patient's medication record by checking it against the doctor's order on his chart.
▶ Wash your hands.
▶ Check the medication label against the patient's medication record.

◆ **ALERT!** Make sure you know which eye to treat because different medications or doses may be ordered for each eye.

▶ Confirm the patient's identity by asking his name and checking the name, room number, and bed number on his wristband.

▶ Explain the procedure to the patient and provide privacy. Put on gloves.
▶ If the patient is wearing an eye dressing, remove it by gently pulling it down and away from his forehead. Take care not to contaminate your hands.
▶ Remove any discharge by cleaning around the eye with sterile gauze pads moistened with warm water or normal saline solution. With the patient's eye closed, clean from the inner to the outer canthus, using a fresh sterile gauze pad for each stroke.
▶ To remove crusted secretions around the eye, moisten a gauze pad with warm water or normal saline solution. Ask the patient to close the eye, and then place the gauze pad over it for 1 or 2 minutes. Remove the pad and then reapply moist sterile gauze pads as necessary, until the secretions are soft enough to be removed without traumatizing the mucosa.
▶ Have the patient sit or lie in the supine position. Instruct him to tilt his head back and toward the side of the affected eye so that excess medication can flow away from the tear duct, minimizing systemic absorption through the nasal mucosa.

### Instilling eyedrops
▶ Remove the dropper cap from the medication container, if necessary, and draw the medication into it. Be careful to avoid contaminating the dropper tip or bottle top.
▶ Before instilling the eyedrops, instruct the patient to look up and away. This moves the cornea away from the lower lid and minimizes the risk of touching the cornea with the dropper if the patient blinks.
▶ You can steady the hand holding the dropper by resting it against the patient's forehead. Then, with your other hand, gently pull down the lower lid of the affected eye and instill the drops in the conjunctival sac. Try to avoid placing the drops directly on the eyeball *to prevent the patient from experiencing discomfort.* (See *Instilling eye medications.*)
▶ If more than one agent is to be instilled, wait 5 or more minutes between each agent.

### Applying eye ointment
▶ Squeeze a small ribbon of medication on the edge of the conjunctival sac from the inner to the outer canthus. Cut off the rib-

# How to insert and remove an eye medication disk

Small and flexible, an oval eye medication disk consists of three layers: two soft outer layers and a middle layer that contains the medication. Floating between the eyelids and the sclera, the disk stays in the eye while the patient sleeps and even during swimming and athletic activities. The disk frees the patient from having to remember to instill his eyedrops. When the disk is in place, ocular fluid moistens it, releasing the medication. Eye moisture or contact lenses don't adversely affect the disk. The disk can release medication for up to 1 week before needing replacement. Pilocarpine, for example, can be administered this way to treat glaucoma.

Contraindications include conjunctivitis, keratitis, retinal detachment, and any condition in which constriction of the pupil should be avoided.

### To insert an eye medication disk

Arrange to insert the disk before the patient goes to bed. This minimizes the blurring that usually occurs immediately after disk insertion.

▶ Wash your hands and put on gloves.

▶ Press your fingertip against the oval disk so that it lies lengthwise across your fingertip. It should stick to your finger. Lift the disk out of its packet.

▶ Gently pull the patient's lower eyelid away from the eye and place the disk in the conjunctival sac. It should lie horizontally, not vertically. The disk will adhere to the eye naturally.

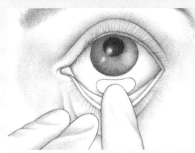

▶ Pull the lower eyelid out, up, and over the disk. Tell the patient to blink several times. If the disk is still visible, pull the lower lid out and over the disk again. Tell the patient that when the disk is in place, he can adjust its position by gently pressing his finger against his closed lid. Caution him against rubbing his eye or moving the disk across the cornea.

▶ If the disk falls out, wash your hands, rinse the disk in cool water, and reinsert it. If the disk appears bent, replace it.

▶ If both the patient's eyes are being treated with medication disks, replace both disks at the same time so that both eyes receive medication at the same rate.

▶ If the disk repeatedly slips out of position, reinsert it under the upper eyelid. To do this, gently lift and evert the upper eyelid and insert the disk in the conjunctival sac. Then gently pull the lid back into position, and tell the patient to blink several times. Again, the patient may press gently on the closed eyelid to reposition the disk. The more the patient uses the disk, the easier it should be for him to retain it. If he can't retain it, notify the doctor.

▶ If the patient will continue therapy with an eye medication disk after discharge, teach him how to insert and remove it himself. To check his mastery of these skills, have him demonstrate insertion and removal for you.

▶ Also, teach the patient about possible adverse reactions. Foreign-body sensation in the eye, mild tearing or redness, increased mucus discharge, eyelid redness, and itchiness can occur with the use of disks. Blurred vision, stinging, swelling, and headaches can occur with pilocarpine, specifically. Mild symptoms are common but should subside within the first 6 weeks of use. Tell the patient to report persistent or severe symptoms to his doctor.

### To remove an eye medication disk

▶ You can remove an eye medication disk with one or two fingers. To use one finger, put on gloves and evert the lower eyelid to expose the disk. Then use the forefinger of your other hand to slide the disk onto the lid and out of the patient's eye. To use two fingers, evert the lower lid with one hand to expose the disk. Then pinch the disk with the thumb and forefinger of your other hand and remove it from the eye.

▶ If the disk is located in the upper eyelid, apply long circular strokes to the patient's closed eyelid with your finger until you can see the disk in the corner of the patient's eye. When the disk is visible, you can place your finger directly on the disk and move it to the lower sclera. Then remove it as you would a disk located in the lower lid.

bon by turning the tube. You can steady the hand holding the medication tube by bracing it against the patient's forehead or cheek.
▶ If more than one ointment is to be instilled, wait 10 minutes before applying the second drug.
▶ If both an ointment and drops have been ordered, the drops should be administered first.

### Using a medication disk
▶ A medication disk can release medication in the eye for up to 1 week before needing to be replaced. Pilocarpine, for example, can be administered this way to treat glaucoma. (For specific instructions, see *How to insert and remove an eye medication disk,* page 115.)

### After instilling eyedrops or eye ointment
▶ Instruct the patient to close his eyes gently, without squeezing the lids shut. If you instilled drops, tell the patient to blink. If you applied ointment, tell him to roll his eyes behind closed lids to help distribute the medication over the surface of the eyeball.
▶ Use a clean tissue to remove any excess solution or ointment leaking from the eye. Remember to use a fresh tissue for each eye to prevent cross-contamination.
▶ Apply a new eye dressing, if necessary.
▶ Return the medication to the storage area. Store it according to the label's instructions.
▶ Wash your hands.

### Special considerations
▶ When giving an eye medication that may be absorbed systemically (such as atropine), gently press your thumb on the inner canthus for 1 to 2 minutes after instilling drops while the patient closes his eyes. This helps prevent medication from flowing into the tear duct.
▶ To maintain the drug container's sterility, never touch the tip of the bottle or dropper to the patient's eyeball, lids, or lashes. Discard any solution remaining in the dropper before returning the dropper to the bottle. If the dropper or bottle tip has become contaminated, discard it and obtain another sterile dropper. To prevent cross-contamination, never use a container of eye medication for more than one patient.

▶ Teach the patient to instill eye medications so that he can continue treatment at home, if necessary. Review the procedure and ask for a return demonstration.

### Complications
Instillation of some eye medications may cause transient burning, itching, and redness. Rarely, systemic effects may also occur.

### Documentation
▶ Record the medication instilled or applied, eye or eyes treated, and date, time, and dose.
▶ Note any adverse effects and the patient's response.

**REFERENCES**
Craven, R., and Hirnle, C.J. *Fundamentals of Nursing: Human Health and Function,* 4th ed. Philadelphia: Lippincott Williams & Wilkins, 2002.
Dogru, M., et al. "Changes in Tear Function and the Ocular Surface After Topical Olopatadine Treatment for Allergic Conjunctivitis: An Open-label Study," *Clinical Therapy* 24(8):1309-21, August 2002.

# Handheld oropharyngeal inhalers

Handheld oropharyngeal inhalers include the metered-dose inhaler (or nebulizer), the turbo-inhaler, and the nasal inhaler. These devices deliver topical medications to the respiratory tract, producing local and systemic effects. The mucosal lining of the respiratory tract absorbs the inhalant almost immediately. Examples of common inhalants are bronchodilators, which are used to improve airway patency and facilitate mucus drainage; mucolytics, which attain a high local concentration to liquefy tenacious bronchial secretions; and corticosteroids, which are used to decrease inflammation.

The use of these inhalers may be contraindicated in patients who can't form an airtight seal around the device and in patients who lack the coordination or clear vision necessary to assemble a turbo-inhaler. Specific inhalant drugs may also be contraindicated. For example, bronchodilators are contraindicated if the patient has tachycar-

# Types of handheld inhalers

Handheld inhalers use air under pressure to produce a mist containing tiny droplets of medication. Drugs delivered in this form (such as mucolytics and bronchodilators) can travel deep into the lungs.

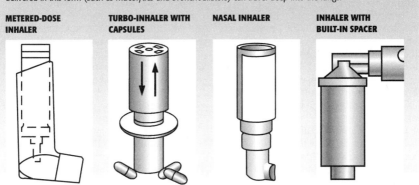

| METERED-DOSE INHALER | TURBO-INHALER WITH CAPSULES | NASAL INHALER | INHALER WITH BUILT-IN SPACER |

dia or a history of cardiac arrhythmias associated with tachycardia.

## Equipment

Patient's medication record and chart ● metered-dose inhaler, turbo-inhaler, or nasal inhaler ● prescribed medication ● normal saline solution (or another appropriate solution) for gargling ● optional: emesis basin (See *Types of handheld inhalers.*)

## Implementation

❱ Verify the order on the patient's medication record by checking it against the doctor's order.
❱ Wash your hands.
❱ Check the label on the inhaler against the order on the medication record. Verify the expiration date.
❱ Confirm the patient's identity by asking his name and by checking his name, room number, and bed number on his wristband.
❱ Explain the procedure to the patient.

### Using a metered-dose inhaler

❱ Shake the inhaler bottle to mix the medication and aerosol propellant.
❱ Remove the mouthpiece and cap. *Note:* Some metered-dose inhalers have a spacer built into the inhaler. Pull the spacer away from the section holding the medication canister until it clicks into place.

❱ Insert the metal stem on the bottle into the small hole on the flattened portion of the mouthpiece. Then turn the bottle upside down.
❱ Have the patient exhale; then place the mouthpiece in his mouth and close his lips around it.
❱ As you firmly push the bottle down against the mouthpiece, ask the patient to inhale slowly and to continue inhaling until his lungs feel full. This action draws the medication into his lungs. Compress the bottle against the mouthpiece only once.
❱ Remove the mouthpiece from the patient's mouth and tell him to hold his breath for several seconds to allow the medication to reach the alveoli. Then instruct him to exhale slowly through pursed lips to keep the distal bronchioles open, allowing increased absorption and diffusion of the drug and better gas exchange.
❱ Have the patient gargle with normal saline solution to remove medication from the mouth and back of the throat. (The lungs retain only about 10% of the inhalant; most of the remainder is exhaled but substantial amounts may remain in the oropharynx.)
❱ Rinse the mouthpiece thoroughly with warm water to prevent accumulation of residue.

## Using a turbo-inhaler

▶ Hold the mouthpiece in one hand, and with the other hand, slide the sleeve away from the mouthpiece as far as possible.

▶ Unscrew the tip of the mouthpiece by turning it counterclockwise.

▶ Firmly press the colored portion of the medication capsule into the propeller stem of the mouthpiece.

▶ Screw the inhaler together securely.

▶ Holding the inhaler with the mouthpiece at the bottom, slide the sleeve all the way down and then up again to puncture the capsule and release the medication. Do this only once.

▶ Have the patient exhale and tilt his head back. Tell him to place the mouthpiece in his mouth, close his lips around it, and inhale once — quickly and deeply — through the mouthpiece.

▶ Tell the patient to hold his breath for several seconds to allow the medication to reach the alveoli. (Instruct him not to exhale through the mouthpiece.)

▶ Remove the inhaler from the patient's mouth and tell him to exhale as much air as possible.

▶ Repeat the procedure until all the medication in the device is inhaled.

▶ Have the patient gargle with normal saline solution to remove medication from the mouth and back of the throat. Make sure you provide an emesis basin if the patient needs one.

▶ Discard the empty medication capsule, put the inhaler in its can, and secure the lid. Rinse the inhaler with warm water at least once per week.

## Using a nasal inhaler

▶ Have the patient blow his nose to clear his nostrils.

▶ Shake the medication cartridge and then insert it in the adapter. (Before inserting a refill cartridge, remove the protective cap from the stem.)

▶ Remove the protective cap from the adapter tip.

▶ Hold the inhaler with your index finger on top of the cartridge and your thumb under the nasal adapter. The adapter tip should be pointing toward the patient.

▶ Have the patient tilt his head back. Tell him to place the adapter tip into one nostril while occluding the other nostril with his finger.

▶ Instruct the patient to inhale gently as he presses the adapter and the cartridge together firmly to release a measured dose of medication. Make sure you follow the manufacturer's instructions. With some medications, such as dexamethasone sodium phosphate (Turbinaire), inhaling during administration isn't desirable.

▶ Tell the patient to remove the inhaler from his nostril and exhale through his mouth.

▶ Shake the inhaler and have the patient repeat the procedure in the other nostril.

▶ Have the patient gargle with normal saline solution to remove medication from his mouth and throat.

▶ Remove the medication cartridge from the nasal inhaler and wash the nasal adapter in lukewarm water. Let the adapter dry thoroughly before reinserting the cartridge.

## Special considerations

▶ When using a turbo-inhaler or nasal inhaler, make sure the pressurized cartridge isn't punctured or incinerated. Store the medication cartridge below 120° F (48.9° C).

▶ If you're using a turbo-inhaler, keep the medication capsules wrapped until needed to keep them from deteriorating.

▶ Spacer inhalers may be recommended to provide greater therapeutic benefit for children and for patients who have difficulty with coordination. A spacer attachment is an extension to the inhaler's mouthpiece that provides more dead-air space for mixing the medication. Some inhalers have built-in spacers.

▶ Teach the patient how to use the inhaler so that he can continue treatments himself after discharge, if necessary. Explain that overdosage — which is common — can cause the medication to lose its effectiveness. Tell him to record the date and time of each inhalation as well as his response to prevent overdosage and to help the doctor determine the drug's effectiveness. Also, note whether the patient uses an unusual amount of medication — for example, more than one cartridge for a metered-dose nebulizer every 3 weeks. Inform the patient of possible adverse reactions.

▶ If more than one inhalation is ordered, advise the patient to wait at least 2 minutes before repeating the procedure.
▶ If the patient is also using a steroid inhaler, instruct him to use the bronchodilator first and then wait 5 minutes before using the steroid. This allows the bronchodilator to open the air passages for maximum effectiveness.

## Documentation
▶ Record the inhalant given, as well as dose and time.
▶ Note significant change in the patient's heart rate and any other adverse reactions.

### REFERENCES
Blanchard, A.R., and Golish, J.A. "Pressurized Metered-dose Inhalers are as Effective as Other Handheld Inhalers For Beta$_2$-Agonist Bronchodilator Use in Asthma," *American College of Physicians Journal Club* 136(3): 111, May-June 2002.
Craven, R., and Hirnle, C.J. *Fundamentals of Nursing: Human Health and Function,* 4th ed. Philadelphia: Lippincott Williams & Wilkins, 2002.

# I.M. injection

Intramuscular (I.M.) injections deposit medication deep into muscle tissue. This route of administration provides rapid systemic action and absorption of relatively large doses (up to 5 ml in appropriate sites). I.M. injections are recommended for patients who can't take medication orally, when I.V. administration is inappropriate, and for drugs that are altered by digestive juices. Because muscle tissue has few sensory nerves, I.M. injection allows less painful administration of irritating drugs.

The site for an I.M. injection must be chosen carefully, taking into account the patient's general physical status and the purpose of the injection. I.M. injections shouldn't be administered at inflamed, edematous, or irritated sites or at sites that contain moles, birthmarks, scar tissue, or other lesions. I.M. injections may also be contraindicated in patients with impaired coagulation mechanisms, occlusive peripheral vascular disease, edema, and shock; after thrombolytic therapy; and during an acute myocardial infarction because these conditions impair peripheral absorption. I.M. injections require sterile technique to maintain the integrity of muscle tissue.

Oral or I.V. routes are preferred for administration of drugs that are poorly absorbed by muscle tissue, such as phenytoin, digoxin, chlordiazepoxide, and diazepam.

## Equipment
Patient's medication record and chart ● prescribed medication ● diluent or filter needle, if needed ● 3- or 5-ml syringe ● 20G to 25G 1″ to 3″ needle ● gloves ● alcohol pads ● optional: gauze pad ● 1″ tape ● ice

The prescribed medication must be sterile. The needle may be packaged separately or already attached to the syringe. Needles used for I.M. injections are longer than subcutaneous needles because they must reach deep into the muscle. Needle length also depends on the injection site, patient's size, and amount of subcutaneous fat covering the muscle. The needle gauge for I.M. injections should be larger to accommodate viscous solutions and suspensions.

### Preparation of equipment
Verify the order on the patient's medication record by checking it against the doctor's order. Also note whether the patient has any allergies, especially before the first dose.

Check the prescribed medication for color and clarity. Also note the expiration date. Never use medication that is cloudy or discolored or contains a precipitate unless the manufacturer's instructions allow it. Remember that for some drugs (such as suspensions), the presence of drug particles is normal. Observe for abnormal changes. If in doubt, check with the pharmacist.

Choose equipment appropriate to the prescribed medication and injection site, and make sure it works properly. The needle should be straight, smooth, and free from burrs.

### For single-dose ampules
Wrap an alcohol pad around the ampule's neck and snap off the top, directing the force away from your body. Attach a filter

needle to the needle and withdraw the medication, keeping the needle's bevel tip below the level of the solution. Tap the syringe to clear air from it. Cover the needle with the needle sheath.

Before discarding the ampule, check the medication label against the patient's medication record. Discard the filter needle and the ampule. Attach the appropriate needle to the syringe.

*For single-dose or multidose vials*
Reconstitute powdered drugs according to instructions. Make sure all crystals have dissolved in the solution. Warm the vial by rolling it between your palms to help the drug dissolve faster.

Wipe the stopper of the medication vial with an alcohol pad and draw up the prescribed amount of medication. Read the medication label as you select the medication, as you draw it up, and after you've drawn it up to verify the correct dosage.

Don't use an air bubble in the syringe. A holdover from the days of reusable syringes, air bubbles can affect the medication dosage by 5% to 100%. Modern disposable syringes are calibrated to administer the correct dose without an air bubble.

Gather all necessary equipment and proceed to the patient's room.

## Implementation
▶ Confirm the patient's identity by asking his name and checking his wristband for name, room number, and bed number.
▶ Provide privacy, explain the procedure to the patient, and wash your hands.
▶ Select an appropriate injection site. The gluteal muscles (gluteus medius and minimus and the upper outer corner of the gluteus maximus) are used most commonly for healthy adults, although the deltoid muscle may be used for a small-volume injection (2 ml or less). Remember to rotate injection sites for patients who require repeated injections.

**ALERT!** For infants and children, the vastus lateralis muscle of the thigh is used most often because it's usually the best developed and contains no large nerves or blood vessels, minimizing the risk of serious injury. The rectus femoris muscle may also be used in infants but is usually contraindicated in adults.

▶ Position and drape the patient appropriately, making sure the site is well exposed and that lighting is adequate.
▶ Loosen the protective needle sheath but don't remove it.
▶ After selecting the injection site, gently tap it to stimulate the nerve endings and minimize pain when the needle is inserted. (See *Locating I.M. injection sites.*)
▶ Clean the skin at the site with an alcohol pad. Move the pad outward in a circular motion to a circumference of about 2″ (5 cm) from the injection site and allow the skin to dry. Keep the alcohol pad for later use.
▶ Put on gloves. With the thumb and index finger of your nondominant hand, gently stretch the skin of the injection site taut.
▶ While you hold the syringe in your dominant hand, remove the needle sheath by slipping it between the free fingers of your nondominant hand and then drawing back the syringe.
▶ Position the syringe at a 90-degree angle to the skin surface with the needle a couple of inches from the skin. Tell the patient that he'll feel a prick as you insert the needle. Then quickly and firmly thrust the needle through the skin and subcutaneous tissue, deep into the muscle.
▶ Support the syringe with your nondominant hand, if desired. Pull back slightly on the plunger with your dominant hand to aspirate for blood. If no blood appears, slowly inject the medication into the muscle. A slow, steady injection rate allows the muscle to distend gradually and accept the medication under minimal pressure. You should feel little or no resistance against the force of the injection.
▶ If blood appears in the syringe on aspiration, the needle is in a blood vessel. If this occurs, stop the injection, withdraw the needle, prepare another injection with new equipment, and inject another site. Don't inject the bloody solution.
▶ After the injection, gently but quickly remove the needle at a 90-degree angle.
▶ Using a gloved hand, cover the injection site immediately with the used alcohol pad, apply gentle pressure and, unless contraindicated, massage the relaxed muscle to help distribute the drug.
▶ Remove the alcohol pad and inspect the injection site for signs of active bleeding or bruising. If bleeding continues, apply pres-

# Locating I.M. injection sites

### Deltoid

Find the lower edge of the acromial process and the point on the lateral arm in line with the axilla. Insert the needle 1″ to 2″ (2.5 to 5 cm) below the acromial process, usually two or three fingerbreadths, at a 90-degree angle or angled slightly toward the process. Typical injection: 0.5 ml (range: 0.5 to 2.0 ml).

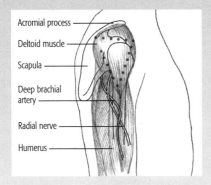

Acromial process
Deltoid muscle
Scapula
Deep brachial artery
Radial nerve
Humerus

### Dorsogluteal

Inject above and outside a line drawn from the posterior superior iliac spine to the greater trochanter of the femur. Or divide the buttock into quadrants and inject in the upper outer quadrant, about 2″ to 3″ (5 to 7.6 cm) below the iliac crest. Insert the needle at a 90-degree angle. Typical injection: 1 to 4 ml (range: 1 to 5 ml).

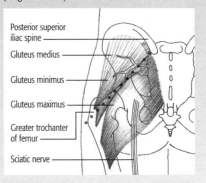

Posterior superior iliac spine
Gluteus medius
Gluteus minimus
Gluteus maximus
Greater trochanter of femur
Sciatic nerve

### Ventrogluteal

Locate the greater trochanter of the femur with the heel of your hand. Then spread your index and middle fingers from the anterior superior iliac spine to as far along the iliac crest as you can reach. Insert the needle between the two fingers at a 90-degree angle to the muscle. (Remove your fingers before inserting the needle.) Typical injection: 1 to 4 ml (range: 1 to 5 ml).

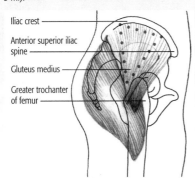

Iliac crest
Anterior superior iliac spine
Gluteus medius
Greater trochanter of femur

### Vastus lateralis

Use the lateral muscle of the quadriceps group, from a handbreadth below the greater trochanter to a handbreadth above the knee. Insert the needle into the middle third of the muscle parallel to the surface on which the patient is lying. You may have to bunch the muscle before insertion. Typical injection: 1 to 4 ml (range: 1 to 5 ml; 1 to 3 ml for infants).

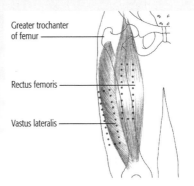

Greater trochanter of femur
Rectus femoris
Vastus lateralis

sure to the site; if bruising occurs, you may apply ice.

▶ Watch for adverse reactions at the site for 10 to 30 minutes after the injection.

**ALERT!** An elderly patient will probably bleed or ooze from the site after the injection because of decreased tissue elasticity. Applying a small pressure bandage may be helpful.

▶ Discard all equipment according to standard precautions and your facility's policy. Don't recap needles; dispose of them in an appropriate sharps container to avoid needle-stick injuries.

### Special considerations

▶ To slow their absorption, some drugs for I.M. administration are dissolved in oil or other special solutions. Mix these preparations well before drawing them into the syringe.

◆ **ALERT!** The gluteal muscles can be used as the injection site only after a toddler has been walking for about 1 year.

▶ Never inject into sensitive muscles, especially those that twitch or tremble when you assess site landmarks and tissue depth. Injections into these trigger areas may cause sharp or referred pain such as the pain caused by nerve trauma.

▶ Keep a rotation record that lists all available injection sites, divided into various body areas, for patients who require repeated injections. Rotate from a site in the first area to a site in each of the other areas. Then return to a site in the first area that is at least 1″ (2.5 cm) away from the previous injection site in that area.

▶ If the patient has experienced pain or emotional trauma from repeated injections, consider numbing the area before cleaning it by holding ice on it for several seconds. If you must inject more than 5 ml of solution, divide the solution and inject it at two separate sites.

▶ Always encourage the patient to relax the muscle you'll be injecting because injections into tense muscles are more painful than usual and may bleed more readily.

▶ I.M. injections can damage local muscle cells, causing elevations in serum enzyme levels (creatine kinase [CK]) that can be confused with elevations resulting from cardiac muscle damage such as in myocardial infarction. To distinguish between skeletal and cardiac muscle damage, diagnostic tests for suspected myocardial infarction must identify the isoenzyme of CK specific to cardiac muscle (CK-MB) and include tests to determine lactate dehydrogenase and aspartate aminotransferase levels. If it's important to measure these enzyme levels, suggest that the doctor switch to I.V.

administration and adjust dosages accordingly.

▶ Dosage adjustments are usually necessary when changing from the I.M. route to the oral route.

### Complications

Accidental injection of concentrated or irritating medications into subcutaneous tissue or other areas where they can't be fully absorbed can cause sterile abscesses to develop. Such abscesses result from the body's natural immune response in which phagocytes attempt to remove the foreign matter.

Failure to rotate sites in patients who require repeated injections can lead to deposits of unabsorbed medications. Such deposits can reduce the desired pharmacologic effect and may lead to abscess formation or tissue fibrosis.

◆ **ALERT!** Because elderly patients have decreased muscle mass, I.M. medications can be absorbed more quickly than expected.

### Documentation

▶ Chart the drug administered, dose, date, time, route of administration, and injection site.

▶ Note the patient's tolerance of the injection and the injection's effects, including any adverse effects.

**REFERENCES**

Edward, D., et al. *Bedside Critical Care Manual.* Philadelphia: Lippincott Williams & Wilkins, 2001.

Petousis-Harris, H. "Needle Angle When Giving I.M. Vaccinations," *Nursing Praxis in New Zealand.* 18(2):52-53, July 2002.

# I.V. bolus injection

The I.V. bolus injection method allows rapid drug administration. It can be used in an emergency to provide an immediate drug effect. It can also be used to administer drugs that can't be given I.M., to achieve peak drug levels in the bloodstream, and to deliver drugs that can't be diluted, such as diazepam, digoxin, and phenytoin. The term bolus usually refers to the concentration or amount of a drug. I.V. push is a technique for rapid I.V. injection.

Bolus doses of medication may be injected directly into a vein, through an existing I.V. line, or through an implanted vascular access port (VAP). The medication administered by these methods usually takes effect rapidly, so the patient must be monitored for an adverse reaction, such as cardiac arrhythmia and anaphylaxis. I.V. bolus injections are contraindicated when rapid drug administration could cause life-threatening complications. For certain drugs, the safe rate of injection is specified by the manufacturer.

Some facilities permit only specially trained nurses (such as emergency department, critical care, and chemotherapy nurses) to give bolus injections.

### Equipment
Patient's medication record and chart ● gloves ● prescribed medication ● 20G needle and syringe ● diluent, if needed ● tourniquet ● povidone-iodine or alcohol pad ● sterile 2″ × 2″ gauze pad ● adhesive bandage ● tape ● optional: winged-tip needle with catheter and second syringe (and needle) filled with normal saline solution and a noncoring needle if used with a VAP.

Winged-tip needles are commonly used for this purpose because they can be quickly and easily inserted. They're ideal for repeated drug administration, such as in weekly or monthly chemotherapy. Another useful dosage form is the ready injectable. (See *Using a ready injectable.*)

#### Preparation of equipment
Verify the order on the patient's medication record by checking it against the doctor's order. Know the actions, adverse effects, and administration rate of the medication to be injected. Draw up the prescribed medication in the syringe and dilute it if necessary.

### Implementation
▶ Confirm the patient's identity, wash your hands, put on gloves, and explain the procedure.

#### Giving direct injections
▶ Select the largest vein suitable for an injection. The larger the vein, the more diluted the drug will become, minimizing vascular irritation.

## Using a ready injectable

A commercially premeasured medication packaged with a syringe and needle, the ready injectable allows for rapid drug administration in an emergency. Usually, preparing a ready injectable takes only 15 to 20 seconds. Other advantages include the reduced risk of breaking sterile technique during administration and the easy identification of medication and dose.

When using a commercially prefilled syringe, make sure you give the precise dose prescribed. For example, if a 50 mg/ml cartridge is supplied but the patient's prescribed dose is 25 mg, you must administer only 0.5 ml – half the volume contained in the cartridge. Be alert for potential medication errors whenever dispensing medications in premeasured dosage forms.

▶ Apply a tourniquet above the injection site to distend the vein.
▶ Clean the injection site with an alcohol or a povidone-iodine pad, working outward from the puncture site in a circular motion to prevent recontamination with skin bacteria.
▶ If you're using the drug syringe's needle, insert it into the vein at a 30-degree angle with the bevel up. The bevel should reach ¼″ (0.6 cm) into the vein. If you're using a winged-tip needle, insert the needle (bevel up), tape the butterfly wings in place when you see blood return in the tubing, and attach the syringe containing the medication.
▶ Pull back on the syringe plunger and check for blood backflow, which indicates that the needle is in the vein.
▶ Remove the tourniquet and inject the medication at the appropriate rate.
▶ Pull back slightly on the syringe plunger and check for blood backflow again. If blood appears, this indicates that the needle remained in place and all the injected medication entered the vein.
▶ Flush the line with the normal saline solution from the second syringe to ensure delivery of all the medication.
▶ Withdraw the needle and apply pressure to the injection site with a sterile gauze pad for at least 3 minutes to prevent hematoma formation.

▶ Apply the adhesive bandage to the site after bleeding has stopped.

### Giving injections through an existing I.V. line
▶ Check the compatibility of the medication with the I.V. solution.
▶ Close the flow clamp, wipe the injection port with an alcohol pad, and inject the medication as you would a direct injection. (Some I.V. lines have a secondary injection port or a T-connector; others have a needleless adapter or latex cap at the end of the I.V. tubing where the needle is attached.)
▶ Open the flow clamp and readjust the flow rate.
▶ If the drug isn't compatible with the I.V. solution, flush the line with normal saline solution before and after the injection.

■ **EVIDENCE BASE** The volume of flush solution should be equal to or twice that of the capacity of the catheter and the add-on device. If the site is used intermittently, it will need to be flushed with normal saline solution (injectable) at established intervals to maintain patency. Flushing will also need to be performed before and after administration of incompatible medications or solutions.

### Giving a bolus injection through a VAP
▶ Wash your hands, put on gloves, and clean the injection site with an alcohol or a povidone-iodine pad, starting at the center of the port and working outward in a circular motion over a 4″ to 5″ (10- to 12.7-cm) diameter. Do this three times.
▶ Attach a 10-ml syringe filled with saline solution to the end of the extension set and remove all the air. Now attach the extension set to the noncoring needle. Check for blood return. Then flush the port with normal saline solution, according to your facility's policy.
▶ Clamp the extension set and remove the saline syringe.
▶ Connect the medication syringe to the extension set. Open the clamp and inject the drug, .
▶ Examine the skin surrounding the needle for signs of infiltration, such as swelling or tenderness. If you note these signs, stop the injection and intervene appropriately.
▶ When the injection is complete, clamp the extension set and remove the medication syringe.

▶ Open the clamp and flush with 5 ml of normal saline solution after each drug injection to minimize drug incompatibility reactions.
▶ Flush with heparin solution according to your facility's policy.

## Special considerations
▶ Because drugs administered by I.V. bolus or push injections are delivered directly into the circulatory system and can produce an immediate effect, an acute allergic reaction or anaphylaxis can develop rapidly. If signs of anaphylaxis (such as dyspnea, cyanosis, seizures, and increasing respiratory distress) occur, notify the doctor immediately and begin emergency procedures, as necessary. Also watch for signs of extravasation (such as redness and swelling). If extravasation occurs, stop the injection, estimate the amount of infiltration, and notify the doctor.
▶ If you're giving diazepam or chlordiazepoxide hydrochloride through a winged-tip needle or an I.V. line, flush with bacteriostatic water instead of normal saline solution to prevent drug precipitation resulting from incompatibility.

## Complications
Excessively rapid administration may cause adverse effects, depending on the medication administered.

## Documentation
▶ Record the amount and type of drug administered, time of injection, appearance of the site, duration of administration, and patient's tolerance of the procedure.
▶ Note the drug's effect and any adverse reactions.

### REFERENCES
Brock-Cascanet, P.H. "Treating Occluded VADs in the Home Setting," *Infusion* 5(4): 18-27, January 1999.
Davis, S.N., et al. "Activity and Dosage of Alteplase Dilution for Clearing Occlusions of Venous-access Devices," *American Journal of Health System Pharmacy* 57(11): 1039-45, 2000.
Heath, J., and Jones, S. "Utilization of an Elastomeric Continuous Infusion Device to Maintain Catheter Patency," *Journal of Intravenous Nursing* 24(2):102-06, March-April 2001.

# Intradermal injection

Because little systemic absorption of intra-dermally injected agents takes place, this type of injection is used primarily to pro-duce a local effect, such as in allergy or tu-berculin testing. Intradermal injections are administered in small volumes (usually 0.5 ml or less) into the outer layers of the skin.

The ventral forearm is the most com-monly used site for intradermal injection because of its easy accessibility and lack of hair. In extensive allergy testing, the outer aspect of the upper arms may be used as well as the area of the back located be-tween the scapulae. (See *Intradermal injec-tion sites.*)

## Equipment

Patient's medication record and chart ● tuberculin syringe with a 26G or 27G ½" to ⅜" needle ● prescribed medication ● gloves ● alcohol pads

### Preparation of equipment

Verify the order on the patient's medication record by checking it against the doctor's orders. Inspect the medication to make sure it isn't abnormally discolored or cloudy and doesn't contain precipitates. Wash your hands.

Choose equipment appropriate to the prescribed medication and injection site and make sure it works properly. Check the medication label against the patient's med-ication record. Read the label again as you draw up the medication for injection.

## Implementation

▸ Verify the patient's identity by asking his name and checking the name, room num-ber, and bed number on his wristband against his medical record.
▸ Tell him where you'll be giving the injec-tion.
▸ Instruct the patient to sit up and to ex-tend his arm and support it on a flat sur-face, with the ventral forearm exposed.
▸ Put on gloves.
▸ With an alcohol pad, clean the surface of the ventral forearm about two or three fin-gerbreadths distal to the antecubital space. Make sure the test site you have chosen is free from hair or blemishes. Allow the skin

## Intradermal injection sites

The most common intradermal injection site is the ventral forearm. Other sites (indicated by dotted areas) include the upper chest, upper arm, and shoulder blades. Skin in these areas is usually light-ly pigmented, thinly keratinized, and relatively hair-less, facilitating detection of adverse reactions.

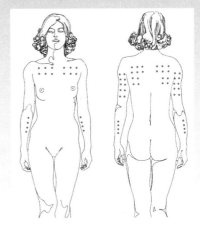

to dry completely before giving the injec-tion.
▸ While holding the patient's forearm in your hand, stretch the skin taut with your thumb.
▸ With your free hand, hold the needle at a 10- to 15-degree angle to the patient's arm, with its bevel up.
▸ Insert the needle about ⅛" (0.3 cm) be-low the epidermis at sites 2" (5 cm) apart. Stop when the needle's bevel tip is under the skin and inject the antigen slowly. You should feel some resistance as you do this, and a wheal should form as you inject the antigen. (See *Giving an intradermal injec-tion,* page 126.)

If no wheal forms, you have injected the antigen too deeply; withdraw the needle, and administer another test dose at least 2" from the first site.
▸ Withdraw the needle at the same angle at which it was inserted. Don't rub the site. This could irritate the underlying tissue, which may affect test results.

## Giving an intradermal injection

Secure the forearm. Insert the needle at a 10- to 15-degree angle so that it just punctures the skin's surface. The antigen should raise a small wheal as it's injected.

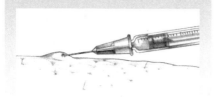

▶ Circle each test site with a marking pen and label each site according to the recall antigen given. Instruct the patient to refrain from washing off the circles until the test is completed.
▶ Dispose of needles and syringes according to your facility's policy.
▶ Remove and discard your gloves and wash your hands.
▶ Assess the patient's response to the skin testing in 24 to 48 hours.

### Special considerations

In patients who are hypersensitive to the test antigens, a severe anaphylactic response can result. This requires immediate epinephrine injection and other emergency resuscitation procedures. Be especially alert after giving a test dose of penicillin or tetanus antitoxin.

### Documentation

▶ Document the type and amount of medication given, the time it was given, and the injection site.
▶ Note skin reactions and other adverse reactions.

**REFERENCES**

Craven, R., and Hirnle, C.J. *Fundamentals of Nursing: Human Health and Function,* 4th ed. Philadelphia: Lippincott Williams & Wilkins, 2002.
Khawplod, P., et al. "Four-site Intradermal Postexposure Boosters in Previously Rabies Vaccinated Subjects," *Journal of Travel Medicine* 9(3):153-55, May-June 2002.

# Intraosseous infusion

When rapid venous infusion is difficult or impossible, intraosseous infusion allows delivery of fluids, medications, or whole blood into the bone marrow. Performed on infants and children, this technique is used in such emergencies as cardiopulmonary arrest, circulatory collapse, hypokalemia from traumatic injury or dehydration, status epilepticus, status asthmaticus, burns, near-drowning, and overwhelming sepsis.

Any drug that can be given I.V. can be given by intraosseous infusion with comparable absorption and effectiveness. Intraosseous infusion has been used as an acceptable alternative for infants and children.

Intraosseous infusion is commonly undertaken at the anterior surface of the tibia. Alternative sites include the iliac crest, spinous process and, rarely, the upper anterior portion of the sternum. Only personnel trained in this procedure should perform it. Usually, a nurse assists. (See *Understanding intraosseous infusion.*)

This procedure is contraindicated in patients with osteogenesis imperfecta, osteopetrosis, and ipsilateral fracture because of the potential for subcutaneous extravasation. Infusion through an area with cellulitis or an infected burn increases the risk of infection.

### Equipment

Bone marrow biopsy needle or specially designed intraosseous infusion needle (cannula and obturator) ● povidone-iodine pads ● sterile gauze pads ● sterile gloves ● sterile drape ● heparin flush solution ● I.V. fluids and tubing ● 1% lidocaine ● 3- or 5-ml syringe ● tape ● sedative, if ordered

### Preparation of equipment

Prepare I.V. fluids and tubing as ordered.

### Implementation

▶ If the patient is conscious, explain the procedure to allay his fears and promote his cooperation. Ensure that the patient or a responsible family member understands the procedure and signs a consent form.
▶ Check the patient's history for hypersensitivity to the local anesthetic. If the patient isn't an infant, tell him which bone site will be infused. Inform him that he'll re-

ceive a local anesthetic and will feel pressure from needle insertion.
▶ Wash your hands.
▶ Provide a sedative, if ordered, before the procedure.
▶ Position the patient based on the selected puncture site.
▶ Using sterile technique, the doctor cleans the puncture site with a povidone-iodine pad and allows it to dry. He then covers the area with a sterile drape.
▶ Using sterile technique, hand the doctor the 3- or 5-ml syringe with 1% lidocaine so that he can anesthetize the infusion site.
▶ The doctor inserts the infusion needle through the skin and into the bone at an angle of 10 to 15 degrees from vertical. He advances it with a forward and backward rotary motion through the periosteum until it penetrates the marrow cavity. The needle should "give" suddenly as it enters the marrow and stand erect when released.
▶ Then the doctor removes the obturator from the needle and attaches a 5-ml syringe. He aspirates some bone marrow to confirm needle placement.
▶ The doctor replaces this syringe with a syringe containing 5 ml of heparin flush solution and flushes the cannula to confirm needle placement and clear the cannula of clots and bone particles.
▶ Next, the doctor removes the syringe of flush solution and attaches I.V. tubing to the cannula to allow infusion of medications and I.V. fluids.
▶ Put on sterile gloves.
▶ Clean the infusion site with povidone-iodine pads and then secure the site with tape and a sterile gauze dressing.
▶ Monitor vital signs and check the infusion site for bleeding and extravasation.

## Special considerations

▶ Intraosseous infusion should be discontinued as soon as conventional vascular access is established (within 2 to 4 hours, if possible). Prolonged infusion significantly increases the risk of infection.
▶ After the needle has been removed, place a sterile dressing over the injection site, and apply firm pressure to the site for 5 minutes.
▶ Intraosseous flow rates are determined by needle size and flow through the bone marrow. Fluids should flow freely if needle placement is correct. Normal saline solution has been given intraosseously at a

### Understanding intraosseous infusion

During intraosseous infusion, the bone marrow serves as a noncollapsible vein; thus, fluid infused into the marrow cavity rapidly enters the circulation by way of an extensive network of venous sinusoids. Here, the needle is shown positioned in the patient's tibia.

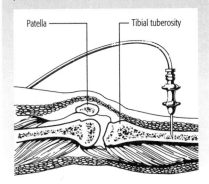

rate of 600 ml/minute and up to 2,500 ml/hour when delivered under pressure of 300 mm Hg through a 13G needle.

## Complications

Common complications include extravasation of fluid into subcutaneous tissue, resulting from incorrect needle placement; subperiosteal effusion, resulting from failure of fluid to enter the marrow space; and clotting in the needle, resulting from delayed infusion or failure to flush the needle after placement. Other complications include subcutaneous abscess, osteomyelitis, and epiphyseal injury.

## Documentation

▶ Record the time, date, location, and patient's tolerance of the procedure.
▶ Document the amount of fluid infused on the input and output record.

### REFERENCES

Craven, R., and Hirnle, C.J. *Fundamentals of Nursing: Human Health and Function*, 4th ed. Philadelphia: Lippincott Williams & Wilkins, 2002.

Reitz, J., et al. "Anesthetic Efficacy of a Repeated Intraosseous Injection Given 30 Minutes Following an Inferior Alveolar Nerve Block/Intraosseous Injection," *Anesthesia Progress* 45(4):143-49, Fall 1998.

# Intrapleural drugs

An intrapleural drug is injected through the chest wall into the pleural space or instilled through a chest tube placed intrapleurally for drainage. Doctors use intrapleural administration to promote analgesia, treat spontaneous pneumothorax, resolve pleural effusions, and administer chemotherapy.

Intrapleurally administered drugs diffuse across the parietal pleura and innermost intercostal muscles to affect the intercostal nerves. During intrapleural injection of a drug, the needle passes through the intercostal muscles and parietal pleura on its way to the pleural space.

The internal intercostal muscle is a key landmark for needle placement. It resists the advancing needle, becoming the posterior intercostal membrane in the posterior chest region.

Drugs commonly given by intrapleural injection include tetracycline, streptokinase, anesthetics, and chemotherapeutic agents (to treat malignant pleural effusion or lung adenocarcinoma).

Contraindications for this route include pleural fibrosis or adhesions, which interfere with diffusion of the drug to the intended site; pleural inflammation; sepsis; and infection at the puncture site. Patients with bullous emphysema and those receiving respiratory therapy using positive endexpiratory pressure also shouldn't have intrapleural injections because the injections may exacerbate an already compromised pulmonary condition.

## Equipment

An intrapleural drug is given through a #16 to #20 or #28 to #40 chest tube if the patient has empyema, pleural effusion, or pneumothorax. Otherwise, it's given through a 16G to 18G blunt-tipped intrapleural (epidural) needle and catheter. Accessory equipment depends on the type of access device the doctor uses. All equipment must be sterile.

*For intrapleural catheter insertion*
Gloves ● gauze ● antiseptic solution such as povidone-iodine ● drape ● local anesthetic such as 1% lidocaine ● 3- or 5-ml syringe with 22G 1″ and 25G ⅝″ needles ● 18G needle or scalpel ● saline-lubricated glass syringe ● dressings ● sutures ● tape

*For chest tube insertion*
Towels ● gloves ● gauze ● antiseptic solution such as povidone-iodine ● 3- or 5-ml syringe ● local anesthetic such as 1% lidocaine ● 18G needle or scalpel ● chest tube with or without trocar (#16 to #20 catheter for air or serous fluid, #28 to #40 catheter for blood, pus, or thick fluid) ● two rubber-tipped clamps ● sutures ● drain dressings ● tape ● thoracic drainage system and tubing

*For drug administration*
Gloves ● sterile gauze pads ● antiseptic solution such as povidone-iodine ● prescribed medication ● appropriate-sized needles and syringes ● 1% lidocaine, if necessary ● dressings ● tape

## Implementation

▶ Explain the procedure to the patient to allay his fears. Encourage him to follow instructions.

### Inserting an intrapleural catheter

▶ The doctor inserts the intrapleural catheter at the patient's bedside with the nurse assisting.

▶ Position the patient on his side with the affected side up. The doctor will insert the catheter into the fourth to eighth intercostal space, 3″ to 4″ (7.5 to 10 cm) from the posterior midline. (See *Giving intrapleural drugs.*)

▶ The doctor puts on sterile gloves, cleans around the puncture site with antiseptic-soaked gauze, and covers the area with a sterile drape. Next, he fills the 3- or 5-ml syringe with local anesthetic and injects it into the skin and deep tissues.

▶ The doctor punctures the skin with the 18G needle or scalpel, which helps the blunt-tipped intrapleural needle penetrate the skin over the superior edge of the lower rib in the chosen interspace. Keeping the bevel tilted upward, he directs the needle medially at a 30- to 40-degree angle to the skin. When the needle tip punctures the posterior intercostal membrane, he removes the stylet and attaches a saline-lubricated glass syringe containing 2 to 4 cc of air to the needle hub.

▶ During puncture, tell the patient to hold his breath (or momentarily disconnect him from mechanical ventilation) until the needle is removed. This helps prevent the needle from injuring lung tissue.

▶ The doctor advances the needle slowly. When the needle punctures the parietal pleura, negative intrapleural pressure moves the plunger outward. He then removes the syringe from the needle and threads the intrapleural catheter through the needle until he has advanced it about 2″ (5 cm) into the pleural space. Without removing the catheter, he carefully withdraws the needle.

▶ Tell the patient that he can breathe again (or reconnect mechanical ventilation).

▶ After inserting the catheter, the doctor coils it to prevent kinking and then sutures it securely to the patient's skin. He confirms placement by aspirating the catheter. Resistance indicates correct placement in the pleural space; aspirated blood means that the catheter probably is misplaced in a blood vessel, and aspirated air means that it's probably in a lung. He'll then order a chest X-ray to detect pneumothorax.

▶ Apply a sterile dressing over the insertion site to prevent catheter dislodgment. Take the patient's vital signs every 15 minutes for the first hour after the procedure and then as needed.

### Inserting a chest tube

▶ The doctor inserts the chest tube with the nurse assisting.

▶ First, position the patient with the affected side up, and drape him with sterile towels.

▶ The doctor puts on gloves and cleans the appropriate site with antiseptic-soaked gauze. If the patient has a pneumothorax, the doctor uses the second intercostal space as the access site because air rises to the top of the pleural space. If the patient has a hemothorax or pleural effusion, the doctor uses the sixth to eighth intercostal space because fluid settles to the bottom of the pleural space.

▶ The doctor fills the 3- or 5-ml syringe with a local anesthetic and injects it into the site. He makes a small incision with the 18G needle or scalpel, inserts the appropriate-sized chest tube, and immediately connects it to the thoracic drainage

---

## Giving intrapleural drugs

In intrapleural administration, the doctor injects a drug into the pleural space using a catheter.

Help the patient lie on one side with the affected side up. The doctor inserts a needle into the fourth to eighth intercostal space, 3″ to 4″ (7.6 to 10 cm) from the posterior midline. He then advances the needle medially over the superior edge of the patient's rib through the intercostal muscles until it tangentially penetrates the parietal pleura, as shown. The catheter is advanced into the pleural space through the needle, which is then removed.

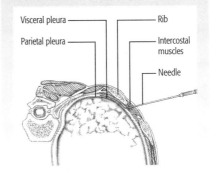

Visceral pleura — Rib
Parietal pleura — Intercostal muscles
— Needle

---

system or clamps it close to the patient's chest. He then sutures the tube to the patient's skin.

▶ Tape the chest tube to the patient's chest distal to the insertion site to help prevent accidental dislodgment. Also tape the junction of the chest tube and drainage tube to prevent their separation. Apply sterile drain dressings and tape them to the site.

▶ After insertion, the doctor checks tube placement with an X-ray. Check the patient's vital signs every 15 minutes for 1 hour and then as needed. Auscultate his lungs at least every 4 hours to assess air exchange in the affected lung. Diminished or absent breath sounds mean that the lung hasn't re-expanded.

### Administering medication

▶ The doctor injects medication through the intrapleural catheter or chest tube with the nurse assisting.

▶ If the patient will receive chemotherapy, expect to give an antiemetic at least 30 minutes beforehand.

▶ Position the patient with the affected side up. Help the doctor move the dressing away from the intrapleural catheter or chest tube and clamp the drainage tube, if present.

▶ The doctor disinfects the access port of the catheter or chest tube with antiseptic-soaked gauze. Draw up the appropriate medication dose and hand it to the doctor with the vial for verification.

▶ The doctor injects the medication. If it's an anesthetic, he gives a bolus or loading dose initially and then a continuous infusion. For tetracycline, he mixes it with an anesthetic, such as lidocaine, to alleviate pain during injection.

▶ Reapply the dressings around the catheter. Monitor the patient closely during and after drug administration to gauge the effectiveness of drug therapy and to check for complications and adverse effects.

## Special considerations

▶ Make sure the patient has signed a consent form.

▶ Before catheter insertion, ask the patient to urinate to reduce the risk of bladder perforation and promote comfort. If the patient is receiving a continuous infusion, label the solution bag clearly. Cover all injection ports so that other drugs aren't injected into the pleural space accidentally.

▶ If the chest tube dislodges, cover the site at once with a sterile gauze pad and tape it in place. Stay with the patient, monitor his vital signs, and observe carefully for signs and symptoms of tension pneumothorax: hypotension, distended neck veins, absent breath sounds, tracheal shift, hypoxemia, dyspnea, tachypnea, diaphoresis, chest pain, and weak, rapid pulse. Have another nurse call the doctor and gather the equipment for reinsertion.

▶ Keep rubber-tipped clamps at the bedside. If a commercial chest tube system cracks or a tube disconnects, use the clamps to clamp the chest tube close to the insertion site temporarily. Make sure to observe the patient closely for signs of tension pneumothorax because no air can escape from the pleural space while the tube is clamped.

▶ You can wrap a piece of petroleum gauze around the chest tube at the insertion site to make an airtight seal; then apply the sterile dressing. After the chest tube is removed, use petroleum gauze to dress the

wound; then cover it with a new piece of sterile gauze.

▶ After the catheter is removed, inspect the skin at the entry site for signs of infection and then cover the wound with a sterile dressing.

## Complications

Pneumothorax or tension pneumothorax may occur if the doctor accidentally injects air into the pleural cavity. These complications are more likely to occur in a patient who is on mechanical ventilation.

Accidental catheter placement in the lung can lead to respiratory distress; catheter placement within a vessel can increase the medication's effects. With catheter fracture, lung puncture may occur. Laceration of intercostal vessels can cause bleeding.

Local anesthetic toxicity can lead to tinnitus, metallic taste, light-headedness, somnolence, visual and auditory disturbances, restlessness, delirium, slurred speech, nystagmus, muscle tremor, seizures, arrhythmias, and cardiovascular collapse. A local anesthetic containing epinephrine can cause tachycardia and hypertension.

Intrapleural chemotherapeutic drugs can irritate the pleura chemically and cause such systemic effects as neutropenia and thrombocytopenia. Administering intrapleural tetracycline without an anesthetic can cause pain.

The insertion site can become infected. However, meticulous skin preparation, strict sterile technique, and sterile dressings usually prevent infection.

## Documentation

▶ Document the drug administered, drug dosage, patient's response to the treatment, and condition of the catheter insertion site.

### REFERENCES

Craven, R., and Hirnle, C.J. *Fundamentals of Nursing: Human Health and Function,* 4th ed. Philadelphia: Lippincott Williams & Wilkins, 2002.

Yellin, A., et al. "Hyperthermic Pleural Perfusion with Cisplatin: Early Clinical Experience," *Cancer* 92(8):2197-203, October 2001.

# Nasal medications

Nasal medications may be instilled by means of drops, a spray (using an atomizer), or an aerosol (using a nebulizer). Most drugs instilled by these methods produce local rather than systemic effects. Drops can be directed at a specific area; sprays and aerosols diffuse medication throughout the nasal passages.

Most nasal medications, such as phenylephrine, are vasoconstrictors, which relieve nasal congestion by coating and shrinking swollen mucous membranes. Because vasoconstrictors may be absorbed systemically, they are usually contraindicated in hypersensitive patients. Other types of nasal medications include antiseptics, anesthetics, and corticosteroids. Local anesthetics may be administered to promote patient comfort during rhinolaryngologic examination, laryngoscopy, bronchoscopy, and endotracheal intubation. Corticosteroids reduce inflammation in allergic or inflammatory conditions and nasal polyps.

## Equipment
Prescribed medication • patient's medication record and chart • emesis basin (with nose drops only) • facial tissues • optional: pillow, small piece of soft rubber or plastic tubing, gloves

## Implementation
▶ Verify the order on the patient's medication record by checking it against the doctor's order. Note the concentration of the medication. Phenylephrine, for example, is available in various concentrations from 0.125% to 1%. Verify the expiration date.
▶ Confirm the patient's identity by asking his name and checking the name, room number, and bed number on his wristband.
▶ Explain the procedure and provide privacy.
▶ Wash your hands. Put on gloves if you notice drainage from the nostrils.

### Instilling nose drops
▶ When possible, position the patient so that the drops flow back into the nostrils, toward the affected area. (See *Positioning the patient for nose drop instillation,* page 132.)
▶ Draw up some medication into the dropper.

▶ Push up the tip of the patient's nose slightly. Position the dropper just above the nostril, and direct its tip toward the midline of the nose so that the drops flow toward the back of the nasal cavity rather than down the throat.
▶ Insert the dropper about ⅜" (1 cm) into the nostril. Don't let the dropper touch the sides of the nostril because this would contaminate the dropper or could cause the patient to sneeze.
▶ Instill the prescribed number of drops, observing the patient carefully for signs of discomfort.
▶ To prevent the drops from leaking out of the nostrils, ask him to keep his head tilted back for at least 5 minutes and to breathe through his mouth. This also allows sufficient time for the medication to constrict mucous membranes.
▶ Keep an emesis basin handy so the patient can expectorate any medication that flows into the oropharynx and mouth. Use a facial tissue to wipe any excess medication from the patient's nostrils and face.
▶ Clean the dropper by separating the plunger and pipette and flushing them with warm water. Allow them to air-dry.

### Using a nasal spray
▶ Have the patient sit upright with his head tilted back slightly. Alternatively, have the patient lie on his back with his shoulders elevated, neck hyperextended, and head tilted back over the edge of the bed. Support his head with one hand to prevent neck strain.
▶ Remove the protective cap from the atomizer.
▶ To prevent air from entering the nasal cavity and to allow the medication to flow properly, occlude one of the patient's nostrils with your finger. Insert the atomizer tip into the open nostril.
▶ Instruct the patient to inhale, and as he does so, squeeze the atomizer once, quickly and firmly. Use just enough force to coat the inside of the patient's nose with medication. Then tell the patient to exhale through his mouth.
▶ If ordered, spray the nostril again. Then repeat the procedure in the other nostril.
▶ Instruct the patient to keep his head tilted back for several minutes and to breathe slowly through his nose so the medication has time to work. Tell him not to blow his nose for several minutes.

# Positioning the patient for nose drop instillation

To reach the ethmoid and sphenoid sinuses, have the patient lie on her back with her neck hyperextended and her head tilted back over the edge of the bed. Support her head with one hand to prevent neck strain.

To reach the maxillary and frontal sinuses, have the patient lie on her back with her head toward the affected side and hanging slightly over the edge of the bed. Ask her to rotate her head laterally after hyperextension, and support her head with one hand to prevent neck strain.

To administer drops to relieve ordinary nasal congestion, help the patient to a reclining or supine position with her head tilted slightly toward the affected side. Aim the dropper upward, toward the patient's eye, rather than downward, toward her ear.

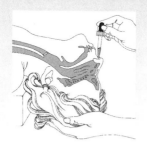 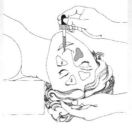 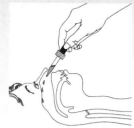

## Using a nasal aerosol

▶ Instruct the patient to blow his nose gently to clear his nostrils.

▶ Insert the medication cartridge according to the manufacturer's directions. With some models, you'll fit the medication cartridge over a small hole in the adapter. When inserting a refill cartridge, first remove the protective cap from the stem. Spacer inhalers may be recommended.

▶ Shake the aerosol well before each use, and remove the protective cap from the adapter tip.

▶ Hold the aerosol between your thumb and index finger, with your index finger positioned on top of the medication cartridge.

▶ Tilt the patient's head back, and carefully insert the adapter tip in one nostril while sealing the other nostril with your finger.

▶ Press the adapter and cartridge together firmly to release one measured dose of medication.

▶ Shake the aerosol and repeat the procedure to instill medication into the other nostril.

▶ Remove the medication cartridge and wash the nasal adapter in lukewarm water daily. Allow the adapter to dry before reinserting the cartridge.

## Special considerations

◆ **ALERT!** Before instilling nose drops in a young child, attach a small piece of tubing to the end of the dropper. Do the same for an uncooperative patient.

▶ If using a metered-dose pump spray system, prime the delivery system with 4 sprays or until a fine mist appears. Reprime the system with 2 sprays or until a fine mist appears if 3 or more days have lapsed since the last use.

▶ When using an aerosol, be careful not to puncture or incinerate the pressurized cartridge. Store it at temperatures below 120° F (48.9° C).

▶ To prevent the spread of infection, label the medication bottle so that it will be used only for that patient.

▶ Teach the patient how to instill nasal medications correctly so that he can continue treatment after discharge, if necessary. Caution him against using nasal medications longer than prescribed because they may cause a rebound effect that worsens the condition. A rebound effect occurs when the medication loses it effectiveness and relaxes the vessels in the nasal turbinates, producing a stuffiness that can be relieved only by discontinuing the medication.

▶ Inform the patient of possible adverse reactions. In addition, explain that when corticosteroids are given by nasal aerosol, therapeutic effects may not appear for 2 days to 2 weeks.

▶ Teach the patient good oral and nasal hygiene.

## Complications

Some nasal medications may cause restlessness, palpitations, nervousness, and other systemic effects. For example, excessive use of corticosteroid aerosols may cause hyperadrenocorticism and adrenal suppression.

## Documentation

▶ Record the medication instilled and its concentration, the number of drops or instillations given, and whether the medication was instilled in one or both nostrils.

▶ Note the time and date of instillation and of any resulting adverse effects.

### REFERENCES

Bachert, C., and El-Akkad, T. "Patient Preferences and Sensory Comparisons of Three Intranasal Corticosteroids for the Treatment of Allergic Rhinitis," *Annals of Allergy Asthma & Immunology* 89(3):292-97, September 2002.

Craven, R., and Hirnle, C.J. *Fundamentals of Nursing: Human Health and Function,* 4th ed. Philadelphia: Lippincott Williams & Wilkins, 2002.

# Nasogastric tube drug instillation

Besides providing an alternate means of nourishment, the nasogastric (NG) tube or gastrostomy tube allows direct instillation of medication into the GI system of patients who can't ingest the drug orally. Before instillation, the patency and positioning of the tube must be carefully checked because the procedure is contraindicated if the tube is obstructed or improperly positioned, if the patient is vomiting around the tube, or if his bowel sounds are absent.

Oily medications and enteric-coated or sustained-release tablets or capsules are contraindicated for instillation through an NG tube. Oily medications cling to the sides of the tube and resist mixing with the irrigating solution, and crushing enteric-coated or sustained-released tablets to facilitate transport through the tube destroys their intended properties.

## Equipment

Patient's medication record and chart ● prescribed medication ● towel or linen-saver pad ● 50- or 60-ml piston-type catheter-tip syringe ● feeding tubing ● two 4″ × 4″ gauze pads ● stethoscope ● gloves ● diluent cup for mixing medication and fluid ● spoon ● 50 ml of water ● rubber band ● gastrostomy tube and funnel, if needed ● optional: mortar and pestle, clamp

For maximum control of suction, use a piston syringe instead of a bulb syringe. The liquid for diluting the medication can be juice, water, or a nutritional supplement.

### Preparation of equipment

Gather equipment for use at the bedside. Liquids should be at room temperature. Administering cold liquids through an NG tube can cause abdominal cramping. Although this is not a sterile procedure, make sure the cup, syringe, spoon, and gauze are clean.

## Implementation

▶ Verify the order on the patient's medication record by checking it against the doctor's order.

▶ Wash your hands and put on gloves.

▶ Check the label on the medication three times before preparing it for administration to make sure you'll be giving the medication correctly.

▶ If the prescribed medication is in tablet form, crush the tablets to ready them for mixing in a cup with the diluting liquid. Request liquid forms of medications, if available. Bring the medication and equipment to the patient's bedside.

▶ Explain the procedure to the patient, if necessary, and provide privacy.

▶ Confirm the patient's identity by asking his name and checking the name, room number, and bed number on his wristband.

▶ Unpin the tube from the patient's gown. To avoid soiling the sheets during the procedure, fold back the bed linens to the patient's waist and drape his chest with a towel or linen-saver pad.

▶ Elevate the head of the bed so that the patient is in Fowler's position, as tolerated.

# Giving medications through an NG tube

Holding the nasogastric (NG) tube at a level somewhat above the patient's nose, pour up to 30 ml of diluted medication into the syringe barrel. To prevent air from entering the patient's stomach, hold the tube at a slight angle and add more medication before the syringe empties. If necessary, raise the tube slightly higher to increase the flow rate.

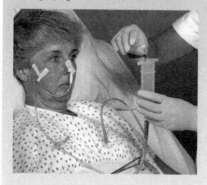

After you've delivered the whole dose, position the patient on her right side, head slightly elevated, to minimize esophageal reflux.

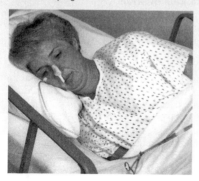

▶ After unclamping the tube, take the 50- or 60-ml syringe and create a 10-cc air space in its chamber. Then attach the syringe to the end of the tube.

▶ Auscultate the patient's abdomen about 3″ (7.6 cm) below the sternum with the stethoscope. Then gently insert 10 cc of air into the tube. When you hear the air bubble entering the stomach, gently draw back on the piston of the syringe. The appearance of gastric contents implies that the tube is patent and in the stomach. (However, only an X-ray can positively confirm the tube's position.) If no gastric contents appear when you draw back on the syringe, the tube may have risen into the esophagus, and you'll have to advance it before proceeding.

▶ If you meet resistance when aspirating, stop the procedure. Resistance may indicate a nonpatent tube or improper tube placement. (Keep in mind that some smaller NG tubes may collapse when aspiration is attempted.) If the tube seems to be in the stomach, resistance probably means the tube is lying against the stomach wall. To relieve resistance, withdraw the tube slightly or turn the patient.

▶ After you have established that the tube is patent and in the correct position, clamp the tube, detach the syringe, and lay the end of the tube on the 4″ × 4″ gauze pad.

▶ Mix the crushed tablets or liquid medication with the diluent. If the medication is in capsule form, open the capsules and empty their contents into the liquid. Pour liquid medications directly into the diluting liquid. Stir well with the spoon. (If the medication was in tablet form, make sure the particles are small enough to pass through the eyes at the distal end of the tube.)

▶ Reattach the syringe, without the piston, to the end of the tube and open the clamp.

▶ Deliver the medication slowly and steadily. (See *Giving medications through an NG tube.*)

▶ If the medication flows smoothly, slowly add more until the entire dose has been given. If the medication does not flow properly, don't force it. If it's too thick, dilute it with water. If you suspect that tube placement is inhibiting the flow, stop the procedure and reevaluate tube placement.

▶ Watch the patient's reaction throughout the instillation. If he shows any sign of discomfort, stop the procedure immediately.

▶ As the last of the medication flows out of the syringe, start to irrigate the tube by adding 30 to 50 ml of water. Irrigation clears medication from the sides of the tube and from the distal end, reducing the risk of clogging.

◆ **ALERT!** For a child, irrigate the tube using only 15 to 30 ml of water.

▶ When the water stops flowing, quickly clamp the tube. Detach the syringe and dispose of it.

▶ Fasten the NG tube to the patient's gown.
▶ Remove the towel or linen-saver pad and replace bed linens.
▶ Leave the patient in Fowler's position, or have him lie on his right side with the head of the bed partially elevated. Have him maintain this position for at least 30 minutes after the procedure to facilitate the downward flow of medication into his stomach and prevent esophageal reflux.
▶ You may be asked to deliver medications through a gastrostomy tube. (See *Giving medications through a gastrostomy tube.*) If medication is prescribed for a patient with a gastrostomy feeding button, ask the doctor to order the liquid form of the drug, if possible. If not, you may give a tablet or capsule if dissolved in 30 to 50 ml of warm water (15 to 30 ml for children). To administer medication this way, use the same procedure as for feeding the patient through the button. Then draw up the dissolved medication into a syringe and inject it into the feeding tube.
▶ Withdraw the medication syringe, and flush the tube with 50 ml of warm water.
◆ **ALERT!** For a child, flush the tube with 30 ml of water.
▶ Then replace the safety plug, and keep the patient upright at a 30-degree angle for 30 minutes after giving the medication.

### Special considerations

▶ To prevent installation of too much fluid (more than 400 ml of liquid at one time for an adult), don't schedule the drug installation with the patient's regular tube feeding, if possible.
▶ If you must schedule a tube feed and medication instillation simultaneously, give the medication first to ensure that the patient receives the prescribed drug therapy even if he can't tolerate an entire feeding. Remember to avoid giving foods that interact adversely with the drug. Tube feedings of Osmolite or Isocal must be held 2 hours before and 2 hours after phenytoin administration.
▶ If the patient receives continuous tube feedings, stop the feeding and check the quantity of residual stomach contents. If it's more than 50% of the previous hour' intake, withhold the medication and feeding and notify the doctor. An excessive amount of residual contents may indicate intestinal obstruction or paralytic ileus.

## Giving medications through a gastrostomy tube

Surgically inserted into the stomach, a gastrostomy tube reduces the risk of fluid aspiration, a constant danger with a nasogastric (NG) tube. To administer medication by this route, prepare the patient and medication as for an NG tube. Then gently lift the dressing around the tube to assess the skin for irritation. Report any irritation to the doctor. If none appears, follow these steps:
▶ Remove the dressing that covers the tube. Then remove the dressing or plug at the tip of the tube, and attach the syringe or funnel to the tip.
▶ Release the clamp and instill about 10 ml of water into the tube through the syringe to check for patency. If the water flows in easily, the tube is patent. If it flows in slowly, raise the funnel to increase pressure. If the water still doesn't flow properly, stop the procedure and notify the doctor.
▶ Pour up to 30 ml of medication into the syringe or funnel. Tilt the tube to allow air to escape as the fluid flows downward. Just before the syringe empties, add medication as needed.
▶ After giving the medication, pour in about 30 ml of water to irrigate the tube.
▶ Tighten the clamp, place a 4″ × 4″ gauze pad on the end of the tube, and secure it with a rubber band.
▶ Cover the tube with two more 4″ × 4″ gauze pads, and secure them firmly with tape.
▶ Keep the head of the bed elevated for at least 30 minutes after the procedure to aid digestion.

▶ If the NG tube is attached to suction, be sure to turn off the suction for 20 to 30 minutes after administering medication.
▶ If possible, teach the patient who requires long-term treatment to instill his medication himself through the NG tube. Have him observe the procedure several times before trying it himself.
▶ Remain with the patient when he performs the procedure for the first few times so that you can provide assistance and answer any questions. Encourage him and correct any errors in technique, as necessary.

## Documentation
▶ Record the instillation of medication, date and time of instillation, dose, and the patient's tolerance of the procedure.
▶ On his intake and output sheet, note the amount of fluid instilled.

### REFERENCES
Bowers, S. "All About Tubes: Your Guide to Enteral Feeding Devices," *Nursing2000* 30(12):41-47, December 2000.

Craven, R., and Hirnle, C.J. *Fundamentals of Nursing: Human Health and Function,* 4th ed. Philadelphia: Lippincott Williams & Wilkins, 2002.

Guenter, P., and Silkroski, M. *Tube Feeding: Practical Guidelines and Nursing Protocols.* Gaithersburg, Md.: Aspen Pubs., Inc., 2001.

# Ommaya reservoir

Also known as a subcutaneous CSF reservoir, the Ommaya reservoir allows delivery of long-term drug therapy to the CSF by way of the brain's ventricles. The reservoir spares the patient repeated lumbar punctures to administer chemotherapeutic drugs, analgesics, antibiotics, and antifungals. It's most commonly used for chemotherapy and pain management, specifically for treating central nervous system (CNS) leukemia, malignant CNS disease, and meningeal carcinomatosis.

The reservoir is a mushroom-shaped silicone apparatus with an attached catheter. It's surgically implanted beneath the patient's scalp in the nondominant lobe, and the catheter is threaded into the ventricle through a burr hole in the skull. (See *How the Ommaya reservoir works.*) Besides providing convenient, comparatively painless access to CSF, the Ommaya reservoir permits consistent and predictable drug distribution throughout the subarachnoid space and CNS. It also allows for measurement of intracranial pressure (ICP).

Before reservoir insertion, the patient may receive a local or general anesthetic, depending on his condition and the doctor's preference. After an X-ray confirms placement of the reservoir, a pressure dressing is applied for 24 hours, followed by a gauze dressing for another day or two. The sutures may be removed in about 10 days. However, the reservoir can be used within 48 hours to deliver drugs, obtain CSF pressure measurements, drain CSF, and withdraw CSF specimens.

The doctor usually injects drugs into the Ommaya reservoir, but a specially trained nurse may perform this procedure if allowed by your facility's policy and the state's nurse practice act. This sterile procedure usually takes 15 to 30 minutes.

## Equipment
Equipment varies but may include the following:
Preservative-free prescribed drug ● gloves ● povidone-iodine solution ● sterile towel ● two 3-ml syringes ● 25G needle or 22G Huber needle ● sterile gauze pad ● collection tubes for CSF, if ordered ● vial of bacteriostatic normal saline solution

### Preparation of equipment
Using the sterile towel, establish a sterile field near the patient. Prepare a syringe with the preservative-free drug to be instilled and place it, the CSF collection tubes, and the normal saline solution on the sterile field.

## Implementation
▶ If your patient is scheduled to receive an Ommaya reservoir, explain the procedure before reservoir insertion. Be sure the patient and his family understand the potential complications, and answer any questions they may have. Reassure the patient that any hair shaved for the implant will grow back and that only a coin-sized patch must remain shaved for injections. (Hair regrowth will be slower if the patient is receiving chemotherapy.)

### Instilling medication
▶ Obtain baseline vital signs.
▶ Position the patient so that he's either sitting or reclining.
▶ Put on gloves and prepare the patient's scalp with the povidone-iodine solution, working in a circular motion from the center outward.
▶ Placing the 25G needle at a 45-degree angle, insert it into the reservoir and aspirate 3 ml of clear CSF into a syringe. (If the aspirate isn't clear, check with the doctor before continuing.)
▶ Continue to aspirate as many milliliters of CSF as you will instill of the drug. Then detach the syringe from the needle hub, at-

tach the drug syringe, and instill the medication slowly, monitoring for headache, nausea, and dizziness. (Some facilities use the CSF instead of a preservative-free diluent to deliver the drug.)

▶ Instruct the patient to lie quietly for about 15 to 30 minutes after the procedure. This may prevent meningeal irritation leading to nausea and vomiting.

▶ Cover the site with a sterile gauze pad, and apply gentle pressure for a moment or two until superficial bleeding stops.

▶ Monitor the patient for adverse drug reactions and signs of increased ICP, such as nausea, vomiting, pain, and dizziness. Assess for adverse reactions every 30 minutes for 2 hours, then every hour for 2 hours, and finally every 4 hours.

### Special considerations

▶ The doctor may prescribe an antiemetic to be administered 30 minutes before the procedure to control nausea and vomiting.

▶ After the reservoir is implanted, the patient may resume normal activities. Instruct him to protect the site from bumps and traumatic injury while the incision heals. Tell him that unless complications develop, the reservoir may function for years.

▶ Instruct the patient and his family to notify the doctor if any signs of infection develop at the insertion site (for example, redness, swelling, tenderness, or drainage) or if the patient develops headache, neck stiffness, or fever, which may indicate a systemic infection.

### Complications

Infection may develop but can usually be treated successfully by injection of antibiotics directly into the reservoir. Persistent infection may require removal of the reservoir.

Catheter migration or blockage may cause symptoms of increased ICP, such as headache and nausea. If the doctor suspects this problem, he may gently push and release the reservoir several times (a technique called pumping). With his finger on the patient's scalp, the doctor can feel the reservoir refill. Slow filling suggests catheter migration or blockage, which must be confirmed by a computed tomography scan. Surgical correction is required.

## How the Ommaya reservoir works

To insert an Ommaya reservoir, the doctor drills a burr hole and inserts the device's catheter through the patient's nondominant frontal lobe into the lateral ventricle. The reservoir, which has a self-sealing silicone injection dome, rests over the burr hole under a scalp flap. This creates a slight, soft bulge on the scalp about the size of a quarter. Usually, drugs are injected into the dome with a syringe.

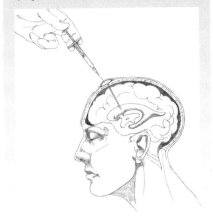

### Documentation

▶ Record the appearance of the reservoir insertion site before and after access, the patient's tolerance of the procedure, the amount of CSF withdrawn and its appearance, and the name and dose of the drug instilled.

### REFERENCES

Craven, R., and Hirnle, C.J. *Fundamentals of Nursing: Human Health and Function,* 4th ed. Philadelphia: Lippincott Williams & Wilkins, 2002.

Park, D.M., and DeAngelis, L.M. "Delayed Infection of the Ommaya Reservoir," *Neurology* 59(6):956-57, September 2002.

## Oral drugs

Because oral administration is usually the safest, most convenient, and least expensive method, most drugs are administered

## Measuring liquid medications

To pour liquids, hold the medication cup at eye level. Use your thumb to mark off the correct level on the cup (see illustration). Then set the cup down and read the bottom of the meniscus at eye level to ensure accuracy. If you've poured too much medication into the cup, discard the excess. Don't return it to the bottle.

Here are a few additional tips:

▶ Hold the container so that the medication flows from the side opposite the label so it won't run down the container and stain or obscure the label. Remove drips from the lip of the bottle first and then from the sides, using a clean, damp paper towel.

▶ For a liquid measured in drops, use only the dropper supplied with the medication.

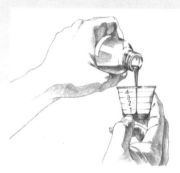

by this route. Drugs for oral administration are available in many forms: tablets, enteric-coated tablets, capsules, syrups, elixirs, oils, liquids, suspensions, powders, and granules. Some require special preparation before administration, such as mixing with juice to make them more palatable; oils, powders, and granules most often require such preparation.

Sometimes oral drugs are prescribed in higher dosages than their parenteral equivalents because after absorption through the GI system they are immediately broken down by the liver before they reach the systemic circulation.

◆ **ALERT!** Oral dosages normally prescribed for adults may be dangerous for elderly patients.

Oral administration is contraindicated for unconscious patients; it may also be contraindicated in patients with nausea and vomiting and in those unable to swallow.

### Equipment

Patient's medication record and chart ● prescribed medication ● medication cup ● optional: appropriate vehicle, such as jelly or applesauce, for crushed pills commonly used with children or elderly patients, and juice, water, or milk for liquid medications; drinking straw; mortar and pestle for crushing pills

### Implementation

▶ Verify the order on the patient's medication record by checking it against the doctor's order.

▶ Wash your hands.

▶ Check the label on the medication three times before administering it to make sure you'll be giving the prescribed medication. Check when you take the container from the shelf or drawer, again before you pour the medication into the medication cup, and again before returning the container to the shelf or drawer. If you're administering a unit-dose medication, check the label for the final time at the patient's bedside immediately after pouring the medication and before discarding the wrapper.

▶ Confirm the patient's identity by asking his name and checking the name, room number, and bed number on his wristband.

▶ Assess the patient's condition, including level of consciousness and vital signs, as needed. Changes in the patient's condition may warrant withholding medication. For example, you may need to withhold a medication that will slow the patient's heart rate if his apical pulse rate is less than 60 beats/minute, but a doctor's order should be obtained if the medication is withheld.

▶ Give the patient his medication and an appropriate vehicle or liquid, as needed, to aid swallowing, minimize adverse effects, or promote absorption. For example, cyclophosphamide is given with fluids to minimize adverse effects; antitussive cough syrup is given without a fluid to avoid diluting its soothing effect on the throat. If appropriate, crush the medication to facilitate swallowing.

Stay with the patient until he has swallowed the drug. If he seems confused or disoriented, check his mouth to make sure he has swallowed it. Return and reassess the patient's response within 1 hour after giving the medication.

## Special considerations

Make sure you have a written order for every medication given. Verbal orders should be signed by the doctor within the specified time period. (Hospitals usually require a signature within 24 hours; long-term-care facilities, within 48 hours.)

Use care in measuring out the prescribed dose of liquid oral medication. (See *Measuring liquid medications.*)

Don't give medication from a poorly labeled or unlabeled container. Don't attempt to label or reinforce drug labels yourself. This must be done by a pharmacist.

Never give a medication poured by someone else. Never allow your medication cart or tray out of your sight. This prevents anyone from rearranging the medications or taking one without your knowledge. Never return unwrapped or prepared medications to stock containers. Instead, dispose of them and notify the pharmacy. Keep in mind that the disposal of any narcotic drug must be cosigned by another nurse, as mandated by law.

If the patient questions you about his medication or the dosage, check his medication record again. If the medication is correct, reassure him. Make sure you tell him about any changes in his medication or dosage. Instruct him, as appropriate, about possible adverse effects. Ask him to report anything he thinks may be an adverse effect.

To avoid damaging or staining the patient's teeth, administer acid or iron preparations through a straw. An unpleasant-tasting liquid can usually be made more palatable if taken through a straw because the liquid contacts fewer taste buds.

If the patient can't swallow a whole tablet or capsule, ask the pharmacist if the drug is available in liquid form or if it can be administered by another route. If not, ask him if you can crush the tablet or open the capsule and mix it with food. Keep in mind that many enteric-coated or time-release medications and gelatin capsules shouldn't be crushed. Remember to contact the doctor for an order to change the administration route when necessary.

Oral medications are relatively easy to give to infants because of their natural sucking instinct and, in infants younger than age 4 months, their undeveloped sense of taste.

## Documentation

Note the drug administered, dose, date and time, and patient's reaction, if any. If the patient refuses a drug, document the refusal and notify the charge nurse and the patient's doctor, as needed.

Note if a drug was omitted or withheld for other reasons, such as radiology or laboratory tests, or if, in your judgment, the drug was contraindicated at the ordered time. Sign out all narcotics given on the appropriate narcotics central record.

### REFERENCES

Ansel, H.C., et al. *Pharmaceutical Dosage Forms and Drug Delivery Systems,* 7th ed. Philadelphia: Lippincott Williams & Wilkins, 1999.

Craven, R., and Hirnle, C.J. *Fundamentals of Nursing: Human Health and Function,* 4th ed. Philadelphia: Lippincott Williams & Wilkins, 2002.

# Pediatric medication administration

Because a child responds to drugs more rapidly and unpredictably than an adult, pediatric drug administration requires special care. Such factors as age, weight, body surface area, and drug form and route may dramatically affect a child's response to a drug. For example, because of his thin epithelium, a neonate or an infant absorbs topical medications much faster than an older child does.

Certain disorders also affect a child's response to medication. For example, gastroenteritis increases gastric motility, which in turn impairs absorption of certain oral medications. Liver or kidney disorders can hinder the metabolism of some medications.

Usual drug administration techniques may need adjustment to account for the child's age, size, and developmental level. A tablet for a young child, for example, may be crushed and mixed with a liquid for oral administration. In addition, the injection site and needle size will vary depending on the child's age and physical development.

## Equipment

*For oral medications*
Prescribed medication ● plastic disposable syringe, plastic medicine dropper, or spoon ● medication cup ● water, syrup, or jelly (for tablets) ● optional: fruit juice

*For injectable medications*
Prescribed medication ● appropriately sized syringe and needle ● alcohol pads or povidone-iodine solution ● gloves ● gauze pad ● adhesive bandage ● optional: cold compress, eutectic mixture of local anesthetic (EMLA), and transparent occlusive dressing

### Preparation of equipment
Check the doctor's order for the prescribed drug, dosage, and route. Compare the order with the drug label, check the drug expiration date, and review the patient's chart for drug allergies.

Carefully calculate the dosage, if necessary, and have another nurse verify it. Typically, you'll double-check dosages for potentially hazardous or lethal drugs, such as insulin, heparin, digoxin, epinephrine, and narcotics. Check your facility's policy to learn which drugs must be calculated and checked by two nurses.

For giving an injection, select the appropriate needle. Typically, for I.M. injections in infants, you'll use a 25G ¾″ needle and, in older children, a 23G 1″ needle. For subcutaneous injections, select a ¾″ or ½″ needle and, for intradermal medications, a 27G ½″ needle. To administer viscous medications, select a larger-gauge needle.

## Implementation
▶ Assess the child's condition to determine the need for the medication and the effectiveness of previous therapy.
▶ Carefully observe the child for a rash, pruritus, cough, or other signs of an adverse reaction to a previously administered drug.
▶ Identify the child by comparing the name on his wristband with that on the medication card. If the child can talk and respond, ask him his name.

▶ Explain the procedure to the child and his parents. Use terms the child can understand. Give the child choices, if possible; for example, ask the child if he wants the medication mixed with chocolate or strawberry syrup.
▶ Provide privacy, especially for an older child.

### Giving oral medication to an infant
▶ Use either a plastic syringe without a needle or a drug-specific medicine dropper to measure the dose. If the medication comes in tablet form, first crush the tablet (if appropriate) and mix it with water or syrup. Then draw the mixture into the syringe or dropper.
▶ Pick up the infant, raising his head and shoulders or turning his head to one side to prevent aspiration. Hold the infant close to your body to help restrain him.
▶ Using your thumb, press down on the infant's chin to open his mouth.
▶ Slide the syringe or medicine dropper into the infant's mouth alongside his tongue. (See *Giving oral medication to an infant.*) Release the medication slowly to let the infant swallow and to prevent choking. If appropriate, allow him to suck on the syringe as you expel the medication.
▶ If not contraindicated, give fruit juice after giving medication.
▶ Place a particularly small or inactive infant on his side or back as recommended by the American Academy of Pediatrics to decrease the risk of sudden infant death syndrome. Allow an active infant to assume a position that is comfortable for him; avoid forcing him into a side-lying position to prevent agitation.

### Giving oral medication to a toddler
▶ Use a plastic, disposable syringe or dropper to measure liquid medication. Then transfer the fluid to a medication cup.
▶ Elevate the toddler's head and shoulders to prevent aspiration.
▶ If possible, ask him to help hold the cup to enlist his cooperation. Otherwise, hold the cup to the toddler's lips or use a syringe or a spoon to administer the liquid. Make sure that the toddler ingests all of the medication.
▶ If the medication is in tablet form, first crush the tablet, if appropriate, and mix it with water, syrup, or jelly. Use a spoon, sy-

ringe, or dropper to administer the medication.

▶ Don't crush enteric-coated or slow- or time-release drugs because doing so may alter absorption, change the taste, or irritate mucus membranes.

### Giving oral medication to an older child

▶ If possible, let the child choose both the liquid medication mixer and a beverage to drink after taking the medication.

▶ If appropriate, allow him to choose where he'll take the medication, for example, sitting in bed or sitting on a parent's lap.

▶ If the medication comes in tablet or capsule form and if the child is old enough (between ages 4 and 6), teach him how to swallow solid medication. (If he already knows how to do this, review the procedure with him for safety's sake.) Tell him to place the pill on the back of his tongue and to swallow it immediately by drinking water or juice. Focus most of your explanation on the water or juice to draw the child's attention away from the pill. Make sure the child drinks enough water or juice to keep the pill from lodging in his esophagus. Afterward, look inside the child's mouth to confirm that he swallowed the pill.

▶ If the child can't swallow the pill whole, crush it (if appropriate) and mix it with water, syrup, or jelly. Or, after checking with the child's doctor, order the medication in liquid form.

### Giving an I.M. injection

▶ Choose an injection site that is appropriate for the child's age and muscle mass. If time allows, place an EMLA cream on the intended skin site at least 1 hour before the procedure. Don't spread the cream or rub it in. Cover with a transparent occlusive dressing.

▶ Immediately before the procedure, remove the dressing and wipe the skin with a gauze pad to remove the cream. (See *I.M. injection sites in children,* page 142.)

▶ Position the patient appropriately for the site chosen and locate key landmarks, for example, the posterior superior iliac spine and the greater trochanter. Have someone help you restrain an infant; seek an older child's cooperation before enlisting assistance.

▶ Put on gloves. Clean the injection site with an alcohol or povidone-iodine pad.

## Giving oral medication to an infant

Use a dropper or syringe without a needle to administer an oral medication to an infant. Place the dropper or syringe at the corner of the infant's mouth so the medication will run into the pocket between the infant's cheek and gum. This keeps him from spitting it out and reduces the risk of aspiration.

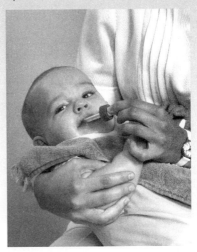

Wipe outward from the center with a spiral motion to avoid contaminating the clean area.

▶ Grasp the tissue surrounding the site between your index finger and thumb to immobilize the site and to create a muscle mass for the injection.

▶ Insert the needle quickly, using a darting motion. If you're using the ventrogluteal site, insert the needle at a 45-degree angle toward the knee.

▶ Aspirate the plunger to ensure that the needle isn't in a blood vessel. If no blood appears, inject the medication slowly so that the muscle can distend to accommodate the volume.

▶ Withdraw the needle and gently massage the area with a gauze pad to stimulate circulation and enhance absorption.

▶ Provide comfort and praise.

# I.M. injection sites in children

When selecting the best site for a child's I.M. injections, consider the child's age, weight, and muscular development; the amount of subcutaneous fat over the injection site; the type of drug you're administering; and the drug's absorption rate.

## Vastus lateralis or rectus femoris muscle

For a child younger than age 3, you'll typically use the vastus lateralis or rectus femoris muscle for an I.M. injection. Constituting the largest muscle mass in this age-group, the vastus lateralis and rectus femoris have fewer major blood vessels and nerves.

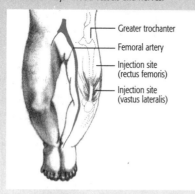

## Ventrogluteal or dorsogluteal muscle

For a child who can walk and is older than age 3, use the ventrogluteal and dorsogluteal muscles. Like the vastus lateralis, the ventrogluteal site is relatively free of major blood vessels and nerves. Before you select either site, make sure that the child has been walking for at least 1 year to ensure sufficient muscle development.

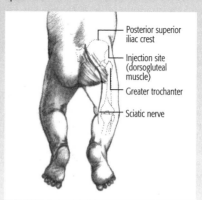

## Deltoid muscle

For a child older than 18 months who needs rapid medication results, consider using the deltoid muscle for the injections. Because blood flows faster in the deltoid muscle than in other muscles, drug absorption should be faster. Be careful if you use this site because the deltoid doesn't develop fully until adolescence. In a younger child, it's small and close to the radial nerve, which may be injured during needle insertion.

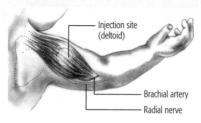

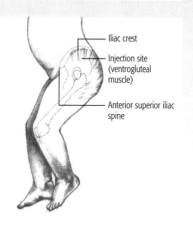

---

Giving a subcutaneous injection

▶ Select from these possible sites: the middle third of the upper outer arm, the middle third of the upper outer thigh, or the abdomen. You may apply a cold compress or EMLA, as described above, to the injection site to minimize pain.

Put on gloves and prepare the injection site with alcohol or povidone-iodine solution according to the patient's needs and your facility's policy.

Pinch the tissue surrounding the site between your index finger and thumb to ensure injection into the subcutaneous tissue. Holding the needle at a 45- to 90-degree angle, quickly insert it into the tissue. Release your grasp on the tissue and slowly inject the medication. Remove the needle quickly to decrease discomfort. Unless contraindicated, gently massage the area to facilitate the drug's absorption.

### Giving an intradermal injection

Put on gloves and pull the patient's skin taut (the site of choice is the inner aspect of the forearm).

Insert the needle, bevel up, at a 10- to 15-degree angle just beneath the outer skin layer.

Slowly inject the medication and watch for a bleb to appear. Quickly remove the needle, being careful to maintain the injection angle. If appropriate—for example, if the injection is related to allergy testing—draw a circle around the bleb and avoid massaging the area to avoid interfering with test results.

## Special considerations

Don't hesitate to consult the parents for tips on successfully giving medication to their child. If possible, have a parent administer a prescribed oral drug while you supervise. However, avoid asking a parent to help with injections because the child may perceive the parent as a cause of pain.

Aim for a trusting relationship with the child and his parents so that you can offer support and promote cooperation even when a medication causes discomfort. If the child will receive one injection, allow him to choose from the appropriate sites. However, if he'll receive numerous injections, remember that site rotation must follow a set pattern. Allow the child to play with a medication cup or syringe and to pretend to give medication to a doll.

When giving medication to an older child, be honest. Reassure him that distaste or discomfort will be brief. Emphasize that he must remain still to promote safety and minimize discomfort. Explain to the child and his parents that an assistant will help

the child remain still, if necessary. Keep your explanations brief and simple.

To divert the child's attention, have him start counting just before the injection and challenge him to try to reach 10 before you finish the injection. If the child cries, don't scold him or allow the parents to scold him. Have one of the parents hold a younger child and praise him for allowing you to give him the injection. You can also apply an adhesive bandage to the injection site as a form of reward or badge.

If the prescribed medication comes only in tablet form, consult the pharmacist (or an appropriate drug reference book) to make sure that crushing the tablet won't invalidate its effectiveness. Avoid adding medication to a large amount of liquid, such as the child's milk or formula, because the child may not drink the entire amount, resulting in an inaccurate dose of medication.

Because infants and toddlers can't tell you what effects they're experiencing from a medication, you must be alert for signs of an adverse reaction. Compile a list of appropriate emergency drugs, calculating the dosages to the patient's weight. Post the list near the patient's bed for reference in an emergency.

If you have any doubt about proper medication dosage, always consult the doctor who ordered the drug. Double-check information in a reliable drug reference.

EMLA cream isn't approved for use in infants less than age 1 month.

## Home care

Teach the parents about the proper dosage and administration of all prescribed medications. If the parents will administer a liquid medication, advise them to use a commercially available, disposable oral syringe to measure the dose. To ensure an accurate dose, advise them to avoid using a teaspoon. Teach them how to use the oral syringe. Use written materials—such as a medication instruction sheet—to reinforce your teaching.

If appropriate, teach the child and his parents about subcutaneous injectors. (See *Using subcutaneous injectors,* page 144.)

## Documentation

Record drug, form, dosage, date, time, administration route and site, effect of

## Using subcutaneous injectors

Currently available for use by patients at home, subcutaneous injectors feature disposable needles or pressure jets to deliver doses of prescribed medication such as short-acting insulin. Appropriate for use in children, these devices deliver medication safely and accurately. The NovoPen, for instance, has disposable needles and replacement cartridges. Preci-jet and MediJector draw their medications from standard bottles. A pressure jet deposits the drug in subcutaneous tissue.

Although still relatively expensive, these devices are easy to use. For example, studies indicate that jet-injected insulin disperses faster and is absorbed more rapidly because it avoids the puddling effect common with needle delivery.

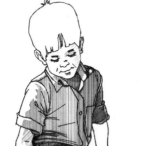

**NEEDLE INJECTION**

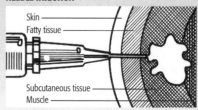

**PRESSURE-JET INJECTION**

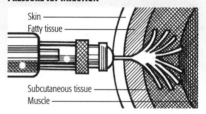

drug, the patient's tolerance of the procedure, complications, and nursing interventions.

▶ Note instructional activities related to medications.

### REFERENCES

Craven, R., and Hirnle, C.J. *Fundamentals of Nursing: Human Health and Function,* 4th ed. Philadelphia: Lippincott Williams & Wilkins, 2002.

Kaushal, R., et al. "Medication Errors and Adverse Drug Events in Pediatric Inpatients," *JAMA* 285(16):2114-20, April 2001.

## Rectal suppositories and ointments

A rectal suppository is a small, solid, medicated mass, usually cone-shaped, with a cocoa butter or glycerin base. It may be inserted to stimulate peristalsis and defecation or to relieve pain, vomiting, and local irritation. Rectal suppositories commonly contain drugs that reduce fever, induce relaxation, interact poorly with digestive enzymes, or have a taste too offensive for oral use. Rectal suppositories melt at body temperature and are absorbed slowly.

Because insertion of a rectal suppository may stimulate the vagus nerve, this procedure is contraindicated in patients with potential cardiac arrhythmias. It may have to be avoided in patients with recent rectal or prostate surgery because of the risk of local trauma or discomfort during insertion.

An ointment is a semisolid medication used to produce local effects. It may be applied externally to the anus or internally to the rectum. Rectal ointments commonly contain drugs that reduce inflammation or relieve pain and itching.

## Equipment

Rectal suppository or tube of ointment and applicator • patient's medication record and chart • gloves • water-soluble lubricant • 4″ × 4″ gauze pads • optional: bedpan

### Preparation of equipment

Store rectal suppositories in the refrigerator until needed to prevent softening and, possibly, decreased effectiveness of the medication. A softened suppository is also difficult to handle and insert. To harden it again, hold the suppository (in its wrapper) under cold running water.

## Implementation

▶ Verify the order on the patient's medication record by checking it against the doctor's order.
▶ Make sure the label on the medication package agrees with the medication order. Read the label again before you open the wrapper and again as you remove the medication. Check the expiration date.
▶ Wash your hands with warm soap and water.
▶ Confirm the patient's identity by asking his name and checking the name, room number, and bed number on his wristband.
▶ Explain the procedure and the purpose of the medication to the patient.
▶ Provide privacy.

### Inserting a rectal suppository

▶ Place the patient on his left side in Sims' position. Drape him with the bedcovers to expose only the buttocks.
▶ Put on gloves. Remove the suppository from its wrapper and lubricate it with water-soluble lubricant.
▶ Lift the patient's upper buttock with your nondominant hand to expose the anus.
▶ Instruct the patient to take several deep breaths through his mouth to help relax the anal sphincters and reduce anxiety or discomfort during insertion.
▶ Using the index finger of your dominant hand, insert the suppository—tapered end first—about 39 (7.5 cm), until you feel it pass the internal anal sphincter. Try to direct the tapered end toward the side of the rectum so that it contacts the membranes. (See *How to administer a rectal suppository or ointment*.)

# How to administer a rectal suppository or ointment

When inserting a suppository, direct its tapered end toward the side of the rectum so that it contacts the membranes (as shown); doing so encourages absorption of the medication.

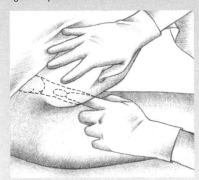

When applying a rectal ointment internally, lubricate the applicator to minimize pain on insertion (as shown). Then direct the applicator tip toward the patient's umbilicus.

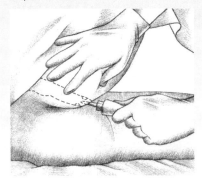

▶ Ensure the patient's comfort. Encourage him to lie quietly and, if applicable, retain the suppository for the appropriate length of time. A suppository administered to relieve constipation should be retained as long as possible (at least 20 minutes) to be effective. Press on the anus with a gauze pad, if necessary, until the urge to defecate passes.
▶ Remove and discard your gloves.

Applying rectal ointment
▶ Put on gloves.
▶ To apply externally, use gloves or a gauze pad to spread medication over the anal area.
▶ To apply internally, attach the applicator to the tube of ointment and coat the applicator with water-soluble lubricant.
▶ Expect to use about 19 (2.5 cm) of ointment. To gauge how much pressure to use during application, squeeze a small amount from the tube before you attach the applicator.
▶ Lift the patient's upper buttock with your nondominant hand to expose the anus.
▶ Instruct the patient to take several deep breaths through his mouth to relax the anal sphincters and reduce anxiety or discomfort during insertion.
▶ Gently insert the applicator, directing it toward the umbilicus.
▶ Slowly squeeze the tube to eject the medication.
▶ Remove the applicator and place a folded 49 2 49 gauze pad between the patient's buttocks to absorb excess ointment.
▶ Detach the applicator from the tube and recap the tube. Then clean the applicator thoroughly with soap and warm water.

### Special considerations
▶ Because the intake of food and fluid stimulates peristalsis, a suppository for relieving constipation should be inserted about 30 minutes before mealtime to help soften the feces in the rectum and facilitate defecation. A medicated retention suppository should be inserted between meals.
▶ Instruct the patient to avoid expelling the suppository. If he has difficulty retaining it, place him on a bedpan.
▶ Make sure the patient's call button is handy and watch for his signal because he may be unable to suppress the urge to defecate. For example, a patient with proctitis has a highly sensitive rectum and may not be able to retain a suppository for long.
▶ Inform the patient that the suppository may discolor his next bowel movement. Anusol suppositories, for example, can give feces a silver-gray pasty appearance.

### Documentation
▶ Record the administration time, dose, and patient's response.

**REFERENCES**
Ansel, H.C., et al. *Pharmaceutical Dosage Forms and Drug Delivery Systems,* 7th ed. Philadelphia: Lippincott Williams & Wilkins, 1999.
Craven, R., and Hirnle, C.J. *Fundamentals of Nursing: Human Health and Function,* 4th ed. Philadelphia: Lippincott Williams & Wilkins, 2002.

# Skin medications

Topical drugs are applied directly to the skin surface. They include lotions, pastes, ointments, creams, powders, shampoos, patches, and aerosol sprays. Topical medications are absorbed through the epidermal layer into the dermis. The extent of absorption depends on the vascularity of the region.

Nitroglycerin, fentanyl, nicotine, and certain supplemental hormone replacements are used for systemic effects. Most other topical medications are used for local effects. Ointments have a fatty base, which is an ideal vehicle for such drugs as antimicrobials and antiseptics. Typically, topical medications should be applied two or three times per day to achieve their therapeutic effect.

### Equipment
Patient's medication record and chart ● prescribed medication ● gloves ● sterile tongue blades ● sterile 4″ × 4″ gauze pads ● transparent semipermeable dressing ● adhesive tape ● solvent (such as cottonseed oil)

### Implementation
▶ Verify the order on the patient's medication record by checking it against the doctor's order in the chart.
▶ Make sure the label on the medication agrees with the medication order. Read the label again before you open the container and as you remove the medication from the container. Check the expiration date.
▶ Confirm the patient's identity by asking his name and checking the name, room number, and bed number on his wristband.
▶ Provide privacy.
▶ Explain the procedure thoroughly to the patient because he may have to apply the medication by himself after discharge.

▶ Wash your hands to prevent cross-contamination and put a glove on your dominant hand. Use gloves on both hands if exposure to body fluids is likely.

▶ Help the patient assume a comfortable position that provides access to the area to be treated.

▶ Expose the area to be treated. Make sure the skin or mucous membrane is intact (unless the medication has been ordered to treat a skin lesion such as an ulcer). Applying medication to broken or abraded skin may cause unwanted systemic absorption and result in further irritation.

▶ If necessary, clean the skin of debris, including crusts, epidermal scales, and old medication. You may have to change the glove if it becomes soiled.

### Applying paste, cream, or ointment

▶ Open the container. Place the lid or cap upside down to prevent contamination of the inside surface.

▶ Remove a tongue blade from its sterile wrapper and cover one end with medication from the tube or jar. Then transfer the medication from the tongue blade to your gloved hand.

▶ Apply the medication to the affected area with long, smooth strokes that follow the direction of hair growth. This technique avoids forcing medication into hair follicles, which can cause irritation and lead to folliculitis. Avoid excessive pressure when applying the medication because it could abrade the skin.

▶ To prevent contamination of the medication, use a new tongue blade each time you remove medication from the container.

### Removing ointment

▶ Wash your hands and apply gloves. Then rub solvent on them and apply it liberally to the ointment-treated area in the direction of hair growth. Alternatively, saturate a sterile gauze pad with the solvent and use the pad to gently remove the ointment. Remove excess oil by gently wiping the area with a sterile gauze pad. Don't rub too hard to remove the medication because you could irritate the skin.

### Applying other topical medications

▶ To apply shampoos, follow package directions. (See *Using medicated shampoos.*)

▶ To apply aerosol sprays, shake the container, if indicated, to completely mix the

---

## Using medicated shampoos

Medicated shampoos include keratolytic and cytostatic agents, coal tar preparations, and lindane (gamma benzene hexachloride) solutions. They can be used to treat such conditions as dandruff, psoriasis, and head lice. However, they're contraindicated in patients with broken or abraded skin.

Because application instructions may vary among brands, check the label on the shampoo before starting the procedure to ensure use of the correct amount. Keep the shampoo away from the patient's eyes. If any shampoo should accidentally get in his eyes, irrigate them promptly with water. Selenium sulfide, used in cytostatic agents, is extremely toxic if ingested.

To apply medicated shampoo, take the following steps:

▶ Prepare the patient for shampoo treatment.

▶ Shake the bottle of shampoo well to mix the solution evenly.

▶ Wet the patient's hair thoroughly and wring out excess water.

▶ Apply the proper amount of shampoo as directed on the label.

▶ Work the shampoo into a lather, adding water as necessary. Part the patient's hair and work the shampoo into his scalp, taking care not to use your fingernails.

▶ Leave the shampoo on the patient's scalp and hair for as long as instructed (usually 5 to 10 minutes). Then rinse his hair thoroughly.

▶ Towel-dry the patient's hair.

▶ After his hair is dry, comb or brush it. Use a fine-tooth comb to remove nits, if necessary.

---

medication. Hold the container 6″ to 12″ (15 to 30.5 cm) from the skin, or follow the manufacturer's recommendation. Spray a thin film of the medication evenly over the treatment area.

▶ To apply powders, dry the skin surface, making sure to spread skin folds where moisture collects. Then apply a thin layer of powder over the treatment area.

▶ To protect applied medications and prevent them from soiling the patient's clothes, tape an appropriate amount of sterile gauze pad or a transparent semipermeable dressing over the treated area. With certain medications (such as topical steroids), semipermeable dressings may be contraindicated. Check medication information and cautions. If you're applying a topical medication to the patient's hands or feet, cover the site with white cotton gloves for the hands or terry cloth scuffs for the feet.

◆ **ALERT!** In children, topical medications (such as steroids) should be covered only loosely with a diaper. Don't use plastic pants.

▶ Assess the patient's skin for signs of irritation, allergic reaction, or breakdown.

### Special considerations

▶ Never apply medication without first removing previous applications to prevent skin irritation from an accumulation of medication.

▶ Wear gloves to prevent absorption by your own skin. If the patient has an infectious skin condition, use sterile gloves and dispose of old dressings according to your facility's policy.

▶ Don't apply ointments to mucous membranes as liberally as you would to skin because mucous membranes are usually moist and absorb ointment more quickly than skin does. Also, don't apply too much ointment to any skin area because it might cause irritation and discomfort, stain clothing and bedding, and make removal difficult.

▶ Never apply ointment to the eyelids or ear canal unless ordered. The ointment might congeal and occlude the tear duct or ear canal.

▶ Inspect the treated area frequently for adverse effects such as signs of an allergic reaction.

### Complications

Skin irritation, a rash, or an allergic reaction may occur.

### Documentation

▶ Record the medication applied; time, date, and site of application; and condition of the patient's skin at the time of application.

▶ Note subsequent effects of the medication, if any.

**REFERENCES**

Ansel, H.C., et al. *Pharmaceutical Dosage Forms and Drug Delivery Systems,* 7th ed. Philadelphia: Lippincott Williams & Wilkins, 1999.

Craven, R., and Hirnle, C.J. *Fundamentals of Nursing: Human Health and Function,* 4th ed. Philadelphia: Lippincott Williams & Wilkins, 2002.

# Subcutaneous injection

When injected into the adipose (fatty) tissues beneath the skin, a drug moves into the bloodstream more rapidly than if given by mouth. Subcutaneous (S.C.) injection allows slower, more sustained drug administration than I.M. injection; it also causes minimal tissue trauma and carries little risk of striking large blood vessels and nerves.

Absorbed mainly through the capillaries, drugs recommended for S.C. injection include nonirritating aqueous solutions and suspensions contained in 0.5 to 2 ml of fluid. Heparin and insulin, for example, are usually administered S.C. (Some diabetic patients, however, may benefit from an insulin infusion pump.)

Drugs and solutions for S.C. injection are injected through a relatively short needle, using meticulous sterile technique. The most common S.C. injection sites are the outer aspect of the upper arm, anterior thigh, loose tissue of the lower abdomen, upper hips, buttocks, and upper back. (See *Locating subcutaneous injection sites.*) Injection is contraindicated in sites that are inflamed, edematous, scarred, or covered by a mole, birthmark, or other lesion. It may also be contraindicated in patients with impaired coagulation mechanisms.

### Equipment

Prescribed medication ● patient's medication record and chart ● 25G to 27G ⅝″ to ½″ needle ● gloves ● 1- or 3-ml syringe ● alcohol pads ● optional: antiseptic cleaning agent, filter needle, and insulin syringe

### Preparation of equipment

Verify the order on the patient's medication record by checking it against the doctor's order. Also, note whether the patient has

# Locating subcutaneous injection sites

Subcutaneous (S.C.) injection sites (as indicated by the dotted areas shown at right) include the fat pads on the abdomen, upper hips, upper back, and lateral upper arms and thighs. For S.C. injections administered repeatedly, such as insulin, rotate sites. Choose one injection site in one area, move to a corresponding injection site in the next area, and so on.

When returning to an area, choose a new site in that area. Preferred injection sites for insulin are the arms, abdomen, thighs, and buttocks. The preferred injection site for heparin is the lower abdominal fat pad just below the umbilicus.

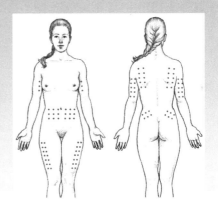

any allergies, especially before the first dose.

Inspect the medication to make sure it isn't abnormally discolored or cloudy and doesn't contain precipitates (unless the manufacturer's instructions allow it).

Wash your hands. Choose equipment appropriate to the prescribed medication and injection site and make sure it works properly.

Check the medication label against the patient's medication record. Read the label again as you draw up the medication for injection.

*For single-dose ampules*
Wrap an alcohol pad around the ampule's neck and snap off the top, directing the force away from your body. Attach a filter needle to the needle and withdraw the medication, keeping the needle's bevel tip below the level of the solution. Tap the syringe to clear any air from it. Cover the needle with the needle sheath.

Before discarding the ampule, check the medication label against the patient's medication record. Discard the filter needle and the ampule. Attach the appropriate needle to the syringe.

*For single-dose or multidose vials*
Reconstitute powdered drugs according to instructions. Make sure all crystals have dissolved in the solution. Warm the vial by rolling it between your palms to help the drug dissolve faster.

Clean the vial's rubber stopper with an alcohol pad. Pull the syringe plunger back until the volume of air in the syringe equals the volume of drug to be withdrawn from the vial.

Without inverting the vial, insert the needle into the vial. Inject the air, invert the vial, and keep the needle's bevel tip below the level of the solution as you withdraw the prescribed amount of medication. Cover the needle with the needle sheath. Tap the syringe to clear any air from it.

Check the medication label against the patient's medication record before discarding the single-dose vial or returning the multidose vial to the shelf.

## Implementation
▶ Confirm the patient's identity by asking his name and checking the name, room number, and bed number on his wristband.
▶ Explain the procedure to the patient and provide privacy.
▶ Select an appropriate injection site. Rotate sites according to a schedule for repeated injections, using different areas of the body unless contraindicated. (Heparin, for example, should be injected only in the abdomen, if possible.)
▶ Put on gloves.
▶ Position the patient and expose the injection site.

## Techniques for subcutaneous injections

Before giving the injection, elevate the subcutaneous tissue at the site by grasping it firmly.

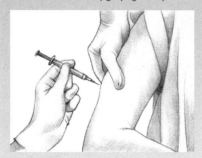

Insert the needle at a 45- or 90-degree angle to the skin surface, depending on needle length and the amount of subcutaneous tissue at the site. Some medications, such as heparin, should always be injected at a 90-degree angle.

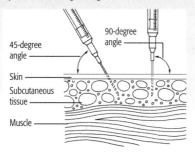

45-degree angle

90-degree angle

Skin

Subcutaneous tissue

Muscle

---

▶ Clean the injection site with an alcohol pad, beginning at the center of the site and moving outward in a circular motion. Allow the skin to dry before injecting the drug to avoid a stinging sensation from introducing alcohol into subcutaneous tissues.

▶ Loosen the protective needle sheath.

▶ With your nondominant hand, grasp the skin around the injection site firmly to elevate the subcutaneous tissue, forming a 1″ (2.5-cm) fat fold.

▶ Holding the syringe in your dominant hand, insert the loosened needle sheath between the fourth and fifth fingers of your other hand while still pinching the skin around the injection site. Pull back the syringe with your dominant hand to uncover the needle by grasping the syringe like a pencil. Don't touch the needle.

▶ Position the needle with its bevel up.

▶ Tell the patient he'll feel a needle prick.

▶ Insert the needle quickly in one motion at a 45- or 90-degree angle. (See *Techniques for subcutaneous injections.*) Release the patient's skin to avoid injecting the drug into compressed tissue and irritating nerve fibers.

▶ Pull back the plunger slightly to check for blood return. If none appears, begin injecting the drug slowly. If blood appears on aspiration, withdraw the needle, prepare another syringe, and repeat the procedure.

▶ Don't aspirate for blood return when giving insulin or heparin. It isn't necessary with insulin and may cause a hematoma with heparin.

▶ After injection, remove the needle gently but quickly at the same angle used for insertion.

▶ Cover the site with an alcohol pad and massage the site gently (unless contraindicated as with heparin and insulin) to distribute the drug and facilitate absorption.

▶ Remove the alcohol pad and check the injection site for bleeding and bruising.

▶ Dispose of injection equipment according to your facility's policy. To avoid needle-stick injuries, don't resheath the needle.

### Special considerations

▶ When using prefilled syringes, adjust the angle and depth of insertion according to needle length.

#### For insulin injections

▶ To establish more consistent blood insulin levels, rotate insulin injection sites within anatomic regions. Preferred insulin injection sites are the arms, abdomen, thighs, and buttocks.

▶ Make sure the type of insulin, unit dosage, and syringe are correct.

▶ When combining insulins in a syringe, make sure they're compatible. Regular insulin can be mixed with all other types. Prompt insulin zinc suspension (semilente insulin) can't be mixed with NPH insulin. Follow your facility's policy regarding which insulin to draw up first.

▶ Before drawing up insulin suspension, gently roll and invert the bottle. Don't

# Types of insulin infusion pumps

A subcutaneous insulin infusion pump provides continuous, long-term insulin therapy for patients with type 1 diabetes mellitus. Complications include infection at the injection site, catheter clogging, and insulin loss from loose reservoir-catheter connections. Insulin pumps work on either an open-loop or a closed-loop system.

### Open-loop system
The open-loop pump is used most commonly. It infuses insulin but can't respond to changes in serum glucose levels. These portable, self-contained, programmable insulin pumps are smaller and less obtrusive than ever – about the size of a credit card – and have fewer buttons.

The pump delivers insulin in small (basal) doses every few minutes and large (bolus) doses that the patient sets manually. The system consists of a reservoir containing the insulin syringe, a small pump, an infusion-rate selector that allows insulin-release adjustments, a battery, and a plastic catheter with an attached needle leading from the syringe to the subcutaneous injection site. The needle is typically held in place with waterproof tape. The patient can wear the pump on his belt or in his pocket – practically anywhere as long as the infusion line has a clear path to the injection site.

The infusion-rate selector automatically releases about half the total daily insulin requirement. The patient releases the remainder in bolus doses before meals and snacks. The patient must change the syringe daily; he must change the needle, catheter, and injection site every other day.

### Closed-loop system
The self-contained closed-loop system detects and responds to changing serum glucose levels. The typical closed-loop system includes a glucose sensor, a programmable computer, a power supply, a pump, and an insulin reservoir. The computer triggers continuous insulin delivery in appropriate amounts from the reservoir.

### Nonneedle catheter system
In the nonneedle delivery system, a tiny plastic catheter is inserted into the skin over a needle using a special insertion device (shown below). The needle is then withdrawn, leaving the catheter in place (shown in the inset). This catheter can be placed in the abdomen, thigh, or flank and should be changed every 2 to 3 days.

**CLOSE-UP OF OPEN-LOOP INFUSION PUMP**

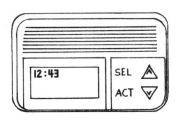

**NONNEEDLE CATHETER INSERTION SYSTEM**

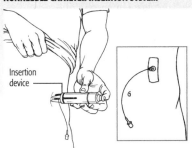

Insertion device

---

shake the bottle because this can cause foam or bubbles to develop in the syringe.
▶ Insulin may be administered through an inserted insulin pump. However, before administering the drug, make sure the patient doesn't already have a pump in place. (See *Types of insulin infusion pumps.*)

## For heparin injections
▶ The preferred site for a heparin injection is the lower abdominal fat pad, 2″ (5 cm) beneath the umbilicus, between the right and left iliac crests. Injecting heparin into this area, which isn't involved in muscle activity, reduces the risk of local capillary bleeding. Always rotate the sites from one side to the other.

▶ Inject the drug slowly into the fat pad. Leave the needle in place for 10 seconds after injection; then withdraw it.

▶ Don't administer an injection within 2″ of a scar, a bruise, or the umbilicus.

▶ Don't aspirate to check for blood return because this can cause bleeding into the tissues at the site.

▶ Don't rub or massage the site after the injection. Rubbing can cause localized minute hemorrhages or bruises.

▶ If the patient bruises easily, apply ice to the site for the first 5 minutes after the injection to minimize local hemorrhage and then apply pressure.

## Complications

Concentrated or irritating solutions may cause sterile abscesses to form. Repeated injections in the same site can cause lipodystrophy. A natural immune response, lipodystrophy can be minimized by rotating injection sites.

## Documentation

▶ Record the time and date of the injection, medication and dose administered, injection site and route, and patient's reaction.

### REFERENCES

Ansel, H.C., et al. *Pharmaceutical Dosage Forms and Drug Delivery Systems,* 7th ed. Philadelphia: Lippincott Williams & Wilkins, 1999.

Craven, R., and Hirnle, C.J. *Fundamentals of Nursing: Human Health and Function,* 4th ed. Philadelphia: Lippincott Williams & Wilkins, 2002.

# Transdermal drugs

Through an adhesive patch or a measured dose of ointment applied to the skin, transdermal drugs deliver constant, controlled medication directly into the bloodstream for a prolonged systemic effect.

Medications available in transdermal form include nitroglycerin, used to control angina; scopolamine, used to treat motion sickness; estradiol, used for postmenopausal hormone replacement; clonidine, used to treat hypertension; nicotine, used for smoking cessation; and fentanyl, a narcotic analgesic used to control chronic pain.

Contraindications for transdermal drug application include skin allergies or skin reactions to the drug. Transdermal drugs shouldn't be applied to broken or irritated skin because they would increase irritation, or to scarred or callused skin, which might impair absorption.

## Equipment

Patient's medication record and chart ● gloves ● prescribed medication (patch or ointment) ● application strip or measuring paper (for nitroglycerin ointment) ● adhesive tape ● plastic wrap (optional for nitroglycerin ointment) or semipermeable dressing

## Implementation

▶ Verify the order on the patient's medication record by checking it against the doctor's order.

▶ Wash your hands and, if necessary, put on gloves.

▶ Check the label on the medication to make sure you're giving the correct drug in the correct dose. Note the expiration date.

▶ Confirm the patient's identity by asking his name and checking the name, room number, and bed number on his wristband.

▶ Explain the procedure to the patient and provide privacy.

▶ Remove any previously applied medication.

### Applying transdermal ointment

▶ Place the prescribed amount of ointment on the application strip or measuring paper, taking care not to get any on your skin. (See *Applying nitroglycerin ointment.*)

▶ Apply the strip to any dry, hairless area of the body. Don't rub the ointment into the skin.

▶ Tape the ointment-filled strip to the skin.

▶ If desired, cover the application strip with the plastic wrap and tape the wrap in place.

### Applying a transdermal patch

▶ Open the package and remove the patch.

▶ Without touching the adhesive surface, remove the clear plastic backing.

▶ Apply the patch to a dry, hairless area — behind the ear, for example, as with scopolamine. (See *Applying a transdermal medication patch,* page 154.)

# Applying nitroglycerin ointment

Unlike most topical medications, nitroglycerin ointment is used for its transdermal systemic effect. It's used to dilate the veins and arteries, thus improving cardiac perfusion in the patient with cardiac ischemia or angina pectoris.

To apply nitroglycerin ointment, start by taking the patient's baseline blood pressure so that you can compare it with later readings. Gather your equipment. Nitroglycerin ointment, which is prescribed by the inch, comes with a rectangular piece of ruled paper to be used in applying the medication. Squeeze the prescribed amount of ointment onto the ruled paper (as shown below). Put on gloves, if desired, to avoid contact with the medication. Nitroglycerin ointment also comes in premeasured single-dose packages.

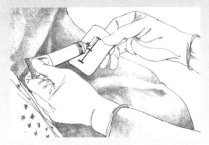

After applying the correct amount of ointment, tape the paper – drug side down – directly to the skin

(as shown below). (Some facilities require you to use the paper to apply the medication to the patient's skin, usually on the chest or arm. Spread a thin layer of the ointment over a 3″ [7.6-cm] area.) For increased absorption, the doctor may request that you cover the site with plastic wrap or a transparent semipermeable dressing.

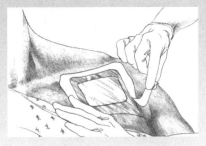

After 5 minutes, record the patient's blood pressure. If it has dropped significantly and he has a headache (from vasodilation of blood vessels in his head), notify the doctor immediately. The doctor may reduce the dose. If the patient's blood pressure has dropped but he has no symptoms, instruct him to lie still until it returns to normal.

Transdermal nitroglycerin should be removed at bedtime to provide a 10- to 12-hour nitrate-free interval, thereby preventing drug tolerance.

---

▸ Write the date, time, and your initials on the patch.

### After applying transdermal medications
▸ Store the medication as ordered.
▸ Instruct the patient to keep the area around the patch or strip as dry as possible.
▸ If you didn't wear gloves, wash your hands immediately after applying the patch or ointment to avoid absorbing the drug yourself.

### Special considerations
▸ Reapply daily transdermal medications at the same time every day to ensure a continuous effect, but alternate the application sites to avoid skin irritation.
▸ When applying a scopolamine or fentanyl patch, instruct the patient not to drive or operate machinery until his response to the drug has been determined.
▸ Warn a patient using a clonidine patch to check with his doctor before taking an over-the-counter cough preparation because such drugs may counteract clonidine's effects.

### Complications
Topical medications may cause skin irritation, such as pruritus and a rash. The patient may also suffer adverse effects of the specific drug administered. For example, transdermal nitroglycerin medications may cause headaches and, in elderly patients, orthostatic hypotension. Scopolamine has various adverse effects; dry mouth and drowsiness are the most common. Transdermal estradiol carries an increased risk of endometrial cancer, thromboembolic

## Applying a transdermal medication patch

If the patient will be receiving medication by transdermal patch, instruct him in its proper use, as described here:

▶ Explain to the patient that the patch consists of several layers. The layer closest to his skin contains a small amount of the drug and allows prompt introduction of the drug into the bloodstream. The next layer controls release of the drug from the main portion of the patch. The third layer contains the main dose of the drug. The outermost layer consists of an aluminized polyester barrier.

▶ Teach the patient to apply the patch to appropriate skin areas, such as the upper arm or chest and behind the ear. Warn him to avoid touching the gel or surrounding tape. Tell him to use a different site for each application to avoid skin irritation. If necessary, he can shave the site. Tell him to avoid any area that may cause uneven absorption, such as skin folds, scars, and calluses, or any irritated or damaged skin areas. Also, tell him not to apply the patch below the elbow or knee.

▶ Instruct the patient to wash his hands after application to remove any medication that may have rubbed off.

▶ Warn the patient not to get the patch wet. Tell him to discard it if it leaks or falls off and then to clean the site and apply a new patch at a different site.

▶ Instruct the patient to apply the patch at the same time at the prescribed interval to ensure continuous drug delivery. Bedtime application is ideal for some transdermal medication patches because body movement is reduced during the night. Finally, tell him to apply a new patch about 30 minutes before removing the old one.

---

disease, and birth defects. Clonidine may cause severe rebound hypertension, especially if withdrawn suddenly.

### Documentation

▶ Record the type of medication; date, time, and site of application; and dose.
▶ Note any adverse effects and the patient's response.

### REFERENCES

Ansel, H.C., et al. *Pharmaceutical Dosage Forms and Drug Delivery Systems,* 7th ed. Philadelphia: Lippincott Williams & Wilkins, 1999.

Craven, R., and Hirnle, C.J. *Fundamentals of Nursing: Human Health and Function,* 4th ed. Philadelphia: Lippincott Williams & Wilkins, 2002.

## Vaginal medications

Vaginal medications include suppositories, creams, gels, and ointments. These medications can be inserted as a topical treatment for infection (particularly *Trichomonas vaginalis* and monilial vaginitis) or inflammation, or as a contraceptive. Suppositories melt when they contact the vaginal mucosa, and their medication diffuses topically (as effectively as creams, gels, and ointments).

Vaginal medications usually come with a disposable applicator that enables placement of medication in the anterior and posterior fornices. Vaginal administration is most effective when the patient can remain lying down afterward to retain the medication.

### Equipment

Patient's medication record and chart ● prescribed medication and applicator ● gloves ● water-soluble lubricant ● small sanitary pad

### Implementation

▶ If possible, plan to insert vaginal medications at bedtime, when the patient is recumbent.
▶ Verify the order on the patient's medication record by checking it against the doctor's order.
▶ Confirm the patient's identity by asking her name and checking the name, room number, and bed number on her wristband.
▶ Wash your hands, explain the procedure to the patient, and provide privacy.
▶ Ask the patient to void.
▶ Ask the patient if she would rather insert the medication herself. If so, provide appropriate instructions. If not, proceed with the following steps.

▶ Help her into the lithotomy position.

▶ Expose only the perineum.

Inserting a suppository

▶ Remove the suppository from the wrapper, and lubricate it with water-soluble lubricant.

▶ Put on gloves and expose the vagina.

▶ With an applicator or the forefinger of your free hand, insert the suppository about 2″ (5 cm) into the vagina. (See *How to insert a vaginal suppository.*)

Inserting ointments, creams, or gels

▶ Insert the plunger into the applicator. Then attach the applicator to the tube of medication.

▶ Gently squeeze the tube to fill the applicator with the prescribed amount of medication. Detach the applicator from the tube, and lubricate the applicator.

▶ Put on gloves and expose the vagina.

▶ Insert the applicator as you would a small suppository, and administer the medication by depressing the plunger on the applicator.

After vaginal insertion

▶ Remove and discard your gloves.

▶ Wash the applicator with soap and warm water and store it, unless it is disposable. If the applicator can be used again, label it so that it will be used only for the same patient.

▶ To prevent the medication from soiling the patient's clothing and bedding, provide a sanitary pad.

▶ Help the patient return to a comfortable position, and advise her to remain in bed as much as possible for the next several hours.

▶ Wash your hands thoroughly.

## Special considerations

▶ Refrigerate vaginal suppositories that melt at room temperature.

▶ If possible, teach the patient how to insert vaginal medication because she may have to administer it herself after discharge. Give her a patient-teaching sheet if one is available.

▶ Instruct the patient not to wear a tampon after inserting vaginal medication because it would absorb the medication and decrease its effectiveness.

▶ Instruct the patient to avoid sexual intercourse during treatment.

# How to insert a vaginal suppository

If the suppository is small, place it in the tip of an applicator. Then lubricate the applicator, hold it by the cylinder, and insert it into the vagina. To ensure the patient's comfort, direct the applicator down initially, toward the spine, and then up and back, toward the cervix (as shown below). When the suppository reaches the distal end of the vagina, depress the plunger.

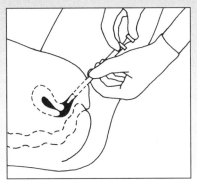

Remove the applicator while the plunger is still depressed.

## Complications

Vaginal medications may cause local irritation.

## Documentation

▶ Document the time of application, name of drug, and dosage.

▶ Document the patient's response to application.

### REFERENCES

Ansel, H.C., et al. *Pharmaceutical Dosage Forms and Drug Delivery Systems,* 7th ed. Philadelphia: Lippincott Williams & Wilkins, 1999.

Craven, R., and Hirnle, C.J. *Fundamentals of Nursing: Human Health and Function,* 4th ed. Philadelphia: Lippincott Williams & Wilkins, 2002.

## Displacing the skin for Z-track injection

By blocking the needle pathway after an injection, the Z-track technique allows I.M. injection while minimizing the risk of subcutaneous irritation and staining from such drugs as iron dextran. The illustrations here show how to perform a Z-track injection.

Before the procedure begins, the skin, subcutaneous fat, and muscle lie in their normal positions.

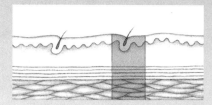

To begin, place your finger on the skin surface and pull the skin and subcutaneous layers out of alignment with the underlying muscle. You should move the skin about ½″ (1.3 cm).

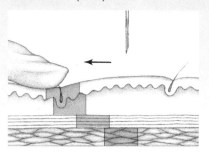

Insert the needle at a 90-degree angle at the site where you initially placed your finger. Inject the drug and withdraw the needle.

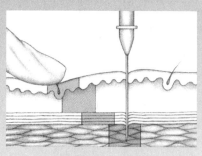

Finally, remove your finger from the skin surface, allowing the layers to return to their normal positions. The needle track (shown by the dotted line) is now broken at the junction of each tissue layer, trapping the drug in the muscle.

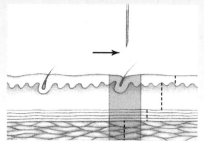

# Z-track injection

The Z-track method of I.M. injection prevents leakage, or tracking, into the subcutaneous tissue. It's typically used to administer drugs that irritate and discolor subcutaneous tissue, primarily iron preparations such as iron dextran.

### Equipment

Patient's medication record and chart ● two 20G 1¼″ to 2″ needles ● prescribed medication ● gloves ● 3- or 5-ml syringe ● two alcohol pads

Preparation of equipment
Verify the order on the patient's medication record by checking it against the doctor's order. Wash your hands.

Make sure the needle you're using is long enough to reach the muscle. As a rule of thumb, a 200-lb (91-kg) patient requires a 2″ needle; a 100-lb (45-kg) patient, a 1¼″ to 1½″ needle.

Attach one needle to the syringe, and draw up the prescribed medication. Then draw 0.2 to 0.5 cc of air (depending on your facility's policy) into the syringe. Remove the first needle and attach the second to prevent tracking the medication through the subcutaneous tissue as the needle is inserted.

## Implementation

▶ Confirm the patient's identity, explain the procedure, and provide privacy.

▶ Place the patient in the lateral position, exposing the gluteal muscle to be used as the injection site.

▶ Clean an area on the upper outer quadrant of the patient's buttock with an alcohol pad.

▶ Put on gloves. Then displace the skin laterally by pulling it away from the injection site. (See *Displacing the skin for Z-track injection.*)

▶ Insert the needle into the muscle at a 90-degree angle.

▶ Aspirate for blood return; if none appears, inject the drug slowly, followed by the air. Injecting air after the drug helps clear the needle and prevents tracking the medication through subcutaneous tissues as the needle is withdrawn.

▶ Wait 10 seconds before withdrawing the needle to ensure dispersion of the medication.

▶ Withdraw the needle slowly. Then release the displaced skin and subcutaneous tissue to seal the needle track. Don't massage the injection site or allow the patient to wear a tight-fitting garment over the site because it could force the medication into subcutaneous tissue.

▶ Encourage the patient to walk or move about in bed to facilitate absorption of the drug from the injection site.

▶ Discard the needles and syringe in an appropriate sharps container. Don't recap needles to avoid needle-stick injuries.

▶ Remove and discard your gloves.

## Special considerations

▶ Never inject more than 5 ml of solution into a single site using the Z-track method. Alternate gluteal sites for repeat injections.

## Complications

Discomfort and tissue irritation may result from drug leakage into subcutaneous tissue. Failure to rotate sites in patients who require repeated injections can interfere with the absorption of medication. Unabsorbed medications may build up in deposits. Such deposits can reduce the desired pharmacologic effect and may lead to abscess formation or tissue fibrosis.

## Documentation

▶ Record the medication, dosage, date, time, and site of injection on the patient's medication record.

▶ Note the patient's response to the injected drug.

### REFERENCES

Craven, R., and Hirnle, C.J. *Fundamentals of Nursing: Human Health and Function,* 4th ed. Philadelphia: Lippincott Williams & Wilkins, 2002.

Engstrom, J.L., et al. "Procedures Used To Prepare and Administer Intramuscular Injections: A Study of Infertility Nurses," *Journal of Obstetric, Gynecologic, and Neonatal Nursing* 29(2):59-68, March-April 2000.

McConnell, E.A. "Administering a Z-track I.M. Injection," *Nursing* 29(1):26, January 1999.

# 4

# Intravascular therapy

**M**ORE THAN 80% OF HOSPITALIZED PATIENTS RECEIVE SOME FORM OF I.V. THERAPY. AL-though you may not be called on to insert all types of I.V. lines, you'll be responsible for maintaining the line and preventing complications throughout therapy. You'll also be responsible for helping the doctor perform minor surgical procedures, such as insertion of central venous and arterial lines.

This chapter explains the administration methods and primary uses of I.V. therapy. You'll review how to prepare for I.V. therapy; how to insert, maintain, and remove specific I.V. lines and devices; how to control infection and maintain flow rates; and how to monitor the patient's response to therapy. You'll also learn about patient teaching responsibilities and home care issues.

This chapter covers the nursing protocols for a patient receiving autologous blood administration, parenteral nutrition, or a massive blood transfusion. You'll learn how to manage the patient having a transfusion reaction and how to maintain a venous access device.

# Protocols

## Managing the patient receiving autotransfusion

### Purpose
To collect, filter, and reinfuse the patient's own blood

### Collaborative level
Interdependent

### Expected patient outcomes
▶ The patient will maintain stabilized fluid volume.
▶ The patient will maintain stable vital signs.
▶ The patient will produce adequate urine output.

### Definition of terms
▶ *Preoperative blood donation:* Donation of blood collected 4 to 6 weeks before surgery. It's recommended for patients scheduled for surgery that may result in large blood loss.
▶ *Perioperative blood donation:* Blood collected during surgery or up to 12 hours afterward.
▶ *Acute normovolemic hemodilution:* Technique used mainly in open-heart

surgery, involving blood collected immediately before or after anesthesia induction. The blood is reinfused immediately after surgery.

### Indications
Treatment
▶ Elective surgery
▶ Nonelective surgery
▶ Perioperative and emergency blood salvage for traumatic injury

Prevention
▶ Bloodborne diseases including AIDS

### Assessment guidance
Signs and symptoms
▶ Fever
▶ Chills
▶ Hypotension
▶ Pain at I.V. site
▶ Back pain
▶ Anxiety

Diagnostic studies
▶ Hemoglobin
▶ Hematocrit
▶ Calcium levels
▶ Coagulation profiles

## Nursing interventions
▶ Identify the patient.
▶ Teach the patient what an autologous transfusion is, how much blood can be donated at one time, and why it's done.
▶ Instruct the patient to increase fluid intake before the procedure to prevent hypovolemia.
▶ Instruct the patient to take iron supplements for at least 1 week before the procedure.
▶ Monitor vital signs, including temperature, before and after the procedure.
▶ Monitor the patient's hemoglobin.
▶ Assist the patient into a supine position.
▶ Clean the needle insertion site (per facility policy).
▶ Apply a tourniquet.
▶ Use a large-bore needle to enter a vein (usually an antecubital vein).
▶ Collect blood and recheck vital signs, including temperature, after the collection procedure is complete.

### Blood reinfusion
▶ Prime the blood filter with sterile normal saline.
▶ Insert spike into the large port on the top of the bottle.
▶ Attach the blood bag to a Y-connector of the blood filter.
▶ Begin the infusion.
▶ Monitor vital signs per facility policy.

## Contraindications
Contraindicated in patients with malignant neoplasms, coagulopathies, anemias, active infections, and excessive hemolysis as well as those receiving antibiotics. Patients with recent weight loss because of malnutrition or disease shouldn't donate.

## Documentation
▶ Document how much blood the patient donated.
▶ Document how much blood was reinfused.
▶ Document how well the patient tolerated each procedure.

## Related procedures
▶ Autotransfusion
▶ Peripheral I.V. line insertion
▶ Peripheral I.V. line maintenance

▶ Standard precautions
▶ Venipuncture

### REFERENCES
*Handbook of Nursing Procedures.* Springhouse, Pa: Springhouse Corp., 2001.
Ignatavicius, D., and Workman, M. *Medical-Surgical Nursing: Thinking for Collaborative Care,* 4th ed. Philadelphia: W.B. Saunders Co., 2002.
Silvestri, L. *Saunders' Comprehensive Review for NCLEX-RN.* Philadelphia: W.B. Saunders Co., 2002.

# Managing the patient receiving parenteral nutrition

## Purpose
To provide nutritional support to patients who can't take feedings via the GI tract

## Collaborative level
Interdependent

## Expected patient outcomes
▶ The patient will maintain or improve nutritional status.
▶ The patient will maintain laboratory values within normal limits.
▶ The patient will meet daily intake of required nutrients.

## Definition of terms
▶ *Hyperalimentation:* Parenteral nutrition therapy; a form of I.V. therapy in which all nutrients (carbohydrates, fats, proteins, vitamins, electrolytes, minerals, and trace elements) are delivered to the patient.
▶ *Partial parenteral nutrition:* Peripheral parenteral nutrition; used when support is needed for fewer than 14 days.
▶ *Total parenteral nutrition* (TPN): Central parenteral nutrition; used when the patient needs intensive nutritional support for an extended period.

## Indications
Treatment
▶ Patients who can't absorb nutrients through the GI tract for at least 10 days
▶ Excessive nitrogen loss from wound infection, fistulas, or abscesses

### Prevention
▶ Nutritional deficits
▶ Growth and development retardation

## Assessment guidance
### Signs and symptoms
▶ Weight gain
▶ Increased temperature
▶ Inflammation
▶ Infection
▶ Increased thirst
▶ Polyuria

### Diagnostic studies
*Laboratory tests*
▶ Electrolytes
▶ CBC
▶ Liver enzymes
▶ Blood glucose

*Other*
▶ Weight assessment
▶ Anthropometric measurements
▶ Assessment for deficiencies or toxicity to specific components in the solution

## Nursing interventions
▶ Assess vital signs at least every 4 hours.
▶ Watch for signs and symptoms of hyperglycemia.
▶ Assess the patient for inflammation and infection at the infusion site.
▶ Perform I.V. site care and dressing changes, per facility policy and as needed.
▶ Explain the purpose of the parenteral nutrition therapy to the patient.
▶ Weigh the patient at the same time each day. Assess for weight gain greater than 1 lb [0.5 kg] per day or 3 lb [1.4 kg] per week. Monitor the patient for fluid imbalance.
▶ Assess for peripheral and pulmonary edema.
▶ Perform physical assessments each day.
▶ Monitor the patient for fluid and electrolyte imbalance.
▶ Monitor the patient for glucose metabolism disturbance.
▶ Monitor blood urea nitrogen and creatinine levels to check kidney function.
▶ Monitor liver enzyme, bilirubin, triglyceride, and cholesterol levels.
▶ Monitor the patient for signs and symptoms of infection and inflammation at the I.V. site.

▶ Monitor emotional status and provide emotional support if needed.
▶ Provide mouth care.
▶ If using a filter, position it close to the access site.
▶ Change TPN bags at least every 24 hours.
▶ Always infuse at a constant rate to avoid glucose fluctuations.

## Contraindications
TPN is contraindicated in patients with a normally functioning GI tract, well-nourished patients whose GI tract will return to normal function within 10 days, and in those patients with a poor prognosis.

## Documentation
▶ Document the condition of the insertion site, including redness, heat, swelling, and drainage.
▶ Document the type and location of the peripheral or central line used.
▶ Document the volume and rate of the infusion.
▶ Document adverse reactions and your nursing interventions.
▶ Document the type and condition of dressing and date and time changed.
▶ Document the time and date of filter and solution changes.
▶ Document the patient's daily weight and physical assessment.

## Related procedures
▶ Central venous line insertion and removal
▶ Patient monitoring during parenteral nutrition
▶ Total parenteral nutrition

### REFERENCES
*Handbook of Nursing Procedures.* Springhouse, Pa: Springhouse Corp., 2001.

Ignatavicius, D., and Workman, M. *Medical-surgical Nursing: Thinking for Collaborative Care,* 4th ed. Philadelphia: W.B. Saunders Co., 2002.

Silvestri, L. *Saunders' Comprehensive Review for NCLEX-RN.* Philadelphia: W.B. Saunders Co., 2002.

# Managing the patient requiring massive blood transfusion

## Purpose
To replenish blood or blood products in patients with a demonstrated deficiency

## Collaborative level
Interdependent

## Expected patient outcomes
▶ The patient will maintain stable vital signs.
▶ The patient will have fluid and blood volume return to normal.
▶ The patient will attain hemodynamic stability.
▶ The patient won't exhibit arrhythmias.

## Definition of terms
▶ *Crossmatching:* Matching the donor's blood and the recipient's blood for compatibility.
▶ *Whole blood:* Red blood cells, plasma, and plasma proteins; primarily used to treat hypovolemic shock resulting from hemorrhage.
▶ *Septicemia:* Infective agents or toxins in the bloodstream.
▶ *Rh factor:* A type of antigen system. Rh-negative blood can be given to either Rh-positive or Rh-negative recipients.
▶ *ABO:* An antigen system. ABO donor and recipient should be compatible.
▶ *Fresh frozen plasma:* Contains no platelets. Used to provide clotting factors or volume expansion.
▶ *Blood warmers:* Used to prevent hypothermia.

## Indications
Treatment
▶ Diminished blood volume and the oxygen carrying capacity of circulating system
▶ Decreased hemoglobin and hematocrit

Prevention
▶ Hypovolemic shock

## Assessment guidance
Signs and symptoms
▶ Increased temperature
▶ Increased heart rate
▶ Pallor

▶ Weak pulse
▶ Weakness
▶ Light-headedness
▶ Confusion

Diagnostic studies
*Laboratory tests*
▶ CBC
▶ Chemistry
▶ ABG analysis
▶ Urinalysis

*Imaging tests*
▶ Dependent on patient's injuries, which may require blood transfusion and may include
　−MRI
　−CT scan
　−X-ray

*Other*
▶ ECG

## Nursing interventions
▶ Obtain doctor's order and signed consent.
▶ Determine if the patient has had a previous reaction to a blood transfusion.
▶ Obtain baseline vital signs (notify doctor if temperature is 100° F [37.8° C] or greater).
▶ Start I.V. if not already started. Use a 20G or larger-diameter catheter.
▶ Avoid obtaining blood until ready to begin infusion.
▶ Check expiration date on the blood bag and observe for abnormalities.
▶ Verify the patient's name and number with those on the blood bag.
▶ Premedicate with acetaminophen (Tylenol) or diphenhydramine (Benadryl).
▶ Put on gloves, gown, and face shield.
▶ Maintain standard precautions.
▶ Use Y-type blood administration set.
▶ Prime tubing with normal saline solution only.
▶ Begin the transfusion slowly during the first 15 minutes. Observe closely.
▶ Change blood administration set every 4 to 6 hours or per facility policy.
▶ Administer blood within 30 minutes of receiving it from blood bank.
▶ Check vital signs, including temperature, and breath sounds before the transfusion begins, 15 minutes after the transfusion begins, then every hour until 1 hour after the

transfusion has been completed. Adhere to facility policy.
▶ Rapid blood replacement may require a pressure bag.
▶ If transfusion reaction occurs, follow facility policy and procedure.

## Contraindications
Blood transfusion is contraindicated if a patient has a religious or cultural bias regarding blood transfusion.

## Documentation
▶ Document the date and time of transfusion.
▶ Document the type and amount of transfusion product.
▶ Document the patient's vital signs, including temperature.
▶ Document identification data.
▶ Document the patient's reaction and responses.
▶ Document any transfusion reaction and responses.

## Related procedures
▶ Peripheral I.V. line insertion
▶ Peripheral I.V. line maintenance
▶ Transfusion of whole blood and packed cells
▶ Venipuncture

### REFERENCES
*Handbook of Nursing Procedures.* Springhouse, Pa.: Springhouse Corp., 2001.
Ignatavicius, D., and Workman, M. *Medicalsurgical Nursing: Thinking for Collaborative Care,* 4th ed. Philadelphia: W.B. Saunders Co., 2002.
Silvestri, L. *Saunders' Comprehensive Review for NCLEX-RN.* Philadelphia: W.B. Saunders Co., 2002.

# Managing the patient with a venous access device

## Purpose
To allow administration of blood and blood components, fluids, electrolytes, enhancing agents for diagnostic imaging, nutrients, and medications; to maintain I.V. access; to sustain patients who can't take substances orally; may be used to measure central venous (CV) pressure; and to provide venous access in emergency situations

## Collaborative level
Interdependent

## Expected patient outcomes
▶ The patient will maintain normal vital signs, temperature, and laboratory values.
▶ The patient will show no signs or symptoms of infection, such as redness, swelling, heat, or drainage at the insertion site.
▶ The patient will achieve medical, diagnostic, or nutritional benefits.
▶ The patient will achieve equal intake and output.
▶ The patient will achieve stable fluid volume.

## Definition of terms
▶ *Peripheral saline lock:* A needleless injection port used for therapy that doesn't require continuous administration of solution.
▶ *Central venous access device:* A catheter that accesses a central vein such as the subclavian vein or the internal jugular vein.
▶ *Phlebitis:* Redness, edema, and pain at the insertion site secondary to inflammation of the vein.
▶ *Implanted infusion port:* A venous access device (VAD) that's placed into the subcutaneous tissue with a catheter that goes into the central venous system.
▶ *Irrigate:* Rinse out with fluid.
▶ *Peripherally inserted central catheter:* A long catheter that's placed in an arm vein leading to the superior vena cava.
▶ *Air embolism:* A bolus of air that enters a vein.
▶ *Infiltration:* The leakage of fluid out of the vein and into the surrounding tissue.

## Indications
Treatment
▶ VADs are indicated for patients who need I.V. therapy, such as:
  –fluid replacement
  –medication administration
  –hyperalimentation
  –lipid emulsion therapy
  –maintenance of venous access.

Prevention
▶ Repeated venipuncture

## Assessment guidance
### Signs and symptoms
▶ Redness, swelling, heat, or drainage at infusion site
▶ Dyspnea
▶ Elevated temperature
▶ Chills
▶ Diaphoresis
▶ Cyanosis
▶ Headache
▶ Nausea and vomiting

### Diagnostic studies
#### Laboratory tests
▶ CBC
▶ Electrolytes
▶ BUN
▶ Creatinine
▶ Peak and trough levels

## Nursing interventions
▶ Watch for redness, swelling, heat, or drainage at the infusion site.
▶ Assess the patient for respiratory distress.
▶ Monitor vital signs, and watch for temperature elevation.
▶ Assess the patient for chills, diaphoresis, or cyanosis.
▶ Watch for headache or nausea and vomiting.
▶ Assess the patient for latex allergy.
▶ Obtain an order to start I.V. therapy, including the specific type of solution, rate, total volume to be infused, and number of hours for infusion.
▶ Determine the best site to insert the catheter if peripheral I.V. therapy is ordered.
▶ Dispose of needles in a biohazard container.
▶ *Caution:* At-risk patients include those who are immunocompromised with diseases such as cancer or acquired immunodeficiency syndrome and elderly patients because of the altered effectiveness of the immune system.
▶ Maintain strict sterile technique when caring for the I.V. site.
▶ Monitor laboratory work, especially white blood cell count.
▶ Check I.V. fluids for cloudiness or contamination.
▶ Change the tubing and dressing according to facility policy.
▶ Change I.V. site according to facility policy.

## Contraindications
Contraindicated in patients with site burns, sclerotic veins, or arteriovenous fistula. Also contraindicated in postmastectomy arm or edematous or impaired arm or hand.

## Documentation
▶ Document the date and time of I.V. insertion.
▶ Document the number of attempts at venipuncture.
▶ Document the location of the insertion site.
▶ Document the gauge and type of needle or catheter used.
▶ Document the flush that was used for catheter patency.
▶ Document the type, amount, and rate of solution infused.
▶ Document the date and time of dressing and tubing change with the name or initials of the person who did the change.
▶ Document the patient's tolerance of the procedure.
▶ Document the status of the I.V. site including any redness, drainage, heat, or swelling.
▶ Document adverse clinical manifestations and actions taken to correct them.
▶ Document how much blood is withdrawn, if any.

## Related procedures
▶ Central venous line insertion and removal
▶ I.V. bolus injection
▶ Pediatric I.V. therapy
▶ Peripheral I.V. line insertion
▶ Peripheral I.V. line maintenance
▶ PICC insertion and removal
▶ Total parenteral nutrition
▶ Transfusion of whole blood and packed cells
▶ Vascular access device maintenance
▶ Venipuncture

### REFERENCES
*Handbook of Nursing Procedures.* Springhouse, Pa: Springhouse Corp., 2001.
Ignatavicius, D., and Workman, M. *Medical-surgical Nursing: Thinking for Collaborative Care,* 4th ed. Philadelphia: W.B. Saunders Co., 2002.

Silvestri, L. *Saunders' Comprehensive Review for NCLEX-RN*. Philadelphia: W.B. Saunders Co., 2002.

# Managing the patient having a transfusion reaction

## Purpose
To provide rapid and effective treatment to prevent or minimize complications of a transfusion reaction

## Collaborative level
Interdependent

## Expected patient outcomes
The patient will:
▶ Preserve renal blood flow and urine output.
▶ Maintain hemodynamic stability.
▶ Maintain adequate ventilation.

## Definition of terms
▶ *Hemolytic transfusion reaction:* Transfusion reaction in which antibodies in the recipient's plasma are directed against antigens on donor cells; ABO incompatibility is the most common cause.
▶ *Nonhemolytic febrile reaction:* Most common type of transfusion reaction; recipient antibodies form against donor white blood cells or platelets.
▶ *Anaphylactic reaction:* Transfusion reaction observed most commonly in patients with a hereditary immunoglobulin (Ig) A deficiency; some of these patients develop complement-binding anti-IgA antibodies that cause anaphylaxis when exposed to donor IgA.

## Indications
### Treatment
▶ Hemolytic transfusion reactions
▶ Nonhemolytic febrile reactions
▶ Anaphylactic reactions

### Prevention
▶ Bronchospasm and respiratory failure
▶ Acute renal failure
▶ Cardiovascular collapse
▶ Disseminated intravascular coagulation

## Assessment guidance
### Signs and symptoms
#### Hemolytic transfusion reaction
▶ Fever
▶ Chills
▶ Nausea
▶ Burning at the I.V. line site
▶ Chest tightness
▶ Restlessness
▶ Apprehension
▶ Joint or back pain
▶ Tachycardia
▶ Tachypnea
▶ In severe cases, hypotension, oozing from the I.V. site or other puncture sites, diffuse bleeding, hemoglobinuria, dark urine, and shock
▶ Oliguria, in renal failure

#### Nonhemolytic febrile reaction
▶ Nonspecific symptoms of fever
▶ Chills
▶ Malaise
▶ Fever

#### Anaphylactic reaction
▶ Rapid development of chills
▶ Abdominal cramps, dyspnea, vomiting, diarrhea
▶ Tachycardia
▶ Flushing
▶ Urticaria (also occurring in minor allergic reactions)
▶ In more severe cases, wheezing, laryngeal edema, and hypotension

### Diagnostic studies
#### Laboratory tests
▶ Hemoglobin (Hb) level
▶ Bilirubin
▶ CBC
▶ Indirect Coombs' test
▶ Serum antibody screen
▶ Prothrombin time
▶ Fibrinogen level
▶ Blood urea nitrogen
▶ Creatinine levels

#### Other
▶ Electrocardiogram

## Nursing interventions
▶ Stop the transfusion immediately; don't discard the blood bag or administration set.
▶ Maintain a patent I.V. line with normal saline solution.

▶ Notify the doctor.

▶ Monitor vital signs every 15 minutes, or as indicated by the severity and type of reaction.

▶ Compare the labels on all blood containers with corresponding patient identification forms to verify that the transfusion was the correct blood or blood product.

▶ Notify the blood bank of possible transfusion reaction and collect blood samples, as ordered. The blood bank should perform a repeat type, crossmatch, antibody screen, and direct and indirect Coombs' tests.

▶ Immediately send the blood samples, all transfusion containers, and the administration set to the blood bank for evaluation. The blood bank needs to determine whether the correct unit of blood was administered to the intended recipient.

▶ Collect the first posttransfusion urine specimen, mark the collection slip "Possible transfusion reaction," and send it to the laboratory immediately; hemoglobinuria indicates a transfusion reaction.

▶ Closely monitor intake and output. Note evidence of oliguria or anuria because hemoglobin deposition in the renal tubules can cause renal damage.

▶ Administer supplemental oxygen or other drugs.

▶ Make the patient as comfortable as possible and provide reassurance as needed.

## Hemolytic transfusion reaction

▶ Begin aggressive fluid resuscitation in order to maximize renal cortical perfusion.

▶ Administer diuretics, such as furosemide (Lasix) or low-dose dopamine, to improve renal blood flow.

▶ Maintain urine output at 30 to 100 ml/hour.

▶ Insert an indwelling urinary drainage catheter to ensure continuous measurement of urine output.

▶ Assist with endotracheal intubation if respiratory insufficiency is present.

## Nonhemolytic febrile reaction

▶ Evaluate the patient for evidence of hemolysis.

## Anaphylactic reaction

▶ Support airway and circulation as necessary.

▶ Assist with endotracheal intubation if respiratory insufficiency is present.

▶ Administer epinephrine, diphenhydramine, and corticosteroids.

▶ Complete the transfusion reaction form, if required by your facility.

## Patient teaching

▶ Be sure to cover these important points with the patient and his family:
  – risks of blood transfusion
  – definition of blood transfusion reaction
  – how to recognize a blood transfusion reaction, and immediate notification of the health care team
  – diagnostic studies performed with suspected transfusion reaction
  – treatment of transfusion reaction and expected outcome
  – prevention of future transfusion reactions, if indicated.

## Precautions

▶ Ensure that informed consent is obtained before blood transfusion.

▶ Carefully examine and compare the patient's name and identification numbers with the label on the unit of blood to ensure administration of correct unit to the intended recipient.

▶ Treat all transfusion reactions as serious until proven otherwise.

▶ Administer leukocyte-poor packed red blood cells (RBCs) in patients who have had two previous febrile nonhemolytic reactions.

▶ Administer frozen deglycerolized packed RBCs or blood from IgA-deficient donors in patients with a history of previous anaphylactic reactions to transfused blood.

## Documentation

▶ Document the transfusion reaction on the patient's medical record, including:
  – the time and date of the transfusion reaction
  – the type and amount of infused blood or blood products
  – subjective symptoms reported by the patient
  – objective signs obtained by nursing assessment
  – samples obtained and sent to the laboratory
  – diagnostic study results
  – nursing interventions
  – doctor notification and intervention
  – the patient's response to treatment.

## Related procedures
▶ Arterial pressure monitoring
▶ Arterial puncture for blood gas analysis
▶ Cardiac monitoring
▶ Cardiopulmonary resuscitation
▶ Central venous pressure monitoring
▶ Electrocardiography
▶ Endotracheal intubation
▶ Endotracheal tube care
▶ End-tidal carbon dioxide monitoring
▶ I.V. bolus injection
▶ Indwelling catheter insertion
▶ Intradermal injection
▶ Manual ventilation
▶ Mechanical ventilation
▶ Oxygen administration
▶ Peripheral I.V. line insertion
▶ Peripheral I.V. line maintenance
▶ Physical assessment
▶ Pulse and ear oximetry
▶ Subcutaneous injection
▶ Tracheal suction
▶ Transfusion of whole blood and packed cells
▶ Urine collection
▶ Venipuncture

## REFERENCES
Braunwald, E., et al., eds. *Harrison's Principles of Internal Medicine,* 15th ed. New York: McGraw-Hill Book Co., 2001.
Uhlmann, E.J., et al., "Prestorage Universal WBC Reduction of RBC Units Does Not Affect the Incidence of Transfusion Reactions," *Transfusion* 41(8):997-1000, August 2001.
Win, N., et al. "Hyperhemolytic Transfusion Reaction in Sickle Cell Disease," *Transfusion* 41(3):323-28, March 2001.
Young, J. "Transfusion Reaction," *Nursing* 30(12):33, December 2000.

## ORGANIZATIONS
American Association of Blood Banks: *www.aabb.org*
Centers for Disease Control and Prevention: *www.cdc.gov*

# Procedures

## Autotransfusion

Also called autologous blood transfusion, autotransfusion is the collection, filtration, and reinfusion of the patient's own blood. Today, with the concern over acquired immunodeficiency syndrome and other blood-borne diseases, the use of autotransfusion is on the rise.

Indications for autotransfusion include:
▶ Elective surgery (blood donated over time)
▶ Nonelective surgery (blood withdrawn immediately before surgery)
▶ Perioperative and emergency blood salvage during and after thoracic or cardiovascular surgery and hip, knee, or liver resection and during surgery for ruptured ectopic pregnancy and hemothorax
▶ Perioperative and emergency blood salvage for traumatic injury of the lungs, liver, chest wall, heart, pulmonary vessels, spleen, kidneys, inferior vena cava, and iliac, portal, or subclavian veins.

Autotransfusion is performed before, during, or after surgery and after traumatic injury. The three techniques used are preoperative blood donation, perioperative blood donation, and acute normovolemic hemodilution.

Preoperative blood donation is commonly recommended for patients scheduled for orthopedic surgery, which causes large blood loss. The donation period begins 4 to 6 weeks before surgery.

Perioperative blood donation (sometimes called intraoperative or postoperative) is used in vascular and orthopedic surgery and in treatment of traumatic injury. Blood may be collected during surgery or up to 12 hours afterward. (Considerable bleeding may follow vascular and orthopedic surgery.) The blood is transfused immediately after collection or processed (washed) before infusion. Blood obtained postoperatively may be collected from chest tubes, mediastinal drains, or wound drains (placed in the surgical wound during surgery). Commonly inserted during orthopedic surgery, wound drains can be used when enough uncontaminated blood is recovered from a closed wound to be reinfused.

Acute normovolemic hemodilution is used mainly in open-heart surgery. One or 2 units of blood are drawn immediately before or after anesthesia induction. The blood is replaced with a crystalloid or colloid solution, such as lactated Ringer's solution or dextran 40, to produce normovolemic anemia. The blood is reinfused right after surgery. The combination of reduced hemoglobin and the replacement solution causes the patient to lose fewer red blood cells during surgery.

The equipment and procedures presented here are for preoperative and perioperative blood donation only. Acute normovolemic hemodilution is performed the same way as preoperative blood donation, and blood collected this way is reinfused the same way as any other transfusion.

## Equipment
### For preoperative blood donation
Ferrous sulfate • povidone-iodine solution • alcohol • tourniquet • rubber ball • large-bore needle for venipuncture • collection bags • I.V. line • in-line filter for reinfusion

### For perioperative blood donation
Autotransfusion system, such as the Davol or Pleur-evac system • anticoagulant citrate dextrose or citrate phosphate dextrose • collection bags • vacuum source regulator • suction tubing • 18G needle • blood administration set with in-line filter • 500 ml of normal saline solution • optional: Hemovac and another autologous transfusion system

## Implementation
The steps to take depend on the circumstances of the autotransfusion.

### For preoperative blood donation
▶ Explain autotransfusion to the patient, including what it is, how it's performed, how often he can donate blood (every 7 days), and how much he can donate (1 unit every week until 3 to 7 days before surgery).
▶ At least 1 week before the first donation, give the patient ferrous sulfate or another iron preparation to take three times a day, as ordered.
▶ To prevent hypovolemia, tell the patient to drink plenty of fluids before donating blood.
▶ Warn him that he may feel light-headed during the donation but that the problem can be treated without further compromise.
▶ Check the patient's hemoglobin level, which must be 11 g/dl or higher to donate blood.
▶ Check vital signs before blood donation.
▶ Help the patient into a supine position.
▶ Clean the needle insertion site (usually the antecubital fossa) with alcohol or povidone-iodine solution.
▶ Apply a tourniquet.
▶ Insert the large-bore needle into the antecubital vein. Have the patient squeeze a rubber ball while you collect blood.
▶ Recheck vital signs after the collection.
▶ If ordered, provide replacement I.V. fluids immediately after the collection.
▶ Send a blood sample to the laboratory to be tested.

### For perioperative blood donation
▶ If you know that the patient will leave surgery with a drain to the autotransfusion device, tell him this beforehand.

### For perioperative blood donation using a Davol system
▶ Open the transfusion unit onto the sterile field. The doctor inserts the drain tube (from the patient) to the connecting tube of the unit.
▶ The doctor injects 25 to 35 ml of ACD or CPD into the injection port on top of the filter and wets the filter with anticoagulant to keep the blood from clotting.
▶ Label the collection bag with the patient's name and the time the transfusion was started so that the reinfusion time is within guidelines.

### After patient arrival in postanesthesia care unit or medical-surgical unit
▶ Note the amount of blood in the bag and on the postoperative sheet.

▶ Attach the tube from the suction source to the port on the suction control module.
▶ Adjust the suction source to between 80 and 100 mm Hg on the wall regulator. Pinch the suction tube. If the regulator exceeds 100 mm Hg, turn the suction down. Suction set at more than 100 mm Hg may cause the collection bag to collapse, resulting in lysis of blood cells. The potential for renal damage renders this blood unsafe. If the collection bag collapses, change the entire collection setup.
▶ If the doctor orders it, start reinfusing the blood when 500 ml has been collected or 4 hours have passed, whichever comes first. Blood reinfusion must be completed within 6 hours of initiating the collection in the operating room.
▶ If less than 200 ml is collected in 4 hours, record the amount on the intake and output sheet and the postoperative sheet. Discard the drainage appropriately because the proportion of anticoagulant (inserted in the operating room) to blood is too great to infuse. If this happens, switch from the container to a closed-wound suction unit. First remove the suction tube from the suction control unit. Clamp the connecting tubing above the filter. Detach the connecting tubing from the patient's tube and cap the patient's tube. Connect a closed-wound suction unit, such as a Hemovac, if you aren't going to collect more blood for reinfusion. If more than 500 ml of blood is collected in the first 4 hours, connect a new autotransfusion unit to the patient. Then reconnect the unit to suction. Monitor and record the drainage on the intake and output sheet.

### For blood reinfusion
▶ Prime the blood filter with 500 ml of normal saline solution.
▶ Twist the suction control module to remove it.
▶ Remove the hanger assembly from the collection bag.
▶ Pull the clear cap from the top of the bag and discard the cap and filter.
▶ Insert a spike adapter into the large port on top of the bottle.
▶ Remove the protective seal to expose the filtered vent.
▶ Attach the blood to the Y-connector of the blood filter.
▶ Invert the bag and hang it.

▶ Obtain vital signs and document them.
▶ Begin the infusion, following your facility's policy.
▶ Be sure to complete the infusion within 2 hours.

### For perioperative blood donation using the Pleur-evac system connected to a chest tube
▶ Establish underwater seal drainage. Following the steps printed on the Pleur-evac unit, connect the patient's chest tube. Inspect the blood collection bag and tubing, making sure that all clamps are open and all connections are airtight.
▶ Before collection, add an anticoagulant, such as heparin or CPD, if prescribed. With CPD, add one part CPD to seven parts blood. Using an 18G (or smaller) needle, inject the anticoagulant through the red self-sealing port on the autotransfusion connector. The system is now ready to use. You should see chest cavity blood begin to collect in the bag.
▶ To collect more than one bag of blood, open a replacement bag when the first one is nearly full. Close the clamps on top of the second bag. Before removing the first collection bag from the drainage unit, reduce excess negativity by using the high-negativity relief valve. Depress the button; release it when negativity drops to the desired level (watch the water seal manometer).
▶ Close the white clamp on the patient tubing. Then close the two white clamps on top of the collection bag.
▶ Disconnect all connectors on the first bag. Attach the red (female) and blue (male) connector sections on top of the autologous transfusion bag.
▶ Remove the protective cap from the collection tubing on the replacement bag. Connect the collection tubing to the patient's chest drainage tube, using the red connectors.
▶ Remove the protective cap from the replacement bag's suction tube and attach the tube to the Pleur-evac unit, using the blue connectors. Make sure all connections are tight. Open all clamps and inspect the system for airtight connections.
▶ Spread the metal support arms and disconnect them. Remove the first bag from the drainage unit by disconnecting the foot hook.

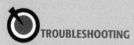

TROUBLESHOOTING

# Managing problems of autotransfusion

| Problem | Cause | Intervention |
|---------|-------|--------------|
| Coagulation | ▶ Not enough anticoagulant<br>▶ Blood not defibrinated in mediastinum | ▶ Add citrate phosphate dextrose (CPD) or another regional anticoagulant at a ratio of 7 parts blood to 1 part anticoagulant. Keep blood and CPD mixed by shaking collection bottle regularly.<br>▶ Check for anticoagulant reversal. |
| Coagulopathies | ▶ Reduced platelet and fibrinogen levels<br>▶ Platelets caught in filters<br>▶ Enhanced levels of fibrin split products | ▶ Transfuse fresh frozen plasma or platelet concentrate as ordered for patients receiving autologous transfusions of more than 4,000 ml of blood. |
| Emboli | ▶ Microaggregate debris<br>▶ Air | ▶ Don't use equipment with roller pumps or pressure infusion systems. Before reinfusion, remove air from blood bags.<br>▶ Reinfuse with a 20- to 40-unit microaggregate filter. |
| Hemolysis | ▶ Trauma to blood caused by turbulence or roller pumps | ▶ Don't skim operative field or use equipment with roller pumps. When collecting blood from chest tubes, keep vacuum below 30 mm Hg; when aspirating from a surgical site, keep vacuum below 60 mm Hg. |
| Sepsis | ▶ Lack of sterile technique<br>▶ Contaminated blood | ▶ Give broad-spectrum antibiotics. Use strict sterile technique. Reinfuse patientthe patient within 4 hours.<br>▶ Don't infuse blood from infected areas or blood that contains feces, urine, or other contaminants. |

▶ Use the foot hook and support arm to attach the replacement bag.
▶ To reinfuse blood from the original collection bag, slide the bag off the support frame; then invert it so that the spike points upward. Reinfuse blood within 6 hours of the start of collection. Never store collected blood.
▶ Remove the protective cap from the spike port and insert a microaggregate filter into the port, using a twisting motion. Prime the filter by gently squeezing the inverted bag. A new filter should be used with each bag.
▶ Continue squeezing until the filter is saturated and the drip chamber is half full. Then close the clamp on the reinfusion line and remove residual air from the bag.

Invert the bag and suspend it from an I.V. pole. After carefully flushing the I.V. line to remove all air, infuse blood according to your facility's policy.

## Special considerations

Autotransfusion is contraindicated in patients with malignant neoplasms, coagulopathies, excessive hemolysis, and active infections. It's also contraindicated in patients taking antibiotics and in those whose blood becomes contaminated by bowel contents. In addition, patients who have recently lost weight because of illness or malnutrition shouldn't donate blood.

## For preoperative blood donation
▶ Monitor the patient closely during and after donation and autotransfusion. Although vasovagal reactions are usually mild and easy to treat, they can quickly progress to severe reactions, such as loss of consciousness and seizures. Also, make sure the patient isn't bacteremic when he donates blood. Bacteria can proliferate in the collection bag and cause sepsis when reinfused.
▶ Clearly label the collection bag AUTOTRANSFUSION USE ONLY. This way the blood won't be subjected to rigorous blood bank testing or be accidentally given to another patient.
▶ Caution the patient to remain in a supine position for at least 10 minutes after donating blood.
▶ Encourage him to drink more fluids than usual for a few hours after blood donation and to eat heartily at his next meal.
▶ Tell him to keep an eye on the needle wound in his arm for a few hours after blood donation. If some bleeding occurs, he should apply firm pressure for 5 to 10 minutes. If the bleeding doesn't stop, he should notify the blood bank or his doctor.
▶ If the patient feels light-headed or dizzy, advise him to sit down immediately and to lower his head between his knees. Or he can lie down with his head lower than the rest of his body until the feeling subsides.
▶ Tell him that he can resume normal activities after resting 15 minutes.

## For all donation methods
▶ Check the patient's laboratory data (coagulation profile, hemoglobin and calcium levels, and hematocrit) after he donates blood and again after reinfusion. Before reinfusion, identify the patient and make sure that the collection bag is clearly marked with his name, his identification number, and an autotransfusion blood label.
▶ Be alert for signs and symptoms of a hemolytic reaction: pain at the I.V. site, fever, chills, back pain, hypotension, and anxiety. If any occurs, stop the transfusion and call the blood bank and doctor. The patient may have received the wrong unit of blood.
▶ Check the patient's laboratory data again after reinfusion.

## Complications
Autotransfusion may cause hemolysis, air and particulate emboli, coagulation, thrombocytopenia, vasovagal reactions (from transient hypotension and bradycardia), and hypovolemia (especially in elderly patients). (See *Managing problems of autotransfusion*.)

## Documentation
▶ Document the amount of blood the patient donated and had reinfused and how he tolerated each procedure.

### REFERENCES
Dalen, T., et al. "Fever and Autologous Blood Retransfusion After Total Knee Arthroplasty: A Prospective Study of 40 Autotransfusion Events in 21 Patients," *Acta Orthopaedica Scandinavica* 73(3):321-25, June 2002.
Henry, D.A., et al. "Pre-Operative Autologous Donation for Minimising Perioperative Allogeneic Blood Transfusion," *Cochrane Database Syst Rev* (2), 2002.
Knichwitz, G., et al. "Intraoperative Washing of Long-stored Packed Red Blood Cells by Using an Autotransfusion Device Prevents Hyperkalemia," *Anesthesia and Analgesia* 95(2):324-25, August 2002.

# Central venous line insertion and removal

A central venous catheter (CVC) is a sterile catheter made of polyurethane, polyvinyl chloride, or silicone rubber. It's inserted through a large vein such as the subclavian vein or, less commonly, the jugular vein. (See *Central venous catheter pathways*, page 172.)
By providing access to the central veins, central venous (CV) therapy offers several benefits. It allows monitoring of CV pressure, which indicates blood volume or pump efficiency and permits aspiration of blood samples for diagnostic tests. It also allows administration of I.V. fluids (in large amounts if necessary) in emergencies or when decreased peripheral circulation makes peripheral vein access difficult; when prolonged I.V. therapy reduces the number of accessible peripheral veins; when solutions must be diluted (for large fluid volumes or for irritating or hypertonic

# Central venous catheter pathways

The illustrations below show several common pathways for central venous catheter (CVC) insertion. Typically, a CVC is inserted in the subclavian vein or in the internal jugular vein. The catheter typically terminates in the superior vena cava. The CVC is tunneled when long-term placement is required.

**Insertion:** Subclavian vein
**Termination:** Superior vena cava

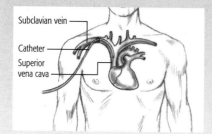

**Insertion:** Internal jugular vein
**Termination:** Superior vena cava

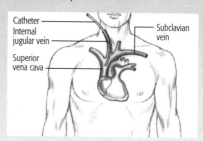

**Insertion:** Basilic vein (peripheral)
**Termination:** Superior vena cava

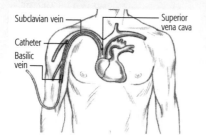

**Insertion:** Through a subcutaneous tunnel to the subclavian vein (Dacron cuff helps hold catheter in place.)
**Termination:** Superior vena cava

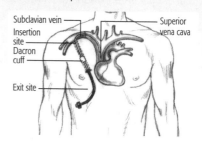

fluids, such as total parenteral nutrition solutions); and when a patient requires long-term venous access. Because multiple blood samples can be drawn through it without repeated venipuncture, the CV line decreases the patient's anxiety and preserves or restores peripheral veins.

A variation of CV therapy, peripheral CV therapy involves the insertion of a catheter into a peripheral vein instead of a central vein, but with the catheter tip still lying in the CV circulation. A peripherally inserted central catheter (PICC) usually enters at the basilic vein and terminates in the superior vena cava. PICCs may be inserted by a specially trained nurse. New catheters have longer needles and smaller lumens, facilitating this procedure. PICCs are commonly used in home I.V. therapy but may also be used with chest injury; chest, neck, or shoulder burns; compromised respiratory function; proximity of a surgical site to the CV line placement site; and if a doctor isn't available to insert a CV line.

CV therapy increases the risk of complications, such as pneumothorax, sepsis, thrombus formation, and vessel and adjacent organ perforation (all life-threatening conditions). Also, the CVC may decrease patient mobility, is difficult to insert, and costs more than a peripheral I.V. catheter.

Removal of a CVC—a sterile procedure—usually is performed by a doctor or nurse either at the end of therapy or at the onset of complications. A peripherally inserted central line may be removed by a specially trained nurse. If the patient may have an infection, the removal procedure includes collection of the catheter tip as a specimen for culture.

## Equipment

*For insertion of a CVC*
Skin preparation kit, if necessary • sterile gloves and gowns • blanket • linen-saver pad • sterile towel • sterile drape • masks • an alcohol applicator or an applicator that contains povidone-iodine solution or other approved antimicrobial solution • alcohol pads • 10% povidone-iodine pads or other approved antimicrobial solution, such as 70% isopropyl alcohol or tincture of iodine 2% • normal saline solution • antibiotic ointment, if necessary • 3-ml syringe with 25G 1″ needle • 1% or 2% injectable lidocaine • dextrose 5% in water • syringes for blood sample collection • suture material • two 14G or 16G CVCs • I.V. solution with administration set prepared for use • infusion pump or controller, as needed • sterile 4″ × 4″ gauze pads • 1″ adhesive tape • sterile scissors • heparin or normal saline flushes as needed • portable X-ray machine • optional: transparent semipermeable dressing

The type of catheter selected depends on the type of therapy to be used. (See *Guide to central venous catheters,* pages 174 to 177.)

Some facilities have prepared trays containing most of the equipment for catheter insertion.

*For flushing a catheter*
Normal saline solution or heparin flush solution • alcohol pad • 70% alcohol solution

*For changing an injection cap*
Alcohol or povidone-iodine pad • injection cap • padded clamp

*For removing a CVC*
Clean gloves and sterile gloves • sterile suture removal set • alcohol pads • povidone-iodine • povidone-iodine ointment • sterile 4″ × 4″ gauze • forceps • tape • sterile, plastic adhesive-backed dressing or transparent semipermeable dressing • agar plate or culture tube, if necessary for culture

### Preparation of equipment

Before insertion of a CV catheter, confirm catheter type and size with the doctor; usually, a 14G or 16G catheter is selected. Set up the I.V. solution and prime the administration set using strict aseptic technique. Attach the line to the infusion pump or controller if ordered. Recheck all connections to make sure they're tight. As ordered, notify the radiology department that a portable X-ray machine will be needed.

## Implementation

▶ Wash your hands thoroughly to prevent the spread of microorganisms.

### Inserting a CVC

▶ Reinforce the doctor's explanation of the procedure and answer the patient's questions. Ensure that the patient has signed a consent form, if necessary, and check his history for hypersensitivity to iodine, latex, or the local anesthetic.
▶ Place the patient in Trendelenburg's position to dilate the veins and reduce the risk of air embolism.
▶ For subclavian insertion, place a rolled blanket lengthwise between the shoulders to increase venous distention. For jugular insertion, place a rolled blanket under the opposite shoulder to extend the neck, making anatomic landmarks more visible. Place a linen-saver pad under the patient to prevent soiling the bed.
▶ Turn the patient's head away from the site to prevent possible contamination from airborne pathogens and to make the site more accessible. Or, if dictated by facility policy, place a mask on the patient unless this increases his anxiety or is contraindicated because of his respiratory status.
▶ Prepare the insertion site. Make sure the skin is free from hair because hair can harbor microorganisms. Infection-control health care providers recommend clipping the hair close to the skin rather than shaving. Shaving may cause skin irritation and create multiple small open wounds, in-

# Guide to central venous catheters

| Type | Description | Indications |
|------|-------------|-------------|
| Groshong catheter | ▶ Silicone rubber<br>▶ About 35″ (88.9 cm) long<br>▶ Closed end with pressure-sensitive two-way valve<br>▶ Dacron cuff<br>▶ Single or double lumen<br>▶ Tunneled | ▶ Long-term central venous (CV) access<br>▶ Patient with heparin allergy |

| | | |
|------|-------------|-------------|
| Short-term single-lumen catheter | ▶ Polyvinyl chloride (PVC) or polyurethane<br>▶ About 8″ (20.3 cm) long<br>▶ Lumen gauge varies<br>▶ Percutaneously placed | ▶ Short-term CV access<br>▶ Emergency access<br>▶ Patient who needs only one lumen |

| | | |
|------|-------------|-------------|
| Short-term multilumen catheter | ▶ PVC or polyurethane<br>▶ Two, three, or four lumens exiting at ¾″ (1.9 cm) intervals<br>▶ Lumen gauges vary<br>▶ Percutaneously placed | ▶ Short-term CV access<br>▶ Patient with limited insertion sites who requires multiple infusions |

creasing the risk of infection. (If the doctor orders that the area be shaved, try shaving it the evening before catheter insertion; this allows minor skin irritations to heal par-

tially.) You may also need to wash the skin with soap and water first.

▶ Establish a sterile field on a table, using a sterile towel or the wrapping from the instrument tray.

| Advantages and disadvantages | Nursing considerations |
|---|---|
| **Advantages**<br>▶ Less thrombogenic<br>▶ Pressure-sensitive two-way valve eliminates frequent heparin flushes.<br>▶ Dacron cuff anchors catheter and prevents bacterial migration.<br>**Disadvantages**<br>▶ Requires surgical insertion<br>▶ Tears and kinks easily<br>▶ Blunt end makes it difficult to clear substances from its tip. | ▶ Two surgical sites require dressing after insertion.<br>▶ Handle catheter gently.<br>▶ Check the external portion frequently for kinks and leaks.<br>▶ Repair kit is available.<br>▶ Remember to flush with enough saline solution to clear the catheter, especially after drawing or administering blood. |
| **Advantages**<br>▶ Easily inserted at bedside<br>▶ Easily removed<br>▶ Stiffness aids central venous pressure (CVP) monitoring.<br>**Disadvantages**<br>▶ Limited functions<br>▶ PVC is thrombogenic and irritates inner lumen of vessel.<br>▶ Should be changed every 3 to 7 days (frequency may depend on facility's CV line infection rate) | ▶ Minimize patient movement.<br>▶ Assess frequently for signs of infection and clot formation. |
| **Advantages**<br>▶ Same as single-lumen catheter<br>▶ Allows infusion of multiple (even incompatible) solutions through the same catheter<br>**Disadvantages**<br>▶ Same as single-lumen catheter | ▶ Know gauge and purpose of each lumen.<br>▶ Use the same lumen for the same task. |

*(continued)*

▶ Put on a mask and sterile gloves and a gown and clean the area around the insertion site with an alcohol applicator or an applicator that contains povidone-iodine solution or other approved antimicrobial solution, working in a circular motion outward from the site. If the patient is sensitive to iodine, use alcohol.

▶ After the doctor puts on a sterile mask, a sterile gown, and sterile gloves and drapes

## Guide to central venous catheters *(continued)*

| Type | Description | Indications |
|------|-------------|-------------|
| Hickman catheter | ▶ Silicone rubber<br>▶ About 35″ (88.9 cm) long<br>▶ Open end with clamp<br>▶ Dacron cuff 1¾″ (4.4 cm) from hub<br>▶ Single lumen or multilumen<br>▶ Tunneled | ▶ Long-term CV access<br>▶ Home therapy |
| Broviac catheter | ▶ Identical to Hickman except smaller inner lumen | ▶ Long-term CV access<br>▶ Patient with small central vessels (pediatric or geriatric) |
| Hickman/Broviac catheter | ▶ Hickman and Broviac catheters combined<br>▶ Tunneled | ▶ Long-term CV access<br>▶ Patient who needs multiple infusions |
| Peripherally inserted central catheter | ▶ Silicone rubber<br>▶ 20″ (50.8 cm) long<br>▶ Available in 16G, 18G, 20G, and 22G<br>▶ Can be used as midline catheter<br>▶ Percutaneously placed | ▶ Long-term CV access<br>▶ Patient with poor CV access<br>▶ Patient at risk for fatal complications from CV catheter insertion<br>▶ Patient who needs CV access but is scheduled for or has had head or neck surgery |

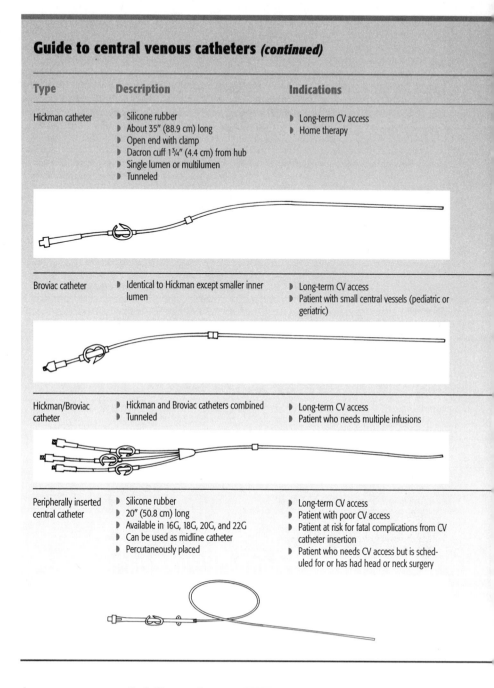

the area to create a sterile field, open the packaging of the 3-ml syringe and 25G needle and give the syringe to him using sterile technique.

**EVIDENCE BASE** Evidence-based studies show that infections and sepsis present a major problem with CV catheter usage. Complications of infection may be

| Advantages and disadvantages | Nursing considerations |
|---|---|
| **Advantages** | ▶ Two surgical sites require dressing after insertion. |
| ▶ Less thrombogenic | ▶ Handle catheter gently. |
| ▶ Dacron cuff prevents excess motion and bacterial migration. | ▶ Observe frequently for kinks and tears. |
| ▶ Clamps eliminate need for Valsalva's maneuver. | ▶ Repair kit is available. |
| **Disadvantages** | ▶ Clamp catheter with a nonserrated clamp any time it becomes disconnected or opens. |
| ▶ Requires surgical insertion | |
| ▶ Open end | |
| ▶ Requires doctor for removal | |
| ▶ Tears and kinks easily | |
| **Advantages** | ▶ Check your facility's policy before drawing blood or administering blood or blood products. |
| ▶ Smaller lumen | |
| **Disadvantages** | |
| ▶ Small lumen may limit uses. | |
| ▶ Single lumen | |
| **Advantages** | ▶ Know the purpose and function of each lumen. |
| ▶ Double-lumen Hickman catheter allows sampling and administration of blood. | ▶ Label lumens to prevent confusion. |
| ▶ Broviac lumen delivers I.V. fluids, including total parenteral nutrition. | |
| **Disadvantages** | |
| ▶ Same as Hickman catheter | |
| **Advantages** | ▶ Check frequently for signs of phlebitis and thrombus formation. |
| ▶ Peripherally inserted | ▶ Insert catheter above the antecubital fossa. |
| ▶ Easily inserted at bedside with minimal complications | ▶ Basilic vein is preferable to cephalic vein. |
| ▶ May be inserted by a specially trained nurse in some states | ▶ Use arm board, if necessary. |
| **Disadvantages** | ▶ Length of catheter may alter CVP measurements. |
| ▶ Catheter may occlude smaller peripheral vessels. | |
| ▶ May be difficult to keep immobile | |
| ▶ Long path to CV circulation | |

minimized through the use of maximum sterile barriers (while inserting CV catheters), antibiotic impregnated catheters, and highly permeable transparent dressings. In addition, the use of real-time ultrasound guidance during CV catheter insertion may help prevent complications of misplaced lines.

# Teaching Valsalva's maneuver

Increased intrathoracic pressure reduces the risk of air embolus during insertion and removal of a central venous catheter. A simple way to achieve this is to ask the patient to perform Valsalva's maneuver: forced exhalation against a closed airway. Instruct the patient to take a deep breath and hold it and then to bear down for 10 seconds. Then tell the patient to exhale and breathe quietly.

Valsalva's maneuver raises intrathoracic pressure from its normal level of 3 to 4 mm Hg to levels of 60 mm Hg or higher. It also slows the pulse rate, decreases the return of blood to the heart, and increases venous pressure.

This maneuver is contraindicated in patients with increased intracranial pressure. It shouldn't be taught to patients who aren't alert or cooperative.

---

▶ Wipe the top of the lidocaine vial with an alcohol pad and invert it. The doctor then fills the 3-ml syringe and injects the anesthetic into the site (as shown below).

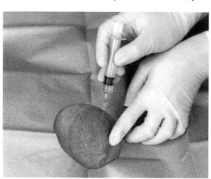

▶ Open the catheter package and give the catheter to the doctor using aseptic technique. The doctor then inserts the catheter.
▶ During this time, prepare the I.V. administration set for immediate attachment to the catheter hub. Ask the patient to perform Valsalva's maneuver while the doctor attaches the I.V. line to the catheter hub. This increases intrathoracic pressure, reducing the possibility of an air embolus. (See *Teaching Valsalva's maneuver.*)
▶ After the doctor attaches the I.V. line to the catheter hub, set the flow rate at a keep-vein-open rate to maintain venous access. (Alternatively, the catheter may be capped and flushed with heparin.) The doctor then sutures the catheter in place.
▶ After an X-ray confirms correct catheter placement in the midsuperior vena cava, set the flow rate as ordered.
▶ Use normal saline solution to remove dried blood that could harbor microorganisms. Secure the catheter with adhesive tape, and apply a sterile 4″ × 4″ gauze pad. You may also use a transparent semipermeable dressing either alone or placed over the gauze pad (as shown below).

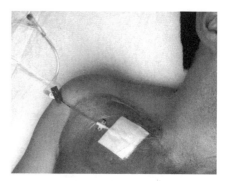

▶ Expect some serosanguineous drainage during the first 24 hours. Label the dressing with the time and date of catheter insertion and catheter length and gauge (as shown below), if not imprinted on the catheter.

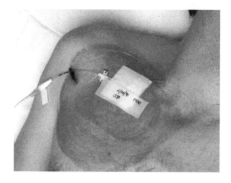

▶ Place the patient in a comfortable position and reassess his status.

## Flushing the catheter
▶ To maintain patency, flush the catheter routinely according to your facility's policy. If the system is being maintained as a

heparin lock and the infusions are intermittent, the flushing procedure will vary according to policy, the medication administration schedule, and the type of catheter.
▶ All lumens of a multilumen catheter must be flushed regularly. Most facilities use a heparin flush solution available in premixed 10-ml multidose vials. Recommended concentrations vary from 10 to 100 units of heparin per milliliter. Use normal saline solution instead of heparin to maintain patency in two-way valved devices, such as the Groshong type, because research suggests that heparin isn't always needed to keep the line open.
▶ The recommended frequency for flushing CVCs varies from once every 12 hours to once weekly.
▶ The recommended amount of flushing solution also varies. Facilities recommend using twice the volume of the capacity of the cannula and the add-on devices if this volume is known. If the volume is unknown, most facilities recommend 3 to 5 ml of solution to flush the catheter, although some facility policies call for as much as 10 ml of solution. Different catheters require different amounts of solution.
▶ To perform the flushing procedure, start by cleaning the cap with an alcohol pad. Allow the cap to dry. If using the needleless system, follow the manufacturer's guidelines.
▶ Access the cap and aspirate to confirm the patency of the CVC.
▶ Inject the recommended type and amount of flush solution.
▶ After flushing the catheter, maintain positive pressure by keeping your thumb on the plunger of the syringe while withdrawing the needle. This prevents blood backflow and clotting in the line. If flushing a valved catheter, close the clamp just before the last of the flush solution leaves the syringe.

## Changing the injection cap
▶ CVCs used for intermittent infusions have needle-free injection caps (short luer-lock devices similar to the heparin lock adapters used for peripheral I.V. infusion therapy). These caps must be luer-lock types to prevent inadvertent disconnection and an air embolism. Unlike heparin lock adapters, these caps contain a minimal amount of empty space, so you don't have to preflush the cap before connecting it.
▶ The frequency of cap changes varies according to your facility's policy and how often the cap is used. Use strict aseptic technique when changing the cap.
▶ Clean the connection site with an alcohol pad or a povidone-iodine pad.
▶ Instruct the patient to perform Valsalva's maneuver while you quickly disconnect the old cap and connect the new cap using aseptic technique. If he can't perform this maneuver, use a padded clamp to prevent air from entering the catheter.

## Removing a CVC
▶ If you'll be removing the CVC, first check the patient's record for the most recent placement (confirmed by an X-ray) to trace the catheter's path as it exits the body. Make sure that assistance is available if a complication (such as uncontrolled bleeding) occurs during catheter removal. (Some vessels, such as the subclavian vein, can be difficult to compress.) Before you remove the catheter, explain the procedure to the patient.
▶ Place the patient in a supine position to prevent an embolism.
▶ Wash your hands and put on clean gloves and a mask.
▶ Turn off all infusions and prepare a sterile field, using a sterile drape.
▶ Remove and discard the old dressing and change to sterile gloves.
▶ Clean the site with an alcohol pad or a gauze pad soaked in povidone-iodine solution. Inspect the site for signs of drainage and inflammation.
▶ Clip the sutures and, using forceps, remove the catheter in a slow, even motion. Have the patient perform Valsalva's maneuver as the catheter is withdrawn to prevent an air embolism.
▶ Apply pressure with a sterile gauze pad immediately after removing the catheter.
▶ Apply povidone-iodine ointment to the insertion site to seal it. Cover the site with a gauze pad and place a transparent semipermeable dressing over the gauze. Label the dressing with the date and time of the removal and your initials. Keep the site covered for 48 hours.
▶ Inspect the catheter tip and measure the length of the catheter to ensure that the catheter has been completely removed. If

# Key steps in changing a central venous dressing

Expect to change your patient's central venous dressing every 3 to 7 days. Many facilities specify dressing changes whenever the dressing becomes soiled, moist, or loose. The following illustrations show the key steps you'll perform.

First, put on clean gloves and remove the old dressing by pulling it toward the exit site of a long-term catheter or toward the insertion site of a short-term catheter. This technique helps you avoid pulling out the line. Remove and discard your gloves.

Next, put on sterile gloves and clean the skin around the site three times using a new applicator soaked in povidone-iodine solution. Start at the center and move outward, using a circular motion (as shown below).

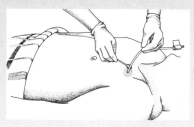

After the solution has dried, cover the site with a dressing, such as a gauze dressing or the transparent semipermeable dressing shown here. Write the time and date on the dressing

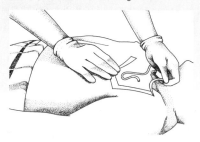

you suspect that the catheter hasn't been completely removed, notify the doctor immediately and monitor the patient closely for signs of distress. If you suspect an infection, swab the catheter on a fresh agar plate and send to the laboratory for culture.

▶ Dispose of the I.V. tubing and equipment properly.

## Special considerations

▶ While you're awaiting chest X-ray confirmation of proper catheter placement, infuse an I.V. solution such as dextrose 5% in water or normal saline solution at a keep-vein-open rate until correct placement is ensured. Or use heparin to flush the line. Infusing an isotonic solution avoids the risk of vessel wall thrombosis.

■ **ALERT!** Be alert for such signs of air embolism as sudden onset of pallor, cyanosis, dyspnea, coughing, and tachycardia, progressing to syncope and shock. If any of these signs occur, place the patient on his left side in Trendelenburg's position and notify the doctor.

▶ After insertion, also watch for signs and symptoms of pneumothorax, such as shortness of breath, uneven chest movement, tachycardia, and chest pain. Notify the doctor immediately if such signs and symptoms appear.

▶ Change the dressing at least every 48 hours if a gauze dressing is used or every 3 to 7 days if a transparent semipermeable dressing is used, according to your facility's policy, or whenever it becomes moist or soiled. Change the tubing every 48 hours and the solution every 24 hours or according to your facility's policy while the CVC is in place. Dressing, tubing, and solution changes for a CVC should be performed using aseptic technique. (See *Key steps in changing a central venous dressing*.) Assess the site for signs and symptoms of infection, such as discharge, inflammation, and tenderness.

▶ To prevent an air embolism, close the catheter clamp or have the patient perform Valsalva's maneuver each time the catheter hub is open to air. (A Groshong catheter doesn't require clamping because it has an internal valve.)

## Home care

Long-term use of a CVC allows patients to receive caustic fluids and blood infusions at home. These catheters have a much longer life because they are less thrombogenic and less prone to infection than short-term devices.

A candidate for home therapy must have a family member or friend who can safely and competently administer the I.V. fluids, a backup helper, a suitable home environment, a telephone, transportation, adequate reading skills, and the ability to prepare, handle, store, and dispose of the equipment. The care procedures used in the home are the same as those used in the facility, except that the home therapy patient uses clean instead of aseptic technique.

The overall goal of home therapy is patient safety, so your patient teaching must begin well before discharge. After discharge, a home therapy coordinator will provide follow-up care until the patient or someone close to him can provide catheter care and infusion therapy independently. Many home therapy patients learn to care for the catheter themselves and infuse their own medications and solution.

### Complications

Complications can occur at any time during infusion therapy. Traumatic complications such as pneumothorax typically occur on catheter insertion but may not be noticed until after the procedure is completed. Systemic complications such as sepsis typically occur later during infusion therapy. Other complications include phlebitis (especially in peripheral CV therapy), thrombus formation, and air embolism.

### Documentation

▶ Record the time and date of insertion, length and location of the catheter, solution infused, doctor's name, and patient's response to the procedure.
▶ Document the time of the X-ray, its results, and your notification of the doctor.
▶ Also record the time and date of removal and the type of antimicrobial ointment and dressing applied. Note the condition of the catheter insertion site and collection of a culture specimen.

### REFERENCES

Ely, E.W, et al. "Venous Air Embolism from Central Venous Catheterization: A Need for Increased Physician Awareness," *Critical Care Medicine* 27(10):2113-17, October 1999.
Vengelen-Tyler, V., ed. *American Association of Blood Banks Technical Manual,* 13th ed. Bethesda, Md.: AABB, 1999.

Weinstein, S.M. *Plumer's Principles and Practice of Infusion Therapy,* 7th ed. Philadelphia: Lippincott Williams & Wilkins, 2001.

# Lipid emulsion administration

Typically given as separate solutions in conjunction with parenteral nutrition, lipid emulsions are a source of calories and essential fatty acids. A deficiency in essential fatty acids can hinder wound healing, adversely affect the production of red blood cells, and impair prostaglandin synthesis.

Lipid emulsions may also be given alone. They can be administered through either a peripheral or a central venous line.

Lipid emulsions are contraindicated in patients who have a condition that disrupts normal fat metabolism, such as pathologic hyperlipidemia, lipid nephrosis, or acute pancreatitis. They must be used cautiously in patients who have liver disease, pulmonary disease, anemia, or coagulation disorders and in those who are at risk for developing a fat embolism.

### Equipment

Lipid emulsion ● I.V. administration set with vented spike (a separate adapter may be used if an administration set with vented spike isn't available) ● access pin with reflux valve ● tape ● time tape ● alcohol pads

If administering the lipid emulsion as part of a 3-in-1 solution, also obtain a filter that is 1.2 microns or greater because lipids will clog a smaller filter.

#### Preparation of equipment

Inspect the lipid emulsion for opacity and consistency of color and texture. If the emulsion looks frothy or oily or contains particles or if you think its stability or sterility is questionable, return the bottle to the pharmacy. To prevent aggregation of fat globules, don't shake the lipid container excessively. Protect the emulsion from freezing and never add anything to it. Make sure you have the correct lipid emulsion and verify the doctor's order and the patient's name.

## Implementation

▶ Explain the procedure to the patient to promote his cooperation.

### Connecting the tubing

▶ First, connect the I.V. tubing to the access pin. Access pins with reflux valves take the place of needles when connecting piggyback tubing to primary tubing.
▶ Close the flow clamp on the I.V. tubing. If the tubing doesn't contain luer-lock connections, tape all connections securely to prevent accidental separation, which can lead to air embolism, exsanguination, and sepsis.
▶ Using sterile technique, remove the protective cap from the lipid emulsion bottle and wipe the rubber stopper with an alcohol pad.
▶ Hold the bottle upright and, using strict sterile technique, insert the vented spike through the inner circle of the rubber stopper.
▶ Invert the bottle and squeeze the drip chamber until it fills to the level indicated in the tubing package instructions.
▶ Open the flow clamp and prime the tubing. Gently tap the tubing to dislodge air bubbles trapped in the Y-ports. If necessary, attach a time tape to the lipid emulsion container to allow accurate measurement of fluid intake.
▶ Label the tubing, noting the date and time the tubing was hung.

### Starting the infusion

▶ If this is the patient's first lipid infusion, administer a test dose at the rate of 1 ml/minute for 30 minutes.
▶ Monitor the patient's vital signs and watch for signs and symptoms of an adverse reaction, such as fever; flushing, sweating, or chills; a pressure sensation over the eyes; nausea; vomiting; headache; chest and back pain; tachycardia; dyspnea; and cyanosis. An allergic reaction is usually due either to the source of lipids or to eggs, which occur in the emulsion as egg phospholipids, which is an emulsifying agent.
▶ If the patient has no adverse reactions to the test dose, begin the infusion at the prescribed rate. Use an infusion pump if you'll be infusing the lipids at less than 20 ml/hour. The maximum infusion rate is 125 ml/hour for a 10% lipid emulsion and 60 ml/hour for a 20% lipid emulsion.

## Special considerations

▶ Always maintain strict sterile technique while preparing and handling equipment.
▶ Observe the patient's reaction to the lipid emulsion. Most patients report a feeling of satiety; some complain of an unpleasant metallic taste.
▶ Change the I.V. tubing and the lipid emulsion container every 24 hours.
▶ Monitor the patient for hair and skin changes. Also, closely monitor his lipid tolerance rate. Cloudy plasma in a centrifuged sample of citrated blood indicates that the lipids haven't been cleared from the patient's bloodstream.
▶ A lipid emulsion may clear from the blood at an accelerated rate in patients with full-thickness burns, multiple traumatic injuries, or a metabolic imbalance. This is because catecholamines, adrenocortical hormones, thyroxine, and growth hormone enhance lipolysis and embolization of fatty acids.
▶ Obtain weekly laboratory tests as ordered. The usual tests include liver function studies, prothrombin time, platelet count, and serum triglyceride levels. Whenever possible, draw blood for triglyceride levels at least 6 hours after the completion of the lipid emulsion infusion to avoid falsely elevated results.
▶ A lipid emulsion is an excellent medium for bacterial growth. Therefore, never rehang a partially empty bottle of emulsion.

## Complications

Immediate or early adverse reactions to lipid emulsion therapy, which occur in fewer than 1% of patients, include fever, dyspnea, cyanosis, nausea, vomiting, headache, flushing, diaphoresis, lethargy, syncope, chest and back pain, slight pressure over the eyes, irritation at the infusion site, hyperlipidemia, hypercoagulability, and thrombocytopenia.

◆ **ALERT!** Thrombocytopenia has been reported in infants receiving a 20% I.V. lipid emulsion.

Delayed but uncommon complications associated with prolonged administration of lipid emulsion include hepatomegaly, splenomegaly, jaundice secondary to central lobular cholestasis, and blood dyscrasias (such as thrombocytopenia, leukopenia, and transient increases in liver function studies). Dry or scaly skin, thinning hair, abnormal liver function studies, and thrombocytopenia may indicate a deficiency of essential fatty acids. For unknown reasons, some patients develop brown pigmentation in the reticuloendothelial system.

◆ **ALERT!** In premature or low-birth-weight infants, peripheral parenteral nutrition with a lipid emulsion may cause lipids to accumulate in the infants' lungs.

Report any adverse reactions to the patient's doctor so that he can change the parenteral nutrition regimen as needed.

## Documentation
▶ Record the times of all dressing changes and solution changes, the condition of the catheter insertion site, your observations of the patient's condition, and any complications and resulting treatments.

### REFERENCES
Chanson, N.F., et al. "LDL Binding to Lipid Emulsion Particles: Effects of Incubation Duration, Temperature, and Addition of Plasma Subfractions," *Lipids* 37(6):573-80, June 2002.

Driscoll, D.F., et al. "The Influence of Medium-chain Triglycerides on the Stability of All-in-one Formulations," *International Journal of Pharmaceutics* 240(1-2):1-10, June 2002.

Lim, S., and Kim, C. "Formulation Parameters Determining the Physicochemical Characteristics of Solid Lipid Nanoparticles Loaded with All-trans Retinoic Acid. *International Journal of Pharmaceutics* 243(1-2):135, August 2002.

# Patient monitoring during parenteral nutrition

Total parenteral nutrition (TPN) requires careful monitoring. Because the typical patient is in a protein-wasting state, TPN therapy causes marked changes in fluid and electrolyte status and in glucose, amino acid, mineral, and vitamin levels. If the patient displays an adverse reaction or signs of complications, the TPN regimen can be changed as needed.

Assessment of the patient's nutritional status includes a physical examination, anthropometric measurements, biochemical determinations, and tests of cell-mediated immunity. Assessment of the patient's condition to detect complications requires recognition of the signs and symptoms of possible complications, understanding of laboratory test results, and careful record keeping.

Because the TPN solution is high in glucose content, the infusion must start slowly to allow the patient's pancreatic beta cells to adapt to it by increasing insulin output. Within the first 3 to 5 days of TPN, the typical adult patient can tolerate 3 L of solution daily without adverse reactions. Lipid emulsions also require monitoring.

## Equipment
TPN solution and administration equipment ● blood glucose meter ● stethoscope ● sphygmomanometer ● watch with second hand ● thermometer ● scale ● intake and output chart ● time tape ● additional equipment for nutritional assessment as ordered

### Preparation of equipment
Attach a time tape to the TPN container to allow approximate measurement of fluid intake. Make sure each bag or bottle has a label listing the expiration date, glucose concentration, and total volume of solution. (If the bag or bottle is damaged and you don't have an immediate replacement, hang a bag of dextrose 10% in water until the new container is ready.)

## Implementation
▶ Explain the procedure to the patient to diminish his anxiety and encourage cooperation. Instruct him to inform you if he experiences any unusual sensations during the infusion.
▶ Record vital signs every 4 hours or more often if necessary because increased temperature is one of the earliest signs of catheter-related sepsis.
▶ Perform I.V. site care and dressing changes at least three times a week (once a week for transparent semipermeable dressings) or whenever the dressing becomes wet, soiled, or nonocclusive. Use strict sterile technique.
▶ Physically assess the patient daily. If ordered, measure arm circumference and skin-fold thickness over the triceps.
▶ Weigh the patient at the same time each morning (after voiding), in similar clothing, and on the same scale. Compare this data with his fluid intake and output record.

Weight gain, especially early in treatment, may indicate fluid overload rather than increasing fat and protein stores. A patient shouldn't gain more than 3 lb (1.5 kg) a week; a gain of 1 lb (0.5 kg) a week is a reasonable goal for most patients. Suspect fluid imbalance if the patient gains more than 1 lb daily. Assess for peripheral and pulmonary edema.

▶ Monitor the patient for signs and symptoms of glucose metabolism disturbance, fluid and electrolyte imbalances, and nutritional aberrations. Remember that some patients may require supplemental insulin for the duration of TPN; the pharmacy usually adds insulin directly to the TPN solution.

▶ Monitor levels of electrolytes and protein frequently — daily at first for electrolytes and twice weekly for serum albumin. Later, as the patient's condition stabilizes, you won't need to monitor these values quite as closely. (Be aware that in a severely dehydrated patient, albumin levels may drop initially as treatment restores hydration.)

Pay close attention to magnesium and calcium levels. If these electrolytes have been added to the TPN solution, the dose may need adjusting to maintain normal serum levels. Assess the patient for signs and symptoms of magnesium and calcium imbalances.

▶ Monitor serum glucose levels every 6 hours initially and then once a day and stay alert for signs and symptoms of hyperglycemia, such as thirst and polyuria. Periodically confirm blood glucose meter readings with laboratory tests.

▶ Check kidney function by monitoring blood urea nitrogen and creatinine levels; increases can indicate excess amino acid intake. Also assess nitrogen balance with 24-hour urine collection.

▶ Assess liver function by periodically monitoring liver enzyme, bilirubin, triglyceride, and cholesterol levels. Abnormal values may indicate an intolerance or excess of lipid emulsions or a problem with metabolizing the protein or glucose in the TPN formula.

▶ Change I.V. administration sets every 24 hours using sterile technique. Because the risk of contamination is so high with TPN, each facility should continuously evaluate protocols based on quality-control findings.

▶ Monitor for signs of inflammation, infection, and sepsis, the most common complications of TPN. Microbial contamination of the venous access device is the usual cause. Watch for redness and drainage at the venous access site and monitor the patient for fever and other signs and symptoms of sepsis.

▶ Provide emotional support. Keep in mind that patients often associate eating with positive feelings and become disturbed when eating is prohibited.

▶ Provide frequent mouth care.

▶ Keep the patient active to enable him to use nutrients more fully.

▶ When discontinuing TPN, decrease the infusion rate slowly, depending on the patient's current glucose intake, to minimize the risk of hyperinsulinemia and resulting hypoglycemia. Weaning usually takes place over 24 to 48 hours but can be completed in 4 to 6 hours if the patient receives sufficient oral or I.V. carbohydrates.

## Special considerations

▶ Always maintain strict sterile technique when handling the equipment used to administer therapy. Because the TPN solution serves as a medium for bacterial growth and the central venous (CV) line provides systemic access, the patient risks infection and sepsis.

▶ When using a filter, position it as close to the access site as possible. Check the filter's porosity and pounds-per-square-inch (psi) capacity to make sure it exceeds the number of pounds per square inch exerted by the infusion pump.

▶ Don't let TPN solutions hang for more than 24 hours.

▶ Be careful when using the TPN line for other functions. If using a single-lumen CV catheter, don't use the line to infuse blood or blood products, to give a bolus injection, to administer simultaneous I.V. solutions, to measure CV pressure, or to draw blood for laboratory tests. Never add medication to a TPN solution container. Also, don't use a three-way stopcock, if possible, because add-on devices increase the risk of infection.

## Complications

Catheter-related, metabolic, and mechanical complications can occur during TPN administration.

## Documentation

▶ Record serial monitoring indexes on the appropriate flowchart to determine the patient's progress and response.

▶ Note any abnormal, adverse, or altered responses. While weaning from TPN, document his dietary intake.

### REFERENCES

"ASPEN Standards of Practice: Standards for Home Nutrition Support," *Nutrition in Clinical Practice* 14(3):151-62, June 1999.

Bliss, D.Z., and Dysart, M. "Using Needleless Intravenous Access Devices for Administering Total Parenteral Nutrition (TPN): Practice Update," *Nutrition in Clinical Practice* 14(6):299-303, December 1999.

Duerksen, D.R., et al. "Peripherally Inserted Central Catheters for Parenteral Nutrition: A Comparison of Centrally Inserted Catheters," *Journal of Parenteral and Enteral Nutrition* 23(2):85-90, March-April 1999.

Trissel, L.A., et al. "Compatibility of Medications with 3-in-1 Parenteral Nutrition Admixtures," *Journal of Parenteral and Enteral Nutrition* 23(2):67-74, March-April 1999.

## Pediatric I.V. therapy

In children, I.V. therapy may be prescribed to administer medications or to correct a fluid deficit, improve serum electrolyte balance, or provide nourishment. Primary nursing concerns related to pediatric I.V. therapy include correlating the I.V. site and equipment with the reason for therapy and the patient's age, size, and activity level. For example, a scalp vein is a typical I.V. site for infants, whereas a peripheral hand, wrist, or foot vein may suit older children.

During I.V. therapy, the nurse must continually assess the patient and the infusion to prevent fluid overload and other complications.

### Equipment

Prescribed I.V. fluid ● volume-control set with microdrip tubing ● infusion pump ● I.V. pole ● normal saline solution or sterile dextrose 5% in water ($D_5W$) for injection ● povidone-iodine solution ● alcohol pads ● 3-ml syringe ● child-sized butterfly needle or I.V. catheter ● tourniquet ● ½" or 1" tape ● gloves ● transparent semipermeable dressing ● optional: arm board and insulated foam or medicine cup

## Easing the pain of venipuncture

For some patients, receiving a needle stick – especially during venipuncture – can be a traumatic experience. You can lessen your patient's anxiety, reduce his pain, and improve compliance during the procedure by applying a transdermal anesthesia cream before the venipuncture. Here are a few guidelines for the use of this cream:

▶ Transdermal anesthesia cream (commonly known by the brand name EMLA Cream) is supplied in a eutectic mixture of lidocaine 2.5% and prilocaine 2.5%. A eutectic mixture has a melting point below room temperature, allowing it to penetrate intact skin as far as the fat layer. The onset, depth, and duration of the anesthesia depend on how long the cream is allowed to stay on the skin. The minimum duration of application is 60 minutes; the maximum is 180 minutes.

▶ Apply the cream in a thick layer to clean, dry, intact skin at the intended venipuncture site. Then cover it with a transparent occlusive dressing, being careful not to spread the cream.

▶ Note the time of application on the dressing with a marking pen. When you're ready to perform the venipuncture, carefully remove the dressing. Wipe off the cream, clean the site with an antiseptic solution, and perform the venipuncture as usual.

▶ EMLA Cream is also indicated for pain relief for various other procedures, including lumbar puncture, port access, bone marrow aspiration, insertion of a peripherally inserted central venous catheter, withdrawal of blood samples for arterial blood gas analysis and other laboratory tests, I.M. injection, and superficial skin surgery. It can be used on adults and on children who are at least 1 month old. Local reactions may include erythema and edema. Avoid administering EMLA Cream to individuals with a known sensitivity to lidocaine or prilocaine.

Whenever possible, use a catheter instead of a needle. A flexible catheter is less likely to perforate the vein wall. To promote compliance and reduce the discomfort associated with catheter insertion, consider using a transdermal anesthetic cream. (See *Easing the pain of venipuncture*.)

## Common pediatric I.V. sites

The most common sites for I.V. therapy in infants and children are shown below. Peripheral hand, wrist, or foot veins (until the child starts to walk) are typically used with older children, whereas scalp veins are used with an infant.

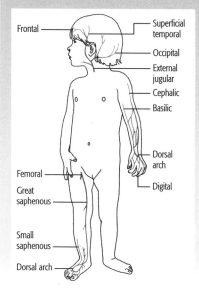

Frontal — Superficial temporal — Occipital — External jugular — Cephalic — Basilic — Dorsal arch — Digital — Femoral — Great saphenous — Small saphenous — Dorsal arch

### Preparation of equipment

Gather the I.V equipment and take it to the patient's bedside. Check the expiration date on the I.V. fluid and inspect the I.V. container (an I.V. bag for leakage and a bottle for cracks). Examine the I.V. tubing for defects or cracks. Make sure that the packaging surrounding the I.V. catheter or needle remains intact.

Open the wrappings on the I.V. solution and the volume-control tubing set. Close all clamps on the tubing set; then insert the tip of the tubing set into the entry port of the I.V. bag or bottle. (If you're using an I.V. bag, make sure you hold the bag upright when attaching the tubing. This will keep the sterile air inside the bag from escaping and making the fluid level difficult to read.)

Hang the bottle or bag from the I.V. pole. Open the clamp between the bag and the volume-control set and allow 30 to 50 ml of solution to flow into the calibrated chamber. Close the clamp.

Squeeze the drip chamber located below the calibrated chamber or volume-control set to create a vacuum. Release the drip chamber and allow it to fill halfway with solution. Then release the clamp below the drip chamber so that fluid flows into the remaining tubing, removing any air. After the tubing fills, close the clamp.

If you're using an infusion pump, attach the I.V. tubing to the infusion cassette and insert the cassette into the infusion pump. Prime the cassette tubing according to the manufacturer's instructions. If you're using an air eliminator I.V. filter, attach the filter to the end of the cassette tubing. To prevent any air bubbles from entering the patient's circulatory system, place the filter as close to the patient as possible. To minimize the risk of infection, maintain sterility at the tip of the I.V. tubing until you connect it to the I.V. needle.

Cut as many strips of ½" or 1" tape as you'll need to secure the I.V. line. Prepare a syringe with 3 ml of flush solution — either the normal saline solution or $D_5W$.

### Implementation

▶ Match the name on the patient's wristband with the name on the doctor's order (or on the medication card). Ask the patient (or his parents) whether he's allergic to povidone-iodine solution or to any type of tape.
▶ Explain the reason for the I.V. therapy. Reassure the parents and enlist their assistance in explaining the procedure to the patient in terms he can understand.
▶ Make sure you have a staff member available to assist you. Inform the parents that the staff member will help the patient remain still, if necessary, during the procedure.
▶ Wash your hands and put on gloves.
▶ Select the insertion site for the butterfly needle or catheter. (See *Common pediatric I.V. sites.*) Aim for the most distal site possible and avoid placing the I.V. line in the patient's dominant arm or in areas of flexion if possible. Avoid previously used or sclerotic veins.
▶ To locate an appropriate scalp vein, carefully palpate the site for arterial pulsations. If you feel these pulsations, select another

site. Before inserting the I.V. line, prepare the selected site as ordered.

▶ To find an appropriate peripheral site, apply a tourniquet to the patient's arm or leg and palpate a suitable vein.

▶ If you're inserting a butterfly needle, flush the tubing connected to the butterfly with $D_5W$ or normal saline solution.

▶ Clean the insertion site. Unless contraindicated, use a povidone-iodine pad. Wipe with a circular motion from the insertion site's center to the outer rim. Let the solution dry.

▶ Insert the I.V. needle into the vein. Watch for blood to flow backward through the catheter or butterfly tubing, which confirms that the needle is in the vein.

▶ Loosen the tourniquet and attach the I.V. tubing to the hub of the needle or catheter. Begin the infusion.

▶ Secure the device by applying a piece of sterile ½″ tape over the hub. Next, place a piece of sterile tape, adhesive side up, underneath and perpendicular to the device. Lift the ends of the tape and crisscross them over the device; then cover the insertion site and device with a sterile transparent semipermeable dressing. Further secure and protect the I.V. line as needed making sure that any tape that is used under the transparent dressing is sterile. (See *Protecting a child's I.V. site,* page 188.)

▶ Adjust the infusional flow, as ordered, by using the clamp on the I.V. volume-control tubing or by setting the infusion rate on the infusion pump.

▶ Add solution hourly (or as needed) from the I.V. bag to the volume-control set.

▶ Assess the I.V. site frequently for signs of infiltration and check the I.V. bottle or bag for the amount of solution infused.

▶ Change the I.V. dressing every 24 hours or as needed to prevent infection. Also change the I.V. tubing every 48 to 72 hours and the I.V. solution bottle or bag every 24 hours. Label the I.V. bottle or bag, tubing, and volume control set with the time and date of change.

▶ Change the I.V. insertion site every 72 hours, if possible, to minimize the risk of infection. If you inserted the I.V. line without proper skin preparation (during an emergency, for example), change the site sooner.

## Special considerations

▶ When selecting an I.V. site, try not to use a site that impairs the child's ability to seek comfort. For example, if an infant typically sucks his right thumb, avoid placing the I.V. needle or catheter in his right arm.

▶ Forewarn parents if you'll start the I.V. infusion in a scalp vein. Also tell them that you may have to shave hair from a small section of the infant's head.

▶ Ask an older child to participate in selecting the I.V. site, if possible, to give him a sense of control. If the child is mobile, aim for an I.V. site on the upper extremity so that he can still get out of bed. Avoid starting the I.V. infusion in the same arm as the patient's identification band, unless you first remove the band and replace it on the other arm, to prevent potential circulatory impairment.

▶ Evaluate the need for restraints after inserting the I.V. line. Apply them only if I.V. needle displacement seems imminent. If you must use restraints, assess the patient's skin integrity and provide hourly skin care to prevent skin breakdown. Remove the restraints at frequent intervals to let the patient move freely. Encourage the parents to hold and comfort the patient when he's unrestrained.

▶ For precise regulation of the I.V. infusion, use a volumetric infusion pump. These pumps infuse fluids at a predetermined rate regardless of temperature fluctuations, vessel variations, or fluid volume changes. Before using an infusion pump, review the operator's manual.

▶ After inserting the I.V. needle or catheter, reward preschool and school-age patients. Popular rewards are colorful stickers to wear on clothes or on the I.V. dressing.

## Home care

Children who require long-term I.V. medications or nourishment may continue receiving I.V. therapy at home. Assess for conditions that promote successful home I.V. therapy—first and foremost, a patient and a parent (or other caregiver) who can and want to participate in home I.V. therapy. Other factors include the availability of relief caregivers to provide occasional assistance (especially in an emergency) and a conducive home environment with electricity, running water, a telephone, refrigeration, storage space for supplies, and an

# Protecting a child's I.V. site

Protecting a child's I.V. site can be a challenge. An active child can easily dislodge an I.V. line, which will necessitate your reinserting it, thus causing him further discomfort; or he may injure himself.

To prevent a child from dislodging an I.V. line, you'll first need to secure the needle or catheter carefully. Tape the I.V. site as you would for an adult, so that the skin over the tip of the venipuncture device is easily visible. However, avoid overtaping the site; doing so makes it harder to inspect the site and the surrounding tissue.

If the child is old enough to understand, warn him not to play with or jostle the equipment and teach him how to walk with an I.V. pole to minimize tension on the line. If necessary, you can restrain the extremity.

You should also create a protective barrier between the I.V. site and the environment using one of the following methods.

### Paper cup

Consider using a small paper cup to protect a scalp site. First, cut off the cup's bottom. (Make sure there are no sharp edges that could damage the child's skin.)

Next, cut a small slot through the top rim to accommodate the I.V. tubing. Place the cup upside down over the insertion site, so the I.V. tubing extends through the slot. Secure the cup with strips of tape (as shown below). The opening you cut in the cup allows you to examine the site.

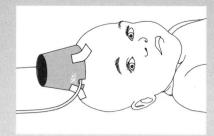

### Stockinette

Place the child's arm on an arm board and secure the arm board to the child's arm with tape. Cut a piece of 4″ (10.2 cm) stockinette the same length as the patient's arm. Slip the stockinette over the patient's arm, as shown.

*Note:* You may also protect a scalp site by placing a stockinette on the patient's head, leaving a hole to allow access to the site.

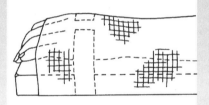

### I.V. shield

Peel off the strips covering the adhesive backing on the bottom of the shield. Position the shield over the site so that the I.V. tubing runs through one of the shield's two slots. Then firmly press the shield's adhesive backing against the patient's skin. The shield's clear plastic composition allows you to see the I.V. site clearly.

If the shield is too large to fit securely over the site, just cut off the shield's narrow end below the two air holes. Now you can easily shape the device to the patient's arm.

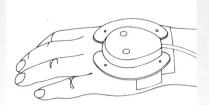

area set up for solution and tubing changes and I.V. site care. Additionally, a hospital should be accessible should the patient need emergency assistance or routine reinsertion of an I.V. line.

Teach the parents (and the patient, if appropriate) how to identify and manage complications, such as site infiltration and clotting in the I.V. needle. Show them how to operate equipment such as the infusion pump. Supplement verbal instructions with written patient-teaching materials for later reference. Before discharge, watch the parents operate the infusion pump for 24 hours so that you can identify areas in which they need further instruction and skills that require refinement.

At discharge, arrange for a home health nurse to visit the patient daily for 2 to 3 days to support and guide initial home therapy. Inform the parents that after her daily visits, the home health nurse will probably visit every 2 to 3 days to assess the I.V. site, provide care, and answer questions.

## Complications
Infection, fluid overload, electrolyte imbalance, infiltration, and circulatory impairment are complications of I.V. therapy.

## Documentation
▶ Record the date and time of the I.V. infusion, the insertion site, and the type and size of I.V. needle or catheter.
▶ Note the patient's tolerance of the procedure. Describe patient- and parent-teaching activities.
▶ Document the condition of the I.V. site according to facility policy. If infiltration affects the I.V. site, document the condition of the site at every shift change until the condition resolves.

### REFERENCES
Frey, A.M., "1999 Pediatric and Neonatal PICC Complications," *Journal of Vascular Access Devices* 4(Suppl. 2):4, 1999.
Pettit, J., and Hughes, K. "1999 Neonatal Intravenous Therapy Practices," *Journal of Vascular Access Devices* 4(1):7-15, 1999.
Weinstein, S.M. *Plumer's Principles and Practices of Intravenous Therapy,* 7th ed. Philadelphia: Lippincott Williams & Wilkins, 2001.

# Peripheral I.V. line insertion

Peripheral I.V. line insertion involves selection of a venipuncture device and an insertion site, application of a tourniquet, preparation of the site, and venipuncture. Selection of a venipuncture device and site depends on the type of solution to be used; frequency and duration of infusion; patency and location of accessible veins; the patient's age, size, and condition; and, when possible, the patient's preference.

If possible, choose a vein in the nondominant arm or hand. Preferred venipuncture sites are the cephalic and basilic veins in the lower arm and the veins in the dorsum of the hand; least favorable are the leg and foot veins because of the increased risk of thrombophlebitis and infection. Antecubital veins can be used if no other venous access is available, to accommodate a large-bore needle, or to administer drugs that require large-volume dilution.

A peripheral line allows administration of fluids, medication, blood, and blood components and maintains I.V. access to the patient. Insertion is contraindicated in a sclerotic vein, an edematous or impaired arm or hand, or a postmastectomy arm and in patients with a mastectomy, burns, or an arteriovenous fistula. Subsequent venipunctures should be performed proximal to a previously used or injured vein.

◆ **ALERT!** Patient allergies influence the selection and preparation of equipment for I.V. therapy. If the patient is allergic to latex, a life-threatening reaction may occur if you use latex-based products. It's recommended that the facility keep a latex-free cart to be used for patients identified with true latex allergies to avoid hypersensitivity reactions.

## Equipment
Alcohol pads or an approved antimicrobial solution, such as tincture of iodine 2% or 10% povidone-iodine ● gloves ● tourniquet (rubber tubing or a blood pressure cuff) ● I.V. access devices ● I.V. solution with attached and primed administration set ● I.V. pole ● sharps container ● sterile 2″ × 2″ gauze pads or a transparent semipermeable dressing ● 1″ hypoallergenic tape ● optional: arm board, roller gauze, tube gauze, warm packs, scissors

Commercial venipuncture kits come with or without an I.V. access device. (See *Comparing venous access devices,* page 190.) In many facilities, venipuncture equipment is kept on a tray or cart, allowing choice of correct access devices and easy replacement of contaminated items.

# Comparing venous access devices

Most I.V. infusions are delivered through one of three basic types of venous access devices: an over-the-needle cannula, a through-the-needle cannula, or a winged infusion set. To improve I.V. therapy and guard against accidental needle sticks, you can use a needle-free system.

### Over-the-needle cannula
**Purpose:** Long-term therapy for an active or agitated patient
**Advantages:** Makes accidental puncture of the vein less likely than with a needle; more comfortable for the patient when it's in place; contains radiopaque thread for easy location. Some units come with a syringe that permits easy check of blood return; some units include wings.
**Disadvantage:** More difficult to insert than other devices

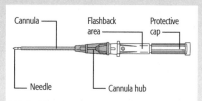

### Through-the-needle cannula
**Purpose:** Long-term therapy for an active or agitated patient
**Advantages:** Makes accidental puncture of the vein less likely than with a needle; more comfortable for the patient when it's in place; available in many lengths; most plastic cannulas contain radiopaque thread for easy location. One variant, the peripherally inserted central catheter, is commonly inserted in the antecubital vein by a specially trained nurse.

**Disadvantages:** Leaking at the site, especially in an elderly patient. The cannula may be severed during insertion if pulled back through the needle.

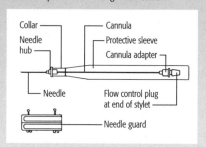

### Winged infusion set
**Purpose:** Short-term therapy for a cooperative adult patient; therapy of any duration for an infant, child, or elderly patient with fragile or sclerotic veins
**Advantages:** Less painful to insert; ideal for I.V. push drugs
**Disadvantages:** May easily cause infiltration if a rigid-needle winged infusion device is used

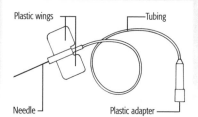

## Preparation of equipment
Check the information on the label of the I.V. solution container, including the patient's name and room number, type of solution, time and date of its preparation, preparer's name, and ordered infusion rate. Compare the doctor's orders with the solution label to verify that the solution is the correct one. Then select the smallest-gauge device that is appropriate for the infusion (unless subsequent therapy will require a larger one). Smaller gauges cause less trauma to veins, allow greater blood flow around their tips, and reduce the clotting risk.

If you're using a winged infusion set, connect the adapter to the administration set, and unclamp the line until fluid flows from the open end of the needle cover. Then close the clamp and place the needle on a sterile surface, such as the inside of its packaging. If you're using a catheter device, open its package to allow easy access.

## Implementation

▶ Place the I.V. pole in the proper slot in the patient's bed frame. If you're using a portable I.V. pole, position it close to the patient.

▶ Hang the I.V. solution with attached primed administration set on the I.V. pole.

▶ Verify the patient's identity by comparing the information on the solution container with the patient's wristband.

▶ Wash your hands thoroughly. Then explain the procedure to the patient to ensure his cooperation and reduce anxiety. Anxiety can cause a vasomotor response resulting in venous constriction.

### Selecting the site

▶ Select the puncture site. If long-term therapy is anticipated, start with a vein at the most distal site so that you can move proximally as needed for subsequent I.V. insertion sites. For infusion of an irritating medication, choose a large vein distal to any nearby joint. Make sure the intended vein can accommodate the cannula.

▶ Place the patient in a comfortable, reclining position, leaving the arm in a dependent position to increase capillary fill of the lower arms and hands. If the patient's skin is cold, warm it by rubbing and stroking the arm, or cover the entire arm with warm packs for 5 to 10 minutes.

### Applying the tourniquet

▶ Apply a tourniquet about 4″ to 6″ (10 cm to 15 cm) above the intended puncture site to dilate the vein (as shown below). Check for a radial pulse. If it isn't present, release the tourniquet and reapply it with less tension to prevent arterial occlusion.

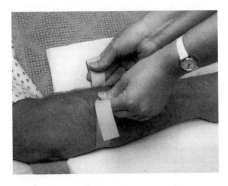

▶ Lightly palpate the vein with the index and middle fingers of your nondominant

hand. Stretch the skin to anchor the vein. If the vein feels hard or ropelike, select another.

▶ If the vein is easily palpable but not sufficiently dilated, one or more of the following techniques may help raise the vein. Place the extremity in a dependent position for several seconds, and gently tap your finger over the vein or rub or stroke the skin upward toward the tourniquet. If you have selected a vein in the arm or hand, tell the patient to open and close his fist several times.

▶ Leave the tourniquet in place for no longer than 3 minutes. If you can't find a suitable vein and prepare the site in that time, release the tourniquet for a few minutes. Then reapply it and continue the procedure.

### Preparing the site

▶ Put on gloves. Clip the hair around the insertion site if needed. Clean the site with alcohol pads or an approved antimicrobial solution, according to your facility's policy.

◆ **ALERT!** Don't apply alcohol after applying 10% povidone-iodine because the alcohol negates the beneficial effect of the povidone-iodine.

Work in a circular motion outward from the site to a diameter of 2″ to 4″ (5 to 10 cm) (as shown below) to remove flora that would otherwise be introduced into the vascular system with the venipuncture. Allow the antimicrobial solution to dry.

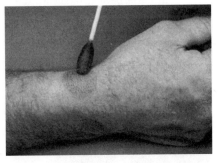

▶ If ordered, administer a local anesthetic. Make sure the patient isn't sensitive to lidocaine.

▶ Lightly press the vein with the thumb of your nondominant hand about ½″ (4 cm) from the intended insertion site. The vein should feel round, firm, fully engorged, and resilient.

▶ Grasp the access cannula. If you're using a winged infusion set, hold the short edges of the wings (with the needle's bevel facing upward) between the thumb and forefinger of your dominant hand. Then squeeze the wings together. If you're using an over-the-needle cannula, grasp the plastic hub with your dominant hand, remove the cover, and examine the cannula tip. If the edge isn't smooth, discard and replace the device. If you're using a through-the-needle cannula, grasp the needle hub with one hand, and unsnap the needle cover. Rotate the access device until the bevel faces upward.

▶ Using the thumb of your nondominant hand, stretch the skin taut below the puncture site to stabilize the vein (as shown below).

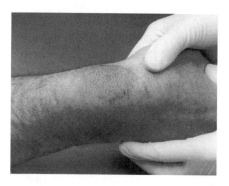

▶ Tell the patient that you are about to insert the device.

▶ Hold the needle bevel up and enter the skin directly over the vein at a 15- to 25-degree angle (as shown below).

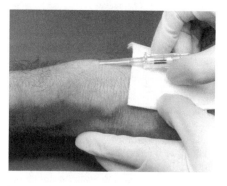

▶ Aggressively push the needle directly through the skin and into the vein in one motion. Check the flashback chamber behind the hub for blood return, signifying that the vein has been properly accessed. (You may not see a blood return in a small vein.)

▶ Then level the insertion device slightly by lifting the tip of the device up to prevent puncturing the back wall of the vein with the access device.

▶ If you're using a winged infusion set, advance the needle fully, if possible, and hold it in place. Release the tourniquet, open the administration set clamp slightly, and check for free flow or infiltration.

▶ If you're using an over-the-needle cannula, advance the device 2 to 3 mm to ensure that the cannula itself—not just the introducer needle—has entered the vein. Then remove the tourniquet.

▶ Grasp the cannula hub to hold it in the vein, and withdraw the needle. As you withdraw it, press lightly on the catheter tip to prevent bleeding (as shown below).

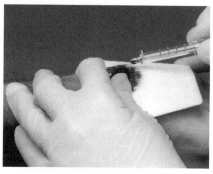

▶ Advance the cannula up to the hub or until you meet resistance.

▶ To advance the cannula while infusing I.V. solution, release the tourniquet and remove the inner needle. Using sterile technique, attach the I.V. tubing and begin the infusion. While stabilizing the vein with one hand, use the other to advance the catheter into the vein. When the catheter is advanced, decrease the I.V. flow rate. This method reduces the risk of puncturing the vein's opposite wall because the catheter is advanced without the steel needle and because the rapid flow dilates the vein.

▶ To advance the cannula before starting the infusion, first release the tourniquet. While stabilizing the vein with one hand, use the other to advance the catheter up to the hub (as shown below).

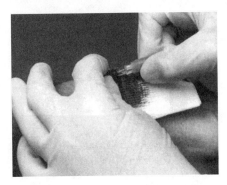

Next, remove the inner needle and, using sterile technique, quickly attach the I.V. tubing. This method commonly results in less blood being spilled.

▶ If you're using a through-the-needle cannula, remove the tourniquet, hold the needle in place with one hand and, with your opposite hand, grasp the cannula through the protective sleeve. Then slowly thread the cannula through the needle until the hub is within the needle collar. Never pull back on the cannula without pulling back on the needle to avoid severing and releasing the cannula into the circulation, causing an embolus. If you feel resistance from the valve, withdraw the cannula and needle slightly and reinsert them, rotating the cannula as you pass the valve. Then withdraw the metal needle, split the needle along the perforated edge (according to the manufacturer's instructions), and carefully remove it from around the cannula. Dispose of the needle pieces appropriately. Remove the stylet and protective sleeve, and attach the administration set to the cannula hub. Open the administration set clamp slightly, and check for free flow or infiltration.

### Dressing the site

▶ After the venous access device has been inserted, clean the skin completely. If necessary, dispose of the stylet in a sharps container. Then regulate the flow rate.

▶ You may use a transparent semipermeable dressing to secure the device. (See *How to apply a transparent semipermeable dressing*.)

## How to apply a transparent semipermeable dressing

To secure the I.V. insertion site, you can apply a transparent semipermeable dressing as follows:

▶ Make sure the insertion site is clean and dry.

▶ Remove the dressing from the package and, using sterile technique, remove the protective seal. Avoid touching the sterile surface.

▶ Place the dressing directly over the insertion site and the hub, as shown. Don't cover the tubing. Also, don't stretch the dressing; doing so may cause itching.

▶ Tuck the dressing around and under the cannula hub to make the site impervious to microorganisms.

▶ To remove the dressing, grasp one corner and then lift and stretch it. If removal is difficult, try loosening the edges with alcohol or water.

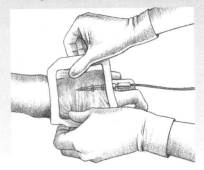

▶ If you don't use a transparent dressing, cover the site with a sterile gauze pad or small adhesive bandage.

▶ Loop the I.V. tubing on the patient's limb, and secure the tubing with tape. The loop allows some slack to prevent dislodgment of the cannula from tension on the line. (See *Methods of taping a venous access site*, pages 194 and 195.)

▶ Label the last piece of tape with the type, gauge of needle, and length of cannula; date and time of insertion; and your initials. Adjust the flow rate as ordered.

▶ If the puncture site is near a movable joint, place a padded arm board under the joint and secure it with roller gauze or tape

# Methods of taping a venous access site

When using tape to secure the access device to the insertion site, use one of the basic methods described below. Use only sterile tape under a transparent, semipermeable dressing.

### Chevron method

▶ Cut a long strip of ½" tape and place it sticky side up under the cannula and parallel to the short strip of tape.

▶ Cross the ends of the tape over the cannula so that the tape sticks to the patient's skin (as shown below).

▶ Apply a piece of 1" tape across the two wings of the chevron.

▶ Loop the tubing and secure it with another piece of 1" tape. When the dressing is secured, apply a label. On the label, write the date and time of the insertion, type and gauge of the needle, and your initials

### U method

▶ Cut a 3" (7.6 cm) strip of ½" tape. With the sticky side up, place it under the hub of the cannula.

▶ Bring each side of the tape up. Folding it over the wings of the cannula in a U shape (as shown below). Press it down parallel to the hub.

▶ Apply tape to stabilize the catheter.

▶ When the dressing is secured, apply a label. On the label, write the date and time of the insertion, type and gauge of the needle, and your initials.

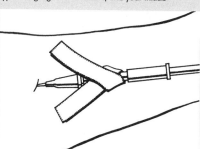
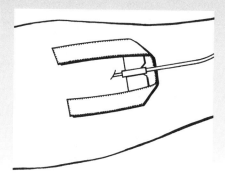

to provide stability because excessive movement can dislodge the venous access device and increase the risk of thrombophlebitis and infection.

▶ Check frequently for impaired circulation distal to the infusion site anytime an armboard is used.

## Removing a peripheral I.V. line

▶ A peripheral I.V. line is removed on completion of therapy, for cannula site changes, and for suspected infection or infiltration; the procedure usually requires gloves, a sterile gauze pad, and an adhesive bandage.

▶ To remove the I.V. line, first clamp the I.V. tubing to stop the flow of solution. Then gently remove the transparent dressing and all tape from the skin.

▶ Using sterile technique, open the gauze pad and adhesive bandage and place them within reach. Put on gloves. Hold the sterile gauze pad over the puncture site with one hand, and use your other hand to withdraw the cannula slowly and smoothly, keeping it parallel to the skin. (Inspect the cannula tip; if it isn't smooth, assess the patient immediately and notify the doctor.)

▶ Using the gauze pad, apply firm pressure over the puncture site for 1 to 2 minutes after removal or until bleeding has stopped.

▶ Clean the site and apply the adhesive bandage or, if blood oozes, apply a pressure bandage.

▶ If drainage appears at the puncture site, send the tip of the device and a sample of the drainage to the laboratory to be cultured according to your facility's policy. (A draining site may or may not be infected.)

### H method

▶ Cut three strips of 1" tape.
▶ Place one strip of tape over each wing, keeping the tape parallel to the cannula (as shown below).
▶ Now place the other strip of tape perpendicular to the first two. Put it either directly on top of the wings or just below the wings, directly on top of the tubing.
▶ Make sure the cannula is secure; then apply a dressing and label. On the label, write the date and time of the insertion, type and gauge of the needle, and your initials.

### X method

▶ Place a transparent semipermeable dressing over the insertion site.
▶ Cut two 2" (5.1 cm) strips of ½" tape.
▶ Place one strip diagonal over the hub of the cannula.
▶ Now place the second strip diagonal to the hub in the opposite direction, forming an X with the first strip (as shown below).

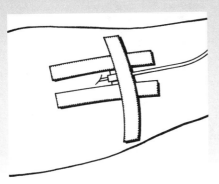

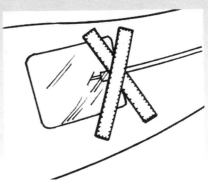

Then clean the area, apply a sterile dressing, and notify the doctor.
▶ Instruct the patient to restrict activity for about 10 minutes and to leave the dressing in place for at least 1 hour. If the patient experiences lingering tenderness at the site, apply warm packs and notify the doctor.

### Special considerations

⬥ **ALERT!** Apply the tourniquet carefully to avoid pinching the skin. If necessary, apply it over the patient's gown. Make sure skin preparation materials are at room temperature to avoid vasoconstriction resulting from lower temperatures.
▶ If the patient is allergic to iodine-containing compounds, clean the skin with alcohol.
▶ If you fail to see blood flashback after the needle enters the vein, pull back slightly

and rotate the device. If you still fail to see flashback, remove the cannula and try again or proceed according to your facility's policy.
▶ Change a gauze or transparent dressing whenever you change the administration set (every 48 to 72 hours or according to your facility's policy).
▶ Be sure to rotate the I.V. site, usually every 48 to 72 hours or according to your facility's policy.

### Home care

Most patients who receive I.V. therapy at home have a central venous line. But if you're caring for a patient going home with a peripheral line, you should teach him how to care for the I.V. site and identify certain complications. If the patient must
*(Text continues on page 200.)*

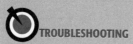

TROUBLESHOOTING

# Risks of peripheral I.V. therapy

| Complication | Signs and symptoms | Possible causes | Nursing interventions |
|---|---|---|---|
| **Local complications** | | | |
| Phlebitis | ▶ Tenderness at tip of and proximal to venous access device<br>▶ Redness at tip of cannula and along vein<br>▶ Puffy area over vein<br>▶ Vein hard on palpation<br>▶ Elevated temperature | ▶ Poor blood flow around venous access device<br>▶ Friction from cannula movement in vein<br>▶ Venous access device left in vein too long<br>▶ Clotting at cannula tip (thrombophlebitis)<br>▶ Drug or solution with high or low pH or high osmolarity | ▶ Remove venous access device.<br>▶ Apply warm soaks.<br>▶ Notify the doctor if the patient has a fever.<br>▶ Document the patient's condition and your interventions.<br>**Prevention**<br>▶ Restart infusion using larger vein for irritating solution, or restart with smaller-gauge device to ensure adequate blood flow.<br>▶ Use filter to reduce risk of phlebitis.<br>▶ Tape device securely to prevent motion. |
| Infiltration | ▶ Swelling at and above I.V. site (may extend along entire limb)<br>▶ Discomfort, burning or pain at site (may be painless)<br>▶ Tight feeling at site<br>▶ Decreased skin temperature around site<br>▶ Blanching at site<br>▶ Continuing fluid infusion even when vein is occluded (although rate may decrease)<br>▶ Absent backflow of blood | ▶ Venous access device dislodged from vein, or perforated vein | ▶ Stop infusion. If extravasation is likely, infiltrate the site with an antidote.<br>▶ Apply warm soaks to aid absorption. Elevate limb.<br>▶ Check for pulse and capillary refill periodically to assess circulation.<br>▶ Restart infusion above infiltration site or in another limb.<br>▶ Document the patient's condition and your interventions.<br>**Prevention**<br>▶ Check I.V. site frequently.<br>▶ Don't obscure area above site with tape.<br>▶ Teach the patient to observe I.V. site and report pain or swelling. |
| Cannula dislodgment | ▶ Loose tape<br>▶ Cannula partly backed out of vein<br>▶ Solution infiltrating | ▶ Loosened tape, or tubing snagged in bed linens, resulting in partial retraction of cannula; pulled out by a confused patient | ▶ If no infiltration occurs, retape without pushing cannula back into vein. If pulled out, apply pressure to I.V. site with sterile dressing.<br>**Prevention**<br>▶ Tape venipuncture device securely on insertion. |

# Risks of peripheral I.V. therapy (continued)

| Complication | Signs and symptoms | Possible causes | Nursing interventions |
|---|---|---|---|
| Occlusion | ▶ No increase in flow rate when I.V. container is raised<br>▶ Blood backflow in line<br>▶ Discomfort at insertion site | ▶ I.V. flow interrupted<br>▶ Heparin lock not flushed<br>▶ Blood backflow in line when the patient walks<br>▶ Line clamped too long | ▶ Use mild flush injection. Don't force it. If unsuccessful, remove I.V. line and insert a new one.<br>**Prevention**<br>▶ Maintain I.V. flow rate.<br>▶ Flush promptly after intermittent piggyback administration.<br>▶ Have the patient walk with his arm bent at the elbow to reduce risk of blood backflow. |
| Vein irritation or pain at I.V. site | ▶ Pain during infusion<br>▶ Possible blanching if vasospasm occurs<br>▶ Red skin over vein during infusion<br>▶ Rapidly developing signs of phlebitis | ▶ Solution with high or low pH or high osmolarity, such as 40 mEq/L of potassium chloride, phenytoin, and some antibiotics (vancomycin, erythromycin, and nafcillin) | ▶ Decrease the flow rate.<br>▶ Try using an electronic flow device to achieve a steady flow.<br>**Prevention**<br>▶ Dilute solutions before administration. For example, give antibiotics in 250-ml solution rather than 100-ml solution. If drug has low pH, ask pharmacist if drug can be buffered with sodium bicarbonate. (Refer to your facility's policy.)<br>▶ If long-term therapy of irritating drug is planned, ask the doctor to use central I.V. line. |
| Hematoma | ▶ Tenderness at venipuncture site<br>▶ Bruised area around site<br>▶ Inability to advance or flush I.V. line | ▶ Vein punctured through opposite wall at time of insertion<br>▶ Leakage of blood from needle displacement<br>▶ Inadequate pressure applied when cannula is discontinued | ▶ Remove venous access device.<br>▶ Apply pressure and warm soaks to affected area.<br>▶ Recheck for bleeding.<br>▶ Document the patient's condition and your interventions.<br>**Prevention**<br>▶ Choose a vein that can accommodate the size of venous access device.<br>▶ Release tourniquet as soon as insertion is successful. |
| Severed cannula | ▶ Leakage from cannula shaft | ▶ Cannula inadvertently cut by scissors<br>▶ Reinsertion of needle into cannula | ▶ If broken part is visible, attempt to retrieve it. If unsuccessful, notify the doctor.<br>▶ If portion of cannula enters bloodstream, place tourniquet above I.V. site to prevent progression of broken part.<br>▶ Notify the doctor and radiology department. |

(continued)

# Risks of peripheral I.V. therapy *(continued)*

| Complication | Signs and symptoms | Possible causes | Nursing interventions |
|---|---|---|---|
| Severed cannula *(continued)* | | | ▶ Document the patient's condition and your interventions. **Prevention** ▶ Don't use scissors around I.V. site. ▶ Never reinsert needle into cannula. ▶ Remove unsuccessfully inserted cannula and needle together. |
| Venous spasm | ▶ Pain along vein ▶ Flow rate sluggish when clamp completely open ▶ Blanched skin over vein | ▶ Severe vein irritation from irritating drugs or fluids ▶ Administration of cold fluids or blood ▶ Very rapid flow rate (with fluids at room temperature) | ▶ Apply warm soaks over vein and surrounding area. ▶ Decrease flow rate. **Prevention** ▶ Use a blood warmer for blood or packed red blood cells. |
| Thrombosis | ▶ Painful, reddened, and swollen vein ▶ Sluggish or stopped I.V. flow | ▶ Injury to endothelial cells of vein wall, allowing platelets to adhere and thrombi to form | ▶ Remove venous access device; restart infusion in opposite limb if possible. ▶ Apply warm soaks. ▶ Watch for I.V. therapy–related infection; thrombi provide an excellent environment for bacterial growth. **Prevention** ▶ Use proper venipuncture techniques to reduce injury to vein. |
| Thrombophlebitis | ▶ Severe discomfort ▶ Reddened, swollen, and hardened vein | ▶ Thrombosis and inflammation | ▶ Same as for thrombosis. **Prevention** ▶ Check site frequently. Remove venous access device at first sign of redness and tenderness. |
| Nerve, tendon, or ligament damage | ▶ Extreme pain (similar to electric shock when nerve is punctured) ▶ Numbness and muscle contraction ▶ Delayed effects, including paralysis, numbness, and deformity | ▶ Improper venipuncture technique, resulting in injury to surrounding nerves, tendons, or ligaments ▶ Tight taping or improper splinting with arm board | ▶ Stop procedure. **Prevention** ▶ Repeatedly penetrate tissues with venous access device. ▶ Don't apply excessive pressure when taping; don't encircle limb with tape. ▶ Pad arm boards and tape securing arm boards if possible. |

# Risks of peripheral I.V. therapy *(continued)*

| Complication | Signs and symptoms | Possible causes | Nursing interventions |
|---|---|---|---|
| *Systemic complications* | | | |
| Systemic infection (septicemia or bacteremia) | ▶ Fever, chills, and malaise for no apparent reason<br>▶ Contaminated I.V. site, usually with no visible signs of infection at site | ▶ Failure to maintain sterile technique during insertion or site care<br>▶ Severe phlebitis, which can set up ideal conditions for organism growth<br>▶ Poor taping that permits venous access device to move, which can introduce organisms into bloodstream<br>▶ Prolonged indwelling time of device<br>▶ Weak immune system | ▶ Notify the doctor.<br>▶ Administer medications as prescribed.<br>▶ Culture the site and device.<br>▶ Monitor vital signs.<br>***Prevention***<br>▶ Use scrupulous sterile technique when handling solutions and tubing, inserting venous access device, and discontinuing infusion.<br>▶ Secure all connections.<br>▶ Change I.V. solutions, tubing, and venous access device at recommended times.<br>▶ Use I.V. filters. |
| Vasovagal reaction | ▶ Sudden collapse of vein during venipuncture<br>▶ Sudden pallor, sweating, faintness, dizziness, and nausea<br>▶ Decreased blood pressure | ▶ Vasospasm from anxiety or pain | ▶ Lower head of bed.<br>▶ Have the patient take deep breaths.<br>▶ Check vital signs.<br>***Prevention***<br>▶ Prepare the patient for therapy to relieve his anxiety.<br>▶ Use local anesthetic to prevent pain. |
| Allergic reaction | ▶ Itching<br>▶ Watery eyes and nose<br>▶ Bronchospasm<br>▶ Wheezing<br>▶ Urticarial rash<br>▶ Edema at I.V. site<br>▶ Anaphylactic reaction (flushing, chills, anxiety, itching, palpitations, paresthesia, wheezing, seizures, cardiac arrest) up to 1 hour after exposure | ▶ Allergens such as medications | ▶ If reaction occurs, stop infusion immediately.<br>▶ Maintain a patent airway.<br>▶ Notify the doctor.<br>▶ Administer antihistaminic steroid, anti-inflammatory, and antipyretic drugs, as prescribed.<br>▶ Give 0.2 to 0.5 ml of 1:1,000 aqueous epinephrine subcutaneously as prescribed. Repeat at 3-minute intervals and as needed and prescribed.<br>***Prevention***<br>▶ Obtain the patient's allergy history. Be aware of cross-allergies.<br>▶ Assist with test dosing and document any new allergies. |

*(continued)*

## Risks of peripheral I.V. therapy *(continued)*

| Complication | Signs and symptoms | Possible causes | Nursing interventions |
|---|---|---|---|
| Allergic reaction *(continued)* | | | ▶ Monitor the patient carefully during first 15 minutes of administration of a new drug. |
| Circulatory overload | ▶ Discomfort<br>▶ Neck vein engorgement<br>▶ Respiratory distress<br>▶ Increased blood pressure<br>▶ Crackles<br>▶ Increased difference between fluid intake and output | ▶ Roller clamp loosened to allow run-on infusion<br>▶ Flow rate too rapid<br>▶ Miscalculation of fluid requirements | ▶ Raise the head of the bed.<br>▶ Administer oxygen as needed.<br>▶ Notify the doctor.<br>▶ Administer medications (probably furosemide) as prescribed.<br>**Prevention**<br>▶ Use pump, controller, or rate minder for elderly or compromised patients.<br>▶ Recheck calculations of fluid requirements.<br>▶ Monitor infusion frequently. |
| Air embolism | ▶ Respiratory distress<br>▶ Unequal breath sounds<br>▶ Weak pulse<br>▶ Increased central venous pressure<br>▶ Decreased blood pressure<br>▶ Loss of consciousness | ▶ Solution container empty<br>▶ Solution container empties, and added container pushes air down the line (if line not purged first) | ▶ Discontinue infusion.<br>▶ Place the patient on his left side in Trendelenburg's position to allow air to enter right atrium and disperse by way of pulmonary artery.<br>▶ Administer oxygen.<br>▶ Notify the doctor.<br>▶ Document the patient's condition and your interventions.<br>**Prevention**<br>▶ Purge tubing of air completely before starting infusion.<br>▶ Use air-detection device on pump or air-eliminating filter proximal to I.V. site.<br>▶ Secure connections. |

observe movement restrictions, make sure he understands them.

Teach the patient how to examine the site, and instruct him to notify the doctor or home care nurse if redness, swelling, or discomfort develops; if the dressing becomes moist; or if blood appears in the tubing.

Also tell the patient to report any problems with the I.V. line, for instance, if the solution stops infusing or if an alarm goes off on an infusion pump. Explain that the I.V. site will be changed at established intervals by a home care nurse.

If the patient is using an intermittent infusion device, teach him how and when to flush it. Finally, teach the patient to document daily whether the I.V. site is free from pain, swelling, and redness.

## Complications

Peripheral line complications can result from the needle or catheter (infection, phlebitis, and embolism) or from the solution (circulatory overload, infiltration, sepsis, and allergic reaction). (See *Risks of peripheral I.V. therapy,* pages 196 to 200.)

## Documentation

▶ In your notes or on the appropriate I.V. sheets, record the date and time of the venipuncture; type, gauge, and length of the cannula or needle; anatomic location of the insertion site; and reason the site was changed.

▶ Also document the number of attempts at venipuncture (if you made more than one), type and flow rate of the I.V. solution, name and amount of medication in the solution (if any), any adverse reactions and actions taken to correct them, patient teaching and evidence of patient understanding, and your initials.

### REFERENCES

Gritter, M. "Latex Allergy: Prevention is the Key," *Journal of Intravenous Nursing* 22(5): 281-85, September-October 1999.

Tan, M.W. "Reuse of Single-Use Equipment: The Intravenous Nurse Specialist's Role in Institutional Policy Development," *Journal of Intravenous Nursing* 22(1):11-13, January-February 1999.

Weinstein, S.M. *Plumer's Principles and Practices of Intravenous Therapy,* 7th ed. Philadelphia: Lippincott Williams & Wilkins, 2001.

# Peripheral I.V. line maintenance

Routine maintenance of I.V. sites and systems includes regular assessment and rotation of the site and periodic changes of the dressing, tubing, and solution. These measures help prevent complications, such as thrombophlebitis and infection. They should be performed according to your facility's policy.

Typically, gauze I.V. dressings are changed every 48 hours and whenever the dressing becomes wet, soiled, or nonocclusive. Transparent semipermeable dressings are changed whenever I.V. tubing is changed every 48 to 72 hours or according to policy, and I.V. solution is changed every 24 hours or as needed. The site should be assessed every 2 hours if a transparent semipermeable dressing is used or with every dressing change otherwise and should be rotated every 48 to 72 hours. Sometimes limited venous access prevents frequent site changes; if so, be sure to assess the site frequently.

## Equipment

*For dressing changes*
Sterile gloves ● povidone-iodine or alcohol pads ● adhesive bandage, sterile 2″ × 2″ gauze pad, or transparent semipermeable dressing ● 1″ adhesive tape

*For solution changes*
Solution container ● alcohol pad

*For tubing changes*
I.V. administration set ● sterile gloves ● 2″ × 2″ gauze pad ● adhesive tape for labeling ● optional: hemostats

*For I.V. site change*
Commercial kits containing the equipment for dressing changes are available.

### Preparation of equipment

If your facility keeps I.V. equipment and dressings in a tray or cart, have it nearby, if possible, because you may have to select a new venipuncture site, depending on the current site's condition. If you're changing both the solution and the tubing, attach and prime the I.V. administration set before entering the patient's room.

## Implementation

▶ Wash your hands thoroughly to prevent the spread of microorganisms. Remember to wear sterile gloves whenever working near the venipuncture site.

▶ Explain the procedure to the patient to allay his fears and ensure cooperation.

### Changing the dressing

▶ Remove the old dressing, open all supply packages, and put on sterile gloves.

▶ Hold the cannula in place with your nondominant hand to prevent accidental movement or dislodgment, which could puncture the vein and cause infiltration.

▶ Assess the venipuncture site for signs of infection (redness and pain at the puncture site), infiltration (coolness, blanching, and edema at the site), and thrombophlebitis (redness, firmness, pain along the path of the vein, and edema). If any such signs are present, cover the area with a sterile 2″ × 2″ gauze pad and remove the catheter or needle. Apply pressure to the area until the bleeding stops, and apply an adhesive bandage. Then, using fresh equipment and solution, start the I.V. in another appropriate site, preferably on the opposite extremity.

▶ If the venipuncture site is intact, stabilize the cannula and carefully clean around the puncture site with a povidone-iodine or alcohol pad. Work in a circular motion outward from the site to avoid introducing bacteria into the clean area. Allow the area to dry completely.

▶ Cover the site with a transparent semipermeable dressing. The transparent dressing allows visualization of the insertion site and maintains sterility. It's placed over the insertion site to halfway up the hub of the cannula.

### Changing the solution
▶ Wash your hands.

▶ Inspect the new solution container for cracks, leaks, and other damage. Check the solution for discoloration, turbidity, and particulates. Note the date and time the solution was mixed and its expiration date.

▶ Clamp the tubing when inverting it to prevent air from entering the tubing. Keep the drip chamber half full.

▶ If you're replacing a bag, remove the seal or tab from the new bag and remove the old bag from the pole. Remove the spike, insert it into the new bag, and adjust the flow rate.

▶ If you're replacing a bottle, remove the cap and seal from the new bottle and wipe the rubber port with an alcohol pad. Clamp the line, remove the spike from the old bottle, and insert the spike into the new bottle. Then hang the new bottle and adjust the flow rate.

### Changing the tubing
▶ Reduce the I.V. flow rate, remove the old spike from the container, and hang it on the I.V. pole. Place the cover of the new spike loosely over the old one.

▶ Keeping the old spike in an upright position above the patient's heart level, insert the new spike into the I.V. container.

▶ Prime the system. Hang the new I.V. container and primed set on the pole, and grasp the new adapter in one hand. Then stop the flow rate in the old tubing.

▶ Put on sterile gloves.

▶ Place a sterile gauze pad under the needle or cannula hub to create a sterile field. Press one of your fingers over the cannula to prevent bleeding.

▶ Gently disconnect the old tubing (as shown top of next column), being careful not to dislodge or move the I.V. device. If you have trouble disconnecting the old tubing, use a hemostat to hold the hub se-

curely while twisting the tubing to remove it. Or use one hemostat on the venipuncture device and another on the hard plastic end of the tubing. Then pull the hemostats in opposite directions. Don't clamp the hemostats shut; this could crack the tubing adapter or the venipuncture device.

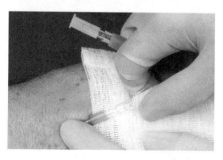

▶ Remove the protective cap from the new tubing, and connect the new adapter to the cannula. Hold the hub securely to prevent dislodging the needle or cannula tip.

▶ Observe for blood backflow into the new tubing to verify that the needle or cannula is still in place. (You may not be able to do this with small-gauge cannulas.)

▶ Adjust the clamp to maintain the appropriate flow rate.

▶ Retape the cannula hub and I.V. tubing, and recheck the I.V. flow rate because taping may alter it.

▶ Label the new tubing and container with the date and time. Label the solution container with a time strip (as shown below).

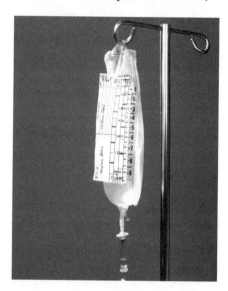

## Special considerations
Check the prescribed I.V. flow rate before each solution change to prevent errors. If you crack the adapter or hub (or if you accidentally dislodge the cannula from the vein), remove the cannula. Apply pressure and an adhesive bandage to stop any bleeding. Perform a venipuncture at another site and restart the I.V.

## Documentation
▶ Record the time, date, and rate and type of solution (and any additives) on the I.V. flowchart.
▶ Record this information, dressing or tubing changes, and appearance of the site in your notes.

### REFERENCES
Mermel, L.A. "Prevention of Intravascular Catheter-related Infections," *Annals of Internal Medicine* 132(5):391-402, March 2000.
Weinstein, S.M. *Plumer's Principles and Practice of Infusion Therapy*, 7th ed. Philadelphia: Lippincott Williams & Wilkins, 2001.
Welk, T. "Clinical and Ethical Considerations of Fluid and Electrolyte Management in the Terminally Ill Client," *Journal of Intravenous Nursing* 22(1):43-47, January-February 1999.

# PICC insertion and removal

For a patient who needs central venous (CV) therapy for 1 to 6 months or who requires repeated venous access, a peripherally inserted central catheter (PICC) may be the best option. The doctor may order a PICC if the patient has suffered trauma or burns resulting in chest injury or if he has respiratory compromise due to chronic obstructive pulmonary disease, a mediastinal mass, cystic fibrosis, or pneumothorax. With any of these conditions, a PICC helps avoid complications that may occur with a CV line.

Made of silicone or polyurethane, a PICC is soft and flexible with increased biocompatibility. It may range from 16G to 23G in diameter and from 16″ to 24″ (40.5 to 61 cm) in length. PICCs are available in single- and double-lumen versions, with or without guide wires. A guide wire stiffens the catheter, easing its advancement through the vein, but can damage the vessel if used improperly.

PICCs are being used increasingly for patients receiving home care. The device is easier to insert than other CV devices and provides safe, reliable access for drug administration and blood sampling. A single catheter may be used for the entire course of therapy with greater convenience and at reduced cost.

Infusions commonly given by PICC include total parenteral nutrition, chemotherapy, antibiotics, narcotics, and analgesics. PICC therapy works best when introduced early in treatment; it shouldn't be considered a last resort for patients with sclerotic or repeatedly punctured veins.

The patient receiving PICC therapy must have a peripheral vein large enough to accept a 14G or 16G introducer needle and a 13.8G to 14.8G catheter. The doctor or nurse inserts a PICC by way of the basilic, median cubital, or cephalic vein. The PICC is then threaded to the superior vena cava or subclavian vein.

PICCs cost from $25 to $60. Insertion may cost from $50 to $300, compared with about $500 for insertion of short-term CV catheters and $1,200 for insertion of long-term CV catheters and implantable CV devices.

If your state nurse practice act permits, you may insert a PICC if you show sufficient knowledge of vascular access devices. To prove your competence in PICC insertion, it's recommended that you complete an 8-hour workshop and demonstrate three successful catheter insertions. You may have to demonstrate competence every year.

## Equipment
Catheter insertion kit • three alcohol pads or an approved antimicrobial solution, such as 10% povidone-iodine or tincture of iodine 2% • povidone-iodine ointment • 3-ml vial of heparin (100 units/ml) • injection port with short extension tubing • sterile and clean measuring tape • vial of normal saline solution • sterile gauze pads • tape • linen-saver pad • sterile drapes • tourniquet • sterile transparent semipermeable dressing • two pairs of sterile gloves • sterile gown • mask • goggles • clean gloves

### Preparation of equipment
Gather the necessary supplies. If you're administering PICC therapy in the patient's home, bring everything with you.

## Implementation

▶ Describe the procedure to the patient and answer her questions.
▶ Wash your hands.

### Inserting a PICC

▶ Place the tourniquet on the patient's arm and assess the antecubital fossa. Select the insertion site.
▶ Remove the tourniquet.
▶ Determine catheter tip placement or the spot at which the catheter tip will rest after insertion.
▶ For placement in the superior vena cava, measure the distance from the insertion site to the shoulder and from the shoulder to the sternal notch. Then add 3″ (7.6 cm) to the measurement (as shown below).

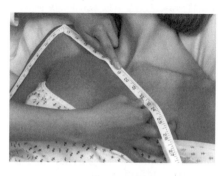

▶ Have the patient lie in a supine position with her arm at a 90-degree angle to her body. Place a linen-saver pad under her arm.
▶ Open the PICC tray and drop the rest of the sterile items onto the sterile field. Put on the sterile gown, mask, goggles, and gloves.
▶ Using the sterile measuring tape, cut the distal end of the catheter according to specific manufacturer's recommendations and guidelines, using the equipment provided by the manufacturer (as shown below).

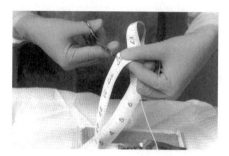

▶ Using sterile technique, withdraw 5 ml of the normal saline solution and flush the extension tubing and the cap.
▶ Remove the needle from the syringe. Attach the syringe to the hub of the catheter and flush (as shown below).

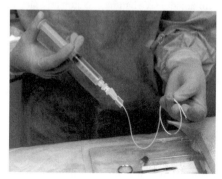

▶ Prepare the insertion site by rubbing it with three alcohol pads or other approved antimicrobial solution. Use a circular motion, working outward from the site about 6″ (15 cm). Allow the area to dry. Be sure not to touch the intended insertion site.
▶ Take your gloves off. Then apply the tourniquet about 4″ (10 cm) above the antecubital fossa.
▶ Put on a new pair of sterile gloves. Then place a sterile drape under the patient's arm and another on top of her arm. Drop a sterile 4″ × 4″ gauze pad over the tourniquet.
▶ Stabilize the patient's vein. Insert the catheter introducer at a 10-degree angle, directly into the vein (as shown below).

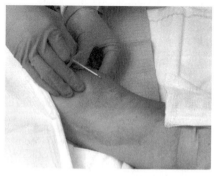

▶ After successful vein entry, you should see a blood return in the flashback chamber. Without changing the needle's position, gently advance the plastic introducer sheath until you're sure the tip is well within the vein.

▶ Carefully withdraw the needle while holding the introducer still. To minimize blood loss, apply finger pressure on the vein just beyond the distal end of the introducer sheath (as shown below).

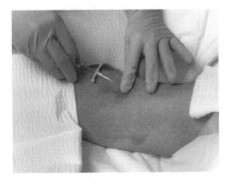

▶ Using sterile forceps, insert the catheter into the introducer sheath, and advance it 2″ to 4″ (5 to 10 cm) into the vein (as shown below).

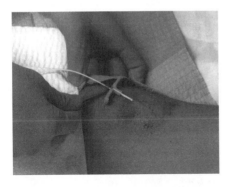

▶ Remove the tourniquet using the 4″ × 4″ gauze pad.

▶ When you have advanced the catheter to the shoulder, ask the patient to turn her head toward the affected arm and place her chin on her chest. This will occlude the jugular vein and ease the catheter's advancement into the subclavian vein.

▶ Advance the catheter until about 4″ remain. Then pull the introducer sheath out of the vein and away from the venipuncture site (as shown top of next column).

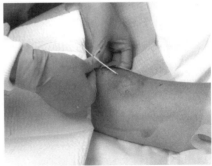

▶ Grasp the tabs of the introducer sheath, and flex them toward its distal end to split the sheath.

▶ Pull the tabs apart and away from the catheter until the sheath is completely split (as shown below). Discard the sheath.

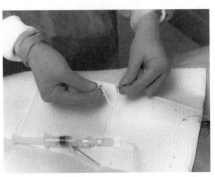

▶ Continue to advance the catheter until it's completely inserted. Flush with normal saline solution followed by heparin, according to your facility's policy.

▶ With the patient's arm below heart level, remove the syringe. Connect the capped extension set to the hub of the catheter.

▶ Apply a sterile 2″ × 2″ gauze pad directly over the site and a sterile transparent semipermeable dressing over that. Leave this dressing in place for 24 hours.

◆ **ALERT!** The tip of the PICC should be in the vena cava. The tip of the catheter can be determined radiologically and should be documented in the patient's medical record before initiation of prescribed therapy. In addition, radiologic confirmation should be performed intermittently as the catheter is no longer considered a central catheter if located outside the vena cava. It will then need to be re-

moved because the location may no longer be appropriate for prescribed therapy.
▶ After the initial 24 hours, apply a new sterile transparent semipermeable dressing. The gauze pad is no longer necessary. You can place Steri-Strips over the catheter wings. Flush with heparin, according to your facility's policy.

### Administering drugs
▶ As with any CV line, be sure to check for blood return and flush with normal saline solution before administering a drug through a PICC line.
▶ Clamp the 7" (17.8 cm) extension tubing, and connect the empty syringe to the tubing. Release the clamp and aspirate slowly to verify blood return. Flush with 3 ml of normal saline solution in a 10-ml syringe, then administer the drug.
▶ After giving the drug, flush again with 3 ml of normal saline solution in a 10-ml syringe. (Remember to flush with normal saline solution between infusions of incompatible drugs or fluids.)

### Changing the dressing
▶ Change the dressing every 3 to 7 days and more frequently if the integrity of the dressing becomes compromised. If possible, choose a transparent semipermeable dressing, which has a high moisture-vapor transmission rate. Use sterile technique.
▶ Wash your hands and assemble the necessary supplies. Position the patient with her arm extended away from her body at a 45- to 90-degree angle so that the insertion site is below heart level to reduce the risk of air embolism. Put on a sterile mask.
▶ Open a package of sterile gloves, and use the inside of the package as a sterile field. Then open the transparent semipermeable dressing and drop it onto the field. Put on clean gloves, and remove the old dressing by holding your left thumb on the catheter and stretching the dressing parallel to the skin. Repeat the last step with your right thumb holding the catheter. Free the remaining section of the dressing from the catheter by peeling toward the insertion site from the distal end to the proximal end to prevent catheter dislodgment. Remove the clean gloves.
▶ Put on sterile gloves. Clean the area thoroughly with three alcohol swabs, starting at the insertion site and working outward

from the site. Repeat the step three times with povidone-iodine swabs and allow to dry.
▶ Apply the dressing carefully. Secure the tubing to the edge of the dressing over the tape with ¼" adhesive tape.

### Removing a PICC
▶ You'll remove a PICC when therapy is complete, if the catheter becomes damaged or broken and can't be repaired or, possibly, if the line becomes occluded. Measure the catheter after you remove it to ensure that the line has been removed intact.
▶ Assemble the necessary equipment at the patient's bedside.
▶ Explain the procedure to the patient. Wash your hands. Place a linen-saver pad under the patient's arm.
▶ Remove the tape holding the extension tubing. Open two sterile gauze pads on a clean, flat surface. Put on clean gloves. Stabilize the catheter at the hub with one hand. Without dislodging the catheter, use your other hand to gently remove the dressing by pulling it toward the insertion site.
▶ Next, withdraw the catheter with smooth, gentle pressure in small increments. It should come out easily. If you feel resistance, stop. Apply slight tension to the line by taping it down. A warm moist pack on the arm may help if a venous spasm is occurring. Try to remove it again in a few minutes. If you still feel resistance after the second attempt, notify the doctor for further instructions.
▶ When you successfully remove the catheter, apply manual pressure to the site with a sterile gauze pad for 1 minute.
▶ Measure and inspect the catheter. If any part has broken off during removal, notify the doctor immediately and monitor the patient for signs of distress.
▶ Cover the site with povidone-iodine ointment, and tape a new folded gauze pad in place. Dispose of used items properly, and wash your hands.

### Special considerations
▶ Be aware that the doctor or nurse probably will place the PICC in the superior vena cava if the patient will receive therapy in the facility.
▶ For a patient receiving intermittent PICC therapy, flush the catheter with 6 ml of normal saline solution and 3 ml of heparin

(100 units/ml) after each use. For catheters that aren't being used routinely, flushing every 12 hours with 3 ml (100 units/ml) heparin will maintain patency.

▶ You can use a declotting agent to clear a clotted PICC, but make sure you read the manufacturer's recommendations first.

▶ Remember to add an extension set to all PICCs so you can start and stop an infusion away from the insertion site. An extension set will also make using a PICC easier for the patient who will be administering infusions herself.

▶ If a patient will be receiving blood or blood products through the PICC, use at least an 18G cannula.

▶ Assess the catheter insertion site through the transparent semipermeable dressing every 24 hours. Look at the catheter and cannula pathway, and check for bleeding, redness, drainage, and swelling. Ask your patient if she's having pain associated with therapy. Although oozing is common for the first 24 hours after insertion, excessive bleeding after that should be evaluated.

◆ **ALERT!** If a portion of the catheter breaks during removal, immediately apply a tourniquet to the upper arm, close to the axilla, to prevent advancement of the catheter piece into the right atrium. Then check the patient's radial pulse. If you don't detect the radial pulse, the tourniquet is too tight. Keep the tourniquet in place until an X-ray can be obtained, the doctor is notified, and surgical retrieval is attempted.

### Complications

PICC therapy causes fewer and less severe complications than conventional CV therapy. Catheter breakage on removal is probably the most common complication. Catheter occlusion is also relatively common. Air embolism, always a potential risk of venipuncture, poses less danger in PICC therapy than in traditional CV therapy because the line is inserted below heart level.

Catheter tip migration may occur with vigorous flushing. Patients receiving chemotherapy are most vulnerable to this complication because of frequent nausea and vomiting and subsequent changes in intrathoracic pressure.

### Documentation

▶ Document the entire procedure, including any problems with catheter placement.
▶ Document the size, length, and type of catheter as well as the insertion location.

### REFERENCES
Camara, D. "Minimizing Risks Associated with Peripherally Inserted Central Catheters in the NICU," *The American Journal of Maternal/Child Nursing* 26(1): 17-21, January-February 2001.
LaRue, G. "Efficacy of Ultrasonography in Peripheral Venous Cannulation," *Journal of Intravenous Nursing* 23(1):29-34, January-February 2000.
Sansivero, G.E. "The Microintroducer Technique for Peripherally Inserted Central Catheter Placement," *Journal of Intravenous Nursing* 23(6):345-51, November-December 2000.
Weinstein, S.M. *Plumer's Principles and Practice of Infusion Therapy*, 7th ed. Philadelphia: Lippincott Williams & Wilkins, 2001.

# Total parenteral nutrition

When a patient can't meet his nutritional needs by oral or enteral feedings, he may require I.V. nutritional support, or parenteral nutrition. The patient's diagnosis, history, and prognosis determine the need for parenteral nutrition. Generally, this treatment is prescribed for any patient who can't absorb nutrients through the GI tract for more than 10 days. More specific indications include:

▶ debilitating illness lasting longer than 2 weeks
▶ loss of 10% or more of pre-illness weight
▶ serum albumin level below 3.5 g/dl
▶ excessive nitrogen loss from wound infection, fistulas, or abscesses
▶ renal or hepatic failure
▶ a nonfunctioning GI tract for 5 to 7 days in a severely catabolic patient.

Parenteral nutrition may be given through a peripheral or central venous (CV) line. Depending on the solution, it may be used to boost the patient's caloric intake, to supply full caloric needs, or to surpass the patient's caloric requirements.

The type of parenteral solution prescribed depends on the patient's condition and metabolic needs and on the administration route. The solution usually contains

# Types of parenteral nutrition

| Type | Solution components | Special considerations |
|---|---|---|
| Standard I.V. therapy | ▶ Dextrose, water, electrolytes in varying amounts; for example: dextrose 5% in water ($D_5W$) = 170 calories/L $D_{10}W$ = 340 calories/L normal saline = 0 calories<br>▶ Vitamins | ▶ Nutritionally incomplete; doesn't provide sufficient calories to maintain adequate nutritional status |
| Total parenteral nutrition (TPN) by way of central venous (CV) line | ▶ $D_{15}W$ or $D_{25}W$ (1 L dextrose 25% = 850 nonprotein calories)<br>▶ Crystalline amino acids 2.5% to 8.5%<br>▶ Electrolytes, vitamins, trace elements, and insulin,<br>▶ Lipid emulsion 10% to 20% (usually infused as a separate solution) | ***Basic solution***<br>▶ Nutritionally complete<br>▶ Requires minor surgical procedure for CV line insertion (can be done at bedside by the doctor)<br>▶ Highly hypertonic solution<br>▶ May cause metabolic complications (glucose intolerance, electrolyte imbalance, essential fatty acid deficiency)<br>***I.V. lipid emulsion***<br>▶ May not be used effectively in severely stressed patients (especially burn patients)<br>▶ May interfere with immune mechanisms; in patients suffering respiratory compromise, reduces carbon dioxide buildup<br>▶ Given by way of CV line; irritates peripheral vein in long-term use |
| Protein-sparing therapy | ▶ Crystalline amino acids in same amounts as TPN<br>▶ Electrolytes, vitamins, minerals, and trace elements | ▶ Nutritionally complete<br>▶ Requires little mixing<br>▶ May be started or stopped any time during the hospital stay<br>▶ Other I.V. fluids, medications, and blood by-products may be administered through the same I.V. line<br>▶ Not as likely to cause phlebitis as peripheral parenteral nutrition<br>▶ Adds a major expense; has limited benefits |
| Total nutrient admixture | ▶ One day's nutrients are contained in a single, 3-L bag (also called 3:1 solution)<br>▶ Combines lipid emulsion with other parenteral solution components | ▶ See TPN (above)<br>▶ Reduces need to handle bag, cutting risk of contamination<br>▶ Decreases nursing time and reduces need for infusion sets and electronic devices, lowering facility costs, increasing patient mobility, and allowing easier adjustment to home care<br>▶ Has limited use because not all types and amounts of components are compatible<br>▶ Precludes use of certain infusion pumps because they can't accurately deliver large volumes of solution; precludes use of standard I.V. tubing filters because a 0.22-micron filter blocks lipid and albumin molecules |

# Types of parenteral nutrition *(continued)*

| Type | Solution components | Special considerations |
|---|---|---|
| Peripheral parenteral nutrition (PPN) | ▶ $D_5W$ or $D_{10}W$ <br> ▶ Crystalline amino acids 2.5% to 5% <br> ▶ Electrolytes, minerals, vitamins, and trace elements <br> ▶ Lipid emulsion 10% or 20% (1 L of dextrose 10% and amino acids 3.5% infused at the same time as 1 L of lipid emulsion = 1,440 nonprotein calories) <br> ▶ Heparin or hydrocortisone | ***Basic solution*** <br> ▶ Nutritionally complete for a short time <br> ▶ Can't be used in nutritionally depleted patients <br> ▶ Can't be used in volume-restricted patients because PPN requires large fluid volume <br> ▶ Doesn't cause weight gain <br> ▶ Avoids insertion and care of CV line but requires adequate venous access; site must be changed every 72 hours <br> ▶ Delivers less hypertonic solutions than CV-line TPN <br> ▶ May cause phlebitis and increases risk of metabolic complications <br> ▶ Less chance of metabolic complications than with CV-line TPN <br> ***I.V. lipid emulsion*** <br> ▶ As effective as dextrose for caloric source <br> ▶ Diminishes phlebitis if infused at the same time as basic nutrient solution <br> ▶ Irritates vein in long-term use <br> ▶ Reduces carbon dioxide buildup when pulmonary compromise is present |

protein, carbohydrates, electrolytes, vitamins, and trace minerals. A lipid emulsion provides the necessary fat. (See *Types of parenteral nutrition*.)

**EVIDENCE BASE** Total parenteral nutrition (TPN) may need to be started early in select populations. Appropriate provision of nutrition with emphasis on early enteral nutrition in the critically ill and surgical patients can enhance wound healing.

Total parenteral nutrition (TPN) refers to any nutrient solution, including lipids, given through a CV line. Peripheral parenteral nutrition (PPN), which is given through a peripheral line, supplies full caloric needs while avoiding the risks that accompany a CV line. To keep from sclerosing the vein through which it's administered, the dextrose in PPN solution must be limited to 10% or less. Therefore, the success of PPN depends on the patient's tolerance for the large volume of fluid necessary to supply his nutritional needs.

Often, you'll need to increase the glucose content beyond the level a peripheral vein can handle. For example, most TPN solutions are six times more concentrated than blood. As a result, they must be delivered into a vein with a high rate of blood flow to dilute the solution.

The most common delivery route for TPN is through a central venous catheter (CVC) into the superior vena cava. The catheter may also be placed through the infraclavicular approach or, less commonly, through the supraclavicular, internal jugular, or antecubital fossa approach.

## Equipment

Bag or bottle of prescribed parenteral nutrition solution ● sterile I.V. tubing with attached extension tubing ● 0.22-micron filter (or 1.2-micron filter if solution contains lipids or albumin) ● reflux valve ● time tape ● alcohol pads ● electronic infusion pump ● portable glucose monitor ● scale ● intake and output record ● sterile gloves ● optional: mask

### Preparation of equipment

Make sure the solution, the patient, and the equipment are ready. Remove the solution from the refrigerator at least 1 hour before use to avoid pain, hypothermia, venous spasm, and venous constriction, which can result from delivery of a chilled solution. Check the solution against the doctor's order for correct patient name, expiration date, and formula components. Observe the container for cracks and the solution for cloudiness, turbidity, and particles. If any of these is present, return the solution to the pharmacy. If you'll be administering a total nutrient admixture solution, look for a brown layer on the solution, which indicates that the lipid emulsion has "cracked," or separated from the solution. If you see a brown layer, return the solution to the pharmacy.

When you're ready to administer the solution, explain the procedure to the patient. Check the name on the solution container against the name on the patient's wristband. Then put on gloves and, if specified by facility policy, a mask. Throughout the procedure, use strict sterile technique.

In sequence, connect the pump tubing, the micron filter with attached extension tubing (if the tubing doesn't contain an inline filter), and the reflux valve. Insert the filter as close to the catheter site as possible. If the tubing doesn't have luer-lock connections, tape all connections to prevent accidental separation, which could lead to air embolism, exsanguination, or sepsis. Next, squeeze the I.V. drip chamber and, holding it upright, insert the tubing spike into the I.V. bag or bottle. Then release the drip chamber. Squeeze the drip chamber before spiking an I.V. bottle to prevent accidental dripping of the parenteral nutrition solution. An I.V. bag, however, shouldn't drip.

Next, prime the tubing. Invert the filter at the distal end of the tubing and open the roller clamp. Let the solution fill the tubing and the filter. Gently tap it to dislodge air bubbles trapped in the Y-ports. If indicated, attach a time tape to the parenteral nutrition container for accurate measurement of fluid intake. Record the date and time you hung the fluid and initial the parenteral nutrition solution container. Next, attach the setup to the infusion pump and prepare it according to the manufacturer's instructions. Remove and discard your gloves.

With the patient in the supine position, put on gloves and clean the catheter injection cap with an alcohol pad and flush the catheter with normal saline solution, according to your facility's policy.

## Implementation

▶ If you'll be attaching the container of parenteral nutrition solution to a CV line, clamp the CV line before disconnecting it to prevent air from entering the catheter. If a clamp isn't available, ask the patient to perform Valsalva's maneuver just as you change the tubing, if possible. Or, if the patient is being mechanically ventilated, change the I.V. tubing immediately after the machine delivers a breath at peak inspiration. Both of these measures increase intrathoracic pressure and prevent air embolism.

▶ Using sterile technique, attach the tubing to the designated luer-locking port. After connecting the tubing, remove the clamp, if applicable.

▶ Make sure the catheter junction is secure. Set the infusion pump at the ordered flow rate and start the infusion.

▶ Tag the tubing with the date and time of change.

### Starting the infusion

▶ Because parenteral nutrition solution often contains a large amount of glucose, you may need to start the infusion slowly to allow the patient's pancreatic beta cells time to increase their output of insulin. Depending on the patient's tolerance, parenteral nutrition is usually initiated at a rate of 40 to 50 ml/hour and then advanced by 25 ml/hour every 6 hours (as tolerated) until the desired infusion rate is achieved. However, when the glucose concentration is low, as occurs in most PPN formulas, you can initiate the rate necessary to infuse the complete 24-hour volume and discontinue the solution without tapering.

▶ You may allow a container of parenteral nutrition solution to hang for 24 hours.

### Changing solutions

▶ Prepare the new solution and I.V. tubing as described earlier. Put on gloves. Remove the protective caps from the solution containers and wipe the tops of the containers with alcohol pads.

▶ Turn off the infusion pump and close the flow clamps. Using strict sterile technique, remove the spike from the solution container that is hanging and insert it into the new container.

▶ Hang the new container and tubing alongside the old. Turn on the infusion pump, set the flow rate, and open the flow clamp completely.

▶ If you'll be attaching the solution to a peripheral line, examine the skin above the insertion site for redness and warmth and assess for pain. If you suspect phlebitis, remove the existing I.V. line and start a line in a different vein. Also insert a new line if the I.V. catheter has been in place for 72 hours or more to reduce the risk of phlebitis and infiltration.

▶ Next, turn off the infusion pump and close the flow clamp on the old tubing. Disconnect the tubing from the catheter hub and connect the new tubing. Open the flow clamp on the new container to a moderately slow rate.

▶ Remove the old tubing from the infusion pump and insert the new tubing according to the manufacturer's instructions. Then turn on the infusion pump, set it to the desired flow rate, and open the flow clamp completely. Remove the old equipment and dispose of it properly.

## Special considerations

▶ Always infuse a parenteral nutrition solution at a constant rate without interruption to avoid blood glucose fluctuations. If the infusion slows, consult the doctor before changing the infusion rate.

▶ Monitor the patient's vital signs every 4 hours or more often if necessary. Watch for an increased temperature, an early sign of catheter-related sepsis. (See *Correcting common parenteral nutrition problems,* page 212.)

▶ Check the patient's blood glucose level every 6 hours. Some patients may require supplementary insulin, which the pharmacist may add directly to the solution. The patient may require additional subcutaneous doses.

▶ Because most patients receiving PPN are in a protein-wasted state, the therapy causes marked changes in fluid and electrolyte status and in levels of glucose, amino acids, minerals, and vitamins. Therefore, record daily intake and output accurately. Specify the volume and type of each fluid and calculate the daily caloric intake.

▶ Monitor the results of routine laboratory tests and report abnormal findings to the doctor to allow for appropriate changes in the parenteral nutrition solution. Such tests typically include measurement of serum electrolyte, calcium, blood urea nitrogen, and creatinine at least three times weekly; serum magnesium and phosphorus levels twice weekly; liver function studies, complete blood count and differential, and serum albumin and transferrin levels weekly; and urine nitrogen balance and creatinine-height index studies weekly. A serum zinc level is obtained at the start of parenteral nutrition therapy. The doctor may also order serum prealbumin levels, total lymphocyte count, amino acid levels, fatty acid-phospholipid fraction, skin testing, and expired gas analysis.

▶ Physically assess the patient daily. If ordered, measure arm circumference and skin-fold thickness over the triceps. Weigh him at the same time each morning after he voids; he should be weighed in similar clothing and on the same scale. Suspect fluid imbalance if he gains more than 1 lb (0.5 kg) daily.

▶ Change the dressing over the catheter according to your facility's policy or whenever the dressing becomes wet, soiled, or nonocclusive. Always use strict sterile technique. When performing dressing changes, watch for signs of phlebitis and catheter retraction from the vein. Measure the catheter length from the insertion site to the hub for verification.

▶ Change the tubing and filters every 24 hours or according to your facility's policy.

▶ Closely monitor the catheter site for swelling, which may indicate infiltration. Extravasation of parenteral nutrition solution can lead to tissue necrosis.

▶ Use caution when using the parenteral nutrition line for other functions. Don't use a single-lumen CVC to infuse blood or blood products, to give a bolus injection, to administer simultaneous I.V. solutions, to measure CV pressure, or to draw blood for laboratory tests.

▶ Provide regular mouth care. Also provide emotional support. Keep in mind that patients commonly associate eating with positive feelings and become disturbed when they can't eat.

▶ Teach the patient the potential adverse effects and complications of parenteral nutrition. Encourage the patient to inspect his mouth regularly for signs of parotitis, glossitis, and oral lesions. Tell him that he may have fewer bowel movements while receiving parenteral nutrition therapy. Encourage

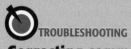

# Correcting common parenteral nutrition problems

| Complications | Signs and symptoms | Interventions |
|---|---|---|
| Hepatic dysfunction | Elevated serum aspartate amino-transferase, alkaline phosphatase, and bilirubin levels | Reduce total caloric intake and dextrose intake, making up lost calories by administering lipid emulsion. Change to cyclical infusion. Use specific hepatic formulations only if the patient has encephalopathy. |
| Hypercapnia | Heightened oxygen consumption, increased carbon dioxide production, measured respiratory quotient of 1 or greater | Reduce total caloric and dextrose intake and balance dextrose and fat calories. |
| Hyperglycemia | Fatigue, restlessness, confusion, anxiety, weakness, polyuria, dehydration, elevated serum glucose levels and, in severe hyperglycemia, delirium or coma | Restrict dextrose intake by decreasing either the rate of infusion or the dextrose concentration. Compensate for calorie loss by administering lipid emulsion. Begin insulin therapy. |
| Hyperosmolarity | Confusion, lethargy, seizures, hyperosmolar hyperglycemic nonketotic syndrome, hyperglycemia, dehydration, and glycosuria | Discontinue dextrose infusion. Administer insulin and half-normal saline solution with 10 to 20 mEq/L of potassium to rehydrate the patient. |
| Hypocalcemia | Polyuria, dehydration, and elevated blood and urine glucose levels | Increase calcium supplements. |
| Hypoglycemia | Sweating, shaking, and irritability after infusion has stopped | Increase dextrose intake or decrease exogenous insulin intake. |
| Hypokalemia | Muscle weakness, paralysis, paresthesia, and arrhythmias | Increase potassium supplements. |
| Hypomagnesemia | Tingling around mouth, paresthesia in fingers, mental changes, and hyperreflexia | Increase magnesium supplements. |
| Hypophosphatemia | Irritability, weakness, paresthesia, coma, and respiratory arrest | Increase phosphate supplements. |
| Metabolic acidosis | Elevated serum chloride level, reduced serum bicarbonate level | Increase acetate and decrease chloride in parenteral nutrition solution. |
| Metabolic alkalosis | Reduced serum chloride level, elevated serum bicarbonate level | Decrease acetate and increase chloride in parenteral nutrition solution. |
| Zinc deficiency | Dermatitis, alopecia, apathy, depression, taste changes, confusion, poor wound healing, and diarrhea | Increase zinc supplements. |

him to remain physically active to help his body use the nutrients more fully.

## Home care

Patients who require prolonged or indefinite parenteral nutrition may be able to receive therapy at home. Home parenteral nutrition reduces the need for long hospitalizations and allows the patient to resume many of his normal activities. Meet with a home care patient before discharge to make sure he knows how to perform the administration procedure and how to handle complications.

## Complications

Catheter-related sepsis is the most serious complication of parenteral nutrition. Although rare, a malpositioned subclavian or jugular vein catheter may lead to thrombosis or sepsis.

An air embolism, a potentially fatal complication, can occur during I.V. tubing changes if the tubing is inadvertently disconnected. It may also result from undetected hairline cracks in the tubing. Extravasation of parenteral nutrition solution can cause necrosis and then sloughing of the epidermis and dermis.

## Documentation

▶ Document the times of the dressing, filter, and solution changes; the condition of the catheter insertion site; your observations of the patient's condition; and any complications and interventions.

### REFERENCES

"ASPEN Standards of Practice: Standards for Home Nutrition Support," *Nutrition in Clinical Practice* 14(3):151-62, June 1999.

Bliss, D.Z., and Dysart, M. "Using Needleless Intravenous Access Devices for Administering Total Parenteral Nutrition (TPN): Practice Update," *Nutrition in Clinical Practice* 14(6):299-303, December 1999.

Duerksen, D.R., et al. "Peripherally Inserted Central Catheters for Parenteral Nutrition: A Comparison of Centrally Inserted Catheters," *Journal of Parenteral and Enteral Nutrition* 23(2):85-90, March-April 1999.

Trissel, L.A., et al. "Compatibility of Medications with 3-in-1 Parenteral Nutrition Admixtures," *Journal of Parenteral and Enteral Nutrition* 23(2):67-74, March-April 1999.

# Transfusion of whole blood and packed cells

Whole blood transfusion replenishes both the volume and the oxygen-carrying capacity of the circulatory system by increasing the mass of circulating red cells. Transfusion of packed red blood cells (RBCs), from which 80% of the plasma has been removed, restores only the oxygen-carrying capacity. After plasma is removed, the resulting component has a hematocrit of 65% to 80% and a usual volume of 300 to 350 ml. (Whole blood without the plasma removed has a hematocrit of about 38%.) Each unit of whole blood or RBCs contains enough hemoglobulin to raise the hemoglobin concentration in an average-sized adult 1 g/dl or by 3%. Both types of transfusion treat decreased hemoglobin levels and hematocrit. Whole blood is usually used only when decreased levels result from hemorrhage; packed RBCs are used when such depressed levels accompany normal blood volume to avoid possible fluid and circulatory overload. (See *Transfusing blood and selected components,* pages 214 and 215.)

◆ **ALERT!** To prevent errors and potential fatal reactions many facilities require that two nurses identify the patient and blood products before administering a transfusion. If the patient is a Jehovah's Witness, a transfusion requires special written permission. Both whole blood and packed RBCs contain cellular debris, requiring in-line filtration during administration. (Washed packed RBCs, commonly used for patients previously sensitized to transfusions, are rinsed with a special solution that removes white blood cells and platelets, thus decreasing the chance of transfusion reaction.)

## Equipment

Blood recipient set (170- to 260-micron filter and tubing with drip chamber for blood, or combined set) ● I.V. pole ● gloves ● gown ● face shield ● multiple-lead tubing ● whole blood or packed RBCs ● 250 ml of normal saline solution ● venipuncture equipment, if necessary (should include 20G or larger catheter) ● optional: ice bag, warm compresses

Straight-line and Y-type blood administration sets are commonly used. The use of these filters can postpone sensitization to transfusion therapy.

# Transfusing blood and selected components

| Blood component | Indications | Crossmatching |
|---|---|---|
| **Whole blood** Complete (pure) blood *Volume: 450 to 500 ml* | ▸ To restore blood volume lost from hemorrhaging, trauma, or burns | ▸ ABO identical: Type A receives A; type B receives B; type AB receives AB; type O receives O ▸ Rh match necessary |
| **Packed red blood cells (RBCs)** Same RBC mass as whole blood but with 80% of the plasma removed *Volume: 250 to 300 ml* | ▸ To restore or maintain oxygen-carrying capacity ▸ To correct anemia and blood loss that occurs during surgery ▸ To increase RBC mass | ▸ Type A receives A or O ▸ Type B receives B or O ▸ Type AB receives AB, A, B, or O ▸ Type O receives O ▸ Rh match necessary |
| **Platelets** Platelet sediment from RBCs or plasma *Volume: 35 to 50 ml/unit; 1 unit of platelets = 7 $\times$ 10$^7$ platelets* | ▸ To treat thrombocytopenia caused by decreased platelet production, increased platelet destruction, or massive transfusion of stored blood ▸ To treat acute leukemia and marrow aplasia ▸ To improve platelet count preoperatively in a patient whose count is 100,000/µl or less | ▸ ABO compatibility unnecessary but preferable with repeated platelet transfusions ▸ Rh match preferred |
| **Fresh frozen plasma (FFP)** Uncoagulated plasma separated from RBCs and rich in coagulation factors V, VIII, and IX *Volume: 180 to 300 ml* | ▸ To expand plasma volume ▸ To treat postoperative hemorrhage or shock ▸ To correct an undetermined coagulation factor deficiency ▸ To replace a specific factor when that factor alone isn't available ▸ To correct factor deficiencies resulting from hepatic disease | ▸ ABO compatibility unnecessary but preferable with repeated platelet transfusions ▸ Rh match preferred |
| **Albumin 5% (buffered saline); albumin 25% (salt poor)** A small plasma protein prepared by fractionating pooled plasma *Volume: 5% = 12.5 g/250 ml; 25% = 12.5 g/50 ml* | ▸ To replace volume lost because of shock from burns, trauma, surgery, or infections ▸ To replace volume and prevent marked hemoconcentration ▸ To treat hypoproteinemia (with or without edema) | ▸ Unneccessary |
| **Factor VIII (cryoprecipitate)** Insoluble portion of plasma recovered from FFP *Volume: approximately 30 ml (freeze-dried)* | ▸ To treat a patient with hemophilia A ▸ To control bleeding associated with factor VIII deficiency ▸ To replace fibrinogen or deficient factor VIII | ▸ ABO compatibility unnecessary but preferable |

Administer packed RBCs with a Y-type set. Using a straight-line set forces you to piggyback the tubing so you can stop the transfusion if necessary but still keep the vein open. Piggybacking increases the chance of harmful microorganisms entering the tubing as you're connecting the blood line to the established line.

## Nursing considerations

- Use a straight-line or Y-type I.V. set to infuse blood over 2 to 4 hours.
- Avoid giving whole blood when the patient can't tolerate the circulatory volume.
- Reduce the risk of a transfusion reaction by adding a microfilter to the administration set to remove platelets.
- Warm blood if giving a large quantity.

- Use a straight-line or Y-type I.V. set to infuse blood over 2 to 4 hours.
- Bear in mind that packed RBCs provide the same oxygen-carrying capacity as whole blood with less risk of volume overload.
- Give packed RBCs, as ordered, to prevent potassium and ammonia buildup, which may occur in stored plasma.
- Avoid administering packed RBCs for anemic conditions correctable by nutritional or drug therapy.

- Use a component drip administration set to infuse 100 ml over 15 minutes.
- As prescribed, premedicate with antipyretics and antihistamines if the patient's history includes a platelet transfusion reaction.
- Avoid administering platelets when the patient has a fever.
- Prepare to draw blood for a platelet count 1 hour after the platelet transfusion to determine platelet transfusion increments.
- Keep in mind that the doctor seldom orders a platelet transfusion for conditions in which platelet destruction is accelerated, such as idiopathic thrombocytopenic purpura and drug-induced thrombocytopenia.

- Use a straight-line I.V. set and administer the infusion rapidly.
- Keep in mind that large-volume transfusions of FFP may require correction for hypocalcemia because citric acid in FFP binds calcium.

- Use a straight-line I.V. set with rate and volume dictated by the patient's condition and response.
- Remember that reactions to albumin (fever, chills, nausea) are rare.
- Avoid mixing albumin with protein hydrolysates and alcohol solutions.
- Consider delivering albumin as a volume expander until the laboratory completes crossmatching for a whole blood transfusion.
- Keep in mind that albumin is contraindicated in severe anemia and administered cautiously in cardiac and pulmonary disease because heart failure may result from circulatory overload.

- Use the administration set supplied by the manufacturer. Administer factor VIII with a filter. Standard dose recommended for treatment of acute bleeding episodes in hemophilia is 15 to 20 units/kg.
- Half-life of factor VIII (8 to 10 hours) necessitates repeated transfusions at specified intervals to maintain normal levels.

Multiple-lead tubing minimizes the risk of contamination, especially when transfusing multiple units of blood (a straight-line set would require multiple piggybacking).

A Y-type set gives you the option of adding normal saline solution to packed cells—decreasing their viscosity—if the patient can tolerate the added fluid volume.

### Preparation of equipment

Avoid obtaining either whole blood or packed RBCs until you're ready to begin the transfusion. Prepare the equipment when you're ready to start the infusion.

## Implementation

▶ Explain the procedure to the patient. Make sure he has signed an informed consent form before transfusion therapy is initiated.

▶ Record the patient's baseline vital signs.

▶ If the patient doesn't have an I.V. line in place, perform a venipuncture, using a 20G or larger-diameter catheter. Avoid using an existing line if the needle or catheter lumen is smaller than 20G. Central venous access devices also may be used for transfusion therapy.

▶ Obtain whole blood or packed RBCs from the blood bank within 30 minutes of the transfusion start time. Check the expiration date on the blood bag and observe for abnormal color, RBC clumping, gas bubbles, and extraneous material. Return outdated or abnormal blood to the blood bank.

▶ Compare the name and number on the patient's wristband with those on the blood bag label. Check the blood bag identification number, ABO blood group, and Rh compatibility. Also, compare the patient's blood bank identification number, if present, with the number on the blood bag. Identification of blood and blood products is performed at the patient's bedside by two licensed professionals, according to the facility's policy.

▶ Put on gloves, a gown, and a face shield. Using a Y-type set, close all the clamps on the set. Then insert the spike of the line you're using for the normal saline solution into the bag of saline solution. Next, open the port on the blood bag and insert the spike of the line you're using to administer the blood or cellular component into the port. Hang the bag of normal saline solution and blood or cellular component on the I.V. pole, open the clamp on the line of saline solution, and squeeze the drip chamber until it's half full. Then remove the adapter cover at the tip of the blood administration set, open the main flow clamp, and prime the tubing with saline solution.

▶ If you're administering packed RBCs with a Y-type set, you can add saline solution to the bag to dilute the cells by closing the clamp between the patient and the drip chamber and opening the clamp from the blood. Then lower the blood bag below the saline container and let 30 to 50 ml of saline solution flow into the packed cells. Finally, close the clamp to the blood bag, rehang the bag, rotate it gently to mix the cells and saline solution, and close the clamp to the saline container.

▶ If you're administering whole blood, gently invert the bag several times to mix the cells.

▶ Attach the prepared blood administration set to the venipuncture device and flush it with normal saline solution. Then close the clamp to the saline solution and open the clamp between the blood bag and the patient. Adjust the flow rate to no greater than 5 ml/ minute for the first 15 minutes of the transfusion to observe for a possible transfusion reaction.

▶ Remain with the patient and watch for signs of a transfusion reaction. If such signs develop, record vital signs and stop the transfusion. Infuse saline solution at a moderately slow infusion rate and notify the doctor at once. If no signs of a reaction appear within 15 minutes, you'll need to adjust the flow clamp to the ordered infusion rate. The rate of infusion should be as rapid as the patient's circulatory system can tolerate. It's undesirable for RBC preparations to remain at room temperature for more than 4 hours. If the infusion rate must be so slow that the entire unit can't be infused within 4 hours, it may be appropriate to divide the unit and keep one portion refrigerated until it can be safely administered.

▶ After completing the transfusion, you'll need to put on gloves and remove and discard the used infusion equipment. Then remember to reconnect the original I.V. fluid, if necessary, or discontinue the I.V. infusion.

▶ Return the empty blood bag to the blood bank, if facility policy dictates, and discard the tubing and filter.

▶ Record the patient's vital signs.

## Special considerations

▶ Although some microaggregate filters can be used for up to 10 units of blood, always replace the filter and tubing if more than 1 hour elapses between transfusions. When administering multiple units of blood under pressure, use a blood warmer to avoid hypothermia. Blood components may be warmed to no more than 107.6° F (42° C).

▶ For rapid blood replacement, you may need to use a pressure bag. Be aware that excessive pressure may develop, leading to broken blood vessels and extravasation, with hematoma and hemolysis of the infusing RBCs.

▶ If the transfusion stops, take these steps as needed:

– Check that the I.V. container is at least 3′ (1 m) above the level of the I.V. site.

– Make sure the flow clamp is open and that the blood completely covers the filter. If it doesn't, squeeze the drip chamber until it does.

– Gently rock the bag back and forth, agitating blood cells that may have settled.

– Untape the dressing over the I.V. site to check cannula placement. Reposition the cannula if necessary.

– Flush the line with saline solution and restart the transfusion. Using a Y-type set, close the flow clamp to the patient and lower the blood bag. Next, open the saline clamp and allow some saline solution to flow into the blood bag. Rehang the blood bag, open the flow clamp to the patient, and reset the flow rate.

– If a hematoma develops at the I.V. site, immediately stop the infusion. Remove the I.V. cannula. Notify the doctor and expect to place ice on the site intermittently for 8 hours; then apply warm compresses. Follow your facility's policy.

– If the blood bag empties before the next one arrives, administer normal saline solution slowly. If you're using a Y-type set, close the blood-line clamp, open the saline clamp, and let the saline run slowly until the new blood arrives. Decrease the flow rate or clamp the line before attaching the new unit of blood.

## Complications

Despite improvements in crossmatching precautions, transfusion reactions can still occur. Unlike a transfusion reaction, an infectious disease transmitted during a transfusion may go undetected until days, weeks, or even months later, when it produces signs and symptoms. Measures to prevent disease transmission include laboratory testing of blood products and careful screening of potential donors, neither of which is guaranteed.

Hepatitis C accounts for most posttransfusion hepatitis cases. The tests that detect hepatitis B and hepatitis C can produce false-negative results and may allow some hepatitis cases to go undetected.

When testing for antibodies to human immunodeficiency virus (HIV), keep in mind that antibodies don't appear until 6 to 12 weeks after exposure. The estimated risk of acquiring HIV from blood products varies from 1 in 40,000 to 1 in 153,000.

Many blood banks screen blood for cytomegalovirus (CMV). Blood with CMV is especially dangerous for an immunosuppressed, seronegative patient. Blood banks also test blood for syphilis, but refrigerating blood virtually eliminates the risk of transfusion-related syphilis.

Circulatory overload and hemolytic, allergic, febrile, and pyogenic reactions can result from any transfusion. Coagulation disturbances, citrate intoxication, hyperkalemia, acid-base imbalance, loss of 2,3-diphosphoglycerate, ammonia intoxication, and hypothermia can result from massive transfusion.

## Documentation

▶ Record the date and time of the transfusion, the type and amount of transfusion product, the patient's vital signs, your check of all identification data, and the patient's response.

▶ Document any transfusion reaction and treatment.

### REFERENCES

Vengelen-Tyler, V., ed. *American Association of Blood Banks. Technical Manual,* 13th ed. Bethesda, Md.: AABB, 1999.

Weinstein, S.M. *Plumer's Principles and Practice of Infusion Therapy,* 7th ed. Philadelphia: Lippincott Williams & Wilkins, 2001.

# Vascular access device management

Surgically implanted under local anesthesia by a doctor, a vascular access device consists of a silicone catheter attached to a reservoir, which is covered with a self-sealing silicone rubber septum. It's used most commonly when an external CVC isn't desirable for long-term I.V. therapy. The most common type of vascular access device is a vascular access port (VAP).

# Understanding vascular access ports

Typically, a vascular access port (VAP) is used to deliver intermittent infusions of medication, chemotherapy, and blood products. Because the device is completely covered by the patient's skin, the risk of extrinsic contamination is reduced. Patients may prefer this type of central line because it doesn't alter the body image and requires less routine catheter care.

The VAP consists of a catheter connected to a small reservoir. A septum designed to withstand multiple punctures seals the reservoir.

Vascular access ports come in two basic designs: top entry and side entry. In a top-entry port, the needle is inserted perpendicular to the reservoir. In a side-entry port, the needle is inserted into the septum nearly parallel to the reservoir. (A needle stop prevents the needle from coming out the other side.)

**TOP-ENTRY VAP**

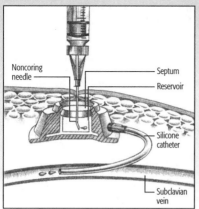

**SIDE-ENTRY VAP**

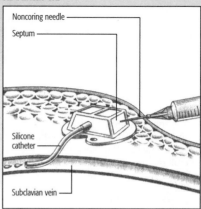

One- and two-piece units with single or double lumens are available. (See *Understanding vascular access ports*.)

VAPs come in two basic types: top entry (such as Med-i-Port, Port-A-Cath, and Infuse-A-Port) and side entry (such as S.E.A. Port). The VAP reservoir can be made of titanium (as with Port-A-Cath), stainless steel (as with Q-Port), or molded plastic (as with Infuse-A-Port). The type and lumen size selected depend on the patient's needs.

Implanted in a pocket under the skin, a VAP functions much like a long-term CVC, except that it has no external parts. The attached indwelling catheter tunnels through the subcutaneous tissue into a vein and the catheter is advanced so that the catheter tip lies in a central vein, for example, the subclavian vein. A VAP can also be used for arterial access or be implanted into the epidural space, peritoneum, or pericardial or pleural cavity.

Typically, VAPs deliver intermittent infusions. Most often used for chemotherapy, a VAP can also deliver I.V. fluids, medications, and blood. It can also be used to obtain blood samples.

VAPs offer several advantages, including minimal activity restrictions, few steps for the patient to perform, and few dressing changes (except when used to maintain continuous infusions or intermittent infusion devices). Implanted devices are easier to maintain than external devices. For instance, they require heparinization only once after each use (or periodically if not in use). They also pose less risk of infection because they have no exit site to serve as an entry for microorganisms.

Because VAPs create only a slight protrusion under the skin, many patients find them easier to accept than external infusion devices. Because the device is implanted, however, it may be harder for the patient to manage, particularly if he'll be administering medication or fluids daily or frequently. And because accessing the device requires inserting a needle through subcutaneous tissue, patients who fear or dislike needle punctures may be uncomfortable using a VAP and may require a local anesthetic. In addition, implantation and removal of the device require surgery and hospitalization. The cost of VAPs makes them worthwhile only for patients who require infusion therapy for at least 6 months.

Implanted VAPs are contraindicated in patients who have been unable to tolerate other implanted devices and in those who may develop an allergic reaction.

## Equipment
*To implant a VAP*
Noncoring needles of appropriate type and gauge (a noncoring needle has a deflected point, which slices the port's septum) • VAP • sterile gloves • mask • alcohol pads • povidone-iodine swabs • extension set • tubing, if needed local anesthetic (lidocaine without epinephrine) • ice pack • 10- and 20-ml syringes • normal saline and heparin flush solutions • I.V. solution • sterile dressings • luer-lock injection cap • clamp • adhesive • skin closures • suture removal set

*To administer a bolus injection*
Extension set • 10-ml syringe filled with normal saline solution • clamp • syringe containing the prescribed medication • optional: sterile syringe filled with heparin flush solution

*To administer a continuous infusion*
Prescribed I.V. solution or drugs • I.V. administration set • filter, if ordered • extension set • clamp • 10-ml syringe filled with normal saline solution • adhesive tape • sterile 2″ × 2″ gauze pad • sterile tape • transparent semipermeable dressing

Some facilities use an implantable port access kit.

### Preparation of equipment
Confirm the size and type of the device and the insertion site with the doctor. Attach the tubing to the solution container, prime the tubing with fluid, fill the syringes with saline or heparin flush solution, and prime

the noncoring needle and extension set. All priming must be done using strict aseptic technique, and all tubing must be free of air. After you've primed the tubing, recheck all connections for tightness. Make sure that all open ends are covered with sealed caps.

## Implementation
❱ Wash your hands to prevent spread of microorganisms.

### Assisting with implantation of a VAP
❱ Reinforce to the patient the doctor's explanation of the procedure, its benefit to the patient, and what's expected of him during and after implantation.
❱ Although the doctor is responsible for obtaining consent for the procedure, make sure the written document is signed, witnessed, and on the chart.
❱ Allay the patient's fears and answer questions about movement restrictions, cosmetic concerns, and management regimens.
❱ Check the patient's history for hypersensitivity to local anesthetics or iodine.
❱ The doctor will surgically implant the VAP, probably using a local anesthetic (similar to insertion of a CVC). Occasionally, a patient may receive a general anesthetic for VAP implantation.
❱ During the implantation procedure, you may be responsible for handing equipment and supplies to the doctor. First, the doctor makes a small incision and introduces the catheter, typically into the superior vena cava through the subclavian, jugular, or cephalic vein. After fluoroscopy verifies correct placement of the catheter tip, the doctor creates a subcutaneous pocket over a bony prominence in the chest wall. Then he tunnels the catheter to the pocket. Next, he connects the catheter to the reservoir, places the reservoir in the pocket, and flushes it with heparin solution. Finally, he sutures the reservoir to the underlying fascia and closes the incision.

### Preparing to access the port
❱ The VAP can be used immediately after placement, although some edema and tenderness may persist for about 72 hours. This makes the device initially difficult to palpate and slightly uncomfortable for the patient.

⊙ TROUBLESHOOTING

# Managing common vascular access port problems

| Problems and possible causes | Nursing interventions |
|---|---|
| **Inability to flush the device or draw blood** | |
| Kinked tubing or closed clamp | ▶ Check tubing or clamp. |
| Catheter lodged against vessel wall | ▶ Reposition the patient.<br>▶ Teach the patient to change his position to free the catheter from the vessel wall.<br>▶ Raise the arm that's on the same side as the catheter.<br>▶ Roll the patient to his opposite side.<br>▶ Have the patient cough, sit up, or take a deep breath.<br>▶ Infuse 10 ml of normal saline solution into the catheter.<br>▶ Regain access to the catheter or vascular access port (VAP) using a new needle. |
| Incorrect needle placement or needle not advanced through septum | ▶ Regain access to the device.<br>▶ Teach the home care patient to push down firmly on the noncoring needle device in the septum and to verify needle placement by aspirating for a blood return |
| Clot formation | ▶ Assess patency by trying to flush the VAP while the patient changes position.<br>▶ Notify the doctor; obtain an order for fibrinolytic agent instillation.<br>▶ Teach the patient to recognize clot formation, to notify the doctor if it occurs, and to avoid forcibly flushing the VAP. |
| Kinked catheter, catheter migration, or port rotation | ▶ Notify the doctor immediately.<br>▶ Tell the patient to notify the doctor if he has trouble using the VAP. |
| **Inability to palpate the device** | |
| Deeply implanted port | ▶ Note portal chamber scar.<br>▶ Use deep palpation technique.<br>▶ Ask another nurse to try locating the VAP.<br>▶ Use a 1½" or 2" (3.8- or 5.1-cm) noncoring needle to gain access to the VAP. |

▶ Prepare to access the port, following the specific steps for top-entry or side-entry ports.
▶ Using aseptic technique, inspect the area around the port for signs of infection or skin breakdown.
▶ Place an ice pack over the area for several minutes to alleviate possible discomfort from the needle puncture. Alternatively, administer a local anesthetic after cleaning the area.

▶ Wash your hands thoroughly. Put on sterile gloves and mask and wear them throughout the procedure.
▶ Clean the area with an alcohol pad, starting at the center of the port and working outward with a firm, circular motion over a 4" to 5" (10- to 12.5-cm) diameter. Repeat this procedure twice. Allow the site to dry, then clean the area with povidone-iodine swabs in the same manner. Repeat this procedure twice.
▶ If facility policy calls for a local anesthetic, check the patient's record for possible

allergies. As indicated, anesthetize the insertion site by injecting 0.1 ml of lidocaine (without epinephrine).

### Accessing a top-entry port
▶ Palpate the area over the port to find its septum.
▶ Anchor the port with your nondominant hand. Then, using your dominant hand, aim the needle at the center of the device.
▶ Insert the needle perpendicular to the port septum. Push the needle through the skin and septum until you reach the bottom of the reservoir.
▶ Check needle placement by aspirating for blood return.
▶ If you can't obtain blood, remove the needle and repeat the procedure. Inability to obtain blood may indicate sludge buildup (from medications) in the port reservoir. If so, you may need to use a fibrinolytic agent to free the occlusion. Ask the patient to raise his arms and perform Valsalva's maneuver. If you still don't get a blood return, notify the doctor; a fibrin sleeve on the distal end of the catheter may be occluding the opening. (See *Managing common vascular access port problems.*)
▶ Flush the device with normal saline solution. If you detect swelling or if the patient reports pain at the site, remove the needle and notify the doctor.

### Accessing a side-entry port
▶ To gain access to a side-entry port, you'll follow the same procedure as with a top-entry port except that you'll insert the needle parallel to the reservoir instead of perpendicular to it.

**■ EVIDENCE BASE** A continuous infusion device may be more cost effective than manually flushing the VAP.

### Administering a bolus injection
▶ Attach the 10-ml syringe filled with saline solution to the end of the extension set and remove all the air. Now attach the extension set to the noncoring needle. Check for blood return. Then flush the port with normal saline solution, according to your facility's policy.
▶ Clamp the extension set and remove the saline syringe.
▶ Connect the medication syringe to the extension set. Open the clamp and inject the drug, as ordered.

▶ Examine the skin surrounding the needle for signs of infiltration, such as swelling or tenderness. If you note these signs, stop the injection and intervene appropriately.
▶ When the injection is complete, clamp the extension set and remove the medication syringe.
▶ Open the clamp and flush with 5 ml of normal saline solution after each drug injection to minimize drug incompatibility reactions.
▶ Flush with heparin solution according to your facility's policy.

### Administering a continuous infusion
▶ Remove all air from the extension set by priming it with an attached syringe of normal saline solution. Now attach the extension set to the noncoring needle.
▶ Flush the port system with normal saline solution. Clamp the extension set and remove the syringe.
▶ Connect the administration set, and secure the connections with sterile tape if necessary.
▶ Unclamp the extension set and begin the infusion.
▶ Affix the needle to the skin. (See *Continuous infusion: Securing the needle,* page 222.)
Then apply a transparent semipermeable dressing.
▶ Examine the site carefully for infiltration. If the patient complains of stinging, burning, or pain at the site, discontinue the infusion and intervene appropriately.
▶ When the solution container is empty, obtain a new I.V. solution container, as ordered.
▶ Flush with normal saline solution followed by heparin solution according to your facility's policy.

## Special considerations
▶ After implantation, monitor the site for signs of hematoma and bleeding. Edema and tenderness may persist for about 72 hours. The incision site requires routine postoperative care for 7 to 10 days. You'll also need to assess the implantation site for signs of infection, device rotation, or skin erosion. You don't need to apply a dressing to the wound site except during infusions or to maintain an intermittent infusion device.
▶ While the patient is hospitalized, a luer-lock injection cap may be attached to the

# Continuous infusion: Securing the needle

When starting a continuous infusion, you must secure the right-angle, noncoring needle to the skin. If the needle hub isn't flush with the skin, place a folded sterile dressing under the hub, as shown. Then apply adhesive skin closures across it.

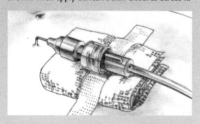

Secure the needle and tubing, using the chevron-taping technique.

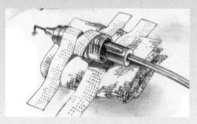

Apply a transparent semipermeable dressing over the entire site.

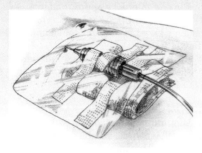

If your patient is receiving a continuous or prolonged infusion, change the dressing and needle every 7 days. You'll also need to change the tubing and solution, as you would for a long-term CV infusion. If your patient is receiving an intermittent infusion, flush the port periodically with heparin solution. When the VAP isn't being used, flush it every weeks. During the course of therapy, you may have to clear a clotted VAP, as ordered.

If clotting threatens to occlude the VAP, the doctor may order a fibrinolytic agent to clear the catheter. Because such agents increase the risk of bleeding, fibrinolytic agents may be contraindicated in patients who have had surgery within the past 10 days; in those who have active internal bleeding such as GI bleeding; and in those who have experienced central nervous system damage, such as infarction, hemorrhage, traumatic injury, surgery, or primary or metastatic disease, within the past 2 months.

Besides performing routine care measures, you must be prepared to handle several common problems that may arise during an infusion with a VAP. These common problems include an inability to flush the VAP, withdraw blood from it, or palpate it.

## Home care

If your patient is going home, he'll need thorough teaching about procedures as well as follow-up visits from a home care nurse to ensure safety and successful treatment. If he'll be accessing the port himself, explain that the most uncomfortable part of the procedure is the actual insertion of the needle into the skin.

Once the needle has penetrated the skin, the patient will feel mostly pressure. Eventually, the skin over the port will become desensitized from frequent needle punctures. Until then, the patient may want to use a topical anesthetic.

Stress the importance of pushing the needle into the port until the patient feels the needle bevel touch the back of the port. Many patients tend to stop short of the back of the port, leaving the needle bevel in the rubber septum.

Also stress the importance of monthly flushes when no more infusions are scheduled. If possible, instruct a family member in all aspects of care.

end of the extension set to provide ready access for intermittent infusions. Besides saving nursing time, a luer-lock cap reduces the discomfort of accessing the port and prolongs the life of the port septum by decreasing the number of needle punctures.

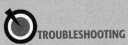

# Risks of vascular access port therapy

| Complications | Signs and symptoms | Possible causes | Nursing interventions |
|---|---|---|---|
| Site infection or skin breakdown | ▶ Erythema and warmth at the port site<br>▶ Oozing or purulent drainage at vascular access port (VAP) site or pocket<br>▶ Fever | ▶ Infected incision or VAP pocket<br>▶ Poor postoperative healing | ▶ Assess the site daily for redness; note any drainage.<br>▶ Notify the doctor.<br>▶ Administer antibiotics as prescribed.<br>▶ Apply warm soaks for 20 minutes four times per day.<br>***Prevention***<br>▶ Teach the patient to inspect for and report redness, swelling, drainage, or skin breakdown at the port site. |
| Extravasation | ▶ Burning sensation or swelling in subcutaneous tissue | ▶ Needle dislodged into subcutaneous tissue<br>▶ Needle incorrectly placed in VAP<br>▶ Needle position not confirmed; needle pulled out of septum<br>▶ Use of vesicant drugs | ▶ Stop the infusion.<br>▶ Notify the doctor; prepare to administer an antidote if ordered.<br>▶ Follow facility protocol for removing the needle.<br>***Prevention***<br>▶ Teach the patient how to gain access to the device, verify its placement, and secure the needle before initiating an infusion. |
| Thrombosis | ▶ Inability to flush port or administer infusion | ▶ Frequent blood sampling<br>▶ Infusion of packed red blood cells (RBCs) | ▶ Notify the doctor; obtain an order to administer a fibrinolytic agent.<br>***Prevention***<br>▶ Flush the VAP thoroughly right after obtaining a blood sample.<br>▶ Administer packed RBCs as a piggyback with normal saline solution and use an infusion pump; flush with saline solution between units. |
| Fibrin sheath formation | ▶ Blocked port and catheter lumen<br>▶ Inability to flush port or administer infusion<br>▶ Possible swelling, tenderness, and erythema in neck, chest, and shoulder | ▶ Adherence of platelets to catheter | ▶ Notify the doctor; add heparin (1,000 to 2,000 units) to continuous infusions. (A fibrinolytic agent may also be ordered.)<br>***Prevention***<br>▶ Use the port only to infuse fluids and medications; don't use it to obtain blood samples.<br>▶ Administer only compatible substances through the port. |

## Complications

A patient who has a VAP faces risks similar to those associated with CVCs. They include infection, thrombus formation, and occlusion. (See *Risks of vascular access port therapy.*)

## REFERENCES

Brock-Cascanet, P.H. "Treating Occluded VADs in the Home Setting," *Infusion* 5(4): 18-27, January 1999.

Davis, S.N., et al. "Activity and Dosage of Alteplase Dilution for Clearing Occlusions of Venous-access Devices," *American Journal of Health System Pharmacy* 57(11): 1039-45, 2000.

Heath, J., and Jones, S. "Utilization of an Elastomeric Continuous Infusion Device to Maintain Catheter Patency," *Journal of Intravenous Nursing* 24(2):102-106, March-April 2001.

Kincaid, E.H. "'Blind' Placement of Long Term Central Venous Access Devices: Report of 589 Consecutive Procedures," *American Surgeon* 65:520-24, June 1999.

# Venipuncture

Performed to obtain a venous blood sample, venipuncture involves piercing a vein with a needle and collecting blood in a syringe or evacuated tube. Typically, venipuncture is performed using the antecubital fossa. If necessary, however, it can be performed on a vein in the dorsal forearm, the dorsum of the hand or foot, or another accessible location.

## Equipment

Tourniquet • gloves • syringe or evacuated tubes and needle holder • alcohol or povidone-iodine sponges • 20G or 21G needle for the forearm or 23 G or 25G needle for the dorsal forearm, hand, and ankle, and for children • color-coded collection tubes containing appropriate additives • labels • laboratory request form • 2″ × 2″ gauze pads • adhesive bandage

### Preparation of equipment

If you're using evacuated tubes, open the needle packet, attach the needle to its holder, and select the appropriate tubes. If you're using a syringe, attach the appropriate needle to it. Be sure to choose a syringe large enough to hold all the blood required for the test but not to exceed a 20 ml size. Label all collection tubes clearly with the patient's name and room number, the doctor's name, and the date and time of collection.

## Implementation

▶ Wash your hands thoroughly and put on gloves.

▶ Tell the patient that you're about to collect a blood sample and explain the procedure to ease his anxiety and ensure his cooperation. Ask him if he has ever felt faint, sweaty, or nauseated when having blood drawn.

▶ If the patient is on bed rest, ask him to lie supine, with his head slightly elevated and his arms at his sides. Ask the ambulatory patient to sit in a chair and support his arm securely on an armrest or a table.

▶ Assess the patient's veins to determine the best puncture site. (See *Common venipuncture sites.*) Observe the skin for the vein's blue color, and palpate the vein for a firm rebound sensation.

▶ Tie a tourniquet 3″ (7.6 cm) proximal to the area chosen. By impeding venous return to the heart while still allowing arterial flow, a tourniquet produces venous dilation. If arterial perfusion remains adequate, you'll be able to feel the radial pulse. (If the tourniquet fails to dilate the vein, have the patient open and close his fist a few times. Then ask him to close his fist loosely as you insert the needle and to open it again when the needle is in place.)

**ALERT!** Opening and closing the fist repeatedly can cause hemoconcentration which may alter complete blood count results.

▶ Clean the venipuncture site with an alcohol or a povidone-iodine pad. Don't wipe off the povidone-iodine with alcohol because alcohol cancels the effect of povidone-iodine. Wipe in a circular motion, spiraling outward from the site to avoid introducing potentially infectious skin flora into the vessel during the procedure. If you use alcohol, apply it with friction for 30 seconds or until the final pad comes away clean. Allow the skin to dry before performing venipuncture.

▶ Immobilize the vein by pressing just below the venipuncture site with your thumb and drawing the skin taut.

▶ Position the needle holder or syringe with the needle bevel up and the shaft parallel to the path of the vein and at a 30-degree angle to the arm. Insert the needle into the vein. If you're using a syringe, venous blood will appear in the hub; withdraw the blood slowly, pulling the plunger

## Common venipuncture sites

The illustrations below show the anatomic locations of veins commonly used for venipuncture. The most commonly used sites are on the forearm, followed by those on the hand.

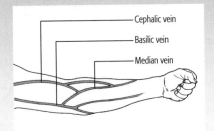

Cephalic vein
Basilic vein
Median vein

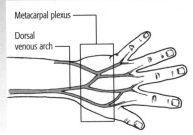

Metacarpal plexus
Dorsal venous arch

of the syringe gently to create steady suction until you obtain the required sample. Pulling the plunger too forcibly may collapse the vein. If you're using a needle holder and an evacuated tube, grasp the holder securely to stabilize it in the vein and push down on the collection tube until the needle punctures the rubber stopper. Blood will flow into the tube automatically.

▶ Remove the tourniquet as soon as blood flows adequately to prevent stasis and hemoconcentration, which can impair test results. If the flow is sluggish, leave the tourniquet in place longer, but always remove it before withdrawing the needle.

▶ Continue to fill the required tubes, removing one and inserting another. Gently rotate each tube as you remove it to help mix the additive with the sample.

▶ After you've drawn the sample, place a gauze pad over the puncture site and slowly and gently remove the needle from the vein. When using an evacuated tube, remove it from the needle holder to release the vacuum before withdrawing the needle from the vein.

▶ Apply gentle pressure to the puncture site for 2 to 3 minutes or until bleeding stops. This prevents extravasation into the surrounding tissue, which can cause a hematoma.

▶ After bleeding stops, apply an adhesive bandage.

▶ If you've used a syringe, transfer the sample to a collection tube. Detach the needle from the syringe, open the collection tube, and gently empty the sample into the tube, being careful to avoid foaming, which can cause hemolysis.

▶ Finally, check the venipuncture site to see if a hematoma has developed. If it has, apply pressure until you are sure bleeding has stopped. Warm soaks may then be applied to help reabsorption.

▶ Discard syringes, needles, and used gloves in the appropriate containers.

### Special considerations

▶ Never collect a venous sample from an arm or a leg that is already being used for I.V. therapy or blood administration because this may affect test results. Check your facility policy if a doctor's order is necessary to obtain a blood specimen from a leg or foot vein. Don't collect a venous sample from an infection site because this may introduce pathogens into the vascular system. Likewise, avoid collecting blood from edematous areas, arteriovenous shunts, and sites of previous hematomas or vascular injury.

▶ If the patient has large, distended, highly visible veins, perform venipuncture without a tourniquet to minimize the risk of hematoma formation. If the patient has a clotting disorder or is receiving anticoagulant therapy, maintain firm pressure on the venipuncture site for at least 5 minutes after withdrawing the needle to prevent hematoma formation.

▶ Avoid using veins in the patient's legs for venipuncture, if possible, because this increases the risk of thrombophlebitis and has a higher risk of infection.

## Complications

A hematoma at the needle insertion site is the most common complication of venipuncture. Infection may result from poor technique.

## Documentation

▶ Record the date, time, and site of the venipuncture; the name of the test; the time the sample was sent to the laboratory; the amount of blood collected; the patient's temperature; and any adverse reactions to the procedure.

**REFERENCES**

O'Brien, S., and Arbique, J. "The Community Phlebotomy Response Plan: How Does Your Facility Measure Up?" *Medical Lab Observer.* 34(7):40-42, 45, July 2002.

Weinstein, S.M. *Plumer's Principles and Practice of Infusion Therapy,* 7th ed. Philadelphia: Lippincott Williams & Wilkins, 2001.

# 5

# Cardiovascular care

C ARDIOVASCULAR DISORDERS, THE LEADING CAUSE OF DEATH IN THE UNITED STATES, AFFECT millions of Americans each year. The responsibility of caring for patients with these disorders pervades nearly every area of nursing practice. As a result, cardiovascular care ranks as one of the most rapidly growing areas of nursing. In addition, it's one of the most rapidly changing fields, with the continuing proliferations of new diagnostic tests, new drugs and other treatments, and sophisticated monitoring equipment. Consequently, nurses face a constant challenge to keep up with the latest developments.

Cardiac and hemodynamic monitoring represents critical cardiovascular care responsibilities. Cardiac monitoring is useful not only for assessing cardiac rhythm but also for gauging a patient's response to drug therapy and for preventing complications associated with diagnostic and therapeutic procedures.

Hemodynamic monitoring uses invasive techniques to measure pressure, flow, and resistance within the cardiovascular system. These measurements are used to guide therapy.

This chapter discusses the nursing protocols associated with cardiovascular care including the management of a patient in cardiac arrest, requiring cardiac pacing, undergoing angiography as well as experiencing decreased cardiac output and ineffective myocardial perfusion.

In cardiovascular emergencies, nurses may perform or assist with cardiopulmonary resuscitation, defibrillation, cardioversion, and temporary pacing. Only nurses with up-to-date information and sharpened skills can provide safe, effective patient care.

# Protocols

## Managing the patient in cardiac arrest

### Purpose
To provide rapid and effective treatment to the patient to minimize the complications of cardiac arrest

### Collaborative level
Interdependent

### Expected patient outcomes
▶ The patient will obtain stable hemodynamic status.
▶ The patient will obtain and maintain adequate tissue perfusion.
▶ The patient will obtain and maintain adequate oxygenation.

### Definition of terms
▶ *Arrhythmia:* Disturbance of the normal cardiac rhythm from the abnormal origin, discharge, or conduction of electrical impulses.

▶ *Defibrillation:* Termination of fibrillation by electric shock.
▶ *Cardioversion:* Restoration of normal rhythm by electric shock or drug therapy.
▶ *Diastole:* Phase of the cardiac cycle in which both atria (atrial diastole) or both ventricles (ventricular diastole) are at rest and filling with blood.
▶ *Systole:* Phase of the cardiac cycle in which both the atria (atrial systole) and the ventricles (ventricular systole) are contracting.

### Indications
Treatment
▶ Asystole
▶ Pulseless electrical activity

Prevention
▶ Respiratory failure
▶ Cardiovascular collapse
▶ Renal failure
▶ Brain death

## Assessment guidance
### Signs and symptoms
▶ Restlessness, dizziness
▶ Feeling of doom
▶ Feeling like "I'm going to die"
▶ Dyspnea
▶ Unresponsiveness
▶ Unconsciousness
▶ Apnea

### Diagnostic studies
*Laboratory tests*
▶ Serum chemistry
▶ Electrolyte level
▶ Drug level
▶ Arterial blood gas values
▶ CK-MB
▶ Troponin level

*Imaging tests*
▶ Echocardiogram

*Other*
▶ Electrocardiogram (ECG)

## Nursing interventions
▶ Establish the patient's unresponsiveness. "Look, listen, and feel."
▶ If the patient is monitored, check a second lead and check the gun again to verify that the flat line is truly asystole and not fine ventricular tachycardia. Also verify the monitor leads are connected to the patient.
▶ Activate the emergency response team.
▶ Establish the patient's airway and begin rescue breathing.
▶ Begin cardiopulmonary resuscitation (CPR).
▶ Establish I.V. access.
▶ If transcutaneous pacemaker is available, perform transcutaneous pacing immediately.
▶ After the patient is intubated, the emergency drugs can be given down the endotracheal (ET) tube if I.V. access isn't immediately available.
▶ Follow the algorithms for asystole and pulseless electrical activity according to the American Heart Association guidelines for basic life support and advanced cardiac life support.
▶ Give I.V. fluids wide open.
▶ Try to determine the cause of the arrhythmia (for example, tension pneumothorax, drug overdose, acute myocardial infarction, cardiac tamponade, hypokalemia, hyperkalemia).
▶ Notify the family of the patient's condition and keep them informed during the resuscitation attempt.
▶ Establish the criteria for terminating the resuscitation.
▶ If necessary, provide postmortem care.

## Patient teaching
▶ Teach the patient and his family about advance directives and do-not-resuscitate (DNR) orders.
▶ Provide the patient and family with appropriate treatment and medication information if the patient is resuscitated.
▶ Remember to support the family at this time. Give them privacy and keep them updated on the patient's condition. If needed, provide any spiritual support the family might need.

## Precautions
▶ If the patient is intubated, confirm placement of ET tube by measuring end-tidal carbon dioxide ($ETCO_2$) and by physical examination.
▶ When performing CPR, maintain proper hand placement to prevent breaking the patient's ribs.
▶ Before initiating CPR, establish that the rhythm is truly asystole by checking that the leads are attached to the patient.
▶ If mouth-to-mouth rescue breathing must be performed, be sure to use a face shield or face mask to avoid contact with the patient's body fluids.
▶ If the patient vomits, turn his head to the side to prevent aspiration.
▶ Before resuscitation efforts are begun, establish whether the patient has a DNR order.

## Contraindications
Contraindicated if DNR order is in place.

## Documentation
▶ Document the time of start and finish of resuscitative efforts and the outcome.
▶ Record the drugs used and the dosages.
▶ Document the size of the ET tube, time of placement, and verification of correct placement.
▶ Document personnel present during the resuscitative effort.

▶ Document the use of a temporary pacemaker and its effect.
▶ Record the I.V. fluids used and the amounts.
▶ Record the results of any blood work.
▶ Document how the patient responded to the resuscitative efforts and to the drugs given, and record the rhythms used during the code.

## Related procedures
▶ Arterial puncture for blood gas analysis
▶ Automated external defibrillation
▶ Cardiac monitoring
▶ Cardiopulmonary resuscitation
▶ Care of the dying patient
▶ Central venous line insertion and removal
▶ Defibrillation
▶ Electrocardiography
▶ Endotracheal intubation
▶ Endotracheal tube care
▶ End-tidal carbon dioxide monitoring
▶ I.V. bolus injection
▶ Indwelling catheter care and removal
▶ Indwelling catheter insertion
▶ Manual ventilation
▶ Mechanical ventilation
▶ Medication therapy
▶ Nasogastric tube insertion and removal
▶ Peripheral I.V. line insertion
▶ Peripheral I.V. line maintenance
▶ Physical assessment
▶ Postmortem care
▶ Pulse and ear oximetry
▶ Spiritual care
▶ Standard precautions
▶ Temporary pacemaker insertion and care
▶ Venipuncture

## REFERENCES
*ACLS Provider Manual.* American Heart Association, 2001.
Asselin, M.E., and Cullen, H.A. "A New Beat for BLS and ACLS Guidelines," *Nursing Management* 33(2): February 2002.
Dries, D.J., and Sample, M.A. "Recent Advances in Emergency Life Support," *Nursing Clinics of North America* 37(10):1-10, March 2002.

## ORGANIZATIONS
American Heart Association:
*www.americanheart.org*

# Managing the patient who needs cardiac pacing

## Purpose
To provide treatment to the patient experiencing hemodynamic instability resulting from symptomatic bradycardia, complete heart block, or symptomatic tachycardia

## Collaborative level
Dependent, independent

## Expected patient outcomes
▶ The patient will maintain adequate tissue perfusion.
▶ The patient will maintain adequate cardiac output.
▶ The patient will maintain stable hemodynamic status.
▶ The patient will increase tolerance for activities of daily living.

## Definition of terms
▶ *Transcutaneous pacemaker:* This type of pacemaker is used in life-threatening situations when rapid initiation of pacing is needed. Two electrodes are attached to the front and back of the patient's chest and the electric current is sent between the two electrodes. This type of pacing should be used only until a transvenous pacemaker can be inserted because it's uncomfortable for the patient.
▶ *Transvenous pacemaker:* Another type of temporary pacemaker in which the doctor threads a pacing catheter through the patient's subclavian or internal jugular vein and into the patient's right atrium or ventricle. The pacing catheter is then attached to an external pulse generator for pacing. This is the most common type of temporary pacemaker.
▶ *Permanent pacemaker:* A self-contained system consisting of pacing electrodes and a pulse generator, implanted surgically in a pocket under the patient's skin, usually in the left pectoral area underneath the clavicle.
▶ *Biventricular pacemaker:* A new type of permanent pacemaker in which pacing leads are placed in the right and left ventricles, enabling both ventricles to be paced together. When used to treat patients with heart failure, these devices improve the activity tolerance of these patients.

## Indications
### Treatment
#### Symptomatic bradycardia
▶ Complete atrioventricular block
▶ Idioventricular rhythm
▶ Sinus bradycardia
▶ Sick sinus syndrome
▶ Drug overdose or toxic levels of therapeutic or recreational drugs
▶ Failure of a permanent pacemaker
▶ Asystole resulting from a drug overdose
▶ Pulseless electrical activity resulting from acidosis or electrolyte imbalances

#### Symptomatic tachycardia
▶ Atrial flutter, atrial fibrillation
▶ Supraventricular tachycardia
▶ Torsades de pointes
▶ Wolff-Parkinson-White syndrome
▶ Ventricular tachycardia

### Prevention
▶ Cardiac arrest
▶ Bleeding
▶ Infection
▶ Progression from a Mobitz II block to complete heart block
▶ Bundle-branch block after an anterior myocardial infarction
▶ Left bundle-branch block in a patient undergoing cardiac catheterization

## Assessment guidance
### Signs and symptoms
▶ Weakness
▶ Fatigue
▶ Dizziness
▶ Unresponsiveness
▶ Hypotension
▶ Bradycardia
▶ Complete heart block
▶ Diaphoresis
▶ Tachycardia
▶ Syncope

### Diagnostic studies
#### Laboratory tests
▶ Electrolyte level and serum chemistries
▶ Drug levels
▶ Complete blood count
▶ CK, CK-MB, troponin levels

#### Imaging tests
▶ Cardiac catheterization
▶ Electrophysiology studies

#### Other
▶ ECG

## Nursing interventions
### Transvenous pacemaker
▶ Establish I.V. access.
▶ Administer oxygen as needed.
▶ Have defibrillator and emergency medications on hand.
▶ Set up the equipment for pacemaker insertion.
▶ Make sure pulse generator is functioning, and then turn it off. The pulse generator must be turned off when the pacing electrodes are attached to it.
▶ Wear gloves to electrically isolate yourself from the patient.
▶ After the doctor has placed the pacing electrodes, attach them to the pulse generator, making sure the positive and negative poles on the pacing electrodes are connected to the positive and negative poles on the pulse generator.
▶ Turn the pacemaker on and establish ventricular capture, using the settings ordered by the doctor. The usual settings to initiate pacing are pulse rate 80 to 100, output of 20 milliamperes (mA), asynchronous mode. After capture is established, decrease the mA to two to three times the minimum pacing threshold.

### Permanent pacemaker
This procedure is performed in either the operating room or the cardiac catheterization laboratory. The nurse's responsibility is for preprocedure and postprocedure care.

#### Preprocedure
▶ Obtain baseline vital signs.
▶ Obtain preoperative laboratory work, chest X-ray, and other tests according to your facility's policy.
▶ Establish I.V. access.
▶ Make sure informed consent is signed, witnessed, and placed in the patient's chart.
▶ Administer preoperative medications, including prophylactic antibiotics if ordered.
▶ Complete operating room checklist.
▶ Make sure the patient is wearing an identification and allergy bracelet and that it's accurate.

## Postprocedure

▶ Place the patient on cardiac monitor and assess pacemaker rhythm and rate. Also assess if the pacemaker is sensing and capturing.

▶ If not done in the operating room, obtain a chest X-ray to confirm lead placement.

▶ Obtain postprocedure laboratory work and medications if ordered.

▶ Examine the subcutaneous pocket for signs of bleeding or infection: redness, swelling, increase in temperature.

▶ Maintain I.V. access.

▶ Instruct the patient to place pacemaker registration card in his wallet.

## Patient teaching

▶ Instruct the patient to not lift his arm above his head on the side of pacemaker insertion for at least 6 weeks.

▶ Be sure to cover with the patient and his family:

  – risks of the procedure
  – risks if the procedure isn't performed
  – informed consent
  – the importance of the patient carrying his pacemaker registration card in his wallet
  – the importance of following up with his doctor and the pacemaker clinic
  – the signs and symptoms of infection of the pacemaker pocket
  – using a cellular phone on the opposite side from the permanent pacemaker
  – the fact that it's no longer necessary to avoid microwave ovens
  – the importance of informing doctors you have a pacemaker if they want you to have magnetic resonance imaging
  – the importance of notifying the doctor if the patient experiences dizziness, palpitations, or fast or slow heart rate
  – discharge teaching.

## Precautions

Temporary pacemaker

▶ Make sure the pacing electrodes and the box are secured. Patient movement could cause the electrode to move away from the ventricular wall, causing loss of capture.

▶ Check the batteries in the pacemaker box at the beginning of every shift.

▶ Make sure the controls on the pacemaker box are covered. Patient movement could accidentally cause the dials to move,

changing the rate or the output and sensitivity to change.

▶ Tape all connections together to prevent accidental disconnection from the pacemaker box.

▶ Assess the patient's rhythm via cardiac monitor every 4 hours for ventricular capture and sensing.

Permanent pacemaker

▶ Make sure informed consent is in the chart.

▶ Watch for signs of infection of the pocket and inform the doctor immediately.

▶ Keep the patient on the cardiac monitor for 12 hours to assess ventricular capture and sensing. If capture or sensing doesn't occur, inform the doctor.

▶ If the patient raises his arm above his shoulder on the same side as the pacemaker insertion, reassess his ECG for capture. It takes 6 weeks for the ventricular lead to adhere permanently to the ventricular wall.

## Contraindications

Contraindicated in the patient with electromagnetic dissociation and ventricular fibrillation.

## Documentation

▶ Document the location and settings of the temporary pacemaker, the condition of the insertion site, the cardiac rhythm, and whether ventricular capture and sensing are occurring. Also document any failure to capture or sense as well as the patient's symptoms.

▶ Document the location and type of permanent pacemaker.

▶ Document the pacemaker setting and manufacturer.

▶ Document the surgical site's condition.

▶ Document the cardiac rhythm and rate and ventricular or atrial capture.

▶ Document patient teaching.

## Related procedures

▶ Cardiac monitoring
▶ Cardiopulmonary resuscitation
▶ Electrocardiography
▶ Oxygen administration
▶ Peripheral I.V. line insertion
▶ Peripheral I.V. line maintenance
▶ Permanent pacemaker insertion and care
▶ Preoperative care

▶ Pulse and ear oximetry
▶ Surgical wound care
▶ Temporary pacemaker insertion and care

## REFERENCES

Boyle, J., and Rost, M.K. "Present Status of Cardiac Pacing: A Nursing Perspective." *Critical Care Nursing Quarterly* 23(1):1-19, May 2000.

Lynn-McHale, D.J. *AACN Procedure Manual for Critical Care.* Philadelphia: W.B. Saunders Co., 2000.

Woods, S.T., et al. *Cardiac Nursing.* Philadelphia: Lippincott Williams & Wilkins, 1999.

## ORGANIZATIONS

American Association of Critical Care Nurses: *www.aacn.org*
American College of Cardiology: *www.acc.org*
Guidant: *www.guidant.com*
Medtronic: *www.medtronic.com*
North American Society of Pacing and Electrophysiology: *www.naspe.org*
St. Jude Medical/Pacesetter: *www.stjudemedical.com*

# Managing the patient undergoing cardiac angiography

## Purpose
To provide effective treatment for the patient undergoing coronary angiography

## Collaborative level
Dependent

## Expected patient outcomes
▶ The patient will maintain hemodynamic status.
▶ The patient will maintain adequate tissue perfusion.
▶ The patient will maintain adequate pulses in all extremities.

## Definition of terms
▶ *Cardiac angiography:* An invasive procedure involving the instillation of radiopaque dye into the coronary arteries to visualize and evaluate blockages within the coronary arteries. Also used to evaluate wall motion, valvular function, and pressures within the heart's chambers.

▶ *Percutaneous transluminal coronary angioplasty:* An invasive procedure in which the cardiologist places a balloon-tipped catheter within a blocked coronary artery and inflates it, causing the artery to open by pressing the plaque against the arterial walls. Also known as PTCA, percutaneous coronary intervention, and balloon angioplasty.

▶ *Coronary stent:* A meshlike metal tube placed at the site of the newly opened arterial blockage and expanded to maintain a patent coronary artery. The stent eventually becomes part of the artery wall. Newer stents may be coated with heparin or certain medications and may help to maintain the patency of the artery for longer periods than uncoated stents. A stented coronary artery will stay patent longer than an artery that has been opened by balloon angioplasty only.

## Indications
Treatment
▶ Acute myocardial infarction
▶ Valvular disease
▶ Unstable angina
▶ Cardiogenic shock

Prevention
▶ Acute coronary artery closure
▶ Bleeding from arterial insertion site
▶ Cardiac arrest
▶ Acute coronary artery rupture
▶ Cardiac tamponade
▶ Stroke
▶ Ventricular tachycardia
▶ Anaphylactic reaction from radiopaque dye

## Assessment guidance
Signs and symptoms
*Preprocedure*
▶ Chest, shoulder, neck, or arm pain or pressure
▶ Nausea or vomiting
▶ Apprehension
▶ Palpitations
▶ Hypotension
▶ Hypertension
▶ Tachycardia
▶ Bradycardia
▶ Diaphoresis
▶ Arrhythmias
▶ Bleeding

### Postprocedure
- Chest pain or pressure
- Dizziness
- Feeling flushed
- Bleeding
- Apprehension
- Location and quality of peripheral pulses
- Color and temperature of extremity used for procedure
- Appearance of arterial insertion site: presence of bleeding or hematoma
- Normal ECG

### Diagnostic studies
#### Laboratory tests
- Preprocedure complete blood count (CBC)
- Serum chemistries and electrolyte level
- Magnesium and calcium levels
- Prothrombin time, partial thromboplastin time (PTT), and International Normalized Ratio (INR)
- Therapeutic drug levels
- Postprocedure CBC
- Electrolyte, blood urea nitrogen, creatinine levels
- CK-MB level
- Troponin level
- Stress test

#### Imaging tests
- Echocardiogram

#### Other
- ECG
- Stress test

## Nursing interventions
### Preprocedure
- Obtain preprocedure laboratory work on admission unless the patient has had preadmission testing performed; place in the patient's chart.
- Make sure consent for the procedure is signed, witnessed, and placed in the patient's chart.
- Complete the nursing assessment and obtain baseline vital signs.
- Assess and mark the dorsalis pedis and posterior tibial pulses bilaterally.
- Start a peripheral I.V. with normal saline or other I.V. solutions according to your facility's policy.
- Inform the doctor of any abnormal laboratory values and the patient's allergies,

especially if the patient is allergic to shellfish and iodine.
- Shave and prepare the patient's groin area according to your facility's policy.
- Administer preprocedure medications or sedation as ordered by the doctor.

### Postprocedure
- Check right groin sheath insertion site for bleeding, hematoma, or retroperitoneal bleeding. Modify instructions according to doctor's orders if an arterial closure device is used.
- Explain to the patient that he must lie flat while the arterial sheath is still in, and for 6 hours after sheath removal.
- Assess quality of distal pulses bilaterally along with the temperature of the extremities.
- Assess vital signs and distal pulses every 15 minutes for the first hour, every 30 minutes for 2 hours, and every hour for 4 hours postprocedure and sheath removal, or according to your facility's policy.
- Maintain I.V. fluids.
- If the patient experiences a vasovagal reaction, keep the I.V. fluids open and notify the doctor. If necessary, administer atropine if ordered by the doctor.
- Maintain cardiac monitoring.
- Obtain postprocedure laboratory work as ordered by the doctor or according to your facility's policy.
- Obtain an ECG as ordered.
- Assess the patient's oxygen saturation and administer supplemental oxygen if needed.
- Maintain adequate fluid intake to minimize the effect of the dye from the kidneys and explain to the patient why he must drink fluids postprocedure.
- If an arterial closure device such as a collagen plug is used, the head of the bed can be elevated to 30 degrees after 30 minutes, provided vital signs are stable and the insertion site is intact. If there's no bleeding from the site and vital signs are stable after 1 hour, the patient is allowed to ambulate.
- If the patient returns to the unit with heparin, maintain PTT and INR within therapeutic limits and watch for signs of bleeding from the sheath site and in the urine, stool, and gums.
- If the patient returns to the unit with a glycoprotein IIb or IIIa receptor-blocking

agent being infused, watch closely for signs of bleeding and assess platelet count.

## Patient teaching
▶ Be sure to cover these important points with the patient and his family:
- —risks of the procedure
- —what to expect during the procedure
- —what to expect after the procedure
- —the importance of informing the staff if the patient experiences any chest pain or bleeding from the insertion site
- —the fact that if the collagen plug is used, the patient may feel a small lump at the insertion site for 5 to 6 weeks
- —discharge teaching.

## Precautions
▶ Ensure informed consent is obtained before procedure.
▶ Monitor the patient closely for evidence of bleeding postprocedure, especially for signs of retroperitoneal bleeding.
▶ Monitor the patient closely for signs and symptoms of coronary artery occlusion: chest pain, ECG changes from baseline, hypotension. Notify the doctor immediately.
▶ Notify the doctor if the patient is allergic to iodine or shellfish.

## Documentation
▶ Document nursing assessment.
▶ Document the quality and character of distal pulses preprocedure and postprocedure.
▶ Document vital signs.
▶ Document the location of the I.V. catheter, gauge, time of insertion, and type of I.V. fluids ordered along with the rate.
▶ Document assessment of the insertion site, and any bleeding, hematoma, or retroperitoneal bleeding.
▶ Document discharge teaching.

## Related procedures
▶ Cardiac monitoring
▶ Cardiopulmonary resuscitation
▶ Electrocardiography
▶ Hand washing
▶ I.V. bolus injection
▶ Oral drugs
▶ Oxygen administration
▶ Percutaneous transluminal coronary angioplasty
▶ Peripheral I.V. line insertion
▶ Peripheral I.V. line maintenance
▶ Physical assessment
▶ Pulse and ear oximetry
▶ Venipuncture

## REFERENCES
Jaffe, R., et al. "Myocardial Perfusion Abnormalities Early (12-24 h) after Coronary Stenting or Balloon Angioplasty: Implications Regarding Pathophysiology and Late Clinical Outcome," *Cardiology* 98(1-2): 60-66, 2002.

Okayama, H., et al. "Usefulness of an Echo-contrast Agent for Assessment of Coronary Flow Velocity and Coronary Flow Velocity Reserve in the Left Anterior Descending Coronary Artery with Transthoracic Doppler Scan Echocardiography," *American Heart Journal* 143(4):668-75, April 2002.

## ORGANIZATIONS
American College of Cardiology: *www.acc.org*
American Heart Association:
    *www.americanheart.org*

# Managing the patient with decreased cardiac output

## Purpose
To provide effective treatment to prevent or minimize the complications of a decreased cardiac output

## Collaborative level
Dependent

## Expected patient outcomes
▶ The patient will maintain hemodynamic stability.
▶ The patient will maintain or improve his activity tolerance.
▶ The patient will maintain or improve his tolerance of activities of daily living.

## Definition of terms
▶ *Cardiac output:* The amount of blood pumped by the heart per minute. The factors that affect cardiac output are: afterload, preload, contractility, and heart rate.
▶ *Stroke volume:* The amount of blood ejected from the heart with each heartbeat.
▶ *Afterload:* The amount of resistance the ventricles must work against to pump the blood into circulation.

▶ *Preload:* The amount of volume in the ventricle at end-diastole.
▶ *Contractility:* The heart's ability to stretch and contract. Damaged heart muscle can't contract, thus decreasing cardiac output.

## Indications
Treatment
▶ Heart failure
▶ Acute myocardial infarction
▶ Arrhythmias
▶ Cardiogenic shock
▶ Cardiomyopathy

Prevention
▶ Pulmonary edema
▶ Cardiogenic shock
▶ Renal failure
▶ Respiratory failure

## Assessment guidance
Sign and symptoms
▶ Coughing
▶ Shortness of breath
▶ Dizziness
▶ Fatigue
▶ Weakness
▶ Sudden weight gain
▶ Edema of the ankles and legs
▶ Venous distention
▶ Bibasilar crackles
▶ Rhonchi
▶ Dyspnea, exertional or at rest
▶ Tachycardia
▶ Hypotension
▶ Diaphoresis
▶ Activity intolerance
▶ Confusion
▶ Nausea
▶ Decreased urine output
▶ $S_3$ and $S_4$
▶ Ascites

Diagnostic studies
*Laboratory tests*
▶ Serum chemistries
▶ Complete blood count
▶ CK-MB
▶ Troponin level
▶ Magnesium level
▶ Electrolyte levels
▶ Calcium level
▶ Arterial blood gas values
▶ B-type natriuretic peptide

*Imaging tests*
▶ Echocardiogram
▶ Cardiac catheterization
▶ Chest X-ray

*Other*
▶ ECG

## Nursing interventions
▶ Nursing interventions should address improving the patient's cardiac output, preload, afterload, and contractility. Inotropic drugs should increase contractility and cardiac output.
▶ Administer oxygen as needed and elevate the head of the bed as tolerated. Be prepared to assist in endotracheal intubation if needed.
▶ Administer diuretics and morphine to decrease pulmonary edema. Monitor the patient's urine output, potassium, and sodium levels.
▶ Place the patient on a cardiac monitor.
▶ If pulmonary artery catheter is placed, obtain cardiac output and hemodynamic pressures upon placement, after changes in the medication regimen, and as per your facility's policy.
▶ Monitor the patient's vital signs. Also perform a respiratory, cardiovascular, and neurologic assessment as needed.
▶ Insert an indwelling urinary catheter to accurately measure the patient's urine output.
▶ If needed, assist in the insertion of an intra-aortic balloon pump (IABP) to help stabilize the patient's vital signs and to decrease afterload.
▶ Administer nitrates as ordered to decrease afterload.
▶ Administer nesiritide as ordered to facilitate diuresis.
▶ Monitor the patient's oxygen saturation.

## Patient teaching
▶ Educate the patient and his family about the medication regimen.
▶ Instruct the patient to check his radial pulse and his weight daily.
▶ Instruct the patient to notify the doctor if he experiences increasing shortness of breath, sudden weight gain, increasing fatigue and activity intolerance, or increased swelling of the feet and ankles.
▶ Instruct the patient and his family on any dietary restrictions and fluid intake restric-

tions. Have the dietitian talk with the patient about dietary changes.

## Precautions

▶ Monitor the patient's serum electrolytes, magnesium, daily weight, and urine output when administering diuretics.

▶ Monitor hourly urine output. If urine output falls below 30 ml per hour, notify the doctor.

▶ If a pulmonary artery catheter is inserted, don't infuse I.V. medications or blood through the balloon port or the pulmonary artery port.

▶ Monitor pulmonary artery waveform to check catheter placement. If the catheter floats into the right ventricle, notify the doctor and monitor the patient for arrhythmias.

▶ Monitor the pulmonary artery wedge pressure waveform. If the waveform flattens out while the balloon is deflated, notify the doctor immediately. The balloon could have floated in the pulmonary artery; if it isn't pulled back, there could be a lack of blood flow to the pulmonary artery.

▶ Make sure the balloon on the pulmonary artery catheter is deflated at all times.

## Contraindications

Contraindicated in patients with aortic insufficiency, severe peripheral vascular disease, aortic aneurysm, or blood coagulopathy.

## Documentation

▶ Document the patient's response to medications.

▶ Document the pulmonary artery catheter insertion and the location and condition of the insertion site.

▶ Record pulmonary artery pressures according to facility policy.

▶ Document discharge teaching.

▶ Document physical assessment, including peripheral pulses and the presence of edema.

## Related procedures

▶ Arterial pressure monitoring
▶ Arterial puncture for blood gas analysis
▶ Cardiac monitoring
▶ Cardiac output monitoring
▶ Central venous pressure monitoring
▶ Electrocardiography
▶ Endotracheal intubation
▶ Hand washing
▶ I.V. bolus injection
▶ Indwelling catheter care and removal
▶ Indwelling catheter insertion
▶ Intra-aortic balloon counterpulsation
▶ Mechanical ventilation
▶ Medication therapy
▶ Nasogastric tube insertion and removal
▶ Oral drugs
▶ Oxygen administration
▶ Peripheral I.V. line insertion
▶ Peripheral I.V. line maintenance
▶ Physical assessment
▶ Pulse and ear oximetry
▶ Standard precautions

## REFERENCES

Carelock, J., and Clark, A. "Heart Failure: Pathophysiologic Mechanisms," *AJN* 101(12):26-33, December 2001.

Holcomb, S.S. "Helping Your Patient Conquer Cardiogenic Shock," *Nursing* 31(9): 32CC1-32CC6, September 2002.

Melander, S.D. *Case Studies in Critical Care Nursing: A Guide for Application and Review,* 2nd ed. Philadelphia: W.B. Saunders Co., 2001.

## ORGANIZATIONS

American College of Cardiology: *www.acc.org*
American Heart Association: *www.americanheart.org*

# Managing the patient with ineffective myocardial perfusion

## Purpose

To prevent complications arising from ineffective myocardial perfusion

## Collaborative level

Dependent

## Expected patient outcomes

▶ The patient will maintain hemodynamic status.

▶ The patient will experience reduction in anginal pain.

▶ The patient will show improvement in activities of daily living.

## Definition of terms

▶ *Bundle branch block:* Slowing or blocking of an impulse as it travels through one of the bundle branches.
▶ *Ischemia:* Inadequate blood supply to a local area as a result of blood vessel blockage.
▶ *Zone of ischemia:* The outermost area of ischemia, which results from interrupted blood flow.
▶ *Infarction:* An area of tissue death after prolonged ischemia.

## Indications

Treatment
▶ Acute myocardial infarction (MI)

Prevention
▶ Cardiovascular collapse
▶ Respiratory failure
▶ Renal insufficiency and failure

## Assessment guidance

Signs and symptoms
▶ Chest pain or tightness or pressure
▶ Arm pain or tightness or pressure
▶ Jaw pain or tightness or pressure
▶ Shortness of breath
▶ Fatigue
▶ Weakness
▶ Dyspnea
▶ Hypotension
▶ Tachycardia
▶ Bradycardia
▶ Diaphoresis
▶ Nausea and vomiting
▶ Arrhythmias

Diagnostic studies
*Laboratory tests*
▶ Serum chemistries
▶ CK-MB level
▶ Troponin level
▶ Magnesium level
▶ Calcium level
▶ CBC
▶ Prothrombin time, partial thromboplastin time (PTT), and International Normalized Ratio (INR)

*Imaging tests*
▶ Chest X-ray
▶ Nuclear perfusion rest or stress test
▶ Echocardiogram
▶ Cardiac catheterization

*Other*
▶ Electrocardiogram (ECG)

## Nursing interventions

▶ If the patient can't be transported to a facility capable of cardiac catheterization or percutaneous transluminal coronary angioplasty (PTCA), consider fibrolytics.
▶ If the patient with persistent symptoms and ST-segment elevation on his ECG goes to a hospital with cardiac catheterization or PTCA capabilities, he should go directly to the catheterization laboratory.
▶ Place the patient on cardiac monitor.
▶ Administer oxygen and monitor oxygen saturation.
▶ Give aspirin, 160 to 325 mg, as soon as possible.
▶ Begin nitrate therapy and adjust to pain relief as long as blood pressure is stable.
▶ Give morphine for pain.
▶ Assist with intra-aortic balloon pump insertion if the patient has persistent pain or hypotension.
▶ Start heparin or low-molecular-weight heparin.
▶ Monitor the patient for reperfusion arrhythmias.
▶ Administer beta-adrenergic blockers to decrease heart rate and heart's workload.
▶ Reassure the patient and his family as needed and explain all procedures to them.
▶ Encourage the patient to get as much rest as possible.
▶ Give antiemetics if the patient has persistent vomiting. Vomiting is a common adverse effect of an inferior wall MI.
▶ Monitor the patient with an anterior wall MI for atrioventricular block.
▶ Monitor all patients for bradycardia and tachycardia.

## Patient teaching

▶ Instruct the patient about his medication regimen.
▶ Instruct the patient to monitor his radial pulse and blood pressure.
▶ Instruct the patient on the signs and symptoms of an MI and to call 911 should they occur.
▶ Explain all procedures to the patient and answer all questions to decrease the patient's anxiety.
▶ Perform discharge teaching.
▶ Encourage patient to participate in an outpatient cardiac rehabilitation program.

## Precautions

▶ Have resuscitation equipment available in case of life-threatening arrhythmias.
▶ If the patient is receiving heparin, monitor and maintain the PTT and INR within therapeutic range. It isn't necessary to obtain PTT and INR with low-molecular-weight heparin.
▶ Monitor the patient for bleeding if fibrinolytics were given.
▶ Maintain serum magnesium, calcium, and potassium levels. Administer supplemental doses as needed.
▶ Monitor the patient for an increase or return of chest pain and ST elevations on the cardiac monitor after PTCA.

## Contraindications

▶ Don't give fibrinolytics to patients with a history of stroke, ulcer disease, aortic aneurysm, uncontrolled hypertension, and coagulopathy.

## Documentation

▶ Document the location, type, quality, and duration of the patient's pain or other cardiac symptoms.
▶ Document the location of I.V. line insertions and medications infusing.
▶ Document the patient's cardiac rhythm.
▶ Document discharge teaching.

## Related procedures

▶ Arterial puncture for blood gas analysis
▶ Cardiac monitoring

▶ Cardiac output measurement
▶ Cardiopulmonary resuscitation
▶ Defibrillation
▶ Electrocardiography
▶ Endotracheal intubation
▶ I.V. bolus injection
▶ Intra-aortic balloon counterpulsation
▶ Mechanical ventilation
▶ Oral drugs
▶ Oxygen administration
▶ Percutaneous transluminal coronary angioplasty
▶ Peripheral I.V. line insertion
▶ Peripheral I.V. line maintenance
▶ Physical assessment
▶ Pulse and ear oximetry
▶ Temporary pacemaker insertion and care

### REFERENCES

Alspach, J. *Core Curriculum for Critical Care Nursing.* Philadelphia: W.B. Saunders Co., 1998.
Melander, S.D. *Case Studies in Critical Care Nursing: A Guide for Application and Review.* Philadelphia: W.B. Saunders Co., 2001.
Woods, S.L., et al. *Cardiac Nursing.* Philadelphia: Lippincott Williams & Wilkins, 1999.

### ORGANIZATIONS

American College of Cardiology: *www.aac.org*
American Heart Association: *www.americanheart.org*
American Association of Critical Care Nursing: *www.aacn.org*

# Procedures

# Arterial pressure monitoring

Direct arterial pressure monitoring permits continuous measurement of systolic, diastolic, and mean pressures and allows arterial blood sampling. Because direct measurement reflects systemic vascular resistance as well as blood flow, it's generally more accurate than indirect methods (such as palpation and auscultation of Korotkoff's, or audible pulse, sounds), which are based on blood flow.

Direct monitoring is indicated when highly accurate or frequent blood pressure measurements are required — for example, in patients with low cardiac output and high systemic vascular resistance. Also, it may be used for patients who are receiving titrated doses of vasoactive drugs or who need frequent blood sampling.

Indirect monitoring, which carries few associated risks, is commonly performed by applying pressure to an artery (such as by inflating a blood pressure cuff around the arm) to decrease blood flow. As pressure is released, flow resumes and can be palpated or auscultated. Korotkoff's sounds presumably result from a combination of blood flow and arterial wall vibrations; with reduced flow, these vibrations may be less pronounced.

## Equipment
*For catheter insertion*
Gloves • sterile gown • mask • protective eyewear • sterile gloves • 16G to 20G catheter (type and length depend on the insertion site, patient's size, and other anticipated uses of the line) • preassembled preparation kit (if available) • sterile drapes • sheet protector • prepared pressure transducer system • ordered local anesthetic • sutures • syringe and 21G to 25G 1" needle • I.V. pole • tubing and medication labels • site care kit (containing sterile dressing and hypoallergenic tape) • arm board and soft wrist restraint (for a femoral site, an ankle restraint) • optional: shaving kit (for femoral artery insertion)

*For blood sample collection*
If an open system is in place: gloves • gown • mask • sterile 4" × 4" gauze pads • protective eyewear • sheet protector • 5- or 10-ml syringe for discard sample • syringes of appropriate size and number for ordered laboratory tests • laboratory request forms and labels • needleless device (depending on your facility's policy) • specimen tubes
If a closed system is in place: gloves • gown • mask • protective eyewear • syringes of appropriate size and number for ordered laboratory tests • laboratory request forms and labels • alcohol pad • blood transfer unit • specimen tubes

*For arterial line tubing changes*
Gloves • gown • mask • protective eyewear • sheet protector • preassembled arterial pressure tubing with flush device and disposable pressure transducer • sterile gloves • 500-ml bag of I.V. flush solution (such as dextrose 5% in water or normal saline solution) • 500 or 1,000 units of heparin • syringe and 21G to 25G 1" needle • alcohol pad • medication label • pressure bag • site care kit • tubing labels

*For arterial catheter removal*
Gloves • mask • gown • protective eyewear • two sterile 4" × 4" gauze pads • sheet protector • sterile suture removal set • dressing • hypoallergenic tape

*For femoral line removal*
Additional sterile 4" × 4" gauze pads • small sandbag (which you may wrap in a towel or place in a pillowcase) • adhesive bandage

*For a catheter-tip culture*
Sterile scissors • sterile container

## Preparation of equipment
Before setting up and priming the monitoring system, wash your hands thoroughly. Maintain asepsis by wearing personal protective equipment throughout preparation.
When you've completed the equipment preparation, set the alarms on the bedside monitor according to your facility's policy.

## Implementation
▶ Explain the procedure to the patient and his family, including the purpose of arterial pressure monitoring and the anticipated duration of catheter placement. Make sure the patient signs a consent form. If he's unable to sign, ask a responsible family member to give written consent.
▶ Check the patient's history for an allergy or a hypersensitivity to iodine, heparin or the ordered local anesthetic.
▶ Maintain asepsis by wearing personal protective equipment throughout all procedures described below.
▶ Position the patient for easy access to the catheter insertion site. Place a sheet protector under the site.
▶ If the catheter will be inserted into the radial artery, perform Allen's test to assess collateral circulation in the hand.

### Inserting an arterial catheter
▶ Using a preassembled preparation kit, the doctor prepares and anesthetizes the insertion site. He covers the surrounding area with sterile drapes. The catheter is then inserted into the artery and attached to the fluid-filled pressure tubing.
▶ While the doctor holds the catheter in place, activate the fast-flush release to flush blood from the catheter. After each fast-flush operation, observe the drip chamber to verify that the continuous flush rate is as

desired. A waveform should appear on the bedside monitor.
▶ The doctor may suture the catheter in place, or you may secure it with hypoallergenic tape. Cover the insertion site with a dressing as specified by facility policy.
▶ Immobilize the insertion site. With a radial or brachial site, use an arm board and soft wrist restraint (if the patient's condition so requires). With a femoral site, assess the need for an ankle restraint and maintain the patient on bed rest, with the head of the bed raised no more than 15 to 30 degrees, to prevent the catheter from kinking. Level the zeroing stopcock of the transducer with the phlebostatic axis. Then zero the system to atmospheric pressure.
▶ Activate monitor alarms as appropriate.

### Obtaining a blood sample from an open system

▶ Assemble the equipment, taking care not to contaminate the dead-end cap, stopcock, and syringes. Turn off or temporarily silence the monitor alarms, depending on your facility's policy. (However, some facilities require that alarms be left on.)
▶ Locate the stopcock nearest the patient. Open a sterile 4″ × 4″ gauze pad. Remove the dead-end cap from the stopcock, and place it on the gauze pad.
▶ Insert the syringe for the discard sample into the stopcock. (This sample is discarded because it's diluted with flush solution.) Follow your facility's policy on how much discard blood to collect. In most cases, you'll withdraw 5 to 10 ml through a 5- or 10-ml syringe.
▶ Next, turn the stopcock off to the flush solution. Slowly retract the syringe to withdraw the discard sample. If you feel resistance, reposition the affected extremity and check the insertion site for obvious problems (such as catheter kinking). After correcting the problem, resume blood withdrawal. Then turn the stopcock halfway back to the open position to close the system in all directions.
▶ Remove the discard syringe, and dispose of the blood in the syringe, observing standard precautions.
▶ Place the syringe for the laboratory sample in the stopcock, turn the stopcock off to the flush solution, and slowly withdraw the required amount of blood. For each additional sample required, repeat this procedure. If the doctor has ordered coagulation

tests, obtain blood for this sample from the final syringe to prevent dilution from the flush device.
▶ After you've obtained blood for the final sample, turn the stopcock off to the syringe and remove the syringe. Activate the fast-flush release to clear the tubing. Then turn off the stopcock to the patient and repeat the fast flush to clear the stopcock port.
▶ Turn the stopcock off to the stopcock port, and replace the dead-end cap. Reactivate the monitor alarms. Attach the needleless device to the filled syringes and transfer the blood samples to the appropriate specimen tubes, labeling them according to facility policy. Send all samples to the laboratory with appropriate documentation.
▶ Check the monitor for return of the arterial waveform and pressure reading. (See *Understanding the arterial waveform,* page 242.)

### Obtaining a blood sample from a closed system

▶ Assemble the equipment, maintaining aseptic technique. Locate the closed-system reservoir and blood sampling site. Deactivate or temporarily silence monitor alarms. (However, some facilities require that alarms be left on.)
▶ Clean the sampling site with an alcohol pad.
▶ Holding the reservoir upright, grasp the flexures and slowly fill the reservoir with blood over 3 to 5 seconds (this blood serves as discard blood). If you feel resistance, reposition the affected extremity and check the catheter site for obvious problems (such as kinking). Then resume blood withdrawal.
▶ Turn the one-way valve off to the reservoir by turning the handle perpendicular to the tubing. Using a syringe with attached cannula, insert the cannula into the sampling site. (Make sure the plunger is depressed to the bottom of the syringe barrel.) Slowly fill the syringe. Then grasp the cannula near the sampling site, and remove the syringe and cannula as one unit. Repeat the procedure as needed to fill the required number of syringes. If the doctor has ordered coagulation tests, obtain blood for those tests from the final syringe to prevent dilution from the flush solution.
▶ After filling the syringes, turn the one-way valve to its original position, parallel to the tubing. Now smoothly and evenly

# Understanding the arterial waveform

Normal arterial blood pressure produces a characteristic waveform, representing ventricular systole and diastole. The waveform has five distinct components: the anacrotic limb, systolic peak, dicrotic limb, dicrotic notch, and end diastole.

The anacrotic limb marks the waveform's initial upstroke, which results as blood is rapidly ejected from the ventricle through the open aortic valve into the aorta. The rapid ejection causes a sharp rise in arterial pressure, which appears as the waveform's highest point. This is called the systolic peak.

As blood continues into the peripheral vessels, arterial pressure falls, and the waveform begins a downward trend. This part is called the dicrotic limb. Arterial pressure usually continues to fall until pressure in the ventricle is less than pressure in the aortic root. When this occurs, the aortic valve closes. This event appears as a small notch (the dicrotic notch) on the waveform's downside. When the aortic valve closes, diastole begins, progressing until the aortic root pressure gradually descends to its lowest point. On the waveform, this is known as end diastole.

NORMAL ARTERIAL WAVEFORM

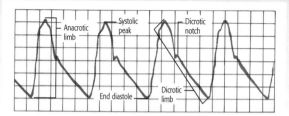

push down on the plunger until the flexures lock in place in the fully closed position and all fluid has been reinfused. The fluid should be reinfused over a 3- to 5-second period. Then activate the fast-flush release to clear blood from the tubing and reservoir.

▶ Clean the sampling site with an alcohol pad. Reactivate the monitor alarms. Using the blood transfer unit, transfer blood samples to the appropriate specimen tubes, labeling them according to facility policy. Send all samples to the laboratory with appropriate documentation.

## Changing arterial line tubing

▶ Wash your hands and follow standard precautions. Assemble the new pressure monitoring system.

▶ Consult your facility's policy and procedure manual to determine how much tubing length to change.

▶ Inflate the pressure bag to 300 mm Hg and check for air leaks. Then release the pressure.

▶ Prepare the I.V. flush solution, and prime the pressure tubing and transducer system checking for air in the tubing and the transducer. At this time, add medication and tubing labels. Apply 300 mm Hg of pressure to the system. Then hang the I.V. bag on a pole.

▶ Place the sheet protector under the affected extremity. Remove the dressing from the catheter insertion site, taking care not to dislodge the catheter or cause vessel trauma. Turn off or temporarily silence the monitor alarms. (However, some facilities require that alarms be left on.)

▶ Turn off the flow clamp of the tubing segment that you'll change. Disconnect the tubing from the catheter hub, taking care not to dislodge the catheter. Immediately insert new tubing into the catheter hub. Secure the tubing and then activate the fast-flush release to clear it.

▶ Reactivate the monitor alarms. Apply an appropriate dressing.

▶ Level the zeroing stopcock of the transducer with the phlebostatic axis, and zero the system to atmospheric pressure.

## Removing an arterial line

▶ Consult facility policy to determine whether you're permitted to perform this procedure.

▶ Explain the procedure to the patient.

▶ Assemble all equipment. Wash your hands. Observe standard precautions, including wearing personal protective equipment, for this procedure.

▶ Record the patient's systolic, diastolic, and mean blood pressures. If a manual, indirect blood pressure hasn't been assessed recently, obtain one now to establish a new baseline.

▶ Turn off the monitor alarms. Then turn off the flow clamp to the flush solution. Deflate the pressure bag.

▶ Carefully remove the dressing over the insertion site. Remove any sutures using the suture removal kit and then carefully check that all sutures have been removed.

▶ Withdraw the catheter using a gentle, steady motion. Keep the catheter parallel to the artery during withdrawal to reduce the risk of traumatic injury.

▶ Immediately after withdrawing the catheter, apply pressure to the site with a sterile 4″ × 4″ gauze pad. Maintain pressure for at least 10 minutes (longer if bleeding or oozing persists). Apply additional pressure to a femoral site or if the patient has coagulopathy or is receiving anticoagulants.

▶ Cover the site with an appropriate dressing and secure the dressing with tape. If stipulated by facility policy, make a pressure dressing for a femoral site by folding in half four sterile 4″ × 4″ gauze pads, and apply the dressing. Cover the dressing with a tight adhesive bandage; then cover the bandage with a sandbag. Maintain the patient on bed rest for 6 hours with the sandbag in place.

▶ If the doctor has ordered a culture of the catheter tip (to diagnose a suspected infection), gently place the catheter tip on a 4″ × 4″ sterile gauze pad. When the bleeding is under control, hold the catheter over the sterile container. Using sterile scissors, cut the tip so it falls into the sterile container. Label the specimen and send it to the laboratory.

▶ Observe the site for bleeding. Assess circulation in the extremity distal to the site by evaluating color, pulses, and sensation. Repeat this assessment every 15 minutes for the first 4 hours, every 30 minutes for the next 2 hours, then hourly for the next 6 hours.

## Special considerations

▶ Observing the pressure waveform on the monitor can enhance assessment of arterial pressure. An abnormal waveform may reflect an arrhythmia (such as atrial fibrillation) or other cardiovascular problems, such as aortic stenosis, aortic insufficiency, pulsus alternans, or pulsus paradoxus. (See *Recognizing abnormal waveforms,* page 244.)

▶ Change the pressure tubing every 2 to 3 days, according to facility policy. Change the dressing at the catheter site at intervals specified by facility policy. Regularly assess the site for signs of infection, such as redness and swelling. Notify the doctor immediately if you note any such signs.

▶ Be aware that erroneous pressure readings may result from a catheter that is clotted or positional, loose connections, an addition of extra stopcocks or extension tubing, inadvertent entry of air into the system, or improper calibration, leveling, or zeroing of the monitoring system. If the catheter lumen clots, the flush system may be improperly pressurized. Regularly assess the amount of flush solution in the I.V. bag and maintain 300 mm Hg of pressure in the pressure bag.

## Complications

Direct arterial pressure monitoring can cause such complications as arterial bleeding, infection, air embolism, arterial spasm, or thrombosis.

## Documentation

▶ Document the date of system setup so that all caregivers will know when to change the components.

▶ Document systolic, diastolic, and mean pressure readings as well.

▶ Record circulation in the extremity distal to the site by assessing color, pulses, and sensation.

▶ Carefully document the amount of flush solution infused to avoid hypervolemia and volume overload, and to ensure accurate assessment of the patient's fluid status.

▶ Make sure the position of the patient is documented when each blood pressure reading is obtained. This is important for determining trends.

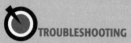

TROUBLESHOOTING

# Recognizing abnormal waveforms

Understanding a normal arterial waveform is relatively straightforward. An abnormal waveform, however, is more difficult to decipher. Abnormal patterns and markings may provide important diagnostic clues to the patient's cardiovascular status, or they may simply signal trouble in the monitor. Use this chart to help you recognize and resolve waveform abnormalities.

| Abnormality | Possible causes | Nursing interventions |
| --- | --- | --- |
| Alternating high and low waves in a regular pattern | Ventricular bigeminy | ▶ Check the patient's electrocardiogram to confirm ventricular bigeminy. The tracing should reflect premature ventricular contractions every second beat. |
| Flattened waveform | Overdamped waveform or hypotensive patient | ▶ Check the patient's blood pressure with a sphygmomanometer. If you obtain a higher reading, suspect overdamping. Correct the problem by trying to aspirate the arterial line and check the pressure on the bag and the patency of the tubing. If you succeed, flush the line and check the pressure on the bag and the patency of the tubing. If the reading is very low or absent, suspect hypotension. |
| Slightly rounded waveform with consistent variations in systolic height | Patient on ventilator with positive end-expiratory pressure | ▶ Check the patient's systolic blood pressure regularly. The difference between the highest and lowest systolic pressure reading should be less than 10 mm Hg. If the difference exceeds that amount, suspect pulsus paradoxus, possibly from cardiac tamponade. |
| Slow upstroke | Aortic stenosis | ▶ Check the patient's heart sounds for signs of aortic stenosis. Also notify the doctor, who will document suspected aortic stenosis in his notes. |
| Diminished amplitude on inspiration | Pulsus paradoxus, possibly from cardiac tamponade, constrictive pericarditis, or lung disease | ▶ Note systolic pressure during inspiration and expiration. If inspiratory pressure is at least 10 mm Hg less than expiratory pressure, call the doctor.<br>▶ If you're also monitoring pulmonary artery pressure, observe for a diastolic plateau. This occurs when the mean central venous pressure (right atrial pressure), mean pulmonary artery pressure, and mean pulmonary artery wedge pressure are within 5 mm Hg of one another. |

**REFERENCES**

Imperial-Perez, F., and McRae, M. "Protocols for Practice: Applying Research at the Bedside. Arterial Pressure Monitoring," *Critical Care Nurse* 19(2):105-107, April 1999.

Kaye, J, et al. "Patency of Radial Arterial Catheters," *American Journal of Critical Care* 10(2):104-11, March 2001.

Keeling, A.W., et al. "Reducing Time in Bed After Cardiac Catheterization (TIBS II),"

*American Journal of Critical Care* 5(4): 277-81, July 1996.

Keeling, A.W., et al. "Reducing Time in Bed After Percutaneous Transluminal Coronary Angioplasty (TIBS III)," *American Journal of Critical Care* 9(3):185-87, May 2000.

Lynn-McHale, D.J., and Carlson, K.K. *AACN Procedure Manual for Critical Care,* 4th ed. Philadelphia: W.B. Saunders Co., 2001.

Rice, W.P., et al. "A Comparison of Hydrostatic Leveling Methods in Invasive Pressure Monitoring," *Critical Care Nurse* 20(6):21-30, December 2000.

# Automated external defibrillation

Automated external defibrillators (AEDs) are commonly used today to meet the need for early defibrillation, which is currently considered the most effective treatment for ventricular fibrillation. Some facilities now require an AED in every noncritical care unit. Their use is also becoming common in such public places as shopping malls, sports stadiums, and airplanes. Instruction in using the AED is already required as part of Basic Life Support (BLS) and Advanced Cardiac Life Support (ACLS) training.

AEDs are being used increasingly to provide early defibrillation—even when no health care provider is present. The AED interprets the victim's cardiac rhythm and gives the operator step-by-step directions on how to proceed if defibrillation is indicated. Most AEDs have a "quick-look" feature that allows visualization of the rhythm with the paddles before electrodes are connected.

The AED is equipped with a microcomputer that senses and analyzes a patient's heart rhythm at the push of a button. Then it audibly or visually prompts you to deliver a shock. AED models all have the same basic function but offer different operating options. For example, all AEDs communicate directions through messages on a display screen, give voice commands, or do both. Some AEDs simultaneously display a patient's heart rhythm.

All devices record your interactions with the patient during defibrillation, either on a cassette tape or in a solid-state memory module. Some AEDs have an integral printer for immediate event documentation. Fa-cility policy determines who is responsible for reviewing all AED interactions; the patient's doctor always has that option. Local and state regulations govern who is responsible for collecting AED case data for reporting purposes.

**■ EVIDENCE BASE** Studies have shown that established Public Access Defibrillation programs (laypersons who are trained to use an AED) have a survival rate as high as 49%, twice the rate reported in the most effective EMS programs.

## Equipment

AED • two prepackaged electrodes

## Implementation

▶ After discovering that your patient is unresponsive to your questions, pulseless, and apneic, follow BLS and ACLS protocols. Then ask a colleague to bring the AED into the patient's room and set it up before the code team arrives.

▶ Open the foil packets containing the two electrode pads. Attach the white electrode cable connector to one pad and the red electrode cable connector to the other. The electrode pads aren't site specific.

▶ Expose the patient's chest. Remove the plastic backing film from the electrode pads, and place the electrode pad attached to the white cable connector on the right upper portion of the patient's chest, just beneath his clavicle.

▶ Place the pad attached to the red cable connector to the left of the heart's apex. To help remember where to place the pads, think "white, right; red, ribs." (Placement for both electrode pads is the same as for manual defibrillation or cardioversion.)

▶ Firmly press the device's on button, and wait while the machine performs a brief self-test. Most AEDs signal their readiness by a computerized voice that says "Stand clear" or by emitting a series of loud beeps. (If the AED isn't functioning properly, it will convey the message "Don't use the AED. Remove and continue CPR.") Remember to report any AED malfunctions in accordance with your facility's procedure.

▶ Now the machine is ready to analyze the patient's heart rhythm. Ask everyone to stand clear and press the analyze button when prompted by the machine. Be careful not to touch or move the patient while the AED is in analysis mode. (If you get the message "Check electrodes," make sure the electrodes are correctly placed and the patient cable is securely attached; then press the analyze button again.)

▶ In 15 to 30 seconds, the AED will analyze the patient's rhythm. When the patient needs a shock, the AED will display a "Stand clear" message and emit a beep that changes into a steady tone as it's charging.

▶ When an AED is fully charged and ready to deliver a shock, it will prompt you to press the shock button. (Some fully automatic AED models automatically deliver a shock within 15 seconds after analyzing the patient's rhythm. If a shock isn't needed, the AED will display "No shock indicated" and prompt you to "Check patient.")

▶ Make sure that no one is touching the patient or his bed and call out "Stand clear." Then press the shock button on the AED. Most AEDs are ready to deliver a shock within 15 seconds.

▶ After the first shock, the AED will automatically reanalyze the patient's heart rhythm. If no additional shock is needed, the machine will prompt you to check the patient. However, if the patient is still in ventricular fibrillation, the AED will automatically begin recharging at a higher joule level to prepare for a second shock. Repeat the steps you performed before delivering a shock to the patient. According to the AED algorithm, the patient can receive up to three shocks at increasing joule levels (200, 200 to 300, and 360 joules).

▶ If the patient is still in ventricular fibrillation after three shocks, resume CPR for 1 minute. Then press the analyze button on the AED to identify the heart rhythm. If the patient is still in ventricular fibrillation, continue the algorithm sequence until the code team leader arrives.

### Special considerations
▶ Defibrillators vary from one manufacturer to the next, so be sure to familiarize yourself with your facility's equipment.
▶ Defibrillator operation should be checked at least every 8 hours and after each use.

### Complications
Defibrillation can cause accidental electric shock to those providing care. Using an in-

sufficient amount of conduction medium can lead to skin burns.

### Documentation
▶ After the code, remove and transcribe the AED's computer memory module or tape, or prompt the AED to print a rhythm strip with code data.
▶ Follow your facility's policy for analyzing and storing code data. Be sure to document the code on the appropriate form.

### REFERENCES
American Heart Association (2000). "Guidelines 2000 for Cardiopulmonary Resuscitation and Emergency Cardiovascular Care: International Consensus on Science," *Circulation* 102(8 Suppl):I-384, August 2000.
Begany, T. "Major Changes Made to ACLS Guidelines," *Pulmonary Reviews* 5(11), November 2000. *www.pulmonaryreviews. com/archives.html.*
Mancini, M.E., and Kaye, W. "In-hospital First-Responder Automated External Defibrillation: What Critical Care Practitioners Need to Know," *American Journal of Critical Care* 7(4):314-19, July 1998.
*Mastering ACLS.* Springhouse, Pa.: Springhouse Corp., 2002.
Riegel, B. "Training Nontraditional Responders to Use Automated External Defibrillators," *American Journal of Critical Care* 7(6):402-10, November 1998.
Robinson, R. "Automated External Defibrillation—Basic." 2001. *www.emcert.com/ tour-courses.asp*

# Cardiac monitoring

Because it allows continuous observation of the heart's electrical activity, cardiac monitoring is used in patients with conduction disturbances and in those at risk for life-threatening arrhythmias. Like other forms of electrocardiography (ECG), cardiac monitoring uses electrodes placed on the patient's chest to transmit electrical signals that are converted into a tracing of cardiac rhythm on an oscilloscope.

Two types of monitoring may be performed: hardwire or telemetry. In hardwire monitoring, the patient is connected to a monitor at the bedside. The rhythm display appears at bedside, but it may also be transmitted to a console at a remote location. Telemetry uses a small transmitter connected to the ambulatory patient to send electrical signals to another location where they're displayed on a monitor screen. Battery-powered and portable, telemetry frees the patient from cumbersome wires and cables and lets him be comfortably mobile and safely isolated from the electrical leakage and accidental shock occasionally associated with hardwire monitoring. Telemetry is especially useful for monitoring arrhythmias that occur during sleep, rest, exercise, or stressful situations. However, unlike hardwire monitoring, telemetry can monitor only heart rate and rhythm.

Regardless of the type, cardiac monitors can display the patient's heart rate and rhythm, produce a printed record of cardiac rhythm, and sound an alarm if the heart rate exceeds or falls below specified limits. Monitors also recognize and count abnormal heartbeats as well as changes. For example, ST-segment monitoring, helps detect myocardial ischemia, electrolyte imbalance, coronary artery spasm, and hypoxic events. The ST segment represents early ventricular repolarization, and any changes in this waveform component reflect alterations in myocardial oxygenation. Any monitoring lead that views an ischemic heart region will reveal ST-segment changes. The monitor's software establishes a template of the patient's normal QRST pattern from the selected leads; then the monitor displays ST-segment changes. Some monitors display such changes continuously, others only on command.

## Equipment

Cardiac monitor • leadwires • patient cable • disposable pregelled electrodes (number of electrodes varies from three to five, depending on patient's needs) • alcohol pads • 4″ × 4″ gauze pads • washcloth • optional: shaving supplies

*For telemetry*
Transmitter • transmitter pouch • telemetry battery pack, leads, and electrodes

### Preparation of equipment
Plug the cardiac monitor into an electrical outlet and turn it on to warm up the unit while you prepare the equipment and the patient. Insert the cable into the appropriate socket in the monitor. Connect the lead-

wires to the cable. In some systems, the leadwires are permanently secured to the cable. Each leadwire should indicate the location for attachment to the patient: right arm (RA), left arm (LA), right leg (RL), left leg (LL), and ground (C or V). This should appear on the leadwire—if it's permanently connected—or at the connection of the leadwires and cable to the patient. Then connect an electrode to each of the leadwires, carefully checking that each leadwire is in its correct outlet.

For telemetry monitoring, insert a new battery into the transmitter. Be sure to match the poles on the battery with the polar markings on the transmitter case. By pressing the button at the top of the unit, test the battery charge and test the unit to ensure that the battery is operational. If the leadwires aren't permanently affixed to the telemetry unit, attach them securely. If they must be attached individually, be sure to connect each one to the correct outlet.

## Implementation
▶ Explain the procedure to the patient, provide privacy, and ask the patient to expose his chest. Wash your hands.
▶ Determine electrode positions on the patient's chest, based on which system and lead you're using. (See *Positioning monitoring leads,* pages 248 and 249.)
▶ If the leadwires and patient cable aren't permanently attached, verify that the electrode placement corresponds to the label on the patient cable.
▶ If necessary, shave an area about 4″ (10 cm) in diameter around each electrode site. Clean the area with an alcohol pad and dry it completely to remove skin secretions that may interfere with electrode function. Gently abrade the dried area by rubbing it briskly until it reddens to remove dead skin cells and to promote better electrical contact with living cells. (Some electrodes have a small, rough patch for abrading the skin; otherwise, use a dry washcloth or a dry gauze pad.)
▶ Remove the backing from the pregelled electrode. Check the gel for moistness. If the gel is dry, discard it and replace it with a fresh electrode.
▶ Apply the electrode to the site and press firmly to ensure a tight seal. Repeat with the remaining electrodes.

# Positioning monitoring leads

These illustrations show the correct electrode positions for some of the monitoring leads you'll use most often. For each lead, you'll see electrode placement for a five-leadwire system, a three-leadwire system, and a telemetry system.

In the two hardwire systems, the electrode positions for one lead may be identical to the electrode positions for another lead. In this case, you simply change the lead selector switch to the setting that corresponds to the lead you want. In some cases, you'll need to reposition the electrodes.

In the telemetry system, you can create the same lead with two electrodes that you do with three, simply by eliminating the ground electrode.

The illustrations below use these abbreviations: RA, right arm; LA, left arm; RL, right leg; LL, Left leg; C, chest; and G, Ground.

| Five-leadwire system | Three-leadwire system | Telemetry system |
| --- | --- | --- |

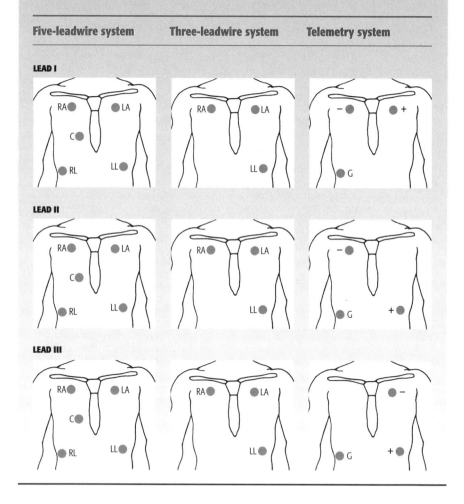

**LEAD I**

**LEAD II**

**LEAD III**

▶ When all the electrodes are in place, check for a tracing on the cardiac monitor. Assess the quality of the ECG. (See *Identifying cardiac monitor problems,* page 250.)

▶ To verify that each beat is being detected by the monitor, compare the digital heart rate display with your count of the patient's heart rate.

## Positioning monitoring leads *(continued)*

| Five-leadwire system | Three-leadwire system | Telemetry system |
| --- | --- | --- |

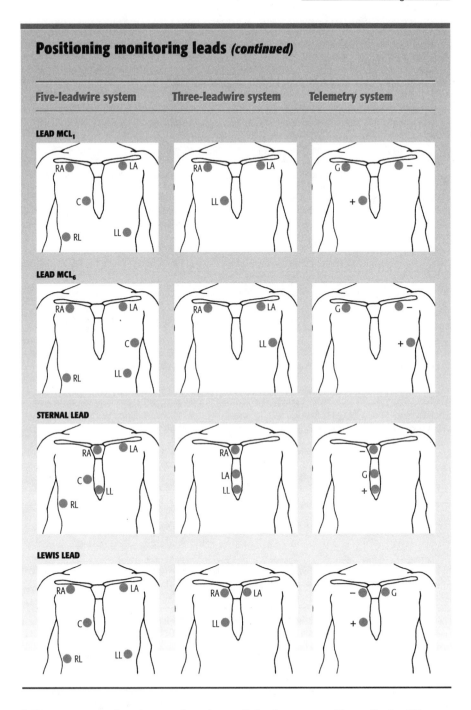

**LEAD MCL₁**

**LEAD MCL₆**

**STERNAL LEAD**

**LEWIS LEAD**

▶ If necessary, use the gain control to adjust the size of the rhythm tracing and use the position control to adjust the waveform position on the recording paper.

▶ Set the upper and lower limits of the heart rate alarm, based on unit policy. Turn the alarm on.

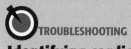

TROUBLESHOOTING

# Identifying cardiac monitor problems

| Problem | Possible causes | Solutions |
|---|---|---|
| False–high-rate alarm | ▶ Monitor interpreting large T waves as QRS complexes, which doubles the rate<br>▶ Skeletal muscle activity | ▶ Reposition electrodes to lead where QRS complexes are taller than T waves.<br>▶ Place electrodes away from major muscle masses. |
| False–low-rate alarm | ▶ Shift in electrical axis from patient movement, making QRS complexes too small to register<br>▶ Low amplitude of QRS<br>▶ Poor contact between electrode and skin | ▶ Reapply electrodes. Set gain so height of complex is greater than 1 millivolt.<br>▶ Increase gain.<br>▶ Reapply electrodes. |
| Low amplitude | ▶ Gain dial set too low<br>▶ Poor contact between skin and electrodes; dried gel; broken or loose leadwires; poor connection between the patient and monitor; malfunctioning monitor; physiologic loss of QRS amplitude | ▶ Increase gain.<br>▶ Check connections on all leadwires and monitoring cable. Replace electrodes as necessary. Reapply electrodes if required. |
| Wandering baseline | ▶ Poor position or contact between electrodes and skin<br>▶ Thoracic movement with respirations | ▶ Reposition or replace electrodes.<br>▶ Reposition electrodes. |
| Artifact (waveform interference) | ▶ Patient having seizures, chills, or anxiety<br><br>▶ Patient movement<br>▶ Electrodes applied improperly<br>▶ Static electricity<br><br>▶ Electrical short circuit in leadwires or cable<br><br>▶ Interference from decreased room humidity | ▶ Notify the doctor and treat the patient as ordered. Keep the patient warm and reassure him.<br>▶ Help the patient relax.<br>▶ Check electrodes and reapply if necessary.<br>▶ Make sure cables don't have exposed connectors. Change static-causing linens.<br>▶ Replace broken equipment. Use stress loops when applying leadwires.<br>▶ Regulate humidity to 40%. |
| Broken leadwires or cable | ▶ Stress loops not used on leadwires<br><br>▶ Cables and leadwires cleaned with alcohol or acetone, causing brittleness | ▶ Replace leadwires and retape them, using stress loops.<br>▶ Clean cable and leadwires with soapy water. Don't allow cable ends to become wet. Replace cable as needed. |
| 60-cycle interference (fuzzy baseline) | ▶ Electrical interference from other equipment in room<br><br>▶ Patient's bed improperly grounded | ▶ Attach all electrical equipment to common ground. Check plugs to make sure prongs aren't loose.<br>▶ Attach bed ground to the room's common ground. |
| Skin excoriation under electrode | ▶ Patient allergic to electrode adhesive<br><br>▶ Electrode on skin too long | ▶ Remove electrodes and apply hypoallergenic electrodes and hypoallergenic tape.<br>▶ Remove electrode, clean site, and reapply electrode at new site. |

## For telemetry monitoring

▶ Wash your hands. Explain the procedure to the patient and provide privacy.

▶ Expose the patient's chest, and select the lead arrangement. Remove the backing from one of the gelled electrodes. Check the gel for moistness. If it's dry, discard the electrode and obtain a new one.

▶ Apply the electrode to the appropriate site by pressing one side of the electrode against the patient's skin, pulling gently, and then pressing the other side against the skin. Press your fingers in a circular motion around the electrode to fix the gel and stabilize the electrode. Repeat for each electrode.

▶ Attach an electrode to the end of each leadwire.

▶ Place the transmitter in the pouch. Tie the pouch strings around the patient's neck and waist, making sure that the pouch fits snugly without causing him discomfort. If no pouch is available, place the transmitter in the patient's bathrobe pocket.

▶ Check the patient's waveform for clarity, position, and size. Adjust the gain and baseline as needed. (If necessary, ask the patient to remain resting or sitting in his room while you locate his telemetry monitor at the central station.)

▶ To obtain a rhythm strip, press the record key at the central station. Label the strip with the patient's name and room number, date, and time. Also, identify the rhythm. Place the rhythm strip in the appropriate location in the patient's chart.

## Special considerations

▶ Make sure that all electrical equipment and outlets are grounded to avoid electric shock and interference (artifacts). Also, ensure that the patient is clean and dry to prevent electric shock.

▶ Avoid opening the electrode packages until just before using to prevent the gel from drying out.

▶ Avoid placing the electrodes on bony prominences, hairy locations, areas where defibrillator pads will be placed, or areas for chest compression.

▶ If the patient's skin is very oily, scaly, or diaphoretic, rub the electrode site with a dry 4″ × 4″ gauze pad before applying the electrode to help reduce interference in the tracing. Have the patient breathe normally during the procedure. If his respirations distort the recording, ask him to hold his breath briefly to reduce baseline wander in the tracing.

▶ Assess skin integrity and reposition the electrodes every 24 hours or as necessary.

▶ If the patient is being monitored by telemetry, show him how the transmitter works. If applicable, show him the button that will produce a recording of his ECG at the central station. Teach him how to push the button whenever he has symptoms. This causes the central console to print a rhythm strip. Tell the patient to remove the transmitter if he takes a shower or bath, but stress that he should tell you before removing the unit.

## Documentation

▶ Record in your nurse's notes the date and time that monitoring begins and the monitoring lead used.

▶ Document a rhythm strip at least every 8 hours and with any changes in the patient's condition (or as stated by your facility's policy).

▶ Label the rhythm strip with the patient's name and room number, the date, and the time.

## REFERENCES

Bickwermert, M. "This Lead, That Lead, What Lead? Lead Placement: Basics Reviewed and Revisited." Presented at National Teaching Institute, American Association of Critical-Care Nurses, 1999.

Chambrin, M.C., et al. "Multicentric Study of Monitoring Alarms in the Adult Intensive Care Unit (ICU): A Descriptive Analysis," *Intensive Care Medicine* 25(12):1360-66, December 1999.

Lynn-McHale, D.J., and Carlson, K.K. *AACN Procedure Manual for Critical Care,* 4th ed. Philadelphia: W.B. Saunders Co., 2001.

Martin, N., and Hendrickson, P. "Telemetry Monitoring in Acute and Critical Care," *Critical Care Nursing Clinics of North America* 11(1):77-85, March 1999.

Schull, M.J., and Redelmeier, D.A. "Continuous Electrocardiographic Monitoring and Cardiac Arrest Outcomes in 8,932 Telemetry Ward Patients," *Academic Emergency Medicine* 7(6):647-52, June 2000.

# Cardiac output measurement

Cardiac output—the amount of blood ejected by the heart—helps evaluate cardiac function. The most widely used method of calculating this measurement is the bolus thermodilution technique. Performed at the patient's bedside, the thermodilution technique is the most practical method of evaluating the cardiac status of critically ill patients and those suspected of having cardiac disease. Other methods include the Fick method and the dye dilution test. (See *Other methods of measuring cardiac output.*)

To measure cardiac output, a quantity of solution colder than the patient's blood is injected into the right atrium via a port on a pulmonary artery (PA) catheter. This indicator solution mixes with the blood as it travels through the right ventricle into the pulmonary artery, and a thermistor on the catheter registers the change in temperature of the flowing blood. A computer then plots the temperature change over time as a curve and calculates flow based on the area under the curve.

Iced or room-temperature injectant may be used. The choice should be based on facility policy as well as the patient's status. The accuracy of the bolus thermodilution technique depends on the computer being able to differentiate the temperature change caused by the injectant in the pulmonary artery and the temperature changes in the pulmonary artery. Because iced injectant is colder than room-temperature injectant, it provides a stronger signal to be detected.

Typically, however, room-temperature injectant is more convenient and provides equally accurate measurements. Iced injectant may be more accurate in patients with high or low cardiac outputs, hypothermic patients, or when smaller volumes of injectant must be used (3 to 5 ml), as in patients with volume restrictions or in children.

## Equipment
*For the thermodilution method*
Thermodilution PA catheter in position • output computer and cables (or a module for the bedside cardiac monitor) • closed or open injectant delivery system • 10-ml syringe • 500-ml bag of dextrose 5% in water or normal saline solution • crushed ice and water (if iced injectant is used)

The newer bedside cardiac monitors measure cardiac output continuously, using either an invasive or a noninvasive method. If your bedside monitor doesn't have this capability, you'll need a free-standing cardiac output computer.

## Preparation of equipment
Wash your hands thoroughly, and assemble the equipment at the patient's bedside. Insert the closed injectant system tubing into the 500-ml bag of I.V. solution. Connect the 10-ml syringe to the system tubing and prime the tubing with I.V. solution until it's free of air. Then clamp the tubing. The steps that follow differ, depending on the temperature of the injectant.

### Room-temperature injectant closed delivery system
After clamping the tubing, connect the primed system to the stopcock of the proximal injectant lumen of the PA catheter. Next, connect the temperature probe from the cardiac output computer to the closed injectant system's flow-through housing device. Connect the cardiac output computer cable to the thermistor connector on the PA catheter and verify the blood temperature reading. Finally, turn on the cardiac output computer and enter the correct computation constant as provided by the catheter's manufacturer. The constant is determined by the volume and temperature of the injectant as well as the size and type of catheter.

◆ **ALERT!** For children, you'll need to adjust the computation constant to reflect a smaller volume and a smaller catheter size.

### Iced injectant closed delivery system
After clamping the tubing, place the coiled segment into the Styrofoam container and add crushed ice and water to cover the entire coil. Let the solution cool for 15 to 20 minutes. The rest of the steps are the same as those for the room-temperature injectant closed delivery system.

## Implementation
▶ Make sure your patient is in a comfortable position. Tell him not to move during the procedure because movement can cause an error in measurement.

# Other methods of measuring cardiac output

In the Fick method (especially useful in detecting low cardiac output [CO] levels), the blood's oxygen content is measured before and after it passes through the lungs. First, blood is removed from the pulmonary and the brachial arteries and analyzed for oxygen content. Then, a spirometer measures oxygen consumption – the amount of air entering the lungs each minute. Next, CO is calculated using this formula:

$$\text{CO (L/minute)} = \frac{\text{oxygen consumption (ml/minute)}}{\text{arterial oxygen content} - \text{venous oxygen content (ml/minute)}}$$

In the dye dilution test, a known volume and concentration of dye is injected into the pulmonary artery and measured by simultaneously sampling the amount of dye in the brachial artery. To calculate CO, these values are entered into a formula or plotted into a time and dilution-concentration curve. A computer, similar to the one used for the thermodilution test, performs the computation. Dye dilution measurements are particularly helpful in detecting intracardiac shunts and valvular insufficiency.

---

▶ Explain to the patient that the procedure will help determine how well his heart is pumping and that he'll feel no discomfort.

### For iced injectant closed delivery system
▶ Unclamp the I.V. tubing and withdraw 5 ml of solution into the syringe.

◆ **ALERT!** For children, use 3 ml or less.

▶ Inject the solution to flow past the temperature sensor, verifying that the injectant temperature registers between 43° and 54° F (6° and 12° C) on the computer.
▶ Verify the presence of a PA waveform on the cardiac monitor.
▶ Withdraw exactly 10 ml of cooled solution before reclamping the tubing.
▶ Turn the stopcock at the catheter injectant hub to open a fluid path between the injectant lumen of the PA catheter and syringe.
▶ Press the start button on the cardiac output computer or wait for the inject message to flash.
▶ Inject the solution smoothly within 4 seconds, making sure it doesn't leak at the connectors.
▶ If available, analyze the contour of the thermodilution washout curve on a strip chart recorder for a rapid upstroke and a gradual, smooth return to baseline.
▶ Wait 1 minute between injections and repeat the procedure until three values are within 10% and 15% of the median value. Compute the average and record the patient's cardiac output.

▶ Return the stopcock to its original position, and make sure the injectant delivery system tubing is clamped.
▶ Verify the presence of a PA waveform on the cardiac monitor.

### For room-temperature injectant closed delivery system
▶ Verify the presence of a PA waveform on the cardiac monitor.
▶ Unclamp the I.V. tubing and withdraw exactly 10 ml of solution. Reclamp the tubing.
▶ Turn the stopcock at the catheter injectant hub to open a fluid path between the injectant lumen of the PA catheter and the syringe.
▶ Press the start button on the cardiac output computer or wait for an inject message to flash.
▶ Inject the solution smoothly within 4 seconds, making sure it doesn't leak at the connectors.
▶ If available, analyze the contour of the thermodilution washout curve on a strip chart recorder for a rapid upstroke and a gradual, smooth return to the baseline.
▶ Repeat these steps until three values are within 10% and 15% of the median value. Compute the average and record the patient's cardiac output.
▶ Return the stopcock to its original position and make sure the injectant delivery system tubing is clamped.
▶ Verify the presence of a PA waveform on the cardiac monitor.

▶ Discontinue cardiac output measurements when the patient is hemodynamically stable and weaned from his vasoactive and inotropic medications. You can leave the PA catheter inserted for pressure measurements.

▶ Disconnect and discard the injectant delivery system and the I.V. bag. Cover any exposed stopcocks with air-occlusive caps.

▶ Monitor the patient for signs and symptoms of inadequate perfusion, including restlessness, fatigue, changes in level of consciousness, decreased capillary refill time, diminished peripheral pulses, oliguria, and pale, cool skin.

## Special considerations

▶ The normal range for cardiac output is 4 to 8 L/minute. The adequacy of a patient's cardiac output is better assessed by calculating his cardiac index (CI), adjusted for his body size.

▶ To calculate the patient's CI, divide his cardiac output by his body surface area (BSA), a function of height and weight. For example, a cardiac output of 4 L/minute might be adequate for a 65″, 120-lb (165-cm, 54-kg) patient (normally a BSA of 1.59 and a CI of 2.5) but would be inadequate for a 74″, 230-lb (188-cm, 104-kg) patient (normally a BSA of 2.26 and a CI of 1.8). The normal CI for adults ranges from 2.5 to 4.2 L/minute/m$^2$; for pregnant women, 3.5 to 6.5 L/minute/m$^2$.

**ALERT!** Normal CI for infants and children is 3.5 to 4 L/minute/m$^2$. Normal CI for elderly adults is 2 to 2.5 L/minute/m$^2$.

▶ Add the fluid volume injected for cardiac output determinations to the patient's total intake. Injectant delivery of 30 ml/hour will contribute 720 ml to the patient's 24-hour intake.

▶ After cardiac output measurement, make sure the clamp on the injectant bag is secured to prevent inadvertent delivery of the injectant to the patient.

**EVIDENCE BASE** There are limitations to the use of the thermodilution method. It can't be used in patients with large intracardiac shunts, in whom a PA catheter may pose a danger. Thermodilution is also contraindicated for patients with a ventricular septal defect because of improper mixing of the thermal indicator with blood, and also can't be used if a patient has tricuspid regurgitation due to blood regurgitation, prolonging the mixing time and movement of the thermal indicator. Due to these limitations, other noninvasive techniques, such as Doppler CO determination, are being developed. The Doppler method uses a transducer placed on the suprasternal notch and aims an ultrasound beam toward the aortic root to measure blood velocity. It's currently still in the evaluative phase, but if it's successful, it will greatly reduce the hazards of CO determination via an invasive line.

## Documentation

▶ Document your patient's cardiac output, CI, and other hemodynamic values and vital signs at the time of measurement.

▶ Note the patient's position during measurement and any other unusual occurrences, such as bradycardia or neurologic changes.

**REFERENCES**

Bridges, E.J. "Monitoring Pulmonary Artery Pressures: Just the Facts," *Critical Care Nurse* 20(6):59-80, December 2000.

Daily, E.K. "Hemodynamic Waveform Analysis," *Journal of Cardiovascular Nursing* 15(2):6-22, January 2001.

Druding, M.C. "Integrating Hemodynamic Monitoring and Physical Assessment," *Dimensions of Critical Care Nursing* 19(4):25-30, July-August 2000.

Keckeisen, M. "Monitoring Pulmonary Artery Pressure," *Critical Care Nurse* 19(6):88-91, December 1999.

Lynn-McHale, D.J., and Carlson, K.K. *AACN Procedure Manual for Critical Care,* 4th ed. Philadelphia: W.B. Saunders Co., 2001.

Ott, K., et al. "New Technologies in the Assessment of Hemodynamic Parameters," *Journal of Cardiovascular Nursing* 15(2):41-55, January 2001.

Quaal, S.J. "Improving the Accuracy of Pulmonary Artery Catheter Measurements," *Journal of Cardiovascular Nursing* 15(2):71-82, January 2001.

Rice, W.P., et al. "A Comparison of Hydrostatic Leveling Methods in Invasive Pressure Monitoring," *Critical Care Nurse* 20(6):20-30, December 2000.

# Cardiopulmonary resuscitation

Cardiopulmonary resuscitation (CPR) seeks to restore and maintain the patient's respiration and circulation after his heartbeat and breathing have stopped. CPR is a basic life support (BLS) procedure performed on victims of cardiac arrest. Another BLS procedure is clearing the obstructed airway.

Most adults in sudden cardiac arrest develop ventricular fibrillation and require defibrillation; CPR alone doesn't improve their chances of survival. Therefore, you must assess the victim and then contact emergency medical services (EMS) or call a code before starting CPR. Timing is critical. Early access to EMS, early CPR, and early defibrillation greatly improve the chances of survival. In most instances, you perform CPR to keep the patient alive until advanced cardiac life support can begin. Basic CPR procedure consists of assessing the victim, calling for help, and then following the ABC protocol: opening the Airway, restoring Breathing, then restoring Circulation. After the airway has been opened and breathing and circulation have been restored, drug therapy, diagnosis by electrocardiogram, or defibrillation may follow. CPR is contraindicated in "no code" patients.

**EVIDENCE BASE** Recent research has contributed to several changes in AHA guidelines for BLS.
▶ Rescuers should phone for help before initiating CPR (except for cases of near-drowning, trauma, or drug overdose). This is in contrast to previous guidelines, which called for 1 minute of CPR before calling for help. This is because it's known that rapid defibrillation is the victim's best chance for survival.
▶ Laryngeal mask airways and the esophageal-tracheal combitube have been added as alternate airway devices.
▶ The following rates have changed: compression rate for adult CPR is 100 per minute (instead of 80 per minute); the compression-ventilation ratio is 15 compressions to 2 ventilations (except when the victim is intubated).

▶ Lay rescuers will no longer be taught management of foreign-body airway obstruction.

## Equipment
CPR requires no special equipment except a hard surface on which to place the patient.

## Implementation
The following illustrated instructions provide a step-by-step guide for CPR as currently recommended by the American Heart Association (AHA).

### One-person rescue
▶ If you're the sole rescuer, expect to open the patient's airway, check for breathing, assess for circulation, and call for help before beginning compressions.
▶ Open the airway
▶ Assess the victim to determine if he's unconscious (as shown below). Gently shake his shoulders and shout, "Are you okay?" This helps ensure that you don't start CPR on a person who is conscious. Check whether he has an injury, particularly to the head or neck. If you suspect a head or neck injury, move him as little as possible to reduce the risk of paralysis.

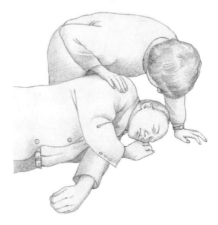

▶ Call out for help. Send someone to contact the EMS or call a code, if appropriate. Place the victim in a supine position on a hard, flat surface. When moving him, roll his head and torso as a unit. Avoid twisting or pulling his neck, shoulders, or hips (as shown below).

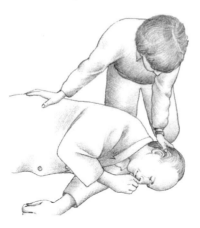

▶ Kneel near his shoulders. This position will give you easy access to his head and chest (as shown below).

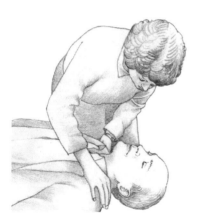

▶ In many cases, the muscles controlling the victim's tongue will be relaxed, causing the tongue to obstruct the airway. If the victim doesn't appear to have a neck injury, use the head-tilt, chin-lift maneuver to open his airway. To accomplish this, first place your hand that's closer to the victim's head on his forehead. Then apply firm pressure. The pressure should be firm enough to tilt the victim's head back. Next place the fingertips of your other hand under the bony part of his lower jaw near the chin. Now lift the victim's chin. At the

same time, keep his mouth partially open (as shown below).

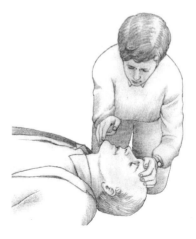

▶ Avoid placing your fingertips on the soft tissue under the victim's chin because this maneuver may inadvertently obstruct the airway you're trying to open.
▶ If you suspect a neck injury, use the jaw-thrust maneuver instead of the head-tilt, chin-lift maneuver. Kneel at the victim's head with your elbows on the ground. Rest your thumbs on his lower jaw near the corners of the mouth, pointing your thumbs toward his feet. Then place your fingertips around the lower jaw. To open the airway, lift the lower jaw with your fingertips (as shown below).

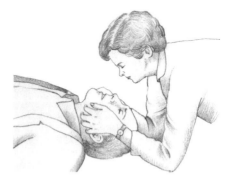

### Check for breathing
▶ While maintaining the open airway, place your ear over the victim's mouth and nose. Now, listen for the sound of air mov-

ing, and note whether his chest rises and falls. You may also feel airflow on your cheek. If he starts to breathe, keep the airway open and continue checking his breathing until help arrives (as shown below).

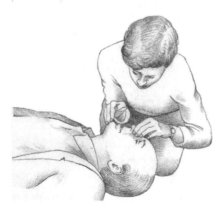

▶ If the victim doesn't start breathing after you open his airway, begin rescue breathing. Pinch his nostrils shut with the thumb and index finger of the hand you've had on his forehead (as shown below).

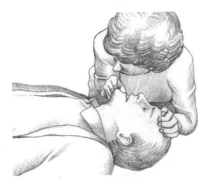

▶ Take a deep breath and place your mouth over the victim's mouth, creating a tight seal (as shown top of next column). Give two full ventilations, taking a deep breath after each to allow enough time for his chest to expand and relax and to prevent gastric distention. Each ventilation should last 1½ to 2 seconds.

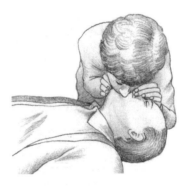

▶ If the first ventilation isn't successful, reposition the victim's head and try again. If you're still not successful, he may have a foreign-body airway obstruction. Check for loose dentures. If dentures or any other objects are blocking the airway, follow the procedure for clearing an airway obstruction.

### Assess circulation

▶ Keep one hand on the victim's forehead so his airway remains open. With your other hand, palpate the carotid artery that's closer to you. To do this, place your index and middle fingers in the groove between the trachea and the sternocleidomastoid muscle. Palpate for 5 to 10 seconds (as shown below).

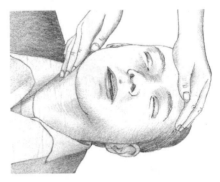

▶ If you detect a pulse, don't begin chest compressions. Instead, perform rescue breathing by giving the victim 12 ventilations per minute (or one every 5 seconds). After every 12 ventilations, recheck his pulse.

▶ If there's no pulse, start giving chest compressions. Make sure your knees are apart for a wide base of support. Using the hand closer to his feet, locate the lower margin of the rib cage (as shown below). Then move your fingertips along the margin to the notch where the ribs meet the sternum.

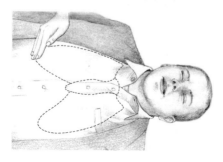

▶ Place your middle finger on the notch and your index finger next to your middle finger. The long axis of the heel of your hand will be aligned with the long axis of the sternum (as shown below).

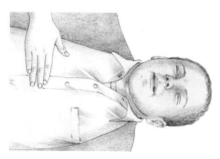

▶ Put the heel of your other hand on the sternum, next to the index finger. The long axis of the heel of your hand will be aligned with the long axis of the sternum (as shown below).

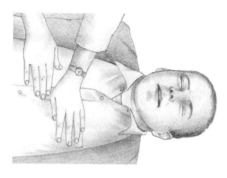

▶ Take the first hand off the notch and put it on top of the hand on the sternum. Make sure you have one hand directly on top of the other and your fingers aren't on his chest (as shown below).

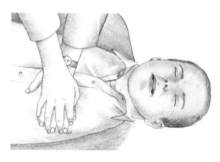

▶ This position will keep the force of the compression on the sternum and reduce the risk of a rib fracture, lung puncture, or liver laceration.

▶ With your elbows locked, arms straight, and your shoulders directly over your hands (as shown below), you're ready to give chest compressions. Using the weight of your upper body, compress the victim's sternum 1½″ to 2″ (3.5 to 5 cm), delivering the pressure through the heels of your hands. After each compression, release the pressure and allow the chest to return to its normal position so that the heart can fill with blood. Don't change your hand position during compressions—you might injure the victim.

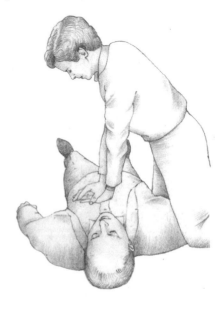

▶ Give 15 chest compressions at a rate of approximately 100 per minute. Count, "One and two and three and..." up to 15. Open the airway and give 2 ventilations. Then find the proper hand position again and deliver 15 more compressions. Do four complete cycles of 15 compressions and 2 ventilations.

▶ Palpate the carotid pulse again. If there's still no pulse, continue performing CPR in cycles of 15 compressions and 2 ventilations. Every few minutes, check for breathing and a pulse at the end of a complete cycle of compressions and ventilations. If you detect a pulse but he isn't breathing, give 12 ventilations per minute and monitor his pulse. If he has a pulse and is breathing, monitor his respirations and pulse closely. You should stop performing CPR only when his respirations and pulse return, he's turned over to the EMS, or you're exhausted.

### Two-person rescue

If another rescuer arrives while you're giving CPR, follow these steps:

▶ If the EMS team hasn't arrived, tell the second rescuer to repeat the call for help. If he's not a health care professional, ask him to stand by. Then, if you become fatigued, he can take over one-person CPR (as shown below).

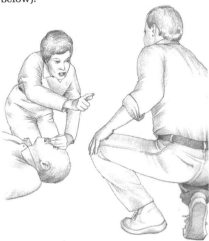

▶ If the rescuer is another health care professional, the two of you can perform two-person CPR. He should start assisting after you've finished a cycle of 15 compressions, two ventilations, and a pulse check.

▶ The second rescuer should get into place opposite you. While you're checking for a pulse, he should be finding the proper hand placement for delivering chest compressions (as shown below).

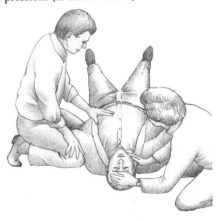

▶ If you don't detect a pulse, say, "No pulse, continue CPR," and give one ventilation. Then the second rescuer should begin delivering compressions at a rate of 100 per minute. Compressions and ventilations should be administered at a ratio of 15 compressions to 2 ventilations. The compressor (at this point, the second rescuer) should count out loud so the ventilator can anticipate when to give ventilations. To ensure that the ventilations are effective, the rescuer performing the chest compressions should stop briefly or at least long enough to observe the victim's chest rise with the air supplied by the rescuer giving ventilations (as shown below).

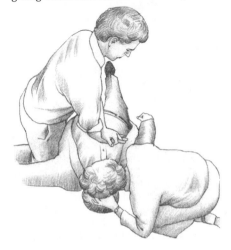

▶ As the ventilator, you must check for breathing and a pulse. Signal the compressor to stop giving compressions for 10 seconds so you can make these assessments (as shown below).

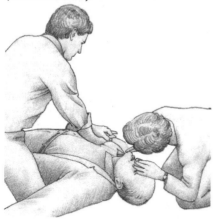

▶ The compressor (second rescuer) may grow tired and call for a switch. This switch should be done carefully, so as not to interrupt CPR. You would then give 2 ventilations and become the compressor by moving down to the victim's chest and placing your hands in the proper position (as shown below).

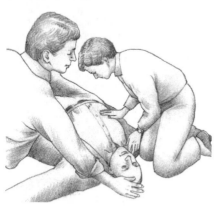

▶ The second rescuer would become the ventilator and move to the victim's head. He'd check the pulse for 10 seconds. If he found no pulse, he'd say, "No pulse" and give a ventilation. You'd then give compressions at a rate of 100 per minute — or 15 compressions for every 2 ventilations. As shown below, both of you should continue giving CPR in this manner until the victim's respirations and pulse return, he's turned over to the EMS, or both of you are exhausted.

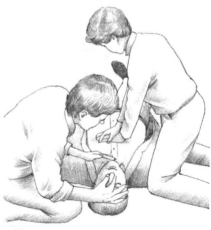

## Special considerations

Although acquired immunodeficiency syndrome (AIDS) isn't known to be transmitted in saliva, some health care professionals may hesitate to give rescue breaths — especially if the victim has AIDS. For this reason, the AHA recommends that all health care professionals learn how to use disposable airway equipment.

## Complications

CPR can cause certain complications — especially if the compressor doesn't place her hands properly on the sternum. These complications include fractured ribs, a lacerated liver, and punctured lungs. Gastric distention, a common complication, results from giving too much air during ventilation. (See *Potential hazards of CPR.*)

### REFERENCES

American Heart Association. "Guidelines 2000 for Cardiopulmonary Resuscitation and Emergency Cardiovascular Care: International Consensus on Science," *Circulation* 102(8 Suppl):I-384, August 2000.

Begany, T. "Major Changes Made to ACLS Guidelines," *Pulmonary Reviews* 5(11), November 2000. *www.pulmonaryreviews.com/archives.html.*

Crawford, M.H., et al. "ACC/AHA Guidelines for Ambulatory Electrocardiography: Executive Summary and Recommendations," *Circulation* 100(8 Suppl):886-93, August 1999.

# Potential hazards of CPR

Cardiopulmonary resuscitation (CPR) can cause various complications, including injury to bones and vital organs. This chart describes the causes of CPR hazards and lists preventive steps.

| Hazard | Causes | Assessment findings | Preventive measures |
|---|---|---|---|
| Sternal and rib fractures | ▶ Osteoporosis<br>▶ Malnutrition<br>▶ Improper hand placement | ▶ Paradoxical chest movement<br>▶ Chest pain or tenderness that increases with inspiration<br>▶ Crepitus<br>▶ Palpation of movable bony fragments over the sternum<br>▶ On palpation, sternum feels unattached to surrounding ribs | *While performing CPR:*<br>▶ Don't rest your hands or fingers on the patient's ribs.<br>▶ Interlock your fingers.<br>▶ Keep your bottom hand in contact with the chest, but release pressure after each compression.<br>▶ Compress the sternum at the recommended depth for the patient's age. |
| Pneumothorax, hemothorax, or both | ▶ Lung puncture from fractured rib | ▶ Chest pain and dyspnea<br>▶ Decreased or absent breath sounds over the affected lung<br>▶ Tracheal deviation from midline<br>▶ Hypotension<br>▶ Hyperresonance to percussion over the affected area along with shoulder pain | ▶ Follow the measures listed for sternal and rib fractures. |
| Injury to the heart and great vessels (pericardial tamponade, atrial or ventricular rupture, vessel laceration, cardiac contusion, punctures of the heart chambers) | ▶ Improperly performed chest compressions<br>▶ Transvenous or transthoracic pacing attempts<br>▶ Central line placement during resuscitation<br>▶ Intracardiac drug administration | ▶ Jugular vein distention<br>▶ Muffled heart sounds<br>▶ Pulsus paradoxus<br>▶ Narrowed pulse pressure<br>▶ Electrical alternans (decreased electrical amplitude of every other QRS complex)<br>▶ Adventitious heart sounds<br>▶ Hypotension<br>▶ Electrocardiogram changes (arrhythmias, ST-segment elevation, T-wave inversion, and marked decrease in QRS voltage) | ▶ Perform chest compressions properly. |
| Organ laceration (primarily liver and spleen) | ▶ Forceful compression<br>▶ Sharp edge of a fractured rib or xiphoid process | ▶ Persistent right upper quadrant tenderness (liver injury)<br>▶ Persistent left upper quadrant tenderness (splenic injury)<br>▶ Increasing abdominal girth | ▶ Follow the measures listed for sternal and rib fractures.<br>▶ Intubate early. |
| Aspiration of stomach contents | ▶ Gastric distention and an elevated diaphragm from high ventilatory pressures | ▶ Fever, hypoxia, and dyspnea<br>▶ Auscultation of wheezes and crackles<br>▶ Increased white blood cell count<br>▶ Changes in color and odor of lung secretions | ▶ Insert a nasogastric tube and apply suction, if gastric distention is marked. |

Heaven, D.J., and Sutton, R. "Syncope," *Critical Care Medicine* 28(10 Suppl.):N116-20, October 2000.

*Mastering ACLS.* Springhouse, Pa.: Springhouse Corp., 2002.

# Central venous pressure monitoring

In central venous pressure (CVP) monitoring, the doctor inserts a catheter through a vein and advances it until its tip lies in or near the right atrium. Because no major valves lie at the junction of the superior vena cava and right atrium, pressure at end diastole reflects back to the catheter. When connected to a manometer, the catheter measures CVP, an index of right ventricular function.

CVP monitoring helps to assess cardiac function, to evaluate venous return to the heart, and to indirectly gauge how well the heart is pumping. The central venous (CV) line also provides access to a large vessel for rapid, high-volume fluid administration and allows frequent blood withdrawal for laboratory samples.

CVP monitoring can be done intermittently or continuously. The catheter is inserted percutaneously or using a cutdown method. To measure the patient's volume status, a disposable plastic water manometer may be attached between the I.V. line and the central catheter with a three- or four-way stopcock. CVP may also be monitored continuously through a CV catheter that is attached to a pressure transducer. CVP is recorded in centimeters of water (cm $H_2O$) or millimeters of mercury (mm Hg).

Normal CVP ranges from 5 to 10 cm $H_2O$. Any condition that alters venous return, circulating blood volume, or cardiac performance may affect CVP. If circulating volume increases (such as with enhanced venous return to the heart), CVP rises. If circulating volume decreases (such as with reduced venous return), CVP drops.

## Equipment

*For intermittent CVP monitoring*
Disposable CVP manometer set • leveling device (such as a rod from a reusable CVP pole holder or a carpenter's level or rule) • additional stopcock (to attach the CVP manometer to the catheter) • extension tub-

ing (if needed) • I.V. pole • I.V. solution • I.V. drip chamber and tubing

*For continuous CVP monitoring*
Pressure monitoring kit with disposable pressure transducer • leveling device • bedside pressure module • continuous I.V. flush solution • pressure bag

*For withdrawing blood samples through the CV line*
Appropriate number of syringes for the ordered tests • 5- or 10-ml syringe for the discard sample (syringe size depends on the tests ordered)

*For using an intermittent CV line*
Syringe with normal saline solution • syringe with heparin flush solution

*For removing a CV catheter*
Sterile gloves • suture removal set • sterile gauze pads • povidone-iodine ointment • dressing • tape

## Implementation

▶ Gather the necessary equipment. Explain the procedure to the patient to reduce his anxiety.

▶ Assist the doctor as he inserts the CV catheter. (The procedure is similar to that used for pulmonary artery pressure monitoring, except that the catheter is advanced only as far as the superior vena cava.)

### Obtaining intermittent CVP readings with a water manometer

▶ With the CV line in place, position the patient flat. Align the base of the manometer with the previously determined zero reference point by using a leveling device. Because CVP reflects right atrial pressure, you must align the right atrium (the zero reference point) with the zero mark on the manometer. To find the right atrium, locate the fourth intercostal space at the midaxillary line. Mark the appropriate place on the patient's chest so that all subsequent recordings will be made using the same location.

▶ If the patient can't tolerate a flat position, place him in semi-Fowler's position. When the head of the bed is elevated, the phlebostatic axis remains constant but the midaxillary line changes. Use the same degree of elevation for all subsequent measurements.

# Measuring CVP with a water manometer

To ensure accurate central venous pressure (CVP) readings, make sure the manometer base is aligned with the patient's right atrium (the zero reference point). The manometer set usually contains a leveling rod to allow you to determine this quickly.

After adjusting the manometer's position, examine the typical three-way stopcock. By turning it to any position shown at right, you can control the direction of fluid flow. Four-way stopcocks also are available.

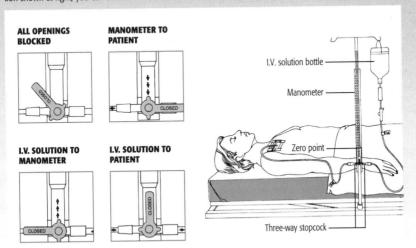

**ALL OPENINGS BLOCKED**

**MANOMETER TO PATIENT**

**I.V. SOLUTION TO MANOMETER**

**I.V. SOLUTION TO PATIENT**

I.V. solution bottle

Manometer

Zero point

Three-way stopcock

---

▶ Attach the water manometer to an I.V. pole or place it next to the patient's chest. Make sure the zero reference point is level with the right atrium. (See *Measuring CVP with a water manometer.*)

▶ Verify that the water manometer is connected to the I.V. tubing. Typically, markings on the manometer range from 12 to 38 cm $H_2O$. However, manufacturer's markings may differ, so be sure to read the directions before setting up the manometer and obtaining readings.

▶ Turn the stopcock off to the patient and slowly fill the manometer with I.V. solution until the fluid level is 10 to 20 cm $H_2O$ higher than the patient's expected CVP value. Don't overfill the tube because fluid that spills over the top can become a source of contamination.

▶ Turn the stopcock off to the I.V. solution and open to the patient. The fluid level in the manometer will drop. When the fluid level comes to rest, it will fluctuate slightly with respirations. Expect it to drop during inspiration and to rise during expiration.

▶ Record CVP at the end of inspiration, when intrathoracic pressure has a negligible effect. Depending on the type of water manometer used, note the value either at the bottom of the meniscus or at the midline of the small floating ball.

▶ After you've obtained the CVP value, turn the stopcock to resume the I.V. infusion. Adjust the I.V. drip rate as required.

▶ Place the patient in a comfortable position.

## Obtaining continuous CVP readings with a water manometer

▶ Make sure the stopcock is turned so that the I.V. solution port, CVP column port, and patient port are open. Be aware that with this stopcock position, infusion of the I.V. solution increases CVP. Therefore, expect higher readings than those taken with the stopcock turned off to the I.V. solution. If the I.V. solution infuses at a constant rate, CVP will change as the patient's condition changes, although the initial reading will be higher. Assess the patient closely for changes.

### Obtaining continuous CVP readings with a pressure monitoring system

▶ Make sure the CV line or the proximal lumen of a pulmonary artery catheter is attached to the system. (If the patient has a CV line with multiple lumens, one lumen may be dedicated to continuous CVP monitoring and the other lumens used for fluid administration.)

▶ Set up a pressure transducer system. Connect pressure tubing from the CVP catheter hub to the transducer. Then connect the flush solution container to a flush device.

▶ To obtain values, position the patient flat. If he can't tolerate this position, use semi-Fowler's position. Locate the level of the right atrium by identifying the phlebostatic axis. Zero the transducer, leveling the transducer air-fluid interface stopcock with the right atrium. Read the CVP value from the digital display on the monitor and note the waveform. Make sure the patient is still when the reading is taken to prevent artifact. (See *Identifying hemodynamic pressure monitoring problems.*) Be sure to use this position for all subsequent readings.

### Removing a CV line

▶ You may assist the doctor in removing a CV line. (In some states, a nurse is permitted to remove the catheter with a doctor's order or when acting under advanced collaborative standards of practice.)

▶ If the head of the bed is elevated, minimize the risk of air embolism during catheter removal—for instance, by placing the patient in Trendelenburg's position, if the line was inserted using a superior approach. If he can't tolerate this, position him flat.

▶ Turn the patient's head to the side opposite the catheter insertion site. The doctor removes the dressing and exposes the insertion site. If sutures are in place, he removes them carefully.

▶ Turn the I.V. solution off.

▶ The doctor pulls the catheter out in a slow, smooth motion and then applies pressure to the insertion site.

▶ Put on sterile gloves. Clean the insertion site, apply povidone-iodine ointment, and cover it with a sterile gauze dressing as ordered. Remove gloves and wash your hands.

▶ Assess the patient for signs of respiratory distress, which may indicate an air embolism.

### Special considerations

▶ As ordered, arrange for daily chest X-rays to check catheter placement.

▶ Care for the insertion site according to your facility's policy. Typically, you'll change the dressing every 24 to 48 hours.

▶ Be sure to wash your hands before performing dressing changes and to use aseptic technique and sterile gloves when redressing the site. When removing the old dressing, observe for signs of infection such as redness and note any patient complaints of tenderness. Apply ointment, if directed by facility policy (use is controversial), and then cover the site with a sterile gauze dressing or a clear occlusive dressing.

▶ After the initial CVP reading, reevaluate readings frequently to establish a baseline for the patient. Authorities recommend obtaining readings at 15-, 30-, and 60-minute intervals to establish a baseline. If the patient's CVP fluctuates by more than 2 cm $H_2O$, suspect a change in his clinical status and report this finding to the doctor.

▶ Change the I.V. solution every 24 hours and the I.V. tubing every 48 hours, according to facility policy. Expect the doctor to change the catheter every 72 hours. Label the I.V. solution, tubing, and dressing with the date, the time, and your initials.

### Complications

Complications of CVP monitoring include pneumothorax (which typically occurs upon catheter insertion), sepsis, thrombus, vessel or adjacent organ puncture, and air embolism.

### Documentation

▶ Document all dressing, tubing, and solution changes.

▶ Document the patient's tolerance of the procedure, the date and time of catheter removal, and the type of dressing applied.

▶ Note the condition of the catheter insertion site and whether a culture specimen was collected.

▶ Note any complications and actions taken.

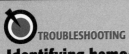

# Identifying hemodynamic pressure monitoring problems

| Problem | Possible causes | Interventions |
|---|---|---|
| No waveform | ▶ Power supply turned off<br>▶ Monitor screen pressure range set too low<br>▶ Loose connection in line<br>▶ Transducer not connected to amplifier<br>▶ Stopcock off to patient<br>▶ Catheter occluded or out of blood vessel | ▶ Check the power supply.<br>▶ Raise the monitor screen pressure range if necessary.<br>▶ Rebalance and recalibrate the equipment.<br>▶ Tighten loose connections.<br>▶ Check and tighten the connection.<br><br>▶ Position the stopcock correctly.<br>▶ Use the fast-flush valve to flush line, or try to aspirate blood from the catheter. If the line remains blocked, notify the doctor and prepare to replace the line. |
| Drifting waveforms | ▶ Improper warm-up<br><br>▶ Electrical cable kinked or compressed<br>▶ Temperature change in room air or I.V. flush solution | ▶ Allow the monitor and transducer to warm up for 10 to 15 minutes.<br>▶ Place the monitor's cable where it can't be stepped on or compressed.<br>▶ Routinely zero and calibrate the equipment 30 minutes after setting it up. This allows I.V. fluid to warm to room temperature. |
| Line fails to flush | ▶ Stopcocks positioned incorrectly<br>▶ Inadequate pressure from pressure bag<br>▶ Kink in pressure tubing<br>▶ Blood clot in catheter | ▶ Make sure stopcocks are positioned correctly.<br>▶ Make sure the pressure bag gauge reads 300 mm Hg.<br>▶ Check the pressure tubing for kinks.<br>▶ Try to aspirate the clot with a syringe. If the line still won't flush, notify the doctor and prepare to replace the line if necessary. *Important:* Never use a syringe to flush a hemodynamic line. |
| Artifact (waveform interference) | ▶ Patient movement<br>▶ Electrical interference<br><br>▶ Catheter fling (tip of pulmonary artery catheter moving rapidly in large blood vessel in heart chamber) | ▶ Wait until the patient is quiet before taking a reading.<br>▶ Make sure electrical equipment is connected and grounded correctly.<br>▶ Notify the doctor, who may try to reposition the catheter. |
| False-high readings | ▶ Transducer balancing port positioned below the patient's right atrium<br>▶ Flush solution flow rate that's too fast<br>▶ Air in system<br>▶ Catheter fling (tip of pulmonary artery catheter moving rapidly in large blood vessel or heart chamber) | ▶ Position the balancing port level with the patient's right atrium.<br><br>▶ Check the flush solution flow rate. Maintain it at 3 to 4 ml/hour.<br>▶ Remove air from the lines and the transducer.<br>▶ Notify the doctor, who may try to reposition the catheter. |

*(continued)*

## Identifying hemodynamic pressure monitoring problems *(continued)*

| Problem | Possible causes | Interventions |
|---|---|---|
| False-low readings | ▶ Transducer balancing port positioned above right atrium | ▶ Position the balancing port level with the patient's right atrium. |
| | ▶ Transducer imbalance | ▶ Make sure the transducer's flow system isn't kinked or occluded and rebalance and recalibrate the equipment. |
| | ▶ Loose connection | ▶ Tighten loose connections. |
| Damped waveform | ▶ Air bubbles | ▶ Secure all connections.<br>▶ Remove air from the lines and the transducer.<br>▶ Check for and replace cracked equipment. |
| | ▶ Blood clot in catheter<br>▶ Blood flashback in line | ▶ Refer to "Line fails to flush" (earlier in this chart).<br>▶ Make sure stopcock positions are correct; tighten loose connections and replace cracked equipment; flush the line with the fast-flush valve; replace the transducer dome if blood backs up into it. |
| | ▶ Incorrect transducer position | ▶ Make sure the transducer is kept at the level of the right atrium at all times. Improper levels give false-high or false-low pressure readings. |
| | ▶ Arterial catheter out of blood vessel or pressed against vessel wall | ▶ Reposition the catheter if it's against the vessel wall.<br>▶ Try to aspirate blood to confirm proper placement in the vessel. If you can't aspirate blood, notify the doctor and prepare to replace the line. *Note:* Bloody drainage at the insertion site may indicate catheter displacement. Notify the doctor immediately. |
| Pulmonary artery wedge pressure tracing unobtainable | ▶ Ruptured balloon | ▶ If you feel no resistance when injecting air, or if you see blood leaking from the balloon inflation lumen, stop injecting air and notify the doctor. If the catheter is left in, label the inflation lumen with a warning not to inflate. |
| | ▶ Incorrect amount of air in balloon | ▶ Deflate the balloon. Check the label on the catheter for correct volume. Reinflate slowly with the correct amount. To avoid rupturing the balloon, never use more than the stated volume. |
| | ▶ Catheter malpositioned | ▶ Notify the doctor. Obtain a chest X-ray. |

**REFERENCES**

Bridges, E.J. "Monitoring Pulmonary Artery Pressures: Just the Facts," *Critical Care Nurse* 20(6):59-80, December 2000.

Daily, E.K. "Hemodynamic Waveform Analysis," *Journal of Cardiovascular Nursing* 15(2):6-22, January 2001.

Druding, M.C. "Integrating Hemodynamic Monitoring and Physical Assessment," *Dimensions of Critical Care Nursing* 19(4):25-30, July-August 2000.

Keckeisen, M. "Monitoring Pulmonary Artery Pressure," *Critical Care Nurse* 19(6):88-91, December 1999.

Lynn-McHale, D.J., and Carlson, K.K. *AACN Procedure Manual for Critical Care,* 4th ed. Philadelphia: W.B. Saunders Co., 2001.

Quaal, S.J. "Improving the Accuracy of Pulmonary Artery Catheter Measurements," *Journal of Cardiovascular Nursing* 15(2):71-82, January 2001.

Rice, W.P., et al. "A Comparison of Hydrostatic Leveling Methods in Invasive Pressure Monitoring," *Critical Care Nurse* 20(6):21-30, December 2000.

# Defibrillation

The standard treatment for ventricular fibrillation, defibrillation involves using electrode paddles to direct an electric current through the patient's heart. The current causes the myocardium to depolarize, which in turn encourages the sinoatrial node to resume control of the heart's electrical activity. The electrode paddles delivering the current may be placed on the patient's chest or, during cardiac surgery, directly on the myocardium.

Because ventricular fibrillation leads to death if not corrected, the success of defibrillation depends on early recognition and quick treatment of this arrhythmia. In addition to treating ventricular fibrillation, defibrillation may also be used to treat ventricular tachycardia that doesn't produce a pulse.

A patient with a history of ventricular fibrillation may be a candidate for an implantable cardioverter-defibrillator (ICD), a sophisticated device that automatically discharges an electric current when it senses a ventricular tachyarrhythmia. (See *Understanding the ICD,* page 268.)

## Equipment

Defibrillator • external paddles • internal paddles (sterilized for cardiac surgery) • conductive medium pads • Electrocardiogram monitor with recorder • oxygen therapy equipment • handheld resuscitation bag • airway equipment • emergency pacing equipment • emergency cardiac medications

## Implementation

▶ Assess the patient to determine if he lacks a pulse. Call for help and perform CPR until the defibrillator and other emergency equipment arrive.
▶ If the defibrillator has "quick-look" capability, place the paddles on the patient's chest to quickly view his cardiac rhythm. Otherwise, connect the monitoring leads of the defibrillator to the patient and assess his cardiac rhythm.
▶ Expose the patient's chest and apply conductive pads at the paddle placement positions. For anterolateral placement, place one paddle to the right of the upper sternum, just below the right clavicle, and the other over the fifth or sixth intercostal space at the left anterior axillary line. For

anteroposterior placement, place the anterior paddle directly over the heart at the precordium, to the left of the lower sternal border. Place the flat posterior paddle under the patient's body beneath the heart and immediately below the scapulae (but not under the vertebral column).
▶ Turn on the defibrillator and, if performing external defibrillation, set the energy level for 200 joules for an adult patient.
▶ Charge the paddles by pressing the charge buttons, which are located either on the machine or on the paddles themselves.
▶ Place the paddles over the conductive pads and press firmly against the patient's chest, using 25 lb (11.3 kg) of pressure.
▶ Reassess the patient's cardiac rhythm.
▶ If the patient remains in ventricular fibrillation or pulseless ventricular tachycardia, instruct all personnel to stand clear of the patient and the bed.
▶ Discharge the current by pressing both paddle charge buttons simultaneously.
▶ Leaving the paddles in position on the patient's chest, reassess the patient's cardiac rhythm and have someone else assess the pulse.
▶ If necessary, prepare to defibrillate a second time. Instruct someone to reset the energy level on the defibrillator to 200 to 300 joules. Announce that you're preparing to defibrillate and follow the procedure described above.
▶ Reassess the patient. If defibrillation is again necessary, instruct someone to reset the energy level to 360 joules. Then follow the same procedure as before.
▶ Perform the three countershocks in rapid succession, reassessing the patient's rhythm before each defibrillation.
▶ If the patient still has no pulse after three initial defibrillations, resume CPR, give supplemental oxygen, and begin administering appropriate medications such as epinephrine. Also consider possible causes for failure of the patient's rhythm to convert, such as acidosis and hypoxia.
▶ If defibrillation restores a normal rhythm, check the patient's central and peripheral pulses and obtain a blood pressure reading, heart rate, and respiratory rate. Assess the patient's level of consciousness, cardiac rhythm, breath sounds, skin color, and urine output. Obtain baseline arterial blood gas levels and a 12-lead electrocardiogram (ECG). Provide supplemental oxygen, ventilation, and medications as needed. Check

## Understanding the ICD

The implantable cardioverter-defibrillator (ICD) has a programmable pulse generator and lead system that monitors the heart's activity, detects ventricular bradyarrhythmias and tachyarrhythmias, and responds with appropriate therapies. The range of therapies includes antitachycardia and bradycardia pacing, cardioversion, and defibrillation. Newer defibrillators can also pace the atrium and the ventricle.

Implantation of the ICD is similar to that of a permanent pacemaker. The cardiologist positions the lead (or leads) transvenously in the endocardium of the right ventricle (and in the right atrium, if both chambers require pacing). The lead connects to a generator box, which is implanted in the right or left upper chest near the clavicle.

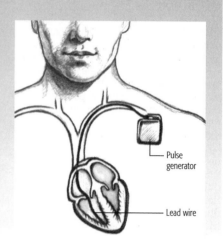

Pulse generator

Lead wire

---

the patient's chest for electrical burns and treat them as ordered with corticosteroid or lanolin-based creams. Also prepare the defibrillator for immediate reuse.

### Special considerations

▶ Defibrillators vary from one manufacturer to the next, so familiarize yourself with your facility's equipment. Defibrillator operation should be checked at least every 8 hours and after each use.

▶ Defibrillation can be affected by several factors, including paddle size and placement, condition of the patient's myocardium, duration of the arrhythmia, chest resistance, and the number of countershocks.

### Complications

Defibrillation can cause accidental electric shock to those providing care. Use of an insufficient amount of conductive medium can lead to skin burns.

### Documentation

▶ Document the procedure, including the patient's ECG rhythms before and after defibrillation; the number of times defibrillation was performed; the voltage used during each attempt; whether a pulse returned; the dosage, route, and time of drug administration; whether CPR was used; how the airway was maintained; and the patient's outcome.

**REFERENCES**
American Heart Association. "Guidelines 2000 for Cardiopulmonary Resuscitation and Emergency Cardiovascular Care," *Circulation* 102(8 Suppl): I90-I94, August 2000.

# Electrocardiography

One of the most valuable and frequently used diagnostic tools, an electrocardiogram (ECG) measures the heart's electrical activity as waveforms. Impulses moving through the heart's conduction system create electric currents that can be monitored on the body's surface. Electrodes attached to the skin can detect these electric currents and transmit them to an instrument that produces a record (the ECG) of cardiac activity.

ECG can be used to identify myocardial ischemia and infarction, rhythm and conduction disturbances, chamber enlargement, electrolyte imbalances, and drug toxicity.

The standard 12-lead ECG uses a series of electrodes placed on the extremities and the chest wall to assess the heart from 12 different views (leads). The 12 leads consist of three standard bipolar limb leads (designated I, II, III), three unipolar augmented leads ($aV_R$, $aV_L$, $aV_F$), and six unipolar precordial leads ($V_1$ to $V_6$). The limb leads and augmented leads show the heart from the frontal plane. The precordial leads show the heart from the horizontal plane.

▪ **EVIDENCE BASE** As a result of the AHA and ACC guidelines, most healthcare facilities have instituted in their policy a system to categorize patients for continuous ECG monitoring. ECG classifications include:

▪ Class I: conditions or patients in which there's a general agreement that ECG monitoring is useful

▪ Class II: conditions or patients in which ECG monitoring is frequently used, but there are differences in opinion about its usefulness

▪ Class III: conditions or patients in which there's a general consensus that ECG monitoring is of little or no use

The ECG device measures and averages the differences between the electrical potential of the electrode sites for each lead and graphs them over time. This creates the standard ECG complex, called PQRST. The P wave represents atrial depolarization; the QRS complex, ventricular depolarization; and the T wave, ventricular repolarization. (See *Reviewing ECG waveforms and components,* page 270.)

Variations of standard ECG include exercise ECG (stress ECG) and ambulatory ECG (Holter monitoring). Exercise ECG monitors heart rate, blood pressure, and ECG waveforms as the patient walks on a treadmill or pedals a stationary bicycle. For ambulatory ECG, the patient wears a portable Holter monitor, which records heart activity continually over 24 hours.

Today, ECG is typically accomplished using a multichannel method. All electrodes are attached to the patient at once, and the machine prints a simultaneous view of all leads.

### Equipment
ECG machine ● recording paper ● disposable pregelled electrodes ● 4″ × 4″ gauze pads ● optional: shaving supplies and marking pen

### Preparation of equipment
Place the ECG machine close to the patient's bed and plug the power cord into the wall outlet. If the patient is already connected to a cardiac monitor, remove the electrodes to accommodate the precordial leads and minimize electrical interference on the ECG tracing. Keep the patient away from electrical fixtures and power cords.

### Implementation
▪ As you set up the machine to record a 12-lead ECG, explain the procedure to the patient. Tell him that the test records the heart's electrical activity and that it may be repeated at certain intervals. Emphasize that no electrical current will enter his body. Also, tell him that the test typically takes about 5 minutes.

▪ Have the patient lie supine in the center of the bed with his arms at his sides. You may raise the head of the bed to promote comfort. Expose his arms and legs and cover him appropriately. His arms and legs should be relaxed to minimize muscle trembling, which can cause electrical interference.

▪ If the bed is too narrow, place the patient's hands under his buttocks to prevent muscle tension. Also use this technique if the patient is shivering or trembling. Make sure his feet aren't touching the bed board.

▪ Select flat, fleshy areas to place the electrodes. Avoid muscular and bony areas. If the patient has an amputated limb, choose a site on the stump.

▪ If an area is excessively hairy, shave it. Clean excess oil or other substances from the skin to enhance electrode contact.

▪ Apply the electrode paste or gel or the disposable electrodes to the patient's wrists and to the medial aspects of his ankles. If you're using paste or gel, rub it into the skin. If you're using disposable electrodes, peel off the contact paper and apply them directly to the prepared site as recommended by the manufacturer's instructions. To guarantee the best connection to the leadwire, position disposable electrodes on the legs with the lead connection pointing superiorly.

▪ If you're using paste or gel, secure electrodes promptly after you apply the conductive medium. This prevents drying of the medium, which could impair ECG quality. Never use alcohol or acetone pads in place of the electrode paste or gel because they impair electrode contact with the skin and diminish the transmission quality of electrical impulses.

▪ Connect the limb leadwires to the electrodes. Make sure the metal parts of the electrodes are clean and bright. Dirty or

# Reviewing ECG waveforms and components

An electrocardiogram (ECG) waveform has three basic components: the P wave, QRS complex, and T wave. These elements can be further divided into the PR interval, J point, ST segment, U wave, and QT interval.

### P wave and PR interval

The P wave represents atrial depolarization. The PR interval represents the time it takes an impulse to travel from the atria through the atrioventricular nodes and bundle of His. The PR interval measures from the beginning of the P wave to the beginning of the QRS complex.

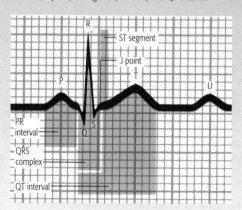

### QRS complex

The QRS complex represents ventricular depolarization (the time it takes for the impulse to travel through the bundle branches to the Purkinje fibers).

The Q wave appears as the first negative deflection in the QRS complex; the R wave, as the first positive deflection. The S wave appears as the second negative deflection or the first negative deflection after the R wave.

### J point and ST segment

Marking the end of the QRS complex, the J point also indicates the beginning of the ST segment. The ST segment represents part of ventricular repolarization.

### T wave and U wave

Usually following the same deflection pattern as the P wave, the T wave represents ventricular repolarization. The U wave follows the T wave, but isn't always seen.

### QT interval

The QT interval represents ventricular depolarization and repolarization. It extends from the beginning of the QRS complex to the end of the T wave.

---

corroded electrodes prevent a good electrical connection.

▸ You'll see that the tip of each leadwire is lettered and color-coded for easy identification. The white or RA leadwire goes to the right arm; the green or RL leadwire, to the right leg; the red or LL leadwire, to the left leg; the black or LA leadwire, to the left arm; and the brown or $V_1$ to $V_6$ leadwires, to the chest.

▸ Now, expose the patient's chest. Put a small amount of electrode gel or paste or a disposable electrode at each electrode position. (See *Positioning chest electrodes.*)

▸ If your patient is a woman, place the chest electrodes below the breast tissue. In a large-breasted woman, you may need to displace the breast tissue laterally.

▸ Check to see that the paper speed selector is set to the standard 25 mm/second and that the machine is set to full voltage. The machine will record a normal standardization mark—a square that is the height of two large squares or 10 small squares on the recording paper. Then, if necessary, enter the appropriate patient identification data.

▸ If any part of the waveform extends beyond the paper when you record the ECG, adjust the normal standardization to halfstandardization. Note this adjustment on the ECG strip because this will need to be considered in interpreting the results.

▶ Now you're ready to begin the recording. Ask the patient to relax and breathe normally. Tell him to lie still and not to talk when you record his ECG. Then press the auto button. Observe the tracing quality. The machine will record all 12 leads automatically, recording three consecutive leads simultaneously. Some machines have a display screen so you can preview waveforms before the machine records them on paper.

▶ When the machine finishes recording the 12-lead ECG, remove the electrodes and clean the patient's skin. After disconnecting the leadwires from the electrodes, dispose of or clean the electrodes as indicated.

### Special considerations

▶ Small areas of hair on the patient's chest or extremities may be shaved, but this usually isn't necessary.

▶ If the patient's skin is exceptionally oily, scaly, or diaphoretic, rub the electrode site with a dry 4″ × 4″ gauze pad before applying the electrode to help reduce interference in the tracing. During the procedure, ask the patient to breathe normally. If his respirations distort the recording, ask him to hold his breath briefly to reduce baseline wander in the tracing.

▶ If the patient has a pacemaker, you can perform an ECG with or without a magnet, according to the doctor's orders. Note the presence of a pacemaker and the use of the magnet (to turn off the pacemaker) on the strip.

### Documentation

▶ Label the ECG recording with the patient's name, room number, and facility identification number.

▶ Document in your notes the test's date and time as well as significant responses by the patient.

▶ Record the date, time, and patient's name and room number on the ECG itself.

▶ Note any appropriate clinical information on the ECG.

### REFERENCES

Lynn-McHale, D.J., and Carlson, K.K. *AACN Procedure Manual for Critical Care,* 4th ed. Philadelphia: W.B. Saunders Co., 2001.

## Positioning chest electrodes

To ensure accurate test results, position chest electrodes as follows:

$V_1$: Fourth intercostal space at right sternal border
$V_2$: Fourth intercostal space at left sternal border
$V_3$: Halfway between $V_2$ and $V_4$
$V_4$: Fifth intercostal space at midclavicular line
$V_5$: Fifth intercostal space at anterior axillary line (halfway between $V_4$ and $V_6$)
$V_6$: Fifth intercostal space at midaxillary line, level with $V_4$

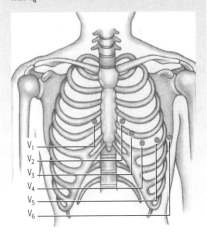

Roberts, A., et al. "ECGs: How To Recognize an Abnormal Reading," *Nursing Times* 98(21):40-41, May 2002.

## Intra-aortic balloon counterpulsation

Providing temporary support for the heart's left ventricle, intra-aortic balloon counterpulsation (IABC) mechanically displaces blood within the aorta by means of an intra-aortic balloon attached to an external pump console. The balloon is usually inserted through the common femoral artery and positioned with its tip just distal to the left subclavian artery. It monitors myocardial perfusion and the effects of drugs on myocardial function and perfusion. When used correctly, IABC improves two key aspects of myocardial physiology: It increases the supply of oxygen-rich blood to the myocardium, and it decreases myocardial oxygen demand.

IABC is recommended for patients with a wide range of low-cardiac-output disorders or cardiac instability, including refractory anginas, ventricular arrhythmias associated with ischemia, and pump failure caused by cardiogenic shock, intraoperative myocardial infarction (MI), or low cardiac output after bypass surgery. IABC is also indicated for patients with low cardiac output secondary to acute mechanical defects after MI (such as ventricular septal defect, papillary muscle rupture, or left ventricular aneurysm).

Perioperatively, the technique is used to support and stabilize patients with a suspected high-grade lesion who are undergoing such procedures as angioplasty, thrombolytic therapy, cardiac surgery, and cardiac catheterization.

IABC is contraindicated in patients with severe aortic regurgitation, aortic aneurysm, or severe peripheral vascular disease.

## Equipment

IABC console and balloon catheters • insertion kit • Dacron graft (for surgically inserted balloon) • ECG monitor and electrodes • sedative • pain medication • pulmonary artery (PA) catheter setup • temporary pacemaker setup • 18G angiography needle • sterile drape • sterile gloves • gown • mask • sutures • povidone-iodine solution • suction setup • oxygen setup and ventilator, if necessary • defibrillator and emergency medications • fluoroscope • indwelling urinary catheter • urinometer • arterial blood gas (ABG) kits and tubes for laboratory studies • povidone-iodine swabs • dressing materials • 4″ × 4″ gauze pads • shaving supplies • optional: I.V. heparin

### Preparation of equipment

Depending on your facility's policy, you or a perfusionist must balance the pressure transducer in the external pump console and calibrate the oscilloscope monitor to ensure accuracy.

## Implementation

◗ Explain to the patient that the doctor will place a special balloon catheter in his aorta to help his heart pump more easily. Briefly explain the insertion procedure, and mention that the catheter will be connected to a large console next to his bed. Tell him that the balloon will temporarily reduce his heart's workload to promote rapid healing of the ventricular muscle. Let him know that it will be removed after his heart can resume an adequate workload. (See *How the intra-aortic balloon pump works.*)

### Preparing for intra-aortic balloon insertion

◗ Make sure the patient or a family member understands and signs a consent form. Verify that the form is attached to his chart.

◗ Obtain the patient's baseline vital signs, including pulmonary artery pressure (PAP). (A PA line should already be in place.) Attach the patient to an electrocardiogram (ECG) machine for continuous monitoring. Apply chest electrodes in a standard lead II position—or in whatever position produces the largest R wave—because the R wave triggers balloon inflation and deflation. Obtain a baseline ECG.

◗ Attach another set of ECG electrodes to the patient unless the ECG pattern is being transmitted from the patient's bedside monitor to the balloon pump monitor through a phone cable. Administer oxygen as ordered and as necessary.

◗ Make sure the patient has an arterial line, a PA line, and a peripheral I.V. line in place. The arterial line is used for withdrawing blood samples, monitoring blood pressure, and assessing the timing and effectiveness of therapy. The PA line allows measurement of PAP, aspiration of blood samples, and cardiac output studies. Increased PAP indicates increased myocardial workload and ineffective balloon pumping. Cardiac output studies are usually performed with and without the balloon to check the patient's progress. The central lumen of the intra-aortic balloon, which is used to monitor central aortic pressure, produces an augmented pressure waveform that allows you to check for proper timing of the inflation-deflation cycle and demonstrates the effects of counterpulsation, elevated diastolic pressure, and reduced end-diastolic and systolic pressures. (See *Interpreting intra-aortic balloon waveforms,* page 274.)

◗ Insert an indwelling urinary catheter with a urinometer so you can measure the patient's urine output and assess his fluid balance and renal function. To reduce the

# How the intra-aortic balloon pump works

Made of polyurethane, the intra-aortic balloon is attached to an external pump console by means of a large-lumen catheter. The illustrations here show the direction of blood flow when the pump inflates and deflates the balloon.

### Balloon inflation
The balloon inflates as the aortic valve closes and diastole begins. Diastole increases perfusion to the coronary arteries.

### Balloon deflation
The balloon deflates before ventricular ejection, when the aortic valve opens. This permits ejection of blood from the left ventricle against a lowered resistance. As a result, aortic end-diastolic pressure and afterload decrease and cardiac output rises.

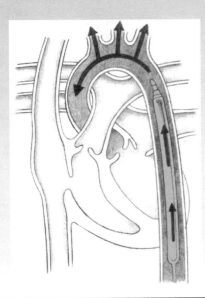

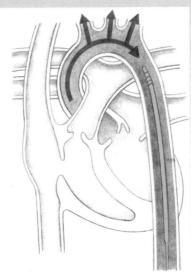

risk of infection, shave or clip hair bilaterally from the lower abdomen to the lower thigh, including the pubic area.
▶ Observe and record the patient's peripheral leg pulse and document sensation, movement, color, and temperature of the legs.
▶ Administer a sedative as ordered. Shave the insertion site if needed.
▶ Have the defibrillator, suction setup, temporary pacemaker setup, and emergency medications readily available in case the patient develops complications during insertion, such as an arrhythmia.
▶ Before the doctor inserts the balloon, he puts on sterile gloves, gown, and mask. He cleans the site with povidone-iodine solution, and drapes the area using a sterile drape.

### Inserting the intra-aortic balloon percutaneously
▶ The doctor may insert the balloon percutaneously through the femoral artery into the descending thoracic aorta, using a modified Seldinger technique. First, he accesses the vessel with an 18G angiography needle and removes the inner stylet.
▶ Then he passes the guide wire through the needle and removes the needle.
▶ Next, the doctor passes an introducer (dilator and sheath assembly) over the guide wire into the vessel until about 1″ (2.5 cm) remains above the insertion site. He then removes the inner dilator, leaving the introducer sheath and guide wire in place.
▶ After passing the balloon over the guide wire into the introducer sheath, the doctor

# Interpreting intra-aortic balloon waveforms

During intra-aortic balloon counterpulsation, you can use electrocardiogram and arterial pressure waveforms to determine whether the balloon pump is functioning properly.

### Normal inflation-deflation timing

Balloon inflation occurs after aortic valve closure; deflation, during isovolumetric contraction, just before the aortic valve opens. In a properly timed waveform, like the one shown at right, the inflation point lies at or slightly above the dicrotic notch. Both inflation and deflation cause a sharp V. Peak diastolic pressure exceeds peak systolic pressure; peak systolic pressure exceeds assisted peak systolic pressure.

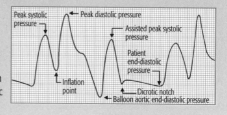

### Early inflation

With early inflation, the inflation point lies before the dicrotic notch. Early inflation dangerously increases myocardial stress and decreases cardiac output.

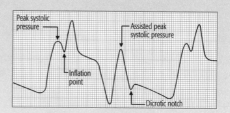

### Early deflation

With early deflation, a U shape appears and peak systolic pressure is less than or equal to assisted peak systolic pressure. This won't decrease afterload or myocardial oxygen consumption.

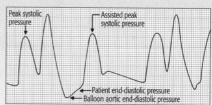

### Late inflation

With late inflation, the dicrotic notch precedes the inflation point, and the notch and the inflation point create a W shape. This can lead to a reduction in peak diastolic pressure, coronary and systemic perfusion augmentation time, and augmented coronary perfusion pressure.

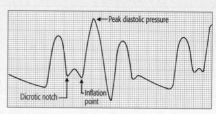

### Late deflation

With late deflation, peak systolic pressure exceeds assisted peak systolic pressure. This threatens the patient by increasing afterload, myocardial oxygen consumption, cardiac workload, and preload. It occurs when the balloon has been inflated for too long.

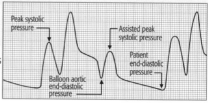

advances the catheter into position, ⅜" to
¾" (1 to 2 cm) distal to the left subclavian
artery under fluoroscopic guidance.
▶ The doctor attaches the balloon to the
control system to initiate counterpulsation.
The balloon catheter then unfurls.

### Inserting the intra-aortic balloon surgically
▶ If the doctor chooses not to insert the
catheter percutaneously, he usually inserts
it by femoral arteriotomy. (See *Surgical insertion sites for the intra-aortic balloon.*)
▶ After making an incision and isolating
the femoral artery, the doctor attaches a
Dacron graft to a small opening in the arterial wall.
▶ He then passes the catheter through this
graft. Using fluoroscopic guidance as necessary, he advances the catheter up the descending thoracic aorta and places the
catheter tip between the left subclavian
artery and the renal arteries.
▶ The doctor sews the Dacron graft around
the catheter at the insertion point and connects the other end of the catheter to the
pump console.
▶ If the balloon can't be inserted through
the femoral artery, the doctor inserts it in
an antegrade direction through the anterior
wall of the ascending aorta. He positions it
⅜" to ¾" (1 to 2 cm) beyond the left subclavian artery and brings the catheter out
through the chest wall.

### Monitoring the patient after balloon insertion
**ALERT!** If the control system malfunctions or becomes inoperable,
don't let the balloon catheter remain
dormant for more than 30 minutes. Get another control system and attach it to the
balloon; then resume pumping. In the
meantime, inflate the balloon manually, using a 60-ml syringe and room air a minimum of once every 5 minutes, to prevent
thrombus formation in the catheter.
▶ The doctor will clean the insertion site
with povidone-iodine swabs and apply a
sterile dressing.
▶ Obtain a chest X-ray to verify correct balloon placement.
▶ Assess and record pedal and posterior
tibial pulses as well as color, sensation, and
temperature in the affected limb every 15
minutes for 1 hour, then hourly. Notify the
doctor immediately if you detect circulato-

# Surgical insertion sites for the intra-aortic balloon

If an intra-aortic balloon can't be inserted percutaneously, the doctor will insert it surgically, using a
femoral or transthoracic approach.

### Femoral approach
Insertion through the femoral artery requires a cutdown and an arteriotomy. The doctor passes the
balloon through a Dacron graft that has been sewn
to the artery.

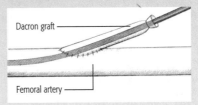

Dacron graft

Femoral artery

### Transthoracic approach
If femoral insertion is unsuccessful, the doctor may
use a transthoracic approach. He inserts the balloon in an antegrade direction through the subclavian artery and then positions it in the descending
thoracic aorta.

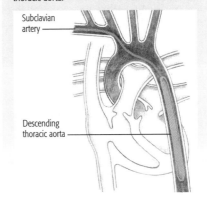

Subclavian
artery

Descending
thoracic aorta

ry changes because the balloon may need
to be removed.
▶ Observe and record the patient's baseline
arm pulses, arm sensation and movement,
and arm color and temperature every 15
minutes for 1 hour after balloon insertion,
then every 2 hours while the balloon is in

place. Loss of left arm pulses may indicate upward balloon displacement. Notify the doctor of any changes.

▶ Monitor the patient's urine output every hour. Note baseline blood urea nitrogen (BUN) and serum creatinine levels, and monitor these levels daily. Changes in urine output, BUN, and serum creatinine levels may signal reduced renal perfusion from downward balloon displacement.

▶ Auscultate and record bowel sounds every 4 hours. Check for abdominal distention and tenderness as well as changes in the patient's elimination patterns.

▶ Measure the patient's temperature every 1 to 4 hours. If it's elevated, obtain blood samples for a culture, send them to the laboratory immediately, and notify the doctor. Culture any drainage at the insertion site.

▶ Monitor the patient's hematologic status. Observe for bleeding gums, blood in the urine or stools, petechiae, and bleeding at the insertion site. Monitor his platelet count, hemoglobin level, and hematocrit daily. Expect to administer blood products to maintain hematocrit at 30%. If the platelet count drops, expect to administer platelets.

▶ Monitor partial thromboplastin time (PTT) every 6 hours while the heparin dose is adjusted to maintain PTT at 1½ to 2 times the normal value, then every 12 to 24 hours while the balloon remains in place.

▶ Measure PAP and pulmonary artery wedge pressure (PAWP) every 1 to 2 hours as ordered. A rising PAWP reflects preload, signaling increased ventricular pressure and workload; notify the doctor if this occurs. Some patients require I.V. nitroprusside during IABC to reduce preload and afterload.

▶ Obtain samples for ABG analysis as ordered.

▶ Monitor serum electrolyte levels — especially sodium and potassium — to assess the patient's fluid and electrolyte balance and help prevent arrhythmias.

▶ Watch for signs and symptoms of a dissecting aortic aneurysm, such as a blood pressure differential between the left and right arms, elevated blood pressure, syncope, pallor, diaphoresis, dyspnea, a throbbing abdominal mass, a reduced red blood cell count with an elevated white blood cell count, and pain in the chest, abdomen, or back. Notify the doctor immediately if you detect any of these complications.

## Weaning the patient from IABC

▶ Assess the cardiac index, systemic blood pressure, and PAWP to help the doctor evaluate the patient's readiness for weaning — usually about 24 hours after balloon insertion. The patient's hemodynamic status should be stable on minimal doses of inotropic agents, such as dopamine (Intropin) or dobutamine (Dobutrex).

▶ To begin weaning, gradually decrease the frequency of balloon augmentation to 1:2 and 1:4, as ordered. Although your facility has its own weaning protocol, be aware that assist frequency is usually maintained for an hour or longer. If the patient's hemodynamic indices remain stable during this time, weaning may continue.

▶ Avoid leaving the patient on a low augmentation setting for more than 2 hours to prevent embolus formation.

▶ Assess the patient's tolerance of weaning. Signs and symptoms of poor tolerance include confusion and disorientation, urine output below 30 ml/hour, cold and clammy skin, chest pain, arrhythmias, ischemic ECG changes, and elevated PAP. If the patient develops any of these problems, notify the doctor at once.

## Removing the intra-aortic balloon

▶ The balloon is removed when the patient's hemodynamic status remains stable after the frequency of balloon augmentation is decreased. The control system is turned off and the connective tubing is disconnected from the catheter to ensure balloon deflation.

▶ The doctor withdraws the balloon until the proximal end of the catheter contacts the distal end of the introducer sheath.

▶ The doctor then applies pressure below the puncture site and removes the balloon and introducer sheath as a unit, allowing a few seconds of free bleeding to prevent thrombus formation.

▶ To promote distal bleedback, the doctor applies pressure above the puncture site.

▶ Apply direct pressure to the site for 30 minutes or until bleeding stops. (In some facilities, this is the doctor's responsibility.)

▶ If the balloon was inserted surgically, the doctor will close the Dacron graft and suture the insertion site. The cardiologist usually removes a percutaneous catheter.

▶ After balloon removal, provide wound care according to your facility's policy. Record the patient's pedal and posterior tibial pulses, and the color, temperature, and sensation of the affected limb. Enforce bed rest as appropriate (usually for 24 hours).

## Special considerations

▶ Before using the IABC control system, make sure you know what the alarms and messages mean and how to respond to them.

 **ALERT!** You must respond immediately to alarms and messages.

▶ Change the dressing at the balloon insertion site every 24 hours or as needed, using strict sterile technique. Don't let povidone-iodine solution come in contact with the catheter.

▶ Make sure the head of the bed is elevated no more than 30 degrees.

▶ Watch for pump interruptions, which may result from loose ECG electrodes or leadwires, static or 60-cycle interference, catheter kinking, or improper body alignment.

▶ Make sure PTT is within normal limits before the balloon is removed to prevent hemorrhage at insertion site.

## Complications

IABC may cause numerous complications. The most common, arterial embolism, stems from clot formation on the balloon surface. Other potential complications include extension or rupture of an aortic aneurysm, femoral or iliac artery perforation, femoral artery occlusion, and sepsis. Bleeding at the insertion site may become aggravated by pump-induced thrombocytopenia caused by platelet aggregation around the balloon.

## Documentation

▶ Document all aspects of patient assessment and management, including the patient's response to therapy.

▶ If you're responsible for the IABC device, document all routine checks, problems, and troubleshooting measures.

▶ If a technician is responsible for the IABC device, record only when and why the technician was notified and the result of his actions on the patient, if any.

▶ Document any teaching of the patient, family, or close friends as well as their responses.

## REFERENCES

Lynn-McHale, D.J., and Carlson, K.K. *AACN Procedure Manual for Critical Care,* 4th ed. Philadelphia: W.B. Saunders Co., 2001.

# Pediatric cardiopulmonary resuscitation

When an adult needs cardiopulmonary resuscitation (CPR), he typically suffers from a primary cardiac disorder or arrhythmia that has stopped the heart. When an infant or child needs CPR, he typically suffers from hypoxia caused by respiratory difficulty or respiratory arrest.

Most pediatric crises requiring CPR are preventable. They include motor vehicle accidents, drowning, burns, smoke inhalation, falls, poisoning, suffocation, and choking (usually from inhaling a plastic bag or small foreign bodies, such as toys or food). Other causes of cardiopulmonary arrest in children include laryngospasm and edema from upper respiratory infections and sudden infant death syndrome. Based on the same principle, CPR in adults, children, and infants aims to restore cardiopulmonary function by ventilating the lungs and pumping the victim's heart until natural function resumes. However, CPR techniques differ depending on whether the patient is an adult, a child, or an infant. For CPR purposes, the American Heart Association defines a patient by age. An infant is under age 1; a child is age 1 to 8; an adult is over age 8. Survival chances improve the sooner CPR begins and the faster advanced life support systems are implemented.

## Equipment

CPR requires no special equipment except a hard surface on which to place the patient.

## Implementation

▶ Gently shake the apparently unconscious child's shoulder and shout at her to elicit a response. If the child is conscious but has difficulty breathing, help her into a position that best eases her breathing—if she hasn't naturally assumed this position already.

▶ Call for help to alert others and to enlist emergency assistance. If you're alone and the child isn't breathing, perform CPR for 1 minute before calling for help.

▶ Position the child supine on a firm, flat surface (usually the ground). The surface should provide the resistance needed for adequate compression of the heart. If you must turn the child from a prone position, support her head and neck and turn her as a unit to avoid injuring her spine (as shown below).

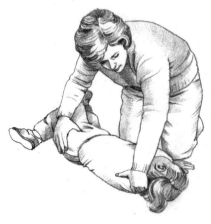

### Establishing a patent airway
▶ Kneel beside the child's shoulder. Place one hand on the child's forehead and gently lift her chin with your other hand to open her airway (as shown below). (In infants, this is called the sniffing position.) Avoid fingering the soft neck tissue to avoid obstructing the airway. Never let the child's mouth close completely.

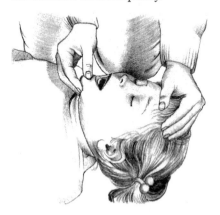

▶ If you suspect a neck injury, use the jaw-thrust maneuver to open the child's airway to keep from moving the child's neck. To do this, kneel beside the child's head. With your elbows on the ground, rest your thumbs at the corners of the child's mouth, and place two or three fingers of each hand under the lower jaw. Lift the jaw upward.

▶ While maintaining an open airway, place your ear near the child's mouth and nose to evaluate her breathing status. Look for chest movement, listen for exhaled air, and feel for exhaled air on your cheek (as shown below).

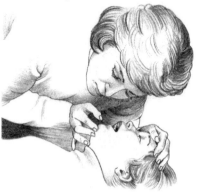

▶ If the child is breathing, maintain an open airway and monitor respirations.

▶ If you suspect that a mechanical airway obstruction blocks respiration (whether the child is conscious or not), attempt to clear the airway as you would in an adult, but with two exceptions: Don't use the blind finger-sweep maneuver (which could compound or relodge the obstruction), and do adjust your technique to the child's size. (For directions, see the section on obstructed airway management.)

### Restoring ventilation
▶ If the child isn't breathing, maintain the open airway position and take a breath. Then pinch the child's nostrils shut and cover the child's mouth with your mouth (as shown top of next page). Give two slow breaths (1 to 1½ seconds/breath), pausing briefly after the first breath.

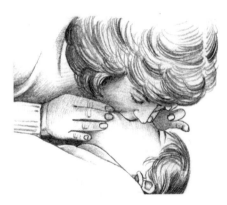

- If your first attempt at ventilation fails to restore the child's breathing, reposition the child's head to open the airway and try again. If you're still unsuccessful, the airway may be obstructed by a foreign body.
- Repeat the steps for airway clearance.
- Once you free the obstruction, check for breathing and pulse. If absent, proceed with chest compressions.

### Restoring heartbeat and circulation
- Assess circulation by palpating the carotid artery for a pulse.
- Locate the carotid artery with two or three fingers of one hand. (You'll need the other hand to maintain the head-tilt position that keeps the airway open.) Place your fingers in the center of the child's neck on the side closest to you, and slide your fingers into the groove formed by the trachea and the sternocleidomastoid muscles (as shown below). Palpate the artery for 5 to 10 seconds to confirm the child's pulse status.

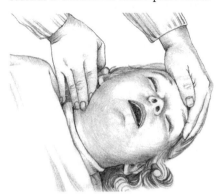

- If you feel the child's pulse, continue rescue breathing, giving one breath every 3 seconds (20 breaths/minute).
- If you can't feel a pulse, begin cardiac compressions.
- Kneel next to the child's chest. Using the hand closest to her feet, locate the lower border of the rib cage on the side nearest you (as shown below).

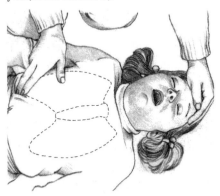

- Hold your middle and index fingers together, and move them up the rib cage to the notch where the ribs and sternum join. Put your middle finger on the notch and your index finger next to it (as shown below).

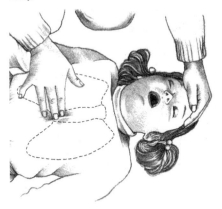

- Lift your hand and place the heel just above the spot where the index finger was (as shown below). The heel of your hand should be aligned with the long axis of the sternum.

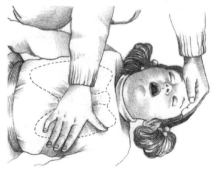

▶ Using the heel of one hand only, apply enough pressure to compress the child's chest downward 1″ to 1½″ (2.5 to 3.5 cm) (as shown below). Deliver five serial compressions at a rate of 100 compressions/minute.

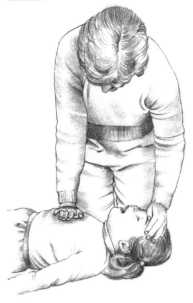

▶ After every five compressions, breathe one breath into the child. Deliver one breath for every five compressions whether you're working alone or with a partner.
▶ After 20 cycles (1 minute) of CPR, feel the pulse for 5 seconds to detect a heartbeat. If you can't detect a pulse, continue chest compressions and rescue breathing.

▶ If you can detect a pulse, check for spontaneous respirations. Without respirations, give one breath every 3 seconds (20 breaths/minute) and continue to monitor the pulse. If the child begins breathing spontaneously, keep the airway open and place the child in a side-lying position to prevent aspiration. If trauma is suspected, logroll the patient to avoid injury. Monitor both the respirations and pulse.

## Special considerations
▶ A child's small airway can be easily blocked by his tongue. If this occurs, simply opening the airway may eliminate the obstruction.
▶ When performing cardiac compressions, take care to ensure smooth motions. Keep your fingers off, and the heel of your hand on, the child's chest at all times. Also, time your motions so that the compression and relaxation phases are equal to promote effective compressions.
▶ If the child has breathing difficulty and a parent is present, find out whether the child recently had a fever or an upper respiratory tract infection. If so, suspect epiglottitis. In this instance, don't attempt to manipulate the airway because laryngospasm may occur and completely obstruct the airway. Allow the child to assume a comfortable position, and monitor his breathing until additional assistance arrives.
▶ Persist in attempts to remove an obstruction. As hypoxia develops, the child's muscles will relax, allowing you to remove the foreign object.
▶ During resuscitation efforts, make sure that someone communicates support and information to the parents.
▶ Be aware that, if available, you can use a one-way valve mask over the child's nose and mouth when performing CPR.

## Documentation
▶ Note where the arrest occurred, and whether it was cardiac or respiratory arrest.
▶ Record all events of resuscitation, names of individuals present, when CPR began and ended, and the outcome.
▶ Record any complications—for example, a fractured rib, bruised mouth, or gastric distention—as well as actions taken to correct them.

▶ If the child received advanced cardiac life support, document which interventions were performed, who performed them, when they were performed, and what equipment was used.

### REFERENCES

Mann, K., et al. "Beneficial Effects of Vasopressin in Prolonged Pediatric Cardiac Arrest: A Case Series," *Resuscitation* 52(2): 149-56, February 2002.

Moyer, M. "Pediatric Advanced Life Support Guidelines," Updated, Part 2. *Air Medical Journal* 21(4):17-19, July-August 2002.

# Percutaneous transluminal coronary angioplasty

A nonsurgical approach to opening coronary vessels narrowed by arteriosclerosis, PTCA uses a balloon-tipped catheter that is inserted into a narrowed coronary artery. This procedure, performed in the cardiac catheterization laboratory under local anesthesia, relieves pain due to angina and myocardial ischemia.

Cardiac catheterization usually accompanies PTCA to assess the stenosis and the efficacy of the angioplasty. Catheterization is used as a visual tool to direct the balloon-tipped catheter through the vessel's area of stenosis. As the balloon is inflated, the plaque is compressed against the vessel wall, allowing coronary blood to flow more freely. (See *Performing PTCA,* page 282.)

PTCA provides an alternative for patients who are poor surgical risks because of chronic medical problems. It's also useful for patients who have total coronary occlusion, unstable angina, and plaque buildup in several areas and for those with poor left ventricular function.

The ideal candidate for PTCA has single- or double-vessel disease excluding the left main coronary artery with at least 50% proximal stenosis. The lesion should be discrete, uncalcified, concentric, and not located near a bifurcation.

Your responsibilities in PTCA include teaching the patient and family about the procedure and assessing for complications afterward.

A newer procedure, laser-enhanced angioplasty, is showing promising results in vaporizing occlusions in atherosclerosis. (See *Laser-enhanced angioplasty,* page 283.)

### Equipment

Povidone-iodine solution ● local anesthetic ● I.V. solution and tubing ● ECG monitor and electrodes ● oxygen ● nasal cannula ● shaving supplies or depilatory cream ● sedative ● PA catheter ● contrast medium ● emergency medications ● heparin for injection ● 5-lb (2.3-kg) sandbag ● introducer kit for PTCA catheter ● sterile gown, gloves, and drapes ● optional: nitroglycerin and collagen plug (Vasoseal or Angioseal), if necessary

### Implementation

▶ Explain the procedure to the patient and family to reduce the patient's fear and promote cooperation.

▶ Inform the patient that the procedure lasts from 1 to 4 hours and that he may feel some discomfort from lying on a hard table for that long.

▶ Tell him that a catheter will be inserted into an artery or a vein in his groin and that he may feel pressure as the catheter moves along the vessel.

▶ Reassure him that although he'll be awake during the procedure, he'll be given a sedative. Explain that the doctor or nurse may ask him how he's feeling and that he should tell them if he experiences any angina.

▶ Explain that the doctor will inject a contrast medium to outline the lesion's location. Warn the patient that he may feel a hot, flushing sensation or transient nausea during the injection.

#### Before angioplasty

▶ Check the patient's history for allergies; if he's had allergic reactions to shellfish, iodine, or contrast media, notify the doctor.

▶ Give 650 mg of aspirin the evening before the procedure, as ordered, to prevent platelet aggregation.

▶ Make sure that the patient signs a consent form.

▶ Restrict food and fluids for at least 6 hours before the procedure or as ordered.

# Performing PTCA

Percutaneous transluminal coronary angioplasty (PTCA) opens an occluded coronary artery without opening the chest. It's performed in the cardiac catheterization laboratory after coronary angiography confirms the presence and location of the occlusion. When the occlusion is located, the doctor threads a guide catheter through the patient's femoral artery and into the coronary artery under fluoroscopic guidance (as shown below).

When the guide catheter's position at the occlusion site is confirmed by angiography, the doctor carefully introduces into the catheter a double-lumen balloon that's smaller than the catheter lumen. He then directs the balloon through the lesion, where a marked pressure gradient will be obvious. The doctor alternately inflates (as shown below) and deflates the balloon until an angiogram verifies successful arterial dilation and the pressure gradient has decreased.

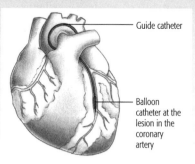

Guide catheter

Balloon catheter at the lesion in the coronary artery

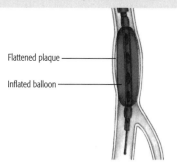

Flattened plaque

Inflated balloon

---

▶ Ensure that the results of coagulation studies, complete blood count, serum electrolyte studies, and blood typing and cross-matching are available.
▶ Insert an I.V. line in case emergency medications are required.
▶ Shave hair from the insertion site (groin or brachial area), or use a depilatory cream. Clean the area with povidone-iodine solution.
▶ Give the patient a sedative as ordered.
▶ Take baseline peripheral pulses in all extremities.

## During angioplasty

▶ When the patient arrives at the cardiac catheterization laboratory, apply ECG electrodes and ensure I.V. line patency.
▶ Administer oxygen through a nasal cannula.
▶ The doctor will put on a sterile gown and gloves. Open the sterile supplies.
▶ The doctor prepares and drapes the site and injects a local anesthetic. If the patient doesn't have a PA catheter in place, the doctor may insert one now.

▶ The doctor inserts a large guide catheter into the artery. Then he threads an angioplasty catheter through the guide catheter. An angioplasty catheter is thinner and longer and has a balloon at its tip. Using a thin, flexible guide wire, he then threads the catheter up through the aorta and into the coronary artery to the area of stenosis.
▶ He injects a contrast medium through the angioplasty catheter and into the obstructed coronary artery to outline the lesion's location and help assess the blockage. He also injects heparin to prevent the catheter from clotting, and intracoronary nitroglycerin to dilate coronary vessels and prevent spasm, if needed.
▶ He inflates the catheter's balloon for a gradually increasing amount of time and pressure. The expanding balloon compresses the atherosclerotic plaque against the arterial wall, expanding the arterial lumen. Because balloon inflation deprives the myocardium distal to the inflation area of blood, the patient may experience angina at this time. If balloon inflation fails to

decrease the stenosis, a larger balloon may be used.

▶ After angioplasty, serial angiograms help determine the effectiveness of treatment.

▶ If the facility uses a collagen plug to promote homeostasis, the doctor will insert it now before removing the sheath. The collagen plug seals the insertion site and prevents bleeding and hematoma formation at the site. If the procedure needs to be repeated, the doctor will suture the guide catheter in place to prevent migration and dislodgement of the catheter.

### After angioplasty

▶ When the patient returns to the unit, he may be receiving I.V. heparin or nitroglycerin.

▶ Monitor the insertion site for bleeding and report and signs of bleeding to the doctor.

▶ Assess the patient's vital signs every 15 minutes for the first hour, then every 30 minutes for 4 hours, unless his condition warrants more frequent checking.

▶ Assess peripheral pulses distal to the catheter insertion site as well as the color, sensation, temperature, and capillary refill of the affected extremity.

▶ Monitor ECG rhythm and arterial pressures.

◆ **ALERT!** Because coronary spasm may occur during or after PTCA, monitor the patient's ECG for ST-segment and T-wave changes, and take vital signs frequently. Coronary artery dissection may occur with no early symptoms, but it can cause restenosis of the vessel. Be alert for symptoms of ischemia, which requires emergency coronary revascularization.

▶ Instruct the patient to keep the affected extremity straight. Elevate the head of the bed 15 to 30 degrees.

▶ Assess the catheter site for hematoma, ecchymosis, and hemorrhage. If an area of expanding hematoma appears, mark the site and alert the doctor. If bleeding occurs, locate the artery and apply manual pressure; then notify the doctor.

▶ Administer I.V. fluids as ordered (usually 100 ml/hour) to promote excretion of the contrast medium. Be sure to assess for signs of fluid overload (distended neck veins, atrial and ventricular gallops, dysp-

## Laser-enhanced angioplasty

Laser-enhanced angioplasty shows great potential for vaporizing occlusions in patients with atherosclerosis. The procedure achieves its best results with thrombotic occlusions, but it may also be used to remove calcified plaques. New lasers that deliver energy in brief pulses have helped solve the problem of thermal or acoustic damage to local tissues. Using the pulsed beam, doctors can dispatch the blockage without destroying the vessel wall.

To perform the procedure, the doctor threads a laser-containing catheter into the diseased artery. When the catheter nears the occlusion, the doctor triggers the laser to emit rapid bursts. Between bursts he rotates the catheter, advancing it until the occlusion is destroyed. The procedure takes about an hour and requires only a local anesthetic. Clearing a completely occluded coronary artery requires ten 1-second bursts of laser energy, followed by balloon angioplasty. After the procedure, angiography may be used to document vessel patency.

Cardiologists have successfully used laser techniques to open totally blocked right main coronary arteries, thereby avoiding bypass surgery. They have also used combinations of direct laser energy, fiber optics, and balloon angioplasty catheters to open totally blocked right main coronary arteries. These advances may make it possible to perform angioplasty in community hospitals in nonsurgical settings.

nea, pulmonary congestion, tachycardia, hypertension, and hypoxemia).

## Special considerations

PTCA is contraindicated in left main coronary artery disease, especially when the patient is a poor surgical risk; in patients with variant angina or critical valvular disease; and in patients with vessels that are occluded at the aortic wall orifice.

## Complications

The most common complication of PTCA is prolonged angina. Others include coronary artery perforation, balloon rupture, reocclusion (necessitating a coronary artery

# Vascular stents

Two serious complications of percutaneous translu-minal coronary angioplasty (PTCA) are acute vessel closure and late restenosis. To prevent these prob-lems, doctors are performing a procedure called stenting. The stent currently used—the Palmaz balloon-expandable stent—consists of a stainless steel tube, the walls of which have a rectangular design. When the stent expands, each rectangle stretches to a diamond shape. The expanded stent supports the artery and helps prevent restenosis.

The stent is used in patients at risk for abrupt clotting after PTCA. Stents may also be inserted after failed PTCA to keep the patient stable until he can undergo coronary artery bypass surgery, or a stent may be used as an alternative to this surgery.

For insertion, the stent is put on a standard bal-loon angioplasty catheter and positioned over a guide wire (as shown below). Fluoroscopy verifies correct placement; then the stent is expanded and the catheter is removed.

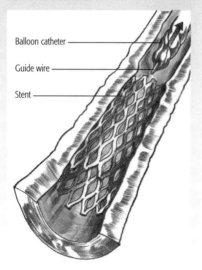

Balloon catheter

Guide wire

Stent

---

bypass graft), myocardial infarction, peri-cardial tamponade, hematoma, hemor-rhage, reperfusion arrhythmias, and clo-sure of the vessel. Vascular stents may be inserted to prevent vessel closure. (See *Vascular stents.*)

## Documentation
▶ Note the patient's tolerance of the proce-dure and his condition after it, including vital signs and the condition of the extrem-ity distal to the insertion site.
▶ Document any complications and inter-ventions.

### REFERENCES
Dietz, U., et al. "Angiographic Analysis of the Angioplasty Versus Rotational Atherecto-my for the Treatment of Diffuse In-stent Restenosis Trial (ARTIST)," *American Jour-nal of Cardiology* 90(8):843, October 2002.
Meils, C.M., et al. "Treatment of the Patient with Acute Myocardial Infarction: Reduc-ing Time Delays," *Journal of Nursing Care Quality* 17(1):83-89, October 2002.

# Permanent pacemaker insertion and care

Designed to operate for 3 to 20 years, a per-manent pacemaker is a self-contained de-vice surgically implanted in a pocket be-neath the patient's skin. This is usually done in the operating room or cardiac catheterization laboratory. Nursing respon-sibilities involve monitoring the ECG and maintaining sterile technique.

Today, permanent pacemakers function in the demand mode, allowing the patient's heart to beat on its own but preventing it from falling below a preset rate. Pacing electrodes can be placed in the atria, in the ventricles, or in both chambers (atrioven-tricular sequential, dual chamber). (See *Understanding pacemaker codes.*) The most common pacing codes are VVI for single-chamber pacing and DDD for dual-chamber pacing.

Candidates for permanent pacemakers include patients with myocardial infarc-tion and persistent bradyarrhythmia and patients with complete heart block or slow ventricular rates stemming from congenital or degenerative heart disease or cardiac surgery. Patients who suffer Stokes-Adams syndrome, as well as those with Wolff-Parkinson-White syndrome or sick sinus syndrome, may also benefit from perma-nent pacemaker implantation.

■ **EVIDENCE BASE** Much research has been done regarding the application of permanent pacemakers in patients other than those with symptomatic bradycardia.

# Understanding pacemaker codes

A permanent pacemaker's three-letter (or sometimes five-letter) code simply refers to how it's programmed. The first letter represents the chamber that's paced; the second letter, the chamber that's sensed; and the third letter, how the pulse generator responds.

| First letter | Second letter | Third letter |
|---|---|---|
| A = atrium | A = atrium | I = inhibited |
| V = ventricle | V = ventricle | T = triggered |
| D = dual (both chambers) | D = dual (both chambers) | D = dual (inhibited and triggered) |
| O = not applicable | O = not applicable | O = not applicable |

### Examples of two common programming codes

| DDD | VVI |
|---|---|
| Pace: atrium and ventricle | Pace: ventricle |
| Sense: atrium and ventricle | Sense: ventricle |
| Response: inhibited and triggered | Response: inhibited |
| This is a fully automatic, or universal, pacemaker. | This is a demand pacemaker that's inhibited when ventricular activity is sensed. |

Permanent pacemakers are also being used in patients with hypertrophic obstructive cardiomyopathy, dilated cardiomyopathy, atrial fibrillation, neurocardiogenic syndrome, and long-QT syndrome.

## Equipment

Sphygmomanometer • stethoscope • ECG monitor and strip-chart recorder • sterile dressing tray • povidone-iodine ointment • shaving supplies • sterile gauze dressing • hypoallergenic tape • sedatives • alcohol pads • emergency resuscitation equipment • sterile gown and mask • optional: I.V. line for emergency medications

## Implementation

▶ Explain the procedure to the patient. Provide and review literature from the manufacturer or the American Heart Association so he can learn about the pacemaker and how it works. Emphasize that the pacemaker merely augments his natural heart rate.
▶ Ensure that the patient or a responsible family member signs a consent form, and ask the patient if he's allergic to anesthetics or iodine.

### Preoperative care

▶ For pacemaker insertion, shave the patient's chest from the axilla to the midline and from the clavicle to the nipple line on the side selected by the doctor.
▶ Establish an I.V. line at a keep-vein-open rate so that you can administer emergency drugs if the patient experiences ventricular arrhythmia.
▶ Obtain baseline vital signs and a baseline ECG.
▶ Provide sedation as ordered.

### Intraoperative care

▶ If you'll be present to monitor arrhythmias during the procedure, put on a gown and mask.
▶ Connect the ECG monitor to the patient, and run a baseline rhythm strip. Make sure that the machine has enough paper to run additional rhythm strips during the procedure.
▶ In transvenous placement, the doctor, guided by a fluoroscope, passes the electrode catheter through the cephalic or external jugular vein and positions it in the right ventricle. He attaches the catheter to the pulse generator, inserts this into the

# Teaching the patient who has a permanent pacemaker

If your patient is going home with a permanent pacemaker, teach him about daily care, safety and activity guidelines, and other precautions..

### Daily care

▶ Clean your pacemaker site gently with soap and water when you take a shower or a bath. Leave the incision exposed to the air.

▶ Inspect your skin around the incision. A slight bulge is normal, but call your doctor if you feel discomfort or notice swelling, redness, a discharge, or other problems.

▶ Check your pulse for 1 minute as your nurse or doctor showed you — on the side of your neck, inside your elbow, or on the thumb side of your wrist. Your pulse rate should be the same as your pacemaker rate or faster. Contact your doctor if you think your heart is beating too fast or too slow.

▶ Take your medications, including those for pain, as prescribed. Even with a pacemaker, you still need the medication your doctor ordered.

### Safety and activity

▶ Keep your pacemaker instruction booklet handy, and carry your pacemaker identification card at all times. This card has your pacemaker model number and other information needed by health care personnel who treat you.

▶ You can resume most of your usual activities when you feel comfortable doing so, but don't drive until the doctor gives you permission. Also avoid heavy lifting and stretching and exercises that involve lifting the same side as the pacemaker for at least 4 weeks or as directed by your doctor.

▶ Try to use both arms equally to prevent stiffness. Check with your doctor before you golf, swim, play tennis, or perform other strenuous activities.

### Electromagnetic interference

▶ Today pacemakers are designed and insulated to eliminate most electrical interference. You can safely operate common household electrical devices, including microwave ovens, razors, and sewing machines. You can ride in or operate a motor vehicle without it affecting your pacemaker.

▶ Take care to avoid direct contact with large running motors, high-powered citizen-band radios and other similar equipment, welding machinery, and radar devices.

▶ If your pacemaker activates the metal detector in an airport, show your pacemaker identification card to the security official.

▶ Because the metal in your pacemaker makes you ineligible for certain diagnostic studies, such as magnetic resonance imaging, be sure to inform your doctors, dentist, and other health care personnel that you have a pacemaker.

▶ When using a cellular phone, use it on the side opposite your pacemaker.

### Special precautions

▶ If you feel light-headed or dizzy when you're near any electrical equipment, moving away from the device should restore normal pacemaker function. Ask your doctor about particular electrical devices.

▶ Notify your doctor if you experience any signs of pacemaker failure, such as palpitations, a fast heart rate, a slow heart rate (5 to 10 beats less than the pacemaker's setting), dizziness, fainting, shortness of breath, swollen ankles or feet, anxiety, forgetfulness, or confusion.

### Checkups

▶ Be sure to schedule and keep regular checkup appointments with your doctor.

▶ If your doctor checks your pacemaker status by telephone, keep your transmission schedule and instructions in a handy place.

---

chest wall, and sutures it closed, leaving a small outlet for a drainage tube.

## Postoperative care

▶ Monitor the patient's ECG to check for arrhythmias and to ensure correct pacemaker functioning.

▶ Monitor the I.V. flow rate; the I.V. line is usually kept in place for 24 to 48 hours postoperatively to allow for possible emergency treatment of arrhythmias.

▶ Check the dressing for signs of bleeding and infection (swelling, redness, or exudate). The doctor may order prophylactic antibiotics for up to 7 days after the implantation.

▶ Change the dressing and apply povidone-iodine ointment at least once every 24 to

48 hours, or according to doctor's orders and facility policy. If the dressing becomes soiled or the site is exposed to air, change the dressing immediately, regardless of when you last changed it.

▶ Check vital signs and level of consciousness (LOC) every 15 minutes for the first hour, every hour for the next 4 hours, every 4 hours for the next 48 hours, and then once every shift.

◆◆ **ALERT!** Confused, elderly patients with second-degree heart block won't show immediate improvement in LOC.

◆◆ **ALERT!** Watch for signs and symptoms of a perforated ventricle, with resultant cardiac tamponade: persistent hiccups, distant heart sounds, pulsus paradoxus, hypotension with narrow pulse pressure, increased venous pressure, cyanosis, distended neck veins, decreased urine output, restlessness, or complaints of fullness in the chest. If the patient develops any of these, notify the doctor immediately.

## Special considerations

▶ If the patient wears a hearing aid, the pacemaker battery is placed on the opposite side accordingly.

▶ Provide the patient with an identification card that lists the pacemaker type and manufacturer, serial number, pacemaker rate setting, date implanted, and doctor's name. (See *Teaching the patient who has a permanent pacemaker.*)

▶ Watch for signs of pacemaker malfunction.

## Complications

Insertion of a permanent pacemaker places the patient at risk for certain complications, such as infection, lead displacement, a perforated ventricle, cardiac tamponade, or lead fracture and disconnection.

## Documentation

▶ Document the type of pacemaker used, the serial number and the manufacturer's name, the pacing rate, the date of implantation, and the doctor's name.

▶ Note whether the pacemaker successfully treated the patient's arrhythmias and the condition of the incision site.

## REFERENCES

American College of Cardiology and the American Heart Association. "1999 Update: ACC/AHA Guidelines for Management of Patients with Acute Myocardial Infarction," *Journal of the American College of Cardiology* 34(3):890-911, September 1999.

Clark, A. "Troubleshooting Cardiac Pacemaker Problems," 2000. *www.nursingceu.com.*

Obias-Manno, D. "Unconventional Applications in Pacemaker Therapy," *AACN Clinical Issues* 12(1):127-39, February 2001.

Shaffer, K.B. "Keeping Pace with Permanent Pacemakers," *Dimensions of Critical Care Nursing* 18(6):2-8, November-December 1999.

# Posterior chest lead electrocardiography

Because of the location of the heart's posterior surface, changes associated with myocardial damage aren't apparent on a standard 12-lead ECG. To help identify posterior involvement, some health care providers recommend adding posterior leads to the 12-lead ECG. Despite lung and muscle barriers, posterior leads may provide clues to posterior wall infarction so that appropriate treatment can begin.

Usually, the posterior lead ECG is performed with a standard ECG and only involves recording the additional posterior leads: $V_7$, $V_8$, and $V_9$.

## Equipment

Multichannel or single-channel ECG machine with recording paper ● disposable pregelled electrodes ● 4″ × 4″ gauze pads or moist cloth ● optional: shaving supplies

## Implementation

▶ Prepare the electrode sites according to the manufacturer's instructions. To ensure good skin contact, shave the site if the patient has considerable back hair.

▶ If you're using a multichannel ECG machine, begin by attaching a disposable electrode to the $V_7$ position on the left posterior axillary line, fifth intercostal space. Then attach the $V_4$ leadwire to the $V_7$ electrode.

▶ Next, attach a disposable electrode to the patient's back at the $V_8$ position on the left midscapular line, fifth intercostal space, and attach the $V_5$ leadwire to this electrode.

▶ Finally, attach a disposable electrode to the patient's back at the $V_9$ position, just left of the spinal column at the fifth intercostal space (as shown below). Then attach the $V_6$ leadwire to the $V_9$ electrode.

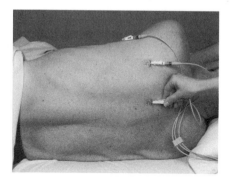

▶ If you're using a single-channel ECG machine, put electrode gel at locations for electrodes $V_7$, $V_8$, and $V_9$. Then connect the brown leadwire to the $V_7$ electrode.

▶ Turn on the machine and make sure that the paper speed is set for 25 mm/second. If necessary, standardize the machine. Press auto and the machine will record.

▶ If you're using a multichannel ECG machine, all leads will print out as a straight line except those labeled $V_4$, $V_5$, and $V_6$. Relabel those leads $V_7$, $V_8$, and $V_9$, respectively.

▶ If you're using a single-channel ECG machine, turn the selector knob to "V" to record the $V_7$ lead. Then stop the machine. Reposition the electrode to the $V_8$ position and record that lead. Repeat the procedure for the $V_9$ position.

▶ When the ECG is complete, remove the electrodes and clean the patient's skin with a gauze pad or a moist cloth. If you think you may need more than one posterior lead ECG, use a marking pen to mark the electrode sites on his skin to permit accurate comparison for future tracings.

### Special considerations

▶ The number of leads may vary according to the cardiologist's preference. (If right posterior leads are requested, position the patient on his left side. These leads, known as $V_{7R}$, $V_{8R}$, and $V_{9R}$, are located at the same landmarks on the right side of the patient's back.)

▶ Some ECG machines won't operate unless you connect all leadwires. In that case, you may need to connect the limb leadwires and the leadwires for $V_1$, $V_2$, and $V_3$.

### Documentation

▶ Document the procedure in your nurse's notes. Make sure that the patient's name, age, and room number, the time and date, and the doctor's name are clearly written on the ECG along with the relabeled lead tracings.

▶ Document any patient teaching you may have performed as well as the patient's tolerance to the procedure.

### REFERENCES

Khaw, K., et al. "Improved Detection of Posterior Myocardial Wall Ischemia with the 15-lead Electrocardiogram," *American Heart Journal* 138(5 Part I):934-40, November 1999.

Wung, S.F., and Drew, B.J. "New Electrocardiographic Criteria for Posterior Wall Acute Myocardial Ischemia Validated by a Percutaneous Transluminal Coronary Angioplasty Model of Acute Myocardial Infarction" *American Journal of Cardiology* 87(8): 970-74, April 2001.

# Right chest lead electrocardiography

Unlike a standard 12-lead ECG, used primarily to evaluate left ventricular function, a right chest lead ECG reflects right ventricular function and provides clues to damage or dysfunction in this chamber. You might need to perform a right chest lead ECG for a patient with an inferior wall myocardial infarction (MI) and suspected right ventricular involvement. Between 25% and 50% of patients with this type of MI have right ventricular involvement. Many of these patients have high creatine kinase levels.

Early identification of a right ventricular MI is essential because its treatment differs from that for other MIs. For instance, in left ventricular MI, treatment involves withholding I.V. fluids or administering them judiciously to prevent heart failure. Conversely, in right ventricular MI, treatment usually requires administration of I.V. fluids to maintain adequate filling pressures on the right side of the heart. This helps the right ventricle eject an adequate volume of blood at an adequate pressure.

## Equipment

Multichannel ECG machine ● paper ● pre-gelled disposable electrodes ● several 4″ × 4″ gauze pads

## Implementation

▶ Take the equipment to the patient's bedside and explain the procedure to him. Inform him that the doctor has ordered a right chest lead ECG, a procedure that involves placing electrodes on his wrists, ankles, and chest. Reassure him that the test is painless and takes only a few minutes, during which he'll need to lie quietly on his back.

▶ Make sure that the paper speed is set at 25 mm/second and the amplitude at 1 mV/10 mm.

▶ Place the patient in a supine position or, if he has difficulty lying flat, in semi-Fowler's position. Provide privacy and expose his arms, chest, and legs. (Cover a female patient's chest with a drape until you apply the chest leads.)

▶ Examine the patient's wrists and ankles for the best areas to place the electrodes. Choose flat and fleshy (not bony or muscular), hairless areas such as the inner aspects of the wrists and ankles. Clean the sites with the gauze pads to promote good skin contact.

▶ Connect the leadwires to the electrodes. The leadwires are color-coded and lettered. Place the white or right arm (RA) wire on the right arm; the black or left arm (LA) wire on the left arm; the green or right leg (RL) wire on the right leg; and the red or left leg (LL) wire on the left leg.

▶ Then examine the patient's chest to locate the correct sites for chest lead placement (as shown below). If the patient is a woman, place the electrodes under the breast tissue.

▶ Use your fingers to feel between the patient's ribs (the intercostal spaces). Start at the second intercostal space on the left (the notch felt at the top of the sternum, where the manubrium joins the body of the sternum). Count down two spaces to the fourth intercostal space. Then apply a disposable electrode to the site and attach leadwire $V_{1R}$ to that electrode.

▶ Move your fingers across the sternum to the fourth intercostal space on the right side of the sternum. Apply a disposable electrode to that site and attach lead $V_{2R}$.

▶ Move your finger down to the fifth intercostal space and over to the midclavicular line. Place a disposable electrode here and attach lead $V_{4R}$.

▶ Visually draw a line between $V_{2R}$ and $V_{4R}$. Apply a disposable electrode midway on this line and attach lead $V_{3R}$.

▶ Move your finger horizontally from $V_{4R}$ to the right midaxillary line. Apply a disposable electrode to this site and attach lead $V_{6R}$.

▶ Move your fingers along the same horizontal line to the midpoint between $V_{4R}$ and $V_{6R}$. This is the right anterior midaxillary line. Apply a disposable electrode to this site and attach lead $V_{5R}$.

▶ Turn on the ECG machine. Ask the patient to breathe normally but to refrain from talking during the recording so that muscle movement won't distort the tracing. Enter any appropriate patient information required by the machine you're using. If necessary, standardize the machine. This will cause a square tracing of 10 mm (two large squares) to appear on the ECG paper when the machine is set for 1 mV (1 mV = 10 mm).

▶ Press the auto key. The ECG machine will record all 12 leads automatically. Check your facility's policy for the number of readings to obtain. (Some facilities require at least two ECGs so that one copy can be sent out for interpretation while the other remains at the bedside.)

▶ When you're finished recording the ECG, turn off the machine. Clearly label the ECG with the patient's name, the date, and the time. Also label the tracing "Right chest ECG" to distinguish it from a standard 12-lead ECG. Remove the electrodes and help the patient get comfortable.

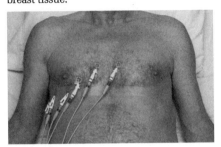

## Special considerations

For best results, place the electrodes symmetrically on the limbs. If the patient's wrist or ankle is covered by a dressing, or if the patient is an amputee, choose an area that is available on both sides.

## Documentation

▶ Document the procedure in your nurse's notes, and document the patient's tolerance to the procedure. Place a copy of the tracing in the patient's chart.

### REFERENCES

Haji, S.A., and Movahed, A. "Right Ventricular Infarction—Diagnosis and Treatment." *Clinical Cardiology* 23(7):473-82, July 2000.

Horan, L.G., and Flowers, N.D. "Right Ventricular Infarction: Specific Requirements of Management," *American Family Physician,* 60(6):1727-34, October 1999.

Kosuge, M., et al. "Implications of the Absence of ST-Segment Elevation in Lead $V_{4R}$ in Patients who Have Inferior Wall Acute Myocardial Infarction with Right Ventricular Involvement," *Clinical Cardiology* 24(3):225-30, March 2001.

# Synchronized cardioversion

Used to treat tachyarrhythmias, synchronized cardioversion delivers an electric charge to the myocardium at the peak of the R wave. This causes immediate depolarization, interrupting reentry circuits, and allowing the sinoatrial node to resume control. Synchronizing the electric charge with the R wave ensures that the current won't be delivered on the vulnerable T wave and thus disrupt repolarization.

Synchronized cardioversion is the treatment of choice for arrhythmias that don't respond to vagal massage or drug therapy, such as atrial tachycardia, atrial flutter, atrial fibrillation, and symptomatic ventricular tachycardia.

Cardioversion may be an elective or urgent procedure, depending on how well the patient tolerates the arrhythmia. For example, if the patient is hemodynamically unstable, he'd require urgent cardioversion. Remember that, when preparing for cardioversion, the patient's condition can deteriorate quickly, necessitating immediate defibrillation.

Indications for cardioversion include stable paroxysmal atrial tachycardia, unstable paroxysmal supraventricular tachycardia, atrial fibrillation, atrial flutter, and ventricular tachycardia.

▪ **EVIDENCE BASE** 2000 AHA guidelines for the treatment of symptomatic (unstable) tachycardias recommend immediate synchronized cardioversion rather than a trial of antiarrhythmics, as was recommended in the past. Treatment must be preceded by rhythm diagnosis and duration and recognizing patients with severely impaired cardiac function (ejection fraction of less than 40% or signs of heart failure). Atrial fibrillation or flutter lasting longer than 48 hours must be anticoagulated before cardioversion.

## Equipment

Cardioverter-defibrillator ● conductive gel pads ● anterior, posterior, or transverse paddles ● ECG monitor with recorder ● sedative ● oxygen therapy equipment ● airway ● handheld resuscitation bag ● emergency pacing equipment ● emergency cardiac medications ● automatic blood pressure cuff (if available) ● pulse oximeter (if available)

## Implementation

▶ Explain the procedure to the patient and make sure he has signed a consent form.
▶ Check the patient's recent serum potassium and magnesium levels and arterial blood gas results. Also, check recent digoxin levels. Although digitalized patients may undergo cardioversion, they tend to require lower energy levels to convert. If the patient takes digoxin, withhold the dose on the day of the procedure.
▶ Withhold all food and fluids for 6 to 12 hours before the procedure. If the cardioversion is urgent, withhold the previous meal.
▶ Obtain a 12-lead ECG to serve as a baseline.
▶ Check to see if the doctor has ordered administration of any cardiac drugs before the procedure. Also, verify that the patient has a patent I.V. site in case drug administration becomes necessary.
▶ Connect the patient to a pulse oximeter and automatic blood pressure cuff, if available.
▶ Consider administering oxygen for 5 to 10 minutes before the cardioversion to pro-

mote myocardial oxygenation. If the patient wears dentures, evaluate whether they support his airway or might cause an airway obstruction. If they might cause an obstruction, remove them.

▶ Place the patient in the supine position and assess his vital signs, level of consciousness (LOC), cardiac rhythm, and peripheral pulses.

▶ Remove any oxygen delivery device just before cardioversion to avoid possible combustion.

▶ Have epinephrine, lidocaine, and atropine at the patient's bedside.

▶ Make sure the resuscitation bag is at the patient's bedside.

▶ Administer a sedative as ordered. The patient should be heavily sedated but still able to breathe adequately.

▶ Carefully monitor the patient's blood pressure and respiratory rate until he recovers.

▶ Press the power button to turn on the defibrillator. Next, push the sync button to synchronize the machine with the patient's QRS complexes. Make sure the sync button flashes with each of the patient's QRS complexes. You should also see a bright green flag flash on the monitor.

▶ Turn the energy select dial to the ordered amount of energy. Advanced Cardiac Life Support protocols call for 50 to 360 joules for a patient with stable paroxysmal atrial tachycardia, 75 to 360 joules for a patient with unstable paroxysmal supraventricular tachycardia, 100 joules for a patient with atrial fibrillation, 50 joules for a patient with atrial flutter, 100 to 360 joules for a patient who has ventricular tachycardia with a pulse, and 200 to 360 joules for a patient with pulseless ventricular tachycardia.

▶ Remove the paddles from the machine and prepare them as you would if you were defibrillating the patient. Place the conductive gel pads or paddles in the same positions as you would to defibrillate.

▶ Make sure everyone stands away from the bed; then push the discharge buttons. Hold the paddles in place and wait for the energy to be discharged—the machine has to synchronize the discharge with the QRS complex.

▶ Check the waveform on the monitor. If the arrhythmia fails to convert, repeat the procedure two or three more times at 3-minute intervals. Gradually increase the energy level with each additional countershock.

▶ After the cardioversion, frequently assess the patient's LOC and respiratory status, including airway patency, respiratory rate and depth, and the need for supplemental oxygen. Because the patient will be heavily sedated, he may require airway support.

▶ Record a postcardioversion 12-lead ECG and monitor the patient's ECG rhythm for 2 hours. Check the patient's chest for electrical burns.

## Special considerations

▶ If the patient is attached to a bedside or telemetry monitor, disconnect the unit before cardioversion. The electric current it generates could damage the equipment.

▶ Be aware that improper synchronization may result if the patient's ECG tracing contains artifact-like spikes, such as peaked T waves or bundle-branch heart blocks when the R8 wave may be taller than the R wave.

▶ Although the electric shock of cardioversion won't usually damage an implanted pacemaker, avoid placing the paddles directly over the pacemaker.

## Complications

Common complications following cardioversion include transient, harmless arrhythmias such as atrial, ventricular, and junctional premature beats. Serious ventricular arrhythmias such as ventricular fibrillation may also occur. However, this type of arrhythmia is more likely to result from high amounts of electrical energy, digitalis toxicity, severe heart disease, electrolyte imbalance, or improper synchronization with the R wave.

## Documentation

▶ Document the procedure, including the voltage delivered with each attempt, rhythm strips before and after the procedure, and how the patient tolerated the procedure.

### REFERENCES

American College of Cardiology and the American Heart Association. "1999 Update: ACC/AHA Guidelines for Management of Patients with Acute Myocardial Infarction," *Journal of the American College of Cardiology* 34(3):890-911, September 1999.

American Heart Association. "Guidelines 2000 for Cardiopulmonary Resuscitation and Emergency Cardiovascular Care: International Consensus on Science," *Circulation* 102(8 Suppl):I-384, August 2000.

Begany, T. "Major Changes Made to ACLS Guidelines," *Pulmonary Reviews* 5(11), November 2000. *www.pulmonaryreviews.com/archives.html.*

*Mastering ACLS.* Springhouse, Pa.: Springhouse Corp., 2002.

# Temporary pacemaker insertion and care

Usually inserted in an emergency, a temporary pacemaker consists of an external, battery-powered pulse generator and a lead or electrode system. Four types of temporary pacemakers exist: transcutaneous, transvenous, transthoracic, and epicardial.

In a life-threatening situation, when time is critical, a transcutaneous pacemaker is the best choice. This device works by sending an electrical impulse from the pulse generator to the patient's heart by way of two electrodes, which are placed on the front and back of the patient's chest. Transcutaneous pacing is quick and effective, but it's used only until the doctor can institute transvenous pacing.

In addition to being more comfortable for the patient, a transvenous pacemaker is more reliable than a transcutaneous pacemaker. Transvenous pacing involves threading an electrode catheter through a vein into the patient's right atrium or right ventricle. The electrode then attaches to an external pulse generator. As a result, the pulse generator can provide an electrical stimulus directly to the endocardium. This is the most common type of pacemaker.

As an elective surgical procedure or as an emergency measure during cardiopulmonary resuscitation (CPR), a doctor may choose to insert a transthoracic pacemaker. To insert this type of pacemaker, the doctor performs a procedure similar to pericardiocentesis, in which he uses a cardiac needle to pass an electrode through the chest wall and into the right ventricle. This procedure carries a significant risk of coronary artery laceration and cardiac tamponade.

During cardiac surgery, the surgeon may insert electrodes through the epicardium of the right ventricle and, if he wants to institute atrioventricular sequential pacing, the right atrium. From there, the electrodes pass through the chest wall, where they remain available if temporary pacing becomes necessary. This is called epicardial pacing.

In addition to helping to correct conduction disturbances, a temporary pacemaker may help diagnose conduction abnormalities. For example, during a cardiac catheterization or electrophysiology study, a doctor may use a temporary pacemaker to localize conduction defects. In the process, he may also learn whether the patient risks developing an arrhythmia.

Among the contraindications to pacemaker therapy are electromechanical dissociation and ventricular fibrillation.

## Equipment
*For transcutaneous pacing*
Transcutaneous pacing generator • cardiac monitor • transcutaneous pacing electrodes

*For all other types of temporary pacing*
Temporary pacemaker generator with new battery • guide wire or introducer • electrode catheter • sterile gloves • sterile dressings • adhesive tape • povidone-iodine solution • nonconducting tape or rubber surgical glove • emergency cardiac drugs • intubation equipment • defibrillator • cardiac monitor with strip-chart recorder • equipment to start a peripheral I.V. line, if appropriate • I.V. fluids • sedative • optional: elastic bandage or gauze strips, restraints

*For transvenous pacing*
All equipment listed for temporary pacing • bridging cable • percutaneous introducer tray or venous cutdown tray • sterile gowns • linen-saver pad • antimicrobial soap • alcohol pads • vial of 1% lidocaine • 5-ml syringe • fluoroscopy equipment, if necessary • fenestrated drape • prepackaged cutdown tray (for antecubital vein placement only) • sutures • receptacle for infectious wastes

*For transthoracic pacing*
All equipment listed for temporary pacing • transthoracic or cardiac needle

*For epicardial pacing*

All equipment listed for temporary pacing • atrial epicardial wires • ventricular epicardial wires • sterile rubber finger cot • sterile dressing materials (if the wires won't be connected to a pulse generator)

## Implementation

▶ If applicable, explain the procedure to the patient.

### For transcutaneous pacing

▶ If necessary, clip the hair over the areas of electrode placement. However, don't shave the area. If you nick the skin, the current from the pulse generator could cause discomfort and the nicks could become irritated or infected after the electrodes are applied.

▶ Attach monitoring electrodes to the patient in lead I, II, or III position. Do this even if the patient is already on telemetry monitoring because you'll need to connect the electrodes to the pacemaker. If you select the lead II position, adjust the LL electrode placement to accommodate the anterior pacing electrode and the patient's anatomy.

▶ Plug the patient cable into the ECG input connection on the front of the pacing generator. Set the selector switch to the monitor on position.

▶ You should see the ECG waveform on the monitor. Adjust the R-wave beeper volume to a suitable level and activate the alarm by pressing the alarm on button. Set the alarm for 10 to 20 beats lower and 20 to 30 beats higher than the intrinsic rate.

▶ Press the START/STOP button for a printout of the waveform.

▶ Now you're ready to apply the two pacing electrodes. First, make sure the patient's skin is clean and dry to ensure good skin contact.

▶ Pull off the protective strip from the posterior electrode (marked back) and apply the electrode on the left side of the back, just below the scapula and to the left of the spine.

▶ The anterior pacing electrode (marked front) has two protective strips — one covering the jellied area and one covering the outer rim. Expose the jellied area and apply it to the skin in the anterior position — to the left side of the precordium in the usual $V_2$ to $V_5$ position. Move this elec-

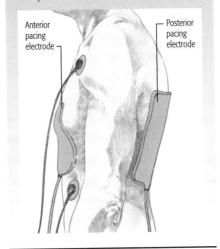
trode around to get the best waveform. Then expose the electrode's outer rim and firmly press it to the skin. (See *Proper electrode placement*.)

▶ Now you're ready to pace the heart. After making sure the energy output in milliamperes (mA) is on 0, connect the electrode cable to the monitor output cable.

▶ Check the waveform, looking for a tall QRS complex in lead II.

▶ Next, turn the selector switch to pacer on. Tell the patient that he may feel a thumping or twitching sensation. Reassure him that you'll give him medication if he can't tolerate the discomfort.

▶ Now set the rate dial to 10 to 20 beats higher than the patient's intrinsic rhythm. Look for pacer artifact or spikes, which will appear as you increase the rate. If the patient doesn't have an intrinsic rhythm, set the rate at 60.

▶ Slowly increase the amount of energy delivered to the heart by adjusting the output mA dial. Do this until capture is achieved — you'll see a pacer spike followed by a widened QRS complex that resembles a premature ventricular contraction. This is the pacing threshold. To ensure consistent capture, increase output by 10%. Don't go any higher because you could cause the patient needless discomfort.

▶ With full capture, the patient's heart rate should be approximately the same as the pacemaker rate set on the machine. The usual pacing threshold is between 40 and 80 mA.

### For transvenous pacing
▶ Check the patient's history for hypersensitivity to local anesthetics. Then attach the cardiac monitor to the patient and obtain a baseline assessment, including the patient's vital signs, skin color, level of consciousness (LOC), heart rate and rhythm, and emotional state. Next, insert a peripheral I.V. line if the patient doesn't already have one. Begin an I.V. infusion at a keep-vein-open rate.

▶ Insert a new battery into the external pacemaker generator, and test it to make sure it has a strong charge. Connect the bridging cable to the generator, and align the positive and negative poles. This cable allows slack between the electrode catheter and the generator, reducing the risk of accidental catheter displacement.

▶ Place the patient in the supine position. If necessary, clip the hair around the insertion site. Next, open the supply tray while maintaining a sterile field. Using sterile technique, clean the insertion site with antimicrobial soap and then wipe the area with povidone-iodine solution. Cover the insertion site with a fenestrated drape. Because fluoroscopy may be used during the placement of leadwires, put on a protective apron.

▶ Provide the doctor with the local anesthetic.

▶ After anesthetizing the insertion site, the doctor will puncture the brachial, femoral, subclavian, or jugular vein. Then he'll insert a guide wire or an introducer and advance the electrode catheter.

▶ As the catheter advances, watch the cardiac monitor. When the electrode catheter reaches the right atrium, you'll notice large P waves and small QRS complexes. Then, as the catheter reaches the right ventricle,

the P waves will become smaller while the QRS complexes enlarge. When the catheter touches the right ventricular endocardium, expect to see elevated ST segments, premature ventricular contractions, or both.

▶ When the electrode catheter is in the right ventricle, it will send an impulse to the myocardium, causing depolarization. If the patient needs atrial pacing, either alone or with ventricular pacing, the doctor may place an electrode in the right atrium.

▶ Meanwhile, continuously monitor the patient's cardiac status and treat any arrhythmias, as appropriate. Also assess the patient for jaw pain and earache; these symptoms indicate that the electrode catheter has missed the superior vena cava and has moved into the neck instead.

▶ When the electrode catheter is in place, attach the catheter leads to the bridging cable, lining up the positive and negative poles.

▶ Check the battery's charge by pressing the battery test button.

▶ Set the pacemaker as ordered.

▶ The doctor will then suture the catheter to the insertion site. Afterward, put on sterile gloves and apply a sterile dressing to the site. Label the dressing with the date and time of application.

### For transthoracic pacing
▶ Clean the skin to the left of the xiphoid process with povidone-iodine solution. Work quickly because CPR must be interrupted for the procedure.

▶ After interrupting CPR, the doctor will insert a transthoracic needle through the patient's chest wall to the left of the xiphoid process into the right ventricle. He'll then follow the needle with the electrode catheter.

▶ Connect the electrode catheter to the generator, lining up the positive and negative poles. Watch the cardiac monitor for signs of ventricular pacing and capture.

▶ After the doctor sutures the electrode catheter into place, use sterile technique to apply a sterile 4″ × 4″ gauze dressing to the site. Tape the dressing securely, and label it with the date and time of application.

▶ Check the patient's peripheral pulses and vital signs to assess cardiac output. If you can't palpate a pulse, continue performing CPR.

▶ If the patient has a palpable pulse, assess the patient's vital signs, ECG, and LOC.

### For epicardial pacing

▶ During your preoperative teaching, inform the patient that epicardial pacemaker wires may be placed during cardiac surgery.

▶ During cardiac surgery, the doctor will hook epicardial wires into the epicardium just before the end of the surgery. Depending on the patient's condition, the doctor may insert either atrial or ventricular wires, or both.

▶ If indicated, connect the electrode catheter to the generator, lining up the positive and negative poles. Set the pacemaker as ordered.

▶ If the wires won't be connected to an external pulse generator, place them in a sterile rubber finger cot. Then cover both the wires and the insertion site with a sterile, occlusive dressing. This will help protect the patient from microshock as well as infection.

### Special considerations

▶ Take care to prevent microshock. This includes warning the patient not to use any electrical equipment that isn't grounded, such as telephones, electric shavers, televisions, or lamps.

▶ Other safety measures you'll want to take include placing a plastic cover supplied by the manufacturer over the pacemaker controls to avoid an accidental setting change. Also, insulate the pacemaker by covering all exposed metal parts, such as electrode connections and pacemaker terminals, with nonconducting tape, or place the pacing unit in a dry, rubber surgical glove. If the patient is disoriented or uncooperative, use restraints to prevent accidental removal of pacemaker wires. If the patient needs emergency defibrillation, make sure the pacemaker can withstand the procedure. If you're unsure, disconnect the pulse generator to avoid damage.

▶ When using a transcutaneous pacemaker, don't place the electrodes over a bony area because bone conducts current poorly. With female patients, place the anterior electrode under the patient's breast but not over her diaphragm. If the doctor inserts the electrode through the brachial or femoral vein, immobilize the patient's arm or leg to avoid putting stress on the pacing wires.

▶ After insertion of any temporary pacemaker, assess the patient's vital signs, skin color, LOC, and peripheral pulses to determine the effectiveness of the paced rhythm. Perform a 12-lead ECG to serve as a baseline, and then perform additional ECGs daily or with clinical changes. Also, if possible, obtain a rhythm strip before, during, and after pacemaker placement; any time that pacemaker settings are changed; and whenever the patient receives treatment because of a complication due to the pacemaker.

▶ Continuously monitor the ECG reading, noting capture, sensing, rate, intrinsic beats, and competition of paced and intrinsic rhythms. If the pacemaker is sensing correctly, the sense indicator on the pulse generator should flash with each beat. (See *When a temporary pacemaker malfunctions,* pages 296 and 297.)

▶ Record the date and time of pacemaker insertion, the type of pacemaker, the reason for insertion, and the patient's response. Note the pacemaker settings. Document any complications and the interventions taken.

▶ If the patient has epicardial pacing wires in place, clean the insertion site with povidone-iodine solution and change the dressing daily. At the same time, monitor the site for signs of infection. Always keep the pulse generator nearby in case pacing becomes necessary.

### Complications

Complications associated with pacemaker therapy include microshock, equipment failure, and competitive or fatal arrhythmias. Transcutaneous pacemakers may also cause skin breakdown and muscle pain and twitching when the pacemaker fires. Transvenous pacemakers may cause such complications as pneumothorax or hemothorax, cardiac perforation and tamponade, diaphragmatic stimulation, pulmonary embolism, thrombophlebitis, and infection. Also, if the doctor threads the electrode through the antecubital or femoral vein, venous spasm, thrombophlebitis, or lead displacement may result.

Complications associated with transthoracic pacemakers include pneumothorax, cardiac tamponade, emboli, sepsis,

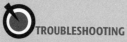

TROUBLESHOOTING

# When a temporary pacemaker malfunctions

Occasionally, a temporary pacemaker may fail to function appropriately. When this occurs, you'll need to take immediate action to correct the problem. Here you'll learn which steps to take when your patient's pacemaker fails to pace, capture, or sense intrinsic beats.

## Failure to pace

Failure to pace occurs when the pacemaker doesn't fire or fires too often. The pulse generator may not be working properly, or it may not be conducting the impulse to the patient.

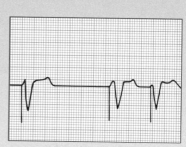

### Nursing interventions

▶ If the pacing or sensing indicator flashes, check the connections to the cable and the position of the pacing electrode in the patient (by X-ray). The cable may have come loose, or the electrode may have been dislodged, pulled out, or broken.

▶ If the pulse generator is turned on but the indicators still aren't flashing, change the battery. If that doesn't help, use a different pulse generator.

▶ Check the settings if the pacemaker is firing too rapidly. If they're correct, or if altering them (according to your facility's policy or the doctor's order) doesn't help, change the pulse generator.

## Failure to capture

In failure to capture, you see pacemaker spikes but the heart isn't responding. This may be caused by changes in the pacing threshold from ischemia, an electrolyte imbalance (high or low potassium or magnesium levels), acidosis, an adverse reaction to a medication, a perforated ventricle, fibrosis, or the position of the electrode.

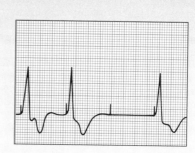

### Nursing interventions

▶ If the patient's condition has changed, notify the doctor and ask him for new settings.

▶ If pacemaker settings are altered by the patient or another, return them to their correct positions. Then make sure the pacemaker's face is covered with a plastic shield. Tell the patient or others not to touch the dials.

▶ If the heart isn't responding, try any or all of these suggestions: Carefully check all connections; increase the milliamperes slowly (according to your facility's policy or the doctor's order); turn the patient on his left side, then on his right (if turning him to the left didn't help); reverse the cable in the pulse generator so the positive electrode wire is in the negative terminal and the negative electrode wire is in the positive terminal; schedule an anteroposterior or lateral chest X-ray to determine the position of the electrode.

---

lacerations of the myocardium or coronary artery, and perforations of a cardiac chamber. Epicardial pacemakers carry a risk of infection, cardiac arrest, and diaphragmatic stimulation.

## Documentation

▶ Record the reason for pacing, the time it started, and the locations of the electrodes. For a transvenous or transthoracic pacemaker, note the date, the time, and reason for the temporary pacemaker.

## When a temporary pacemaker malfunctions *(continued)*

### Failure to sense intrinsic beats

Failure to sense intrinsic beats could cause ventricular tachycardia or ventricular fibrillation if the pacemaker fires on the vulnerable T wave. This could be caused by the pacemaker sensing an external stimulus such as a QRS complex, which could lead to asystole, or by the pacemaker not being sensitive enough, which means it could fire anywhere within the cardiac cycle.

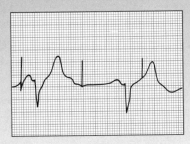

### Nursing interventions

▶ If the pacing is undersensing, turn the sensitivity control completely to the right. If it's oversensing, turn it slightly to the left.

▶ If the pacemaker isn't functioning correctly, change the battery or the pulse generator.

▶ Remove items in the room that could cause electromechanical interference (razors, radios, cautery devices, and so on). Check the ground wires on the bed and other equipment for obvious damage. Unplug each piece and see if the interference stops. When you locate the cause, notify the staff engineer and ask him to check it.

▶ If the pacemaker is still firing on the T wave and all else has failed, turn off the pacemaker. Make sure atropine is available in case the patient's heart rate drops. Be prepared to call a code and institute cardiopulmonary resuscitation, if necessary.

---

▶ For any temporary pacemaker, record the pacemaker settings. Note the patient's response to the procedure, along with any complications and the interventions taken. If possible, obtain rhythm strips before, during, and after pacemaker placement, and whenever pacemaker settings are changed or when the patient receives treatment for a complication caused by the pacemaker. As you monitor the patient, record his response to temporary pacing and note any changes in his condition.

### REFERENCES

American College of Cardiology and the American Heart Association. "1999 Update: ACC/AHA Guidelines for Management of Patients with Acute Myocardial Infarction," *Journal of the American College of Cardiology* 34(3):890-911, September 1999.

## Transducer system setup

The exact type of transducer system used depends on the patient's needs and the doctor's preference. Some systems monitor pressure continuously, whereas others monitor pressure intermittently. Single-pressure transducers monitor only one type of pressure — for example, pulmonary artery pressure (PAP). Multiple-pressure transducers can monitor two or more types of pressure, such as PAP and central venous pressure.

### Equipment

Bag of heparin flush solution (usually 500 ml normal saline solution with 500 or 1,000 units heparin) ● pressure infusion bag ● medication-added label ● preassembled disposable pressure tubing with flush device and disposable transducer ● monitor and monitor cable ● I.V. pole with transducer mount ● carpenter's level

### Preparation of equipment

Turn the monitor on before gathering the equipment to give it sufficient time to warm up. Gather the equipment you'll need. Wash your hands.

### Implementation

To set up and zero a single-pressure transducer system, perform the following steps.

### Setting up the system

▶ Follow your facility's policy on adding heparin to the flush solution. If your patient has a history of bleeding or clotting problems, use heparin with caution. Add the ordered amount of heparin to the solution—usually, 1 to 2 units of heparin/ml of solution—and then label the bag.

▸ Put the pressure module into the monitor, if necessary, and connect the transducer cable to the monitor.

▸ Remove the preassembled pressure tubing from the package. If necessary, connect the pressure tubing to the transducer. Tighten all tubing connections.

▸ Position all stopcocks so the flush solution can flow through the entire system. Then roll the tubing's flow regulator to the off position.

▸ Spike the flush solution bag with the tubing, invert the bag, open the roller clamp, and squeeze all the air through the drip chamber. Then, compress the tubing's drip chamber, filling it no more than halfway with the flush solution.

▸ Place the flush solution bag into the pressure infuser bag. To do this, hang the pressure infuser bag on the I.V. pole and then position the flush solution bag inside the pressure infuser bag.

▸ Open the tubing's flow regulator, uncoil the tube if you haven't already done so, and remove the protective cap at the end of the pressure tubing. Squeeze the continuous flush device slowly to prime the entire system, including the stopcock ports, with the flush solution.

▸ As the solution nears the disposable transducer, hold the transducer at a 45-degree angle (as shown below). This forces the solution to flow upward to the transducer. In doing so, the solution forces any air out of the system.

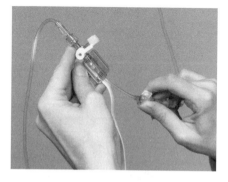

▸ When the solution nears a stopcock, open the stopcock to air, allowing the solution to flow into the stopcock (as shown at top of column). When the stopcock fills, close it

to air and turn it open to the remainder of the tubing. Do this for each stopcock.

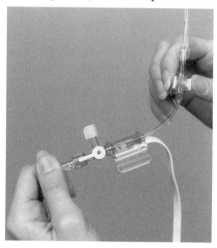

▸ After you've completely primed the system, replace the protective cap at the end of the tubing.

▸ Inflate the pressure infuser bag to 300 mm Hg. This bag keeps the pressure in the arterial line higher than the patient's systolic pressure, preventing blood backflow into the tubing and ensuring a continuous flow rate. When you inflate the pressure bag, take care that the drip chamber doesn't completely fill with fluid. Afterward, flush the system again to remove all air bubbles.

▸ Replace the vented caps on the stopcocks with sterile nonvented caps. If you're going to mount the transducer on an I.V. pole, insert the device into its holder.

### Zeroing the system

▸ Now you're ready for a preliminary zeroing of the transducer. To ensure accuracy, position the patient and the transducer on the same level each time you zero the transducer or record a pressure. Typically, the patient lies flat in bed, if he can tolerate that position.

▸ Next, use the carpenter's level to position the air-reference stopcock or the air-fluid interface of the transducer level with the phlebostatic axis (midway between the posterior chest and the sternum at the fourth intercostal space, midaxillary line). Alternatively, you may level the air-reference stopcock or the air-fluid interface to the same position as the catheter tip.

▶ After leveling the transducer, turn the stopcock next to the transducer off to the patient and open to air. Remove the cap to the stopcock port. Place the cap inside an opened sterile gauze package to prevent contamination.

▶ Now zero the transducer. To do so, follow the manufacturer's directions for zeroing.

▶ When you've finished zeroing, turn the stopcock on the transducer so that it's open to air and open to the patient. This is the monitoring position. Replace the cap on the stopcock. You're now ready to attach the single-pressure transducer to the patient's catheter. Now you've assembled a single-pressure transducer system. The photograph below shows how the system will look.

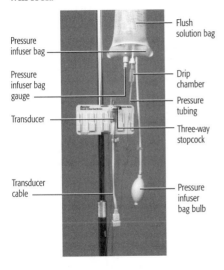

Pressure infuser bag

Pressure infuser bag gauge

Transducer

Transducer cable

Flush solution bag

Drip chamber

Pressure tubing

Three-way stopcock

Pressure infuser bag bulb

### Special considerations

▶ You may use any of several methods to set up a multiple-pressure transducer system. The easiest way is to add to the single-pressure system. You'll also need another bag of heparin flush solution in a second pressure infuser bag. Then you'll prime the tubing, mount the second transducer, and connect an additional cable to the monitor. Finally, you'll zero the second transducer.

### Documentation

▶ Document the patient's position for zeroing so that other health care team members can replicate the placement.

## REFERENCES

Aitken, L.M. "Expert Critical Care Nurses' Use of Pulmonary Artery Pressure Monitoring," *Intensive Critical Care Nurse* 16(4): 209-20, August 2000.

Edward, D., et al. *Bedside Critical Care Manual.* Philadelphia: Lippincott Williams & Wilkins, 2001.

# Ventricular assist device insertion and care

A temporary life-sustaining treatment for a failing heart, the ventricular assist device (VAD) diverts systemic blood flow from a diseased ventricle into a centrifugal pump. It temporarily reduces ventricular work, allowing the myocardium to rest and contractility to improve. Although used most commonly to assist the left ventricle, this device may also assist the right ventricle or both ventricles. (See *VAD: Help for the failing heart*, page 300.)

Candidates for VAD include patients with massive myocardial infarction, irreversible cardiomyopathy, acute myocarditis, an inability to be weaned from cardiopulmonary bypass, valvular disease, bacterial endocarditis, or heart transplant rejection. The device may also be used in those awaiting a heart transplant.

### Equipment

The ventricular assist device is inserted in the operating room.

### Implementation

▶ Before surgery, explain to the patient that food and fluid intake must be restricted and that you will continuously monitor his cardiac function (using an ECG, a pulmonary artery catheter, and an arterial line). Offer the patient reassurance. Before sending him to the operating room, ensure that he has signed a consent form.

▶ If time permits, shave the patient's chest and scrub it with an antiseptic solution.

▶ When the patient returns from surgery, administer analgesics, as ordered.

▶ Frequently monitor vital signs, intake, and output.

▶ Keep the patient immobile to prevent accidental extubation, contamination, or disconnection of the VAD.

▶ Monitor pulmonary artery pressures. If you've been prepared to adjust the pump,

# VAD:
# Help for the failing heart

The ventricular assist device (VAD) functions some-what like an artificial heart. The major difference is that the VAD assists the heart, whereas the artificial heart replaces it. The VAD is designed to aid one or both ventricles. The pumping chambers themselves aren't usually implanted in the patient.

The permanent VAD is implanted in the patient's chest cavity, although it still provides only temporary support. The device receives power through the skin by a belt of electrical transformer coils (worn externally as a portable battery pack). It can also operate off an implanted, rechargeable battery for up to 1 hour at a time.

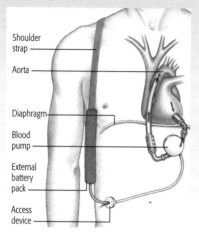

Shoulder strap

Aorta

Diaphragm

Blood pump

External battery pack

Access device

---

maintain cardiac output at about 5 to 8 L/ minute, central venous pressure at about 8 to 16 mm Hg, pulmonary capillary wedge pressure at about 10 to 20 mm Hg, mean arterial pressure at greater than 60 mm Hg, and left atrial pressure between 4 and 12 mm Hg.

▶ Monitor the patient for signs and symp-toms of poor perfusion and ineffective pumping, including arrhythmias, hypoten-sion, slow capillary refill, cool skin, olig-uria or anuria, confusion, anxiety, and rest-lessness.

▶ Administer heparin as ordered to pre-vent clotting in the pump head and throm-bus formation. Check for bleeding, espe-cially at the operative sites. Monitor

laboratory studies, as ordered, especially complete blood count and coagulation studies.

▶ Assess the patient's incisions and the cannula insertion sites for signs of infec-tion. Monitor the patient's white blood cell count and differential daily, and take rectal or core temperatures every 4 hours.

▶ Change the dressing over the cannula sites daily or according to facility policy.

▶ Provide supportive care, including range-of-motion exercises and mouth and skin care.

## Special considerations

▶ If ventricular function fails to improve within 4 days, the patient may need a transplant. If so, provide psychological support for the patient and family as they endure referral. You may also initiate the transplant process by contacting the appro-priate agency.

▶ The psychological effects of the VAD can produce stress in the patient, his family, and his close friends. If appropriate, refer them to other support personnel.

## Complications

▶ The VAD carries a high risk of complica-tions, including damaged blood cells, which can increase the likelihood of thrombus formation and subsequent pul-monary embolism or cerebrovascular acci-dent.

## Documentation

▶ Note the patient's condition following in-sertion of the VAD. Document any pump adjustments as well as any complications and interventions.

**REFERENCES**

Edward, D., et al. *Bedside Critical Care Manu-al.* Philadelphia: Lippincott Williams & Wilkins, 2001.

Kavarana, M.N., et al. "Right Ventricular Dys-function and Organ Failure in Left Ventric-ular Assist Device Recipients: A Continu-ing Problem," *Annals of Thoracic Surgery* 73(3):745-50, March 2002.

# 6

# Pulmonary care

NO MATTER WHERE YOU WORK, YOU'RE SURE TO ENCOUNTER PATIENTS WITH RESPIRATORY conditions. Such conditions may be acute or chronic and may have developed as a primary disorder or resulted from a cardiac or other disorder.

Caring for the patient with a respiratory condition will challenge your nursing skills. The patient's oxygenation is compromised, and he may develop other problems as well. For instance, the patient may experience ineffective airway clearance and impaired gas exchange, altered cardiac output, altered fluid volume, impaired thermoregulation, and decreased mobility. He may be anxious, cope ineffectively, and have an impaired ability to communicate.

To meet your care goals, you need to have a working knowledge of the many therapies available to the patient with a respiratory condition. Many health care facilities have staff members who specialize in respiratory procedures, but you still need to keep your knowledge up-to-date. That way, you'll understand the rationales behind the patient's treatment and be able to perform or assist with procedures, recognize complications, and detect the need for additional therapy.

# Protocols

## Managing the patient requiring ventilatory assistance

### Purpose
To provide ventilation to the patient with an impaired ability to breathe on his own, a supportive measure

### Collaborative level
Interdependent

### Expected patient outcomes
▶ The patient will maintain a patent airway and adequate ventilation.
▶ The patient will maintain acceptable arterial blood gas values (ABGs), hemoglobin, and hemodynamics.
▶ The patient will use an alternate means of communication.

### Definition of terms
▶ *Vital capacity:* The amount of gas expired from the lungs.
▶ *Tidal volume:* The total amount of gas passing in and out of the lungs with each respiratory cycle.
▶ *Pressure support ventilation:* A mode of ventilation that provides positive pressure

in response to spontaneous breath. Used in weaning.
▶ *Intermittent mandatory ventilation:* A mode of ventilation that provides breaths at preset volumes and intervals but allows the patient to breathe spontaneously. Used in weaning.

### Indications
Treatment
▶ Impaired ventilation causing hypercapnia and respiratory distress, as found in patients with:
 —neuromuscular disorders, such as Guillain-Barré syndrome, myasthenia gravis, and poliomyelitis
 —central nervous system disorders, such as cerebral hemorrhage and spinal cord transsection
 —pulmonary edema
 —chronic obstructive pulmonary disease
 —adult respiratory distress syndrome
 —flail chest
 —acute hypoventilation.

Prevention
▶ Respiratory arrest

## Assessment guidance
### Signs and symptoms
▶ Use of accessory muscles to breathe, nasal flaring
▶ Pallid appearance, anxiety, restlessness
▶ Decreased blood pressure
▶ Diaphoresis

### Diagnostic studies
*Laboratory tests*
▶ ABG analysis

*Imaging tests*
▶ Chest X-ray

*Other*
▶ Pulmonary function tests
▶ Pulse oximetry

## Nursing interventions
▶ Verify ventilator type and settings. Check all connections between the ventilator and the patient and make sure all critical alarms are turned on. Make sure the patient can reach call signal.
▶ Assess ABG values when changes are made to ventilator settings, if the patient is unstable, or if there are changes in his hemodynamic, respiratory, or neurologic status.
▶ Assess continuous pulse oximetry and end-tidal or transcutaneous carbon dioxide, when ordered.
▶ Assess the need for suctioning, and suction as needed.
▶ Monitor vital signs: temperature; breath sounds; spontaneous respiratory effort; presence, amount, color, and consistency of sputum; and endotracheal (ET) tube centimeter markings at teeth or gums. Auscultate the patient's lungs and epigastrium to confirm ET tube placement. Decreased breath sounds on the left side may indicate a tube slippage into the right mainstem bronchus.
▶ Evaluate the patient's hydration status by monitoring intake and output, electrolyte balance, and weight.
▶ Monitor the patient's response to respiratory treatments.
▶ Monitor for adequacy of nutritional support by consulting with the dietitian and monitoring parameters, such as weight, electrolytes, glucose, minerals, prealbumin, total protein, transferrin, hemoglobin and hematocrit, nitrogen balance, and triglycerides.

▶ Assess the patient's pain, discomfort, and anxiety levels, and treat as needed.

## Patient teaching
▶ Explain the procedure to the patient and his family to reduce anxiety and fear. Include information related to the rationale for ventilatory support, medications given for sedation and pain control, use of restraints, routine nursing care, and nutritional support.
▶ If the patient requires a ventilator at home, teach him and his family how to use the device and check the settings.
▶ Teach the patient how to use nebulizer and oxygen equipment and care for the humidifier.
▶ Instruct the patient to call the doctor if he has chest pain, fever, shortness of breath, or swollen extremities.
▶ Teach the patient to count his pulse and report changes in rate or rhythm and to report a weight gain of 5 lb (2.3 kg) or more in a week.
▶ Teach the patient how to clean his tracheostomy daily.
▶ Send the patient home with emergency phone numbers as needed.

## Precautions
▶ After intubation, arrange for a chest X-ray to evaluate ET tube placement.
▶ Keep equipment necessary to maintain airway patency and ventilation readily available at the bedside in case of accidental extubation or mechanical ventilator failure. Use soft restraints to prevent the patient from extubating himself, if necessary.
▶ Check the humidifier and refill as needed. Discard collected water from tubing, using care not to drain it into the humidifier or into the patient's airway, as it may be contaminated with bacteria.
▶ Change the humidifier, nebulizer, and ventilator tubing according to facility policy to reduce the risk of ventilator-associated nosocomial pneumonia.
▶ Reposition the patient and perform chest physical therapy as necessary.
▶ Monitor the patient for decreased bowel sounds or distention, which could signify paralytic ileus.
▶ Monitor the patient for stress ulcers by checking nasogastric aspirate and stools for blood.
▶ If the patient is receiving high-pressure ventilation, monitor him for pneumothorax

by assessing for absent or diminished breath sounds, acute chest pain, and possible tracheal deviation or subcutaneous or mediastinal emphysema.

▶ If the patient is receiving high oxygen concentration, watch for oxygen toxicity: substernal chest pain, increased coughing, tachypnea, decreased lung compliance, and vital capacity and decreased partial pressure of carbon dioxide without a change in oxygen concentration.

▶ Assess ABG levels as needed. Overventilation may cause respiratory alkalosis. Inadequate alveolar ventilation or atelectasis and inappropriate tidal volume may cause respiratory acidosis.

▶ If the patient is fighting the ventilator, ineffective ventilation may result. Give him a sedative, anxiolytic, or neuromuscular blocking agent.

▶ Wean the patient from the ventilator when necessary.

## Documentation

▶ Document the date and time mechanical ventilation started.

▶ Record the type of ventilator used and settings, including ventilatory mode, tidal volume, rate, fraction of inspired oxygen, positive end-expiratory pressure, and peak inspiratory flow.

▶ Record the size of the ET tube, centimeter mark of ET tube, and cuff pressure.

▶ Document the patient's subjective and objective responses to treatment, including vital signs, breath sounds, use of accessory muscles, comfort level, and physical appearance.

▶ Describe complications as they occur and interventions required.

▶ Record laboratory data, including ABG values and oxygen saturation.

▶ Document tracheal suctioning and the character of secretions.

▶ Record adjustments made to the ventilator settings as a result of changing ABG levels.

▶ Record ventilator component maintenance, such as draining condensate and changing, cleaning, or discarding tubing.

▶ Document patient teaching and emotional support.

▶ Document the duration of spontaneous breathing and his ability to maintain the weaning schedule, if the patient is receiving pressure support ventilation or using a T-piece or tracheostomy collar.

▶ Record the control breath rate, time of each breath reduction, and rate of spontaneous respirations, if the patient is receiving intermittent mandatory ventilation with or without pressure support ventilation.

## Related procedures

▶ Arterial puncture for blood gas analysis
▶ Endotracheal intubation
▶ Endotracheal tube care
▶ End-tidal carbon dioxide monitoring
▶ I.V. bolus injection
▶ Manual ventilation
▶ Mechanical ventilation
▶ Mixed venous oxygen saturation monitoring
▶ Oxygen administration
▶ Peripheral I.V. line maintenance
▶ Prone positioning
▶ Pulse and ear oximetry
▶ Total parenteral nutrition
▶ Tracheal cuff-pressure measurement
▶ Tracheal suction
▶ Tracheostomy care
▶ Venipuncture

### REFERENCES

*Chart Smart.* Springhouse, Pa.: Springhouse Corporation, 2002.
*Diseases,* 3rd ed. Springhouse, Pa.: Springhouse Corporation, 2001.
*Illustrated Manual of Nursing Practice,* 3rd ed. Springhouse, Pa.: Lippincott Williams & Wilkins, 2002.
SOP: Patients Requiring Ventilatory Assistance, National Institutes of Health, 1999, *www.cc.nih.gov/nursingnew.*

### ORGANIZATIONS

American Association for Respiratory Care: *www.aarc.org*

# Managing the patient with an ineffective breathing pattern

## Purpose

To provide relief from symptoms and return to effective breathing patterns

## Collaborative level

Interdependent

## Expected patient outcomes
▶ The patient will feel comfortable during breathing.
▶ The patient will experience maximum lung expansion and adequate ventilation.
▶ The patient will maintain respiratory rate within 5 breaths/minute of baseline.

## Definition of terms
▶ *Adventitious breath sounds:* Abnormal breath sounds, such as crackles, wheezes, rhonchi, stridor, and pleural friction rub.

## Indications
Treatment
▶ Breathing that may be caused by chronic obstructive pulmonary disease (COPD) and pulmonary embolus

Prevention
▶ Complications, including respiratory distress or respiratory compromise

## Assessment guidance
Signs and symptoms
▶ Dyspnea
▶ Use of accessory muscles while breathing
▶ Decreased breath sounds
▶ Adventitious breath sounds
▶ Bronchospasm

Diagnostic studies
*Laboratory tests*
▶ Arterial blood gas analysis

*Imaging tests*
▶ Chest X-ray

*Other*
▶ Pulmonary function test
▶ Electrocardiogram

## Nursing interventions
▶ Auscultate breath sounds at least every 4 hours.
▶ Assess adequacy of ventilation to detect early signs of respiratory compromise.
▶ Give bronchodilators to relieve wheezing and bronchospasm.
▶ Administer oxygen to relieve hypoxemia and respiratory distress.

## Patient teaching
▶ Teach relaxation and breathing techniques to decrease anxiety and improve ventilation.

## Precautions
▶ Respiratory distress
▶ Respiratory compromise

## Documentation
▶ Record the date and time of start of signs and symptoms of ineffective breathing pattern.
▶ Document assessment data as stated above.
▶ Document the time, dose, and route of administration of bronchodilators and the patient's response.
▶ Record the patient's response to all interventions.
▶ Record the dose, route, and time of oxygen administration and the patient's response.

## Related procedures
▶ Arterial puncture for blood gas analysis
▶ Electrocardiography
▶ Oxygen administration

**REFERENCES**
*Assessment Made Incredibly Easy,* 2nd ed. Springhouse Pa.: Springhouse Corporation, 2002.
*Chart Smart.* Springhouse Pa.: Springhouse Corporation, 2002.
*Illustrated Manual of Nursing Practice,* 3rd. ed. Springhouse Pa.: Lippincott Williams & Wilkins, 2002.

**ORGANIZATIONS**
American Association for Respiratory Care: *www.aarc.org*

# Managing the patient with impaired gas exchange

## Purpose
To improve the oxygen supply or oxygen-carrying capacity of the blood

## Collaborative level
Interdependent

## Expected patient outcomes
▶ The patient will maintain a respiratory rate within 5 breaths/minute of baseline.
▶ The patient will have normal breath sounds.
▶ The patient will maintain arterial blood gas (ABG) values within normal limits.

## Definition of terms
▶ *Continuous positive-airway pressure (CPAP):* Treatment that maintains positive pressure in the airways through the entire respiratory cycle. May be delivered to an intubated or nonintubated patient.
▶ *Positive end-expiratory pressure (PEEP):* A type of mechanical ventilation that provides positive pressure during expiration.

## Indications
Treatment
▶ Acute respiratory failure
▶ Chronic obstructive pulmonary disease
▶ Pneumonia
▶ Pulmonary embolism
▶ Other respiratory problems

Prevention
▶ Respiratory failure

## Assessment guidance
Signs and symptoms
▶ Dyspnea
▶ Pleuritic chest pain
▶ Coughing
▶ Altered respirations
▶ Cyanosis
▶ Crackles, rhonchi, wheezes, or diminished breath sounds
▶ Restlessness, confusion, or irritability
▶ Cardiac arrhythmias, tachycardia, elevated blood pressure
▶ Fever, chills

Diagnostic studies
*Laboratory tests*
▶ ABG levels
▶ Hemoglobin level
▶ Hematocrit
▶ Electrolyte levels
▶ White blood cell count

*Imaging tests*
▶ Chest X-ray

*Other*
▶ Electrocardiogram

## Nursing interventions
▶ Monitor the patient's vital signs and temperature.
▶ Give antibiotics and monitor the patient's response to treat infection and improve alveolar expansion.
▶ Ensure adequate fluid intake and monitor intake and output.

▶ Monitor ABG values and notify the doctor of changes.
▶ Provide CPAP or PEEP to improve the driving pressure of oxygen across the alveolocapillary membrane and enhance arterial blood oxygenation.
▶ Provide emotional support to the patient and his family.

## Patient teaching
▶ Teach incentive spirometry and deep breathing to enhance lung expansion and ventilation.
▶ Explain all procedures and rationales.

## Precautions
▶ Start mechanical ventilation to improve ventilation, if needed. Have an Ambu bag readily available.

## Documentation
▶ Record the date and time of detection of signs and symptoms.
▶ Document assessment findings.
▶ Note interventions and the patient's response.
▶ Use a flow sheet to record vital signs, temperature, intake and output, and ABG findings.
▶ Record medication administration and the patient's response.
▶ Document patient teaching and the patient's response to teaching.

## Related procedures
▶ Arterial puncture for blood gas analysis
▶ Electrocardiography
▶ Incentive spirometry
▶ Mechanical ventilation

**REFERENCES**
*Assessment Made Incredibly Easy,* 2nd ed. Springhouse, Pa.: Springhouse Corporation, 2002.
*Chart Smart.* Springhouse, Pa.: Springhouse Corporation, 2002.
*Illustrated Manual of Nursing Practice,* 3rd ed. Springhouse, Pa.: Lippincott Williams & Wilkins, 2002.

**ORGANIZATIONS**
American Association for Respiratory Care: *www.aarc.org*

# Managing the patient with ineffective airway clearance

## Purpose
To provide treatment to help mobilize and remove secretions, reduce the work of breathing, and improve gas exchange

## Collaborative level
Interdependent

## Expected patient outcomes
▶ The patient will maintain a patent airway.
▶ The patient will have improved breath sounds.
▶ The patient will have a normal rate and depth of respirations.

## Definition of terms
▶ *Positive airway pressure adjuncts—used:* Therapy used to help mobilize secretions and treat atelectasis; always used together with other airway clearance techniques.
▶ *High-frequency compression-oscillation—rapid:* Rapid vibratory movement of small volumes of air back and forth in the respiratory tract to enhance cough clearance of secretions.

## Indications
Treatment
▶ Copious secretions
▶ Acute lobar atelectasis
▶ Acute respiratory failure with retained secretions
▶ Pulmonary infiltrates or consolidations causing ventilation or perfusion abnormalities
▶ Cystic fibrosis
▶ Neuromuscular disorders
▶ Bronchiectasis
▶ Chronic bronchitis

Prevention
▶ Atelectasis
▶ Infection
▶ Mucus plugging
▶ Airway obstruction
▶ Respiratory failure

## Assessment guidance
Signs and symptoms
▶ Shortness of breath, anxiety, cough, fatigue
▶ Tachypnea
▶ Tachycardia
▶ Ineffective cough
▶ Restlessness
▶ Cyanosis
▶ Diaphoresis
▶ Change in level of consciousness
▶ Excessive sputum production or lack of sputum production
▶ Use of accessory muscles to breathe
▶ Abnormal breath sounds (rhonchi, crackles, wheezes, diminished breathing)

Diagnostic studies
*Laboratory tests*
▶ Arterial blood gas (ABG) analysis
▶ Basic metabolic panel
▶ Complete blood count

*Imaging tests*
▶ Chest X-ray

*Other*
▶ Pulse oximetry

## Nursing interventions
▶ Assess the patency of the patient's airway.
▶ Position the patient to optimize breathing.
▶ Assess the patient's respiratory rate, rhythm, and depth.
▶ Watch for signs of hypoxia, such as cyanosis, change in mental status, restlessness, and anxiety.
▶ Assess lung sounds.
▶ Check the patient's vital signs, heart rate and rhythm, and pulse oximetry.
▶ Assess effectiveness of the patient's cough.
▶ Monitor ABG results.
▶ Administer oxygen with humidification when ordered.
▶ Provide nasotracheal or nasopharyngeal suctioning as needed.
▶ Initiate or assist with chest physiotherapy, which may include:
  −postural drainage: monitor patient response to positioning
  −coughing: directed cough
  −positive airway pressure adjuncts (positive end-expiratory pressure [PEEP], continuous positive airway pressure [CPAP],

expiratory positive airway pressure [EPAP])
–high-frequency compression-oscillation: flutter valve
–mobilization and exercise.
▶ Administer medications, which may include:
–bronchodilators: monitor patient response
–corticosteroids: monitor glucose level
–aminophylline: monitor drug levels
–antimicrobials: give after you obtain appropriate cultures.
▶ Force fluids (unless contraindicated) to help liquefy secretions.
▶ Monitor the patient's chest X-ray results.
▶ Assist and teach the patient to cough and deep breathe to maximize air exchange.
▶ Help the patient use incentive spirometry to open alveoli maximally.
▶ Assist and teach the patient to turn and reposition every 2 hours.

### Patient teaching
▶ Explain the need for coughing and deep breathing to remove retained secretions.
▶ Teach the importance of repositioning to maximize alveolar expansion.
▶ Instruct the patient on hydration, which is needed to liquefy secretions to ease removal.

### Precautions
▶ Keep suction equipment, Ambu bag, mask, and oral airway at the bedside.
▶ Obtain blood or sputum cultures before antibiotic administration.

### Contraindications
Some airway clearance techniques, such as postural drainage and directed cough, are contraindicated in patients with increased intracranial pressure; unstable head, neck, or spinal injury; and eye surgery.

### Documentation
▶ Record pulmonary assessment points indicating the need for airway clearance interventions and the patient's response to interventions, including objective and subjective data.

### Related procedures
▶ Oronasopharyngeal suction
▶ Oxygen administration

▶ Pulse and ear oximetry
▶ Sputum collection

### REFERENCES
Rubin, B.K. "Physiology of Airway Mucus Clearance." *Respiratory Care* 47(7):761-68, July 2002.
Scanlan, C.L., et al., eds. *Egan's Fundamentals of Respiratory Care,* 7th ed. St. Louis: Mosby–Year Book, Inc., 1999.
Tucker, S.M., et al. *Patient Care Standards: Collaborative Planning and Nursing Interventions,* 7th ed. St. Louis: Mosby–Year Book, Inc., 2000.

### ORGANIZATIONS
American Association for Respiratory Care: *www.AARC.org*
COPD Professional: *www.COPDprofessional.org*

# Managing the patient with ineffective pulmonary perfusion

### Purpose
To improve oxygenation and ventilation; to prevent extension of pulmonary embolus and cardiovascular compromise

### Collaborative level
Interdependent

### Expected patient outcomes
▶ The patient will maintain adequate oxygen and carbon dioxide exchange, as evidenced by arterial blood gas (ABG) values within normal limits.
▶ The patient will have a normal rate and depth of respirations.
▶ The patient will have normal lung sounds.
▶ The patient won't have complications related to the embolism.

### Definition of terms
▶ *Vena cava filter:* Placed percutaneously in inferior vena cava to prevent peripheral emboli from migrating to pulmonary circulation.
▶ *Plethysmography:* Noninvasive technique for measuring peripheral venous flow by measuring changes in vascular resistance and blood volume.

## Indications

### Treatment
▶ Venous thromboembolism
▶ Fat emboli
▶ Air emboli

### Prevention
▶ Extension of embolism
▶ Hypoxemia
▶ Respiratory failure
▶ Right ventricular failure and shock

## Assessment guidance

### Signs and symptoms
▶ Sudden onset of dyspnea, chest pain, cough, hemoptysis, restlessness, and anxiety
▶ History or current symptoms of deep vein thrombosis (swelling of lower extremities, erythema, warmth, tenderness)
▶ Tachypnea, chest pain, hemoptysis, diaphoresis, cyanosis, and hypotension
▶ Abnormal breath sounds: diminished breathing, crackles, friction rub, wheezes

### Diagnostic studies

*Laboratory tests*
▶ ABG analysis

*Imaging tests*
▶ Lung scan
▶ Computed tomography scan
▶ Pulmonary angiogram
▶ Ultrasound of lower extremities

*Other*
▶ Pulmonary artery pressure
▶ Electrocardiogram (ECG)

## Nursing interventions
▶ Maintain bed rest and limit activity to prevent dislodging additional clots.
▶ Administer oxygen.
▶ Assess the patient's respiratory rate, rhythm, and depth.
▶ Assess the patient's lung sounds.
▶ Observe for signs of hypoxia (cyanosis, change in mental status, restlessness, anxiety).
▶ Position the patient to optimize breathing.
▶ Monitor the patient's pulse oximetry, ABG values, ECG, and vital signs.
▶ Monitor prothrombin time, International Normalized Ratio, and partial thromboplastin time, as indicated.

▶ Administer medications, which may include:
  – anticoagulants
  – heparin, Coumadin
  – thrombolytics
  – streptokinase, urokinase
  – parenteral fluids
  – anxiolytics.
▶ Provide postprocedural care related to the placement of the vena cava filter or embolectomy.

## Patient teaching
▶ Teach rationale for activity limitations.
▶ Explain the diagnostic studies the patient needs to have done, such as chest X-ray, ventilation and perfusion scan, spiral CT, ultrasound, and plethysmography.
▶ Instruct the patient on anticoagulation therapy.
▶ Teach ways to prevent venous pooling.
▶ Explain the risk factors for deep vein thrombosis (oral contraceptives, surgery, long trips by air or automobile, childbirth, cancer, fractures, and orthopedic surgery).

## Precautions
▶ Assess the patient for signs of bleeding secondary to anticoagulation therapy: hematuria, hemoptysis, bruising, bleeding gums, GI (occult, frank).
▶ Encourage bed rest to avoid dislodging clots.
▶ Advise the patient to avoid positions that decrease venous return, such as crossed ankles, prolonged knee bending, or hip flexion.

## Documentation
▶ Record objective signs and symptoms, including pulmonary assessment points.
▶ Document nursing interventions.
▶ Document the patient's response to treatment.
▶ Record monitoring of diagnostic and laboratory results with appropriate doctor notification.

## Related procedures
▶ Cardiac monitoring
▶ Oxygen administration
▶ Pulse and ear oximetry
▶ Subcutaneous injection

**REFERENCES**

Chulay, M., et al. *AACN Handbook of Critical Care Nursing.* Stamford, Conn.: Appleton & Lange, 1997.

Launius, B.K., and Graham, B.D. "Understanding and Preventing Deep Vein Thrombosis and Pulmonary Embolism," *AACN Clinical Issues* 9(1):91-99, February 1998.

Tucker, S.M., et al. *Patient Care Standards: Collaborative Planning and Nursing Interventions,* 7th ed. St. Louis: Mosby–Year Book, Inc., 2000.

**ORGANIZATIONS**

American Academy of Family Physicians: *www.aafp.org*

American Association of Critical Care Nurses: *www.AACN.org*

American Lung Association: *www.lungusa.org*

American Thoracic Society: *www.thoracic.org*

# Procedures

# Arterial puncture for blood gas analysis

Obtaining an arterial blood sample requires percutaneous puncture of the brachial, radial, or femoral artery or withdrawal of a sample from an arterial line. Once collected, the sample can be analyzed to determine arterial blood gas (ABG) values.

ABG analysis evaluates the effectiveness of ventilation by measuring blood pH and the partial pressures of arterial oxygen ($PaO_2$) and carbon dioxide ($PaCO_2$). Blood pH measurement reflects the blood's acid-base state. $PaO_2$ indicates the amount of oxygen that the lungs deliver to the blood, and $PaCO_2$ indicates the lungs' capacity to eliminate carbon dioxide. ABG samples can also be analyzed for oxygen content and saturation and for bicarbonate values.

Typically, ABG analysis is ordered for patients who have chronic obstructive pulmonary disease, pulmonary edema, acute respiratory distress syndrome, myocardial infarction, or pneumonia. It's also performed during episodes of shock and after coronary artery bypass surgery, resuscitation from cardiac arrest, changes in respiratory therapy or status, and prolonged anesthesia.

Most ABG samples are collected by a respiratory technician or specially trained nurse. Collection from the femoral artery, however, is usually performed by a doctor.

Allen's test should be performed before a radial puncture is attempted. (See *Performing Allen's test.*)

## Equipment

10-ml glass syringe or plastic luer-lock syringe specially made for drawing blood for ABG analysis ● 1-ml ampule of aqueous heparin (1:1,000) ● 20G 1¼ " needle ● 22G 1" needle ● gloves ● alcohol or povidone-iodine pad ● two 2" × 2" gauze pads ● rubber cap for syringe hub or rubber stopper for needle ● ice-filled plastic bag ● label ● laboratory request form ● adhesive bandage ● optional: 1% lidocaine solution

Many health care facilities use a commercial ABG kit that contains all the equipment listed above (except the adhesive bandage and ice). If your facility doesn't use such a kit, obtain a sterile syringe specially made for drawing blood for ABG values and use a clean emesis basin filled with ice instead of the plastic bag to transport the sample to the laboratory.

### Preparation of equipment

Prepare the collected equipment before entering the patient's room. Wash your hands thoroughly; then open the ABG kit and remove the sample label and the plastic bag. Record on the label the patient's name and room number, date and collection time, and doctor's name. Fill the plastic bag with ice and set it aside.

## Performing Allen's test

Rest the patient's arm on the mattress or bedside stand, and support his wrist with a rolled towel. Have him clench his fist. Then, using your index and middle fingers, press on the radial and ulnar arteries. Hold this position for a few seconds.

Without removing your fingers from the patient's arteries, ask him to unclench his fist and hold his hand in a relaxed position. The palm will be blanched because pressure from your fingers has impaired the normal blood flow.

Release pressure on the patient's ulnar artery. If the hand becomes flushed, which indicates blood filling the vessels, you can safely proceed with the radial artery puncture. If the hand doesn't flush, perform the test on the other arm.

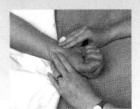 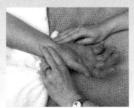 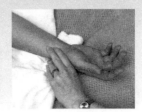

If the syringe isn't heparinized, you'll need to do so. To heparinize the syringe, first attach the 20G needle to the syringe. Then open the ampule of heparin. Draw all the heparin into the syringe to prevent the sample from clotting. Hold the syringe upright, and pull the plunger back slowly to about the 7-ml mark. Rotate the barrel while pulling the plunger back to allow the heparin to coat the inside surface of the syringe. Then slowly force the heparin toward the hub of the syringe and expel all but about 0.1 ml of the heparin.

To heparinize the needle, first replace the 20G needle with the 22G needle. Then hold the syringe upright, tilt it slightly, and eject the remaining heparin. Excess heparin in the syringe alters blood pH and $PaO_2$ values.

### Implementation

▶ Tell the patient you need to collect an arterial blood sample and explain the procedure to help ease anxiety and promote cooperation. Tell him that the needle stick will cause some discomfort but that he must remain still during the procedure.
▶ After washing your hands and putting on gloves, place a rolled towel under the patient's wrist for support. Locate the artery and palpate it for a strong pulse.
▶ Clean the puncture site with an alcohol or a povidone-iodine pad. Don't wipe off the povidone-iodine with alcohol.

▶ Using a circular motion, clean the area, starting in the center of the site and spiraling outward. If you use alcohol, apply it with friction for 30 seconds or until the final sponge comes away clean. Allow the skin to dry.
▶ Palpate the artery with the index and middle fingers of one hand while holding the syringe over the puncture site with the other hand.
▶ Hold the needle bevel up at a 30- to 45-degree angle. When puncturing the brachial artery, hold the needle at a 60-degree angle. (See *Arterial puncture technique,* page 312.)
▶ Puncture the skin and arterial wall in one motion, following the path of the artery.
▶ Watch for blood backflow in the syringe. Don't pull back on the plunger because arterial blood should enter the syringe spontaneously. Fill the syringe to the 5-ml mark.
▶ Withdraw the needle and then press a gauze pad firmly over the puncture site until the bleeding stops—at least 5 minutes. If the patient is receiving anticoagulant therapy or has a blood dyscrasia, apply pressure for 10 to 15 minutes; if necessary, ask a coworker to hold the gauze pad in place while you prepare the sample for transport to the laboratory. Don't ask the patient to hold the pad. If he fails to apply sufficient pressure, a large, painful

## Arterial puncture technique

The angle of needle penetration in arterial blood gas sampling depends on which artery is sampled. For the radial artery, which is used most often, the needle should enter bevel-up at a 30- to 45-degree angle over the radial artery.

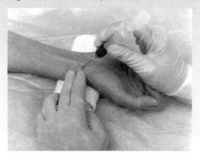

hematoma may form, hindering future arterial punctures at that site.

▶ Check the syringe for air bubbles. If any appear, remove them by holding the syringe upright and slowly ejecting some of the blood onto a 2″ × 2″ gauze pad.

▶ Insert the needle into a rubber stopper or remove the needle and place a rubber cap over the syringe tip. This prevents the sample from leaking and keeps air out of the syringe.

▶ Put the labeled sample in the ice-filled plastic bag or emesis basin. Attach a properly completed laboratory request form and send the sample to the laboratory immediately.

▶ When bleeding stops, apply a small adhesive bandage to the site.

▶ Monitor the patient's vital signs, and observe for signs of circulatory impairment, such as swelling, discoloration, pain, numbness, or tingling in the arm or leg. Watch for bleeding at the puncture site.

### Special considerations

▶ If the patient is receiving oxygen, make sure that his therapy has been in progress for at least 15 minutes before collecting an arterial blood sample.

▶ Unless ordered, don't turn off existing oxygen therapy before collecting arterial blood samples. Be sure to indicate on the laboratory request slip the amount and type of oxygen therapy the patient is receiving.

▶ If the patient isn't receiving oxygen, indicate that he's breathing room air.

▶ If the patient has just received a nebulizer treatment, wait about 20 minutes before collecting the sample.

▶ If necessary, you can anesthetize the puncture site with 1% lidocaine solution. Consider such use of lidocaine carefully because it delays the procedure, the patient may be allergic to the drug, or the resulting vasoconstriction may prevent successful puncture.

▶ When filling out a laboratory request form for ABG analysis, include the following information to help the laboratory staff calibrate the equipment and evaluate results correctly: the patient's current temperature, most recent hemoglobin level, current respiratory rate and, if the patient is on a ventilator, fraction of inspired oxygen and tidal volume and ventilatory frequency.

### Complications

If you use too much force when attempting to puncture the artery, the needle may touch the periosteum of the bone, causing the patient considerable pain, or you may advance the needle through the opposite wall of the artery. If this happens, slowly pull the needle back a short distance and check to see if you obtain a blood return. If blood still fails to enter the syringe, withdraw the needle completely and start with a fresh heparinized needle. Don't make more than two attempts to withdraw blood from the same site. Probing the artery may injure it and the radial nerve. Also, hemolysis will alter test results.

If arterial spasm occurs, blood won't flow into the syringe and you won't be able to collect the sample. If this happens, replace the needle with a smaller one and try the puncture again. A smaller-bore needle is less likely to cause arterial spasm.

### Documentation

▶ Record the results of Allen's test, the time the sample was drawn, the patient's temperature, the site of the arterial puncture, the amount of time that pressure was applied to the site to control bleeding, and the type and amount of oxygen therapy the patient was receiving.

## REFERENCES

Ngan, M.F. "Sonographically Guided Arterial Blood Sampling Using a Handheld Doppler Device," *Journal of Clinical Ultrasound* 30(3):158-60, March-April 2002.

Planes, C., et al. "Arterial Blood Gases During Exercise: Validity of Transcutaneous Measurements," *Archives of Physical Medicine and Rehabilitation* 82(12):1686-91, December 2001.

# Chest tube insertion

The pleural space normally contains a thin layer of lubricating fluid that allows the visceral and parietal pleura to move without friction during respiration. An excess of fluid (hemothorax or pleural effusion), air (pneumothorax), or both in this space alters intrapleural pressure and causes partial or complete lung collapse.

Chest tube insertion allows drainage of air or fluid from the pleural space. Usually performed by a doctor with a nurse assisting, this procedure requires sterile technique. The insertion site varies, depending on the patient's condition and the doctor's judgment. For pneumothorax, the second intercostal space is the usual site because air rises to the top of the intrapleural space. For hemothorax or pleural effusion, the sixth to eighth intercostal spaces are common sites because fluid settles to the lower levels of the intrapleural space. For removal of air and fluid, a chest tube is inserted into a high and a low site.

After insertion, one or more chest tubes are connected to a thoracic drainage system that removes air, fluid, or both from the pleural space and prevents backflow into that space, thus promoting lung reexpansion.

## Equipment

Two pairs of sterile gloves • sterile drape • vial of 1% lidocaine • povidone-iodine solution • 10-ml syringe • alcohol pad • 22G 1" needle • 25G ⅜" needle • sterile scalpel (usually with #11 blade) • sterile forceps • two rubber-tipped clamps for each chest tube inserted • sterile 4" × 4" gauze pads • two sterile 4" × 4" drain dressings (gauze pads with slit) • 3" or 4" sturdy, elastic tape • 1" adhesive tape for connections • chest tube of appropriate size (#16 to #20 French catheter for air or serous fluid; #28 to #40 French catheter for blood, pus, or thick fluid), with or without a trocar • sterile Kelly clamp • suture material (usually 2-0 silk with cutting needle) • thoracic drainage system • sterile drainage tubing • 6" (15.2 cm) long connector • sterile Y-connector (for two chest tubes on the same side) • optional: petroleum gauze

### Preparation of equipment

Check the expiration date on the sterile packages and inspect for tears. In a nonemergency situation, make sure that the patient has signed the appropriate consent form. Then assemble all equipment in the patient's room and set up the thoracic drainage system. Place it next to the patient's bed below the chest level to facilitate drainage.

## Implementation

▶ Explain the procedure to the patient, provide privacy, and wash your hands.
▶ Record baseline vital signs and respiratory assessment.
▶ Position the patient appropriately. If he has a pneumothorax, place him in high Fowler's, semi-Fowler's, or the supine position. The doctor will insert the tube in the anterior chest at the midclavicular line in the second to third intercostal space. If the patient has a hemothorax, have him lean over the overbed table or straddle a chair with his arms dangling over the back. The doctor will insert the tube in the fourth to sixth intercostal space at the midaxillary line. For either pneumothorax or hemothorax, the patient may lie on his unaffected side with arms extended over his head.
▶ When you've positioned the patient properly, place the chest tube tray on the overbed table. Open it using sterile technique.
▶ The doctor puts on sterile gloves and prepares the insertion site by cleaning the area with povidone-iodine solution.
▶ Wipe the rubber stopper of the lidocaine vial with an alcohol pad. Then invert the bottle and hold it for the doctor to withdraw the anesthetic.
▶ After the doctor anesthetizes the site, he makes a small incision and inserts the chest tube. Then he either immediately connects the chest tube to the thoracic drainage system or momentarily clamps the tube close to the patient's chest until he can connect it to the drainage system. He

# Removing a chest tube

After the patient's lung has reexpanded, you may assist the doctor in removing the chest tube. To do so, first obtain the patient's vital signs and perform a respiratory assessment. After explaining the procedure to the patient, administer an analgesic, as ordered, 30 minutes before tube removal. Then follow the steps listed below:

▶ Place the patient in semi-Fowler's position or on his unaffected side.

▶ Place a linen-saver pad under the affected side to protect the linen from drainage and to provide a place to put the chest tube after removal.

▶ Put on clean gloves and remove the chest tube dressings, being careful not to dislodge the chest tube. Discard soiled dressings.

▶ The doctor puts on sterile gloves, holds the chest tube in place with sterile forceps, and cuts the suture anchoring the tube.

▶ Make sure the chest tube is securely clamped and then instruct the patient to perform Valsalva's maneuver by exhaling fully and bearing down. Valsalva's maneuver effectively increases intrathoracic pressure.

▶ The doctor holds an airtight dressing, usually petroleum gauze, so that he can cover the insertion site with it immediately after removing the tube. After he removes the tube and covers the insertion site, secure the dressing with tape. Be sure to cover the dressing completely with tape to make it as airtight as possible.

▶ Dispose of the chest tube, soiled gloves, and equipment according to facility policy.

▶ Take vital signs, as ordered, and assess the depth and quality of the patient's respirations. Assess the patient carefully for signs and symptoms of pneumothorax, subcutaneous emphysema, or infection.

▶ Securely tape the chest tube to the patient's chest distal to the insertion site to help prevent accidental tube dislodgment.

▶ Securely tape the junction of the chest tube and the drainage tube to prevent their separation.

▶ Coil the drainage tubing, and secure it to the bed linen with tape and a safety pin, leaving enough slack for the patient to move and turn. These measures prevent the tubing from getting kinked or dropping to the floor, and they help prevent accidental dislodgment of the chest tube.

▶ Immediately after the drainage system is connected, instruct the patient to take a deep breath, hold it momentarily, and slowly exhale to assist drainage of the pleural space and lung re-expansion.

▶ A portable chest X-ray is then done to check tube position.

▶ Take the patient's vital signs every 15 minutes for 1 hour, then as his condition indicates. Auscultate his lungs at least every 4 hours after the procedure to assess air exchange in the affected lung. Diminished or absent breath sounds indicate that the lung hasn't reexpanded.

▶ Monitor and measure and record pleural fluid drainage.

## Special considerations

▶ If the chest tube comes out, cover the site immediately with 4″ × 4″ gauze pads and tape them in place. Stay with the patient, and monitor his vital signs every 10 minutes. Observe him for signs and symptoms of tension pneumothorax (such as hypotension, distended neck veins, absent breath sounds, tracheal shift, hypoxemia, weak and rapid pulse, dyspnea, tachypnea, diaphoresis, and chest pain). Have another staff member notify the doctor and gather the equipment needed to reinsert the tube.

▶ Place the rubber-tipped clamps at the bedside. If the drainage system cracks or a tube disconnects, clamp the chest tube momentarily as close to the insertion site as possible. Because no air or liquid can escape from the pleural space while the tube is clamped, observe the patient closely for signs and symptoms of tension pneumothorax while the clamp is in place.

▶ Petroleum gauze may be wrapped around the tube at the insertion site to make an airtight seal.

▶ The tube may be clamped with large, smooth, rubber-tipped clamps for several

may then secure the tube to the skin with a suture.

▶ As the doctor is inserting the chest tube, reassure the patient and assist the doctor as necessary.

▶ Open the packages containing the 4″ × 4″ drain dressings and gauze pads and put on sterile gloves. Then place two 4″ × 4″ drain dressings around the insertion site, one from the top and the other from the bottom. Place several 4″ × 4″ gauze pads on top of the drain dressings. Tape the dressings, covering them completely.

hours before removal. This allows time to observe the patient for signs of respiratory distress, an indication that air or fluid remains trapped in the pleural space. A chest tube is usually removed within 7 days of insertion to prevent infection along the tube tract. (See *Removing a chest tube.*)

## Documentation

▶ Record the date and time of chest tube insertion, the insertion site, drainage system used, presence of drainage and bubbling, vital signs and auscultation findings, any complications, and the nursing action taken.

### REFERENCES

Edward, D., et al. *Bedside Critical Care Manual.* Philadelphia: Lippincott Williams & Wilkins, 2001.

Vines, D.L., et al. "Current Respiratory Care, Part 1: Oxygen Therapy, Oximetry, Bronchial Hygiene," *Journal of Critical Illness* 15(9):507-10, 513-15, September 2000.

# Endotracheal intubation

Endotracheal (ET) intubation involves the oral or nasal insertion of a flexible tube through the larynx into the trachea for the purposes of controlling the airway and mechanically ventilating the patient. Performed by a doctor, anesthetist, respiratory therapist, or nurse educated in the procedure, ET intubation usually occurs in emergencies, such as cardiopulmonary arrest or in diseases such as epiglottitis. However, intubation may also occur under more controlled circumstances, such as just before surgery. In such instances, ET intubation requires patient teaching and preparation.

Advantages of the procedure are that it establishes and maintains a patent airway, seals off the trachea from the digestive tract, allows for more effective bronchial suctioning, and provides a route for mechanical ventilation. Disadvantages are that it bypasses normal respiratory defenses against infection, reduces cough effectiveness, and prevents verbal communication.

Oral ET intubation is contraindicated in patients with acute cervical spinal injury and degenerative spinal disorders, whereas nasal intubation is contraindicated in patients with apnea, bleeding disorders, chronic sinusitis, or nasal obstructions.

## Equipment

Two ET tubes (one spare) in appropriate size ● 10-ml syringe ● stethoscope ● gloves ● lighted laryngoscope with a handle and blades of various sizes, curved and straight ● sedative ● local anesthetic spray ● mucosal vasoconstricting agent (for nasal intubation) ● overbed or other table ● water-soluble lubricant ● adhesive or other strong tape or Velcro tube holder ● compound benzoin tincture ● gloves ● oral airway or bite block (for oral intubation) ● suction equipment ● handheld resuscitation bag with sterile swivel adapter ● humidified oxygen source ● optional: prepackaged intubation tray ● sterile gauze pad ● stylet ● Magill forceps ● sterile water ● sterile basin

### Preparation of equipment

Quickly gather the individual supplies or use a prepackaged intubation tray, which will contain most of the necessary supplies. First, select an ET tube of the appropriate size—typically, 2.5 to 5.5 mm, uncuffed, for children and 6 to 10 mm, cuffed, for adults. The typical size of an oral tube is 7.5 mm for women and 9 mm for men. Select a slightly smaller tube for nasal intubation.

Check the light in the laryngoscope by snapping the appropriate-sized blade into place; if the bulb doesn't light, replace the batteries or the laryngoscope (whichever will be quicker).

Using sterile technique, open the package containing the ET tube and, if desired, open the other supplies on an overbed table. Pour the sterile water into the basin. Then, to ease insertion, lubricate 1″ (2.5 cm) of the distal end of the ET tube with the water-soluble lubricant using aseptic technique. Do this by squeezing the lubricant directly on the tube. Use only water-soluble lubricant because it can be absorbed by mucous membranes.

Next, attach the syringe to the port on the tube's exterior pilot balloon. Slowly inflate the cuff, observing for uniform inflation. Then use the syringe to deflate the cuff.

A stylet may be used on oral intubations to stiffen the tube. Lubricate the entire stylet. Insert the stylet into the tube so that its distal tip lies about ½″ (1.5 cm) inside the distal end of the tube. Avoid vocal cord trauma by making sure that the stylet doesn't protrude from the tube. Prepare the humidified oxygen source and the suction equipment for immediate use. If the patient is in bed, remove the headboard to provide easier access.

## Implementation

▶ Administer a sedative, as ordered, to induce amnesia or analgesia and help calm and relax the conscious patient. Remove dentures and bridgework, if present.

▶ Hyperventilate with 100% oxygen via bag-valve-mask before insertion attempt to prevent hypoxia.

▶ Place the patient supine in the sniffing position so that his mouth, pharynx, and trachea are extended. For a blind intubation, place the patient's head and neck in a neutral position.

▶ Put on gloves.

▶ For oral intubation, spray a local anesthetic, such as lidocaine, deep into the posterior pharynx to diminish the gag reflex and reduce patient discomfort. For nasal intubation, spray a local anesthetic and a mucosal vasoconstrictor into the nasal passages to anesthetize the nasal turbinates and reduce the chance of bleeding.

▶ If necessary, suction the patient's pharynx just before tube insertion to improve visualization of the patient's pharynx and vocal cords.

▶ Time each intubation attempt, limiting attempts to less than 30 seconds to prevent hypoxia.

▶ Hyperventilate the patient between attempts if necessary.

### Intubation with direct visualization

▶ Stand at the head of the patient's bed. Using your right hand, hold the patient's mouth open by crossing your index finger over your thumb, placing your thumb on the patient's upper teeth and your index finger on his lower teeth. This technique provides greater leverage.

▶ Grasp the laryngoscope handle in your left hand and gently slide the blade into the right side of the patient's mouth. Center the blade and push the patient's tongue to the left. Hold the patient's lower lip away from his teeth to prevent the lip from being traumatized.

▶ Advance the blade to expose the epiglottis. When using a straight blade, insert the tip under the epiglottis; when using a curved blade, insert the tip between the base of the tongue and the epiglottis.

▶ Lift the laryngoscope handle upward and away from your body at a 45-degree angle to reveal the vocal cords. Avoid pivoting the laryngoscope against the patient's teeth to avoid damaging them.

▶ If desired, have an assistant apply pressure to the cricoid ring to occlude the esophagus and minimize gastric regurgitation.

▶ When performing an oral intubation, insert the ET tube into the right side of the patient's mouth. When performing a nasotracheal intubation, insert the ET tube through the nostril and into the pharynx. Then use Magill forceps to guide the tube through the vocal cords.

▶ Guide the tube into the vertical openings of the larynx between the vocal cords, being careful not to mistake the horizontal opening of the esophagus for the larynx. If the vocal cords are closed because of a spasm, wait a few seconds for them to relax; then gently guide the tube past them to avoid traumatic injury.

▶ Advance the tube until the cuff disappears beyond the vocal cords. Avoid advancing the tube farther to avoid occluding a major bronchus and precipitating lung collapse.

▶ Holding the ET tube in place, quickly remove the stylet, if present.

### Blind nasotracheal intubation

▶ Pass the ET tube along the floor of the nasal cavity. If necessary, use gentle force to pass the tube through the nasopharynx and into the pharynx.

▶ Listen and feel for air movement through the tube as it's advanced to ensure that the tube is properly place in the airway.

▶ Slip the tube between the vocal cords when the patient inhales because the vocal cords separate on inhalation.

▶ When the tube is past the vocal cords, the breath sounds should become louder. If, at any time during tube advancement, breath sounds disappear, withdraw the tube until they reappear.

### After intubation

▶ Inflate the tube's cuff with 5 to 10 cc of air until you feel resistance. When the patient is mechanically ventilated, you'll use the minimal-leak technique or the minimal occlusive volume technique to establish correct inflation of the cuff.

▶ Remove the laryngoscope. If the patient was intubated orally, insert an oral airway or a bite block to prevent him from obstructing airflow or puncturing the tube with his teeth.

▶ To ensure correct tube placement, observe for chest expansion and auscultate for bilateral breath sounds. If the patient is unconscious or uncooperative, use a hand-held resuscitation bag while observing for upper chest movement and auscultating for breath sounds. Feel the tube's tip for warm exhalations and listen for air movement. Observe for condensation forming inside the tube.

▶ If you don't hear any breath sounds, auscultate over the stomach while ventilating with the resuscitation bag. Stomach distention, belching, or a gurgling sound indicates esophageal intubation. Immediately deflate the cuff and remove the tube. After reoxygenating the patient to prevent hypoxia, repeat insertion using a sterile tube to prevent contamination of the trachea.

▶ Auscultate bilaterally to exclude the possibility of endobronchial intubation. If you fail to hear breath sounds on both sides of the chest, you may have inserted the tube into one of the mainstem bronchi (usually the right one because of its wider angle at the bifurcation); such insertion occludes the other bronchus and lung and results in atelectasis on the obstructed side. Or the tube may be resting on the carina, resulting in dry secretions that obstruct both bronchi. (The patient's coughing and fighting the ventilator will alert you to the problem.) To correct these situations, deflate the cuff, withdraw the tube ⅛″ (1 to 2 mm), auscultate for bilateral breath sounds, and reinflate the cuff.

▶ When you've confirmed correct tube placement, administer oxygen or initiate mechanical ventilation and suction, if indicated.

▶ To secure tube position, apply compound benzoin tincture to each cheek and let it dry. Tape the tube firmly with adhesive or other strong tape or use a Velcro tube holder. (See *Three methods to secure an ET tube,* pages 318 and 319.)

▶ Inflate the cuff with the minimal-leak or minimal occlusive volume technique. For the minimal-leak technique, attach a 10-ml syringe to the port on the tube's exterior pilot balloon and place a stethoscope on the side of the patient's neck. Inject small amounts of air with each breath until you hear no leak. Then aspirate 0.1 cc of air from the cuff to create a minimal air leak. Record the amount of air needed to inflate the cuff. For the minimal occlusive volume technique, follow the first two steps of the minimal-leak technique but place the stethoscope over the trachea instead. Aspirate until you hear a small leak on inspiration and add just enough air to stop the leak. Record the amount of air needed to inflate the cuff for subsequent monitoring of tracheal dilation or erosion.

▶ Clearly note the centimeter marking on the tube where it exits the patient's mouth or nose. By periodically monitoring this mark, you can detect tube displacement.

▶ Make sure that a chest X-ray is taken to verify tube position.

▶ Place a swivel adapter between the tube and the humidified oxygen source to allow for intermittent suctioning and to reduce tube tension.

▶ Place the patient on his side with his head in a comfortable position to avoid tube kinking and airway obstruction.

▶ Auscultate both sides of the chest and watch chest movement as indicated by the patient's condition to ensure correct tube placement and full lung ventilation. Provide frequent oral care to the orally intubated patient and position the ET tube to prevent formation of pressure ulcers and avoid excessive pressure on the sides of the mouth. Provide frequent nasal and oral care to the nasally intubated patient to prevent formation of pressure ulcers and drying of oral mucous membranes.

▶ Suction secretions through the ET tube as the patient's condition indicates to clear secretions and prevent mucus plugs from obstructing the tube.

## Special considerations

▶ Orotracheal intubation is preferred in emergencies because insertion is easier and faster than it is with nasotracheal intubation. However, maintaining exact tube placement is more difficult, and the tube must be well secured to avoid kinking and prevent bronchial obstruction or accidental extubation. Orotracheal intubation is also poorly tolerated by the conscious patient because it stimulates salivation, coughing, and retching.

# Three methods to secure an ET tube

Before taping an endotracheal (ET) tube in place, make sure the patient's face is clean, dry, and free from beard stubble. If possible, suction his mouth and dry the tube just before taping. Also, check the reference mark on the tube to ensure correct placement. After taping, always check for bilateral breath sounds to ensure that the tube hasn't been displaced by manipulation.

To tape the tube securely, use one of these three methods.

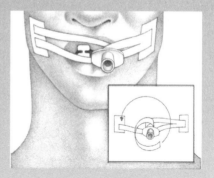

### Method 1

Cut two 2" (5.1-cm) strips and two 15" (38.1-cm) strips of 1" cloth adhesive tape. Then cut a 13" (33-cm) slit in one end of each 15" strip (as shown below).

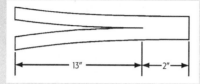

Apply compound benzoin tincture to the patient's cheeks. Place the 2" strips on his cheeks, creating a new surface on which to anchor the tape securing the tube. When frequent retaping is necessary, this helps preserve the patient's skin integrity. If the patient's skin is excoriated or at risk, you can use a transparent semipermeable dressing to protect the skin.

Apply the benzoin tincture to the tape on the patient's face and to the part of the tube where you'll be applying the tape. On the side of the mouth where the tube will be anchored, place the unslit end of the long tape on top of the tape on the patient's cheek.

Wrap the top half of the tape around the tube twice, pulling the tape tightly around the tube. Then, directing the tape over the patient's upper lip, place the end of the tape on his other cheek. Cut off excess tape. Use the lower half of the tape to secure an oral airway, if necessary (as shown above).

Or, twist the lower half of the tape around the tube twice and attach it to the original cheek (as shown below). Taping in opposite directions places equal traction on the tube.

If you've taped in an oral airway or are concerned about the tube's stability, apply the other 15" strip of tape in the same manner, starting on the other side of the patient's face. If the tape around the tube is too bulky, use only the upper part of the tape and cut off the lower part. If the patient has copious oral secretions, seal the tape by cutting a 1" piece of paper tape, coating it with benzoin tincture, and placing the paper tape over the adhesive tape.

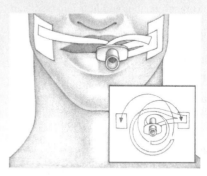

❱ Nasotracheal intubation is preferred for elective insertion when the patient is capable of spontaneous ventilation for a short period. Blind intubation is typically used in conscious patients who risk imminent respiratory arrest or who have cervical spinal injury.

❱ Although nasotracheal intubation is more comfortable than oral intubation, it's also more difficult to perform. Because the tube passes blindly through the nasal cavity, the procedure causes greater tissue trauma, increases the risk of infection by nasal bacteria introduced into the trachea, and

# Three methods to secure an ET tube *(continued)*

## Method 2

Cut one piece of 1" cloth adhesive tape long enough to wrap around the patient's head and overlap in front. Then cut an 8" (20.3-cm) piece of tape and center it on the longer piece, sticky sides together. Next, cut a 5" (12.7-cm) slit in each end of the longer tape (as shown below).

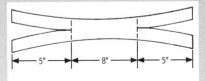

Apply benzoin tincture to the patient's cheeks, under his nose, and under his lower lip. (Don't spray benzoin directly on his face because the vapors can be irritating if inhaled and can also harm his eyes.)

Place the top half of one end of the tape under the patient's nose and wrap the lower half around the ET tube. Place the lower half of the other end of the tape along his lower lip and wrap the top half around the tube (as shown below).

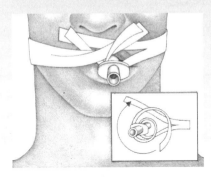

## Method 3

Cut a tracheostomy tie in two pieces, one a few inches longer than the other, and cut two 6" (15.2-cm) pieces of 1" cloth adhesive tape. Then cut a 2" slit in one end of both pieces of tape. Fold back the other end of the tape ½" (1.3 cm) so that the sticky sides are together, and cut a small hole in it (as shown below).

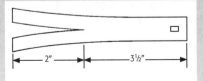

Apply benzoin tincture to the part of the ET tube that will be taped. Wrap the split ends of each piece of tape around the tube, one piece on each side. Overlap the tape to secure it.

Apply the free ends of the tape to both sides of the patient's face. Then insert tracheostomy ties through the holes in the tape and knot the ties (as shown below).

Bring the longer tie behind the patient's neck. Knotting the ties on the side prevents him from lying on the knot and developing a pressure ulcer.

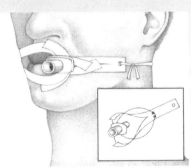

risks pressure necrosis of the nasal mucosa. However, exact tube placement is easier, and the risk of dislodgment is lower. The cuff on the ET tube maintains a closed system that permits positive-pressure ventilation and protects the airway from aspiration of secretions and gastric contents.

▶ Although low-pressure cuffs have significantly reduced the incidence of tracheal erosion and necrosis caused by cuff pres-

sure on the tracheal wall, overinflation of a low-pressure cuff can negate the benefit. Use the minimal-leak technique to avoid these complications. Inflating the cuff a bit more to make a complete seal with the least amount of air is the next most desirable method.

▶ Always record the volume of air needed to inflate the cuff. A gradual increase in this volume indicates tracheal dilatation or

# Retrograde intubation:
# An alternative method to establish an artificial airway

When a patient's airway can't be secured using conventional oral or nasal intubation, retrograde intubation should be considered. In this technique, a wire is inserted through the trachea and out the mouth and is then used to guide the insertion of an endotracheal (ET) tube (as shown below).

Only doctors, nurses, and paramedics who have been specially trained may perform retrograde intubation. However, the procedure has numerous advantages: It requires little or no head movement; it's less invasive than cricothyrotomy or tracheotomy

and doesn't leave a permanent scar; and it doesn't require direct visualization of the vocal cords.

Retrograde intubation is contraindicated in patients with complete airway obstruction, a thyroid tumor, an enlarged thyroid gland that overlies the cricothyroid ligament, or coagulopathy and in those whose mouths can't open wide enough to allow the guide wire to be retrieved. Possible complications include minor bleeding and hematoma formation at the puncture site, subcutaneous emphysema, hoarseness, and bleeding into the trachea.

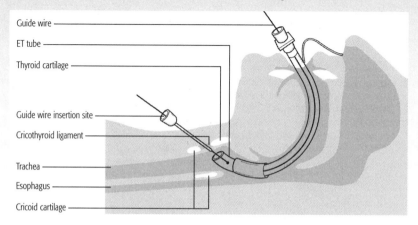

Guide wire
ET tube
Thyroid cartilage
Guide wire insertion site
Cricothyroid ligament
Trachea
Esophagus
Cricoid cartilage

---

erosion. A sudden increase in volume indicates rupture of the cuff and requires immediate reintubation if the patient is being ventilated or if he requires continuous cuff inflation to maintain a high concentration of delivered oxygen. When the cuff has been inflated, measure its pressure at least every 8 hours to avoid overinflation. Normal cuff pressure is about 18 mm Hg.
◗ When neither method of ET intubation is possible, consider the alternative of retrograde intubation. (See *Retrograde intubation: An alternative method to establish an artificial airway.*)

## Complications

ET intubation can result in apnea caused by reflex breath-holding or interruption of oxygen delivery; bronchospasm; aspiration of blood, secretions, or gastric contents; tooth damage or loss; and injury to the lips,

mouth, pharynx, or vocal cords. It can also result in laryngeal edema and erosion and in tracheal stenosis, erosion, and necrosis. Nasotracheal intubation can result in nasal bleeding, laceration, sinusitis, and otitis media.

## Documentation

◗ Record the date and time of the procedure.
◗ Document indication for the procedure and its success or failure.
◗ Write down the tube type and size.
◗ Note cuff size, amount of inflation, and inflation technique.
◗ Document administration of medication.
◗ Record initiation of supplemental oxygen or ventilation therapy.
◗ Record results of chest auscultation and of chest X-ray.

▶ Document any complications and interventions

▶ Record the patient's reaction to the procedure.

## REFERENCES

American Heart Association in Collaboration with the International Liaison Committee on Resuscitation. "Guidelines 2000 for Cardiopulmonary Resuscitation and Emergency Cardiovascular Care," *Circulation* 102(8 Suppl):I1-384, August 2000.

Asselin, M.E., and Cullen, H.A. "What You Need to Know about the New ACLS Guidelines," *Nursing2001* 31(4):48-50, April 2001.

Kern, K.B., et al. "New Guidelines for Cardiopulmonary Resuscitation and Emergency Cardiac Care: Changes in the Management of Cardiac Arrest," *JAMA* 285(10): 1267-69, March 2001.

Wong, E., et al. "Confirmation of Endotracheal Tube Placement: Analysis of 6,294 Emergency Department Intubations," *Annals of Emergency Medicine* 36(4 Pt 2):S53, October 2000.

# Endotracheal tube care

The intubated patient requires meticulous care to ensure airway patency and prevent complications until he can maintain independent ventilation. This care includes frequent assessment of airway status, maintenance of proper cuff pressure to prevent tissue ischemia and necrosis, repositioning of the tube to avoid traumatic manipulation, and constant monitoring for complications. Endotracheal (ET) tubes are repositioned for patient comfort or if a chest X-ray shows improper placement. Move the tube from one side of the mouth to the other to prevent pressure ulcers.

## Equipment

*For maintaining the airway*
Stethoscope ● suction equipment ● gloves

*For repositioning the tube*
10-ml syringe ● compound benzoin tincture ● stethoscope ● adhesive or hypoallergenic tape or Velcro tube holder ● suction equipment ● sedative or 2% lidocaine ● gloves ● handheld resuscitation bag with mask (in case of accidental extubation)

*For removing the tube*
10-ml syringe ● suction equipment ● supplemental oxygen source with mask ● coolmist, large-volume nebulizer ● handheld resuscitation bag with mask ● gloves ● equipment for reintubation

## Preparation of equipment
*For repositioning the ET tube*
Assemble all equipment at the patient's bedside. Using sterile technique, set up the suction equipment.

*For removing the ET tube*
Assemble all equipment at the patient's bedside. Set up the suction and supplemental oxygen equipment. Have ready all equipment for emergency reintubation.

## Implementation
▶ Explain the procedure to the patient even if he doesn't appear to be alert. Provide privacy, wash your hands thoroughly, and put on gloves.

## Maintaining airway patency
▶ Auscultate the patient's lungs at any sign of respiratory distress. If you detect an obstructed airway, determine the cause and treat it accordingly. If secretions are obstructing the lumen of the tube, suction the secretions from the tube.

▶ If the ET tube has slipped from the trachea into the right or left mainstem bronchus, breath sounds will be absent over one lung. Obtain a chest X-ray, as ordered, to verify tube placement and, if necessary, carefully reposition the tube. It's best to have another nurse to assist to avoid inadvertent dislodgement.

## Repositioning the ET tube
▶ Get help from a respiratory therapist or another nurse to prevent accidental extubation during the procedure if the patient coughs.

▶ Suction the patient's trachea through the ET tube to remove any secretions, which can cause the patient to cough during the procedure. Coughing increases the risk of trauma and tube dislodgment. Then suction the patient's pharynx to remove any secretions that may have accumulated above the tube cuff. This helps to prevent aspiration of secretions during cuff deflation.

▶ To prevent traumatic manipulation of the tube, instruct the assisting nurse to hold it as you carefully untape the tube or unfasten the Velcro tube holder. When freeing the tube, locate a landmark such as a number on the tube or measure the distance from the patient's mouth to the top of the tube so that you have a reference point when moving the tube.

▶ Next, deflate the cuff by attaching a 10-ml syringe to the pilot balloon port and aspirating air until you meet resistance and the pilot balloon deflates. Deflate the cuff before moving the tube because the cuff forms a seal within the trachea and movement of an inflated cuff can damage the tracheal wall and vocal cords.

▶ Reposition the tube as necessary, noting new landmarks or measuring the length. Then immediately reinflate the cuff. To do this, instruct the patient to inhale and slowly inflate the cuff using a 10-ml syringe attached to the pilot balloon port. As you do this, use your stethoscope to auscultate the patient's neck to determine the presence of an air leak. When air leakage ceases, stop cuff inflation and, while still auscultating the patient's neck, aspirate a small amount of air until you detect a slight leak. This creates a minimal air leak, which indicates that the cuff is inflated at the lowest pressure possible to create an adequate seal. If the patient is being mechanically ventilated, aspirate to create a minimal air leak during the inspiratory phase of respiration because the positive pressure of the ventilator during inspiration will create a larger leak around the cuff. Note the number of cubic centimeters of air required to achieve a minimal air leak.

▶ Measure cuff pressure and compare the reading with previous pressure readings to prevent overinflation. Then use benzoin and tape to secure the tube in place, or refasten the Velcro tube holder.

**EVIDENCE BASE** Studies have shown that adhesive or twill tape has been very effective in preventing an unplanned extubation and maintaining skin integrity of the oral mucosa and face.

▶ Make sure the patient is comfortable and the airway patent. Properly clean or dispose of equipment.

▶ When the cuff is inflated, measure its pressure at least every 8 hours to avoid overinflation.

## Removing the ET tube

**EVIDENCE BASE** When your patient no longer requires mechanical ventilation, his ET tube may be removed. The Agency for Healthcare Research and Quality (AHRQ) selected the McMaster University Evidence-Based Practice Center to investigate issues related to weaning patients from mechanical ventilation. Their recommendations include:

▶ Develop a protocol implemented by nurses and respiratory therapists to begin trials to decrease ventilator support soon after intubation. This ventilator support should be reduced at every opportunity.

▶ When using step-wise reductions in mechanical ventilation, pressure support mode or multiple T-piece trials may be better than using intermittent mandatory ventilation.

▶ When using weaning trials of unassisted breathing, low levels of pressure support may be helpful.

▶ Patients who are alert, cooperative, and ready to breathe without an artificial airway may benefit from early extubation and use of noninvasive positive pressure.

▶ When you're authorized to remove the tube, obtain another nurse's assistance to prevent traumatic manipulation of the tube when it's untaped or unfastened.

▶ Elevate the head of the patient's bed to approximately 90 degrees.

▶ Suction the patient's oropharynx and nasopharynx to remove any accumulated secretions and to help prevent aspiration of secretions when the cuff is deflated.

▶ Using a handheld resuscitation bag or the mechanical ventilator, give the patient several deep breaths through the ET tube to hyperinflate his lungs and increase his oxygen reserve.

▶ Attach a 10-ml syringe to the pilot balloon port and aspirate air until you meet resistance and the pilot balloon deflates. If you fail to detect an air leak around the deflated cuff, notify the doctor immediately and don't proceed with extubation. Absence of an air leak may indicate marked tracheal edema, which can result in total airway obstruction if the ET tube is removed.

▶ If you detect the proper air leak, untape or unfasten the ET tube while the assisting nurse stabilizes the tube.

▶ Insert a sterile suction catheter through the ET tube. Then apply suction and ask

the patient to take a deep breath and to open his mouth fully and pretend to cry out. This causes abduction of the vocal cords and reduces the risk of laryngeal trauma during withdrawal of the tube.
▶ Simultaneously remove the ET tube and the suction catheter in one smooth, outward, and downward motion, following the natural curve of the patient's mouth. Suctioning during extubation removes secretions retained at the end of the tube and prevents aspiration.
▶ Give the patient supplemental oxygen. For maximum humidity, use a cool-mist, large-volume nebulizer to help decrease airway irritation, patient discomfort, and laryngeal edema.
▶ Encourage the patient to cough and breathe deeply. Remind him that a sore throat and hoarseness are to be expected and will gradually subside.
▶ Make sure the patient is comfortable and the airway is patent. Clean or dispose of equipment.
▶ After extubation, auscultate the patient's lungs frequently and watch for signs of respiratory distress. Be especially alert for stridor or other evidence of upper airway obstruction. If ordered, draw an arterial sample for blood gas analysis.

### Special considerations
▶ When repositioning an ET tube, be especially careful in patients with highly sensitive airways. Sedation or direct instillation of 2% lidocaine to numb the airway may be indicated in such patients. Because the lidocaine is absorbed systemically, you must have a doctor's order to use it.
▶ After extubation of a patient who has been intubated for an extended time, keep reintubation supplies readily available for at least 12 hours or until you're sure he can tolerate extubation.
▶ Never extubate a patient unless someone skilled at intubation is readily available.
▶ If you inadvertently cut the pilot balloon on the cuff, immediately call the person responsible for intubation in your facility, who will remove the damaged ET tube and replace it with one that is intact. Don't remove the tube because a tube with an air leak is better than no airway.

### Complications
Traumatic injury to the larynx or trachea may result from tube manipulation, accidental extubation, or tube slippage into the right bronchus. Ventilatory failure and airway obstruction, due to laryngospasm or marked tracheal edema, are the gravest possible complications of extubation.

### Documentation
▶ After tube repositioning, record the date and time of the procedure, reason for repositioning (such as malposition shown by chest X-ray), new tube position, total amount of air in the cuff after the procedure, any complications and interventions, and the patient's tolerance of the procedure.
▶ After extubation, record the date and time of extubation, presence or absence of stridor or other signs of upper airway edema, type of supplemental oxygen administered, any complications and required subsequent therapy, and the patient's tolerance of the procedure.

### REFERENCES
Agency for Healthcare Research and Quality. *Criteria for Weaning from Mechanical Ventilation.* Evidence Report/Technology Assessment: Number 23. AHRQ Publication No. 00-E028, June 2000. *www.ahrq.gov/clinic/epcsums/mechsumm.htm*
American Association for Respiratory Care. "AARC Clinical Practice Guideline: Removal of the Endotracheal Tube," *Respiratory Care* 44(1):85-90, January 1999.
Moore, A.S. "Clinical Highlights: Does It Matter Whether You Use Twill or Adhesive Tape?" *RN* 62(2):20, February 1999.

# End-tidal carbon dioxide monitoring

Monitoring of end-tidal carbon dioxide ($ETCO_2$) determines the carbon dioxide ($CO_2$) concentration in exhaled gas. In this technique, a photodetector measures the amount of infrared light absorbed by airway gas during inspiration and expiration. (Light absorption increases along with the $CO_2$ concentration.) A monitor converts these data to a $CO_2$ value and a corresponding waveform, or capnogram, if capnography is used. (See *How $ETCO_2$ monitoring works,* page 324.)

$ETCO_2$ monitoring provides information about the patient's pulmonary, cardiac, and metabolic status that aids patient manage-

# How ETco₂ monitoring works

The optical portion of an end-tidal carbon dioxide (ETco₂) monitor contains an infrared light source, a sample chamber, a special carbon dioxide ($CO_2$) filter, and a photodetector. The infrared light passes through the sample chamber and is absorbed in varying amounts, depending on the amount of $CO_2$ the patient has just exhaled. The photodetector measures $CO_2$ content and relays this information to the microprocessor in the monitor, which displays the $CO_2$ value and waveform.

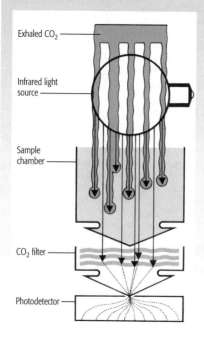

Exhaled CO₂

Infrared light source

Sample chamber

CO₂ filter

Photodetector

ment and helps prevent clinical compromise. This technique has become standard during anesthesia administration and mechanical ventilation.

The sensor, which contains an infrared light source and a photodetector, is positioned at one of two sites in the monitoring setup. With a mainstream monitor, it's positioned directly at the patient's airway with an airway adapter, between the endotracheal (ET) tube and the breathing circuit tubing. With a sidestream monitor, the airway adapter is positioned at the airway (re-

gardless of whether the patient is intubated) to allow aspiration of gas from the patient's airway back to the sensor, which lies either within or close to the monitor.

Some $CO_2$ detection devices provide semiquantitative indications of $CO_2$ concentrations, supplying an approximate range rather than a specific value for ETco₂. Other devices simply indicate whether $CO_2$ is present during exhalation (See *Analyzing CO₂ levels*.)

ETco₂ monitoring may be used to help wean a patient with a stable acid-base balance from mechanical ventilation. It also reduces the need for frequent arterial blood gas (ABG) measurements, especially when combined with pulse oximetry. Other uses for ETco₂ monitoring include assessing resuscitation efforts and identifying the return of spontaneous circulation. Because no $CO_2$ is exhaled when breathing stops, this technique also detects apnea.

When used during ET intubation, ETco₂ monitoring can avert neurologic injury and even death by confirming correct ET tube placement and detecting accidental esophageal intubation because $CO_2$ isn't normally produced by the stomach. Ongoing ETco₂ monitoring throughout intubation can also prove valuable because an ET tube may become dislodged during manipulation or patient movement or transport.

## Equipment

Gloves ● mainstream or sidestream $CO_2$ monitor ● $CO_2$ sensor ● airway adapter as recommended by the manufacturer (a neonatal adapter may have a much smaller dead space, making it appropriate for a smaller patient)

### Preparation of equipment

If the monitor you're using isn't self-calibrating, calibrate it as the manufacturer directs. If you're using a sidestream $CO_2$ monitor, replace the water trap between patients, if directed. The trap allows humidity from exhaled gases to be condensed into an attached container. Newer sidestream models don't require water traps.

## Implementation

▶ If the patient requires ET intubation, an ETco₂ detector or monitor is usually applied immediately after the tube is inserted. If he doesn't require intubation or is already intubated and alert, explain the purpose and expected duration of monitoring. Tell an intubated patient that the monitor will painlessly measure the amount of $CO_2$ he exhales. Inform a nonintubated patient that the monitor will track his $CO_2$ concentration to make sure his breathing is effective.

▶ Wash your hands. After turning on the monitor and calibrating it (if necessary), position the airway adapter and sensor as the manufacturer directs. For an intubated patient, position the adapter directly on the ET tube. For a nonintubated patient, place the adapter at or near the patient's airway. (An oxygen-delivery cannula may have a sample port through which gas can be aspirated for monitoring.)

▶ Turn on all alarms and adjust alarm settings as appropriate for your patient. Make sure the alarm volume is loud enough to hear.

### Special considerations

▶ Wear gloves when handling the airway adapter to prevent cross-contamination. Make sure the adapter is changed with every breathing circuit and ET tube change.

▶ Place the adapter on the ET tube to avoid contaminating exhaled gases with fresh gas flow from the ventilator. If you're using a heat and moisture exchanger, you may be able to position the airway adapter between the exchanger and breathing circuit.

▶ If your patient's $ETCO_2$ values differ from his partial pressure of arterial carbon dioxide, assess him for factors that can influence $ETCO_2$, especially when the differential between arterial and $ETCO_2$ values (the arterial absolute difference of carbon dioxide [a-$ADCO_2$]) is above normal.

◆ **ALERT!** After $ETCO_2$ monitoring begins, obtain an ABG sample to determine baseline values. Note the difference between $ETCO_2$ and partial pressure of arterial carbon dioxide ($PaCO_2$) values (a-$ADCO_2$). Typically, $ETCO_2$ levels are 1 to 6 mm Hg less than $PaCO_2$ levels. As long as a-$ADCO_2$ is normal, you can estimate $PaCO_2$ from $ETCO_2$. Each time an ABG is obtained, note a-$ADCO_2$. If you use $ETCO_2$ values to estimate $PaCO_2$, measure expired ventilation at the same time. If expired ventilation and $ETCO_2$ values are constant, the patient's a-$ADCO_2$ isn't likely to have changed. Avoid estimating $PaCO_2$ from the $ETCO_2$ if the expired ventilation has

## Analyzing $CO_2$ levels

Depending on which end-tidal carbon dioxide ($ETCO_2$) detector you use, the meaning of color changes within the detector dome may differ from the analysis for the Easy Cap detector described below:

▶ The rim of the Easy Cap is divided into four segments (clockwise from the top): CHECK, A, B, and C. The CHECK segment is solid purple, signifying the absence of carbon dioxide ($CO_2$).

▶ The numbers in the other sections range from 0.03 to 5 and indicate the percentage of exhaled $CO_2$. The color should fluctuate during ventilation from purple (in section A) during inspiration to yellow (in section C) at the end of expiration. This indicates that the $ETCO_2$ levels are adequate (above 2%).

▶ An end-expiratory color change from C to the B range may be the first sign of hemodynamic instability.

▶ During cardiopulmonary resuscitation (CPR), an end-expiratory color change from the A or B range to the C range may mean the return of spontaneous ventilation.

▶ During prolonged cardiac arrest, inadequate pulmonary perfusion leads to inadequate gas exchange. The patient exhales little or no $CO_2$, so the color stays in the purple range even with proper intubation. Ineffective CPR also leads to inadequate pulmonary perfusion.

**COLOR INDICATIONS ON END-EXPIRATION**

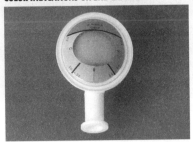

changed. Alert the doctor if your patient's a-$ADCO_2$ level is above the normal range. The patient may have a mismatching or shunting problem. Monitor a-$ADCO_2$ levels throughout therapy to determine the effectiveness of treatment and detect potential problems. If a-$ADCO_2$ increases, the patient may have reduced pulmonary perfusion.

# CO₂ waveform

The carbon dioxide ($CO_2$) waveform, or capnogram, produced in end-tidal carbon dioxide ($ETCO_2$) monitoring, reflects the course of $CO_2$ elimination during exhalation. A normal capnogram (shown below) consists of several segments, which reflect the various stages of exhalation and inhalation.

Normally, gas eliminated from the airway during early exhalation is dead-space gas, which hasn't undergone exchange at the alveolocapillary membrane. Measurements taken during this period contain no $CO_2$. As exhalation continues, $CO_2$ concentration rises sharply and rapidly. The sensor now detects gas that has undergone exchange, producing measurable quantities of $CO_2$.

The final stages of alveolar emptying occur during late exhalation. During the alveolar plateau phase, $CO_2$ concentration rises more gradually because alveolar emptying is more constant.

The point at which the $ETCO_2$ value is derived is at the end of exhalation, when $CO_2$ concentration peaks. Unless an alveolar plateau is present, this value doesn't accurately estimate alveolar $CO_2$. During inhalation, the $CO_2$ concentration declines sharply to zero.

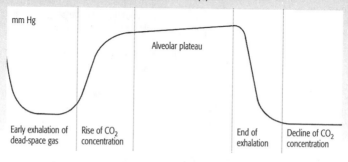

mm Hg

Alveolar plateau

Early exhalation of dead-space gas | Rise of $CO_2$ concentration | End of exhalation | Decline of $CO_2$ concentration

▶ The a-ADCO₂ value, if correctly interpreted, provides useful information about your patient's status. For example, an increased a-ADCO₂ may mean that your patient has worsening dead space, especially if his tidal volume remains constant.

▶ Remember that $ETCO_2$ monitoring doesn't replace ABG measurements because it doesn't assess oxygenation or blood pH. Supplementing $ETCO_2$ monitoring with pulse oximetry may provide more complete information.

▶ If the $CO_2$ waveform is available, assess it for height, frequency, rhythm, baseline, and shape to help evaluate gas exchange. Make sure you know how to recognize a normal waveform and can identify any abnormal waveforms and their possible causes. If a printer is available, record and document any abnormal waveforms in the patient's medical record. (See *CO₂ waveform*.)

▶ In a nonintubated patient, use $ETCO_2$ values to establish trends. Be aware that in a nonintubated patient, exhaled gas is more likely to mix with ambient air, and exhaled $CO_2$ may be diluted by fresh gas flow from the nasal cannula.

▶ $ETCO_2$ monitoring commonly is discontinued when the patient has been weaned effectively from mechanical ventilation or when he's no longer at risk for respiratory compromise. Carefully assess your patient's tolerance for weaning. After extubation, continuous $ETCO_2$ monitoring may detect the need for reintubation.

▶ Disposable $ETCO_2$ detectors are available. When using a disposable $ETCO_2$ detector, always check its color under fluorescent or natural light because the dome looks pink under incandescent light. (See *Precautions when using a disposable ETCO₂ detector.*)

## Complications

Inaccurate measurements, such as from poor sampling technique, calibration drift, contamination of optics with moisture or secretions, or equipment malfunction, can lead to misdiagnosis and improper treatment.

The effects of manual resuscitation or ingestion of alcohol or carbonated beverages

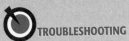

TROUBLESHOOTING

# Precautions when using a disposable ETco₂ detector

When using a disposable end-tidal carbon dioxide (ETco₂) detector, check the instructions and ensure ideal working conditions for the device. Here are some additional guidelines.

### Avoiding high humidity, moisture, and heat

▶ Watch for changes indicating that the ETco₂ detector's life span is decreasing – for example, slug-gish color changes from breath to breath. A detector normally may be used for about 2 hours. However, using it with a ventilator that delivers high-humidity ventilation may shorten its life span to no more than 15 minutes.

▶ Don't use the detector with a heated humidifier or nebulizer.

▶ Keep the detector protected from secretions, which would render the device useless. If secretions enter the dome, remove and discard the detector.

▶ Use a heat and moisture exchanger to protect the detector. In some detectors, this filter fits between the endotracheal (ET) tube and the detector.

▶ If you're using a heat and moisture exchanger, remember that it increases your patient's breathing

effort. Be alert for increased resistance and breathing difficulties and remove the exchanger, if necessary.

### Taking additional precautions

▶ Instilling epinephrine through the ET tube can damage the detector's indicator (the color may stay yellow). If this happens, discard the device.

▶ Take care when using an ETco₂ detector on a child who weighs less than 30 lb (13.6 kg). A small patient who rebreathes air from the dead air space (about 38 cc) will inhale too much of his own carbon dioxide.

▶ Frequently spot-check the ETco₂ detector you're using for effectiveness. If you must transport the patient to another area for testing or treatment, use another method to verify the tube's placement.

▶ Never reuse a disposable ETco₂ detector; it's intended for one-time, one-patient use only.

---

can alter the detector's findings. Color changes detected after fewer than six ventilations can be misleading.

## Documentation

▶ Document the initial ETco₂ value and all ventilator settings. Describe the waveform if one appears on the monitor. If the monitor has a printer, you may want to print out a sample waveform and include it in the patient's medical record.

▶ Document ETco₂ values at least as often as vital signs, whenever significant changes in waveform or patient status occur, and before and after weaning, respiratory, and other interventions.

▶ Periodically obtain samples for ABG analysis as the patient's condition dictates and document the corresponding ETco₂ values.

## REFERENCES

Ahrens, T., et al. "End-Tidal Carbon Dioxide Measurements as a Prognostic Indicator of Outcome of Cardiac Arrest," *American*
*Journal of Critical Care* 10(6):391-98, November 2001.
American Heart Association in Collaboration with the International Liaison Committee on Resuscitation. "Guidelines 2000 for Cardiopulmonary Resuscitation and Emergency Cardiovascular Care," *Circulation* 102(8 Suppl):I1-384, August 2000.
Blonshine, S. "Expanding the Knowledge Base: New Applications of Capnography," *AARC Times* 23(2):51-53, February 1999.
Capovilla, J., et al. "Noninvasive Blood Gas Monitoring," *Critical Care Nursing Quarterly* 23(2):79-86, August 2000.
Carroll, P. "Respiratory Monitoring: Evolutions: Capnography," *RN* 62(5):68-71, 78, May 1999.

# Incentive spirometry

Incentive spirometry involves using a breathing device to help the patient achieve maximal lung expansion. The device measures respiratory flow or respiratory volume and induces the patient to take a deep breath and hold it for several seconds. This deep breath increases lung volume, boosts alveolar inflation, and promotes venous return. This exercise also establishes alveolar hyperinflation for a longer time than is possible with a normal deep breath, thus preventing and reversing the alveolar collapse that causes atelectasis and pneumonitis.

Devices used for incentive spirometry provide a visual incentive to breathe deeply. Some are activated when the patient inhales a certain volume of air; the device then estimates the amount of air inhaled. Others contain plastic floats, which rise according to the amount of air the patient pulls through the device when he inhales.

Patients at low risk for developing atelectasis may use a flow incentive spirometer. Patients at high risk may need a volume incentive spirometer, which measures lung inflation more precisely.

Incentive spirometry benefits the patient on prolonged bed rest, especially the postoperative patient who may tend to hyperventilate due to such predisposing factors as abdominal or thoracic surgery, advanced age, inactivity, obesity, smoking, medications that depress respirations, and decreased ability to cough effectively and expel lung secretions.

### Equipment
Flow or volume incentive spirometer, as indicated, with sterile disposable tube and mouthpiece (the tube and mouthpiece are sterile on first use and clean on subsequent uses) ● stethoscope ● watch ● pencil and paper

### Preparation of equipment
Assemble the ordered equipment at the patient's bedside. Read the manufacturer's instructions for spirometer setup and operation.

Remove the sterile flow tube and mouthpiece from the package and attach them to the device. Set the flow rate or volume goal as determined by the doctor or respiratory therapist and based on the patient's preoperative performance. Turn on the machine if necessary.

### Implementation
▶ Assess the patient's condition.

▶ Explain the procedure to the patient, making sure that he understands the importance of performing incentive spirometry regularly to maintain alveolar inflation. Wash your hands.

▶ Help the patient into a comfortable sitting or semi-Fowler's position to promote optimal lung expansion. If you're using a flow incentive spirometer and the patient is unable to assume or maintain this position, he can perform the procedure in any position as long as the device remains upright. Tilting a flow incentive spirometer decreases the required patient effort and reduces the exercise's effectiveness.

▶ Auscultate the patient's lungs to provide a baseline for comparison with posttreatment auscultation.

▶ Instruct the patient to insert the mouthpiece and close his lips tightly around it because a weak seal may alter flow or volume readings.

▶ Instruct the patient to exhale normally and then inhale as slowly and as deeply as possible. If he has difficulty with this step, tell him to suck as he would through a straw but more slowly. Ask the patient to retain the entire volume of air he inhaled for 3 seconds or, if you're using a device with a light indicator, until the light turns off. This deep breath creates sustained transpulmonary pressure near the end of inspiration and is sometimes called a sustained maximal inspiration.

▶ Tell the patient to remove the mouthpiece and exhale normally. Allow him to relax and take several normal breaths before attempting another breath with the spirometer. Repeat this sequence 5 to 10 times during every waking hour. Note tidal volumes.

▶ Evaluate the patient's ability to cough effectively and encourage him to cough after each effort because full lung inflation may loosen secretions and facilitate their removal. Observe any expectorated secretions.

▶ Auscultate the patient's lungs, and compare findings with the first auscultation.

▶ Instruct the patient to remove the mouthpiece. Wash the device in warm water and shake it dry. Avoid immersing the spirometer itself because this enhances bacterial growth and impairs the internal filter's effectiveness in preventing inhalation of extraneous material.

▶ Place the mouthpiece in a plastic storage bag between exercises and label it and the spirometer, if applicable, with the patient's name to avoid inadvertent use by another patient.

### Special considerations
▶ If the patient is scheduled for surgery, make a preoperative assessment of his respiratory pattern and capability to ensure the development of appropriate postoperative goals. Teach the patient how to use the spirometer before surgery so that he can concentrate on your instructions and practice the exercise. A preoperative evaluation will also help in establishing a postoperative therapeutic goal.
▶ Avoid exercising at mealtime to prevent nausea. Provide paper and pencil so the patient can note exercise times. Exercise frequency varies with condition and ability.
▶ Immediately after surgery, monitor the exercise frequently to ensure compliance and assess achievement.

### Documentation
▶ Record any preoperative teaching you provided.
▶ Document preoperative flow or volume levels, the date and time of the procedure, the type of spirometer, the flow or volume levels achieved, and the number of breaths taken. Also note the patient's condition before and after the procedure, his tolerance of the procedure, and the results of both auscultations.

### REFERENCES
Edwards, D., et al. *Bedside Critical Care Manual.* Philadelphia: Lippincott Williams & Wilkins, 2001.
Vines, D.L., et al. "Current Respiratory Care, Part 1: Oxygen Therapy, Oximetry, Bronchial Hygiene," *Journal of Critical Illness* 15(9):507-10, 513-15, September 2000.

## Manual ventilation

A handheld resuscitation bag is an inflatable device that can be attached to a face mask or directly to an endotracheal (ET) or tracheostomy tube to allow manual delivery of oxygen or room air to the lungs of a patient who can't breathe by himself. Usually used in an emergency, manual ventilation also can be performed while the patient is disconnected temporarily from a mechanical ventilator, such as during a tubing change, during transport, or before suctioning. In such instances, the use of the handheld resuscitation bag maintains ventilation. Oxygen administration with a resuscitation bag can help improve a compromised cardiorespiratory system.

### Equipment
Handheld resuscitation bag ● mask ● oxygen source (wall unit or tank) ● oxygen tubing ● nipple adapter attached to oxygen flowmeter ● optional: suction equipment, oxygen accumulator and positive end-expiratory pressure (PEEP) valve (See *Using a PEEP valve,* page 330.)

#### Preparation of equipment
Unless the patient is intubated or has a tracheostomy, select a mask that fits snugly over the mouth and nose. Attach the mask to the resuscitation bag.

If oxygen is readily available, connect the handheld resuscitation bag to the oxygen. Attach one end of the tubing to the bottom of the bag and the other end to the nipple adapter on the flowmeter of the oxygen source.

Turn on the oxygen and adjust the flow rate according to the patient's condition. For example, if the patient has a low partial pressure of arterial oxygen, he'll need a higher fraction of inspired oxygen ($FIO_2$). To increase the concentration of inspired oxygen, you can add an oxygen accumulator (also called an oxygen reservoir). This device, which attaches to an adapter on the bottom of the bag, permits an $FIO_2$ of up to 100%. Then, if time allows, set up suction equipment.

### Implementation
▶ Before using the handheld resuscitation bag, check the patient's upper airway for foreign objects. If any are present, remove them because this alone may restore spontaneous respirations in some instances. Also, foreign matter or secretions can obstruct the airway and impede resuscitation efforts. Suction the patient to remove any secretions that may obstruct the airway. If necessary, insert an oropharyngeal or nasopharyngeal airway to maintain airway

## Using a PEEP valve

Add positive end-expiratory pressure (PEEP) to manual ventilation by attaching a PEEP valve to the resuscitation bag. This may improve oxygenation if the patient hasn't responded to increased fraction of inspired oxygen levels. Always use a PEEP valve to manually ventilate a patient who has been receiving PEEP on the ventilator.

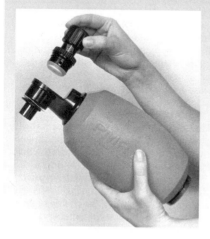

patency. If the patient has a tracheostomy or ET tube in place, suction the tube.

❯ If appropriate, remove the bed's headboard and stand at the head of the bed to help keep the patient's neck extended and to free space at the side of the bed for other activities such as cardiopulmonary resuscitation.

❯ Use the head-tilt chin lift to move the tongue away from the base of the pharynx and prevent obstruction of the airway. If trauma is present, use the jaw thrust method. (See *How to apply a handheld resuscitation bag and mask.*)

**EVIDENCE BASE** New basic life support guidelines recommend delivering a smaller tidal volume of 6 to 7 ml/ kg (about 400 to 600 ml) over 1 to 2 seconds when using a handheld resuscitation bag. Smaller tidal volumes reduce the risk of air entering the stomach and causing regurgitation, aspiration and pneumonia. That's because smaller tidal volumes don't exceed the pressure of the lower esophageal sphincter. Smaller tidal volumes do, however, increase the risk of hypoxia and hypercapnia.

Using supplemental oxygen (minimum flow rate of 8 to 12 L/minute) will improve oxygen saturation when using smaller tidal volumes. Because it's hard to assess tidal volume, use chest expansion and oxygen saturation values to determine the effectiveness of your ventilations.

When supplemental oxygen isn't available, use a larger tidal volume of 10 ml/kg (700 to 1,000 ml) over 2 seconds. You should notice a considerable chest rise when using a larger tidal volume.

❯ Keeping your nondominant hand on the patient's mask, exert downward pressure to seal the mask against his face. For an adult patient, use your dominant hand to compress the bag every 5 seconds to deliver approximately 1 L of air.

**◆ ALERT!** For infants and children, use a pediatric handheld resuscitation bag. For a child, deliver 15 breaths/ minute, or one compression of the bag every 4 seconds; for an infant, 20 breaths/ minute, or one compression every 3 seconds. Infants and children should receive 250 to 500 ml of air with each bag compression.

❯ Deliver breaths with the patient's own inspiratory effort, if any is present. Don't attempt to deliver a breath as the patient exhales.

❯ Observe the patient's chest to ensure that it rises and falls with each compression. If ventilation fails to occur, check the fit of the mask and the patency of the patient's airway; if necessary, reposition his head and ensure patency with an oral airway.

### Special considerations

❯ Avoid neck hyperextension if the patient has a possible cervical injury; instead, use the jaw-thrust technique to open the airway. If you need both hands to keep the patient's mask in place and maintain hyperextension, use the lower part of your arm to compress the bag against your side.

❯ Observe for vomiting through the clear part of the mask. If vomiting occurs, stop the procedure immediately, lift the mask, wipe and suction the vomitus, and resume resuscitation.

❯ Underventilation commonly occurs because the handheld resuscitation bag is difficult to keep positioned tightly on the patient's face while ensuring an open airway. In addition, the volume of air delivered to the patient varies with the type of bag used and the hand size of the person compressing the bag. An adult with a small- or medium-sized hand may not consistently deliver 1 L of air. For these reasons, have someone assist with the procedure, if possible.

### Complications

Aspiration of vomitus can result in pneumonia, and gastric distention may result from air forced into the patient's stomach.

### Documentation

❯ In an emergency, record the date and time of the procedure, manual ventilation efforts, any complications and the nursing action taken, and the patient's response to treatment according to your facility's protocol for respiratory arrest.
❯ In a nonemergency situation, record the date and time of the procedure, reason and length of time the patient was disconnected from mechanical ventilation and received manual ventilation, any complications and the nursing action taken, and the patient's tolerance of the procedure.

### REFERENCES

American Heart Association in Collaboration with the International Liaison Committee on Resuscitation. "Guidelines 2000 for Cardiopulmonary Resuscitation and Emergency Cardiovascular Care," *Circulation* 102(8 Suppl):I1-384, August 2000.

Asselin, M.E., and Cullen, H.A. "What You Need to Know about the New ACLS Guidelines," *Nursing2001* 31(4):48-50, April 2001.

"Don't Intubate for Peds Emergencies," *AJN* 100(5):19, May 2000.

Frakes, M.A. "Pediatric Intubation," *AJN* 100(9):14, September 2000.

Kern, K.B., et al. "New Guidelines for Cardiopulmonary Resuscitation and Emergency Cardiac Care Changes in the Management of Cardiac Arrest," *JAMA* 285(10):1267-69, March 2001.

Little, C. "Manual Ventilation," *Nursing2000* 30(3):50-51, March 2000.

## How to apply a handheld resuscitation bag and mask

Place the mask over the patient's face so that the apex of the triangle covers the bridge of his nose and the base lies between his lower lip and chin.

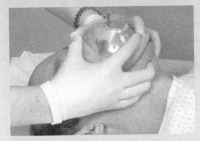

Make sure that the patient's mouth remains open underneath the mask. Attach the bag to the mask and to the tubing leading to the oxygen source.

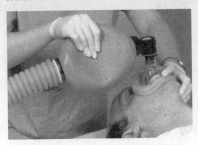

Or, if the patient has a tracheostomy tube or an endotracheal tube in place, remove the mask from the bag and attach the handheld resuscitation bag directly to the tube.

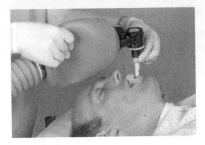

# Mechanical ventilation

A mechanical ventilator moves air in and out of a patient's lungs. Although the equipment serves to ventilate a patient, it doesn't ensure adequate gas exchange. Mechanical ventilators may use either positive or negative pressure to ventilate patients.

Positive-pressure ventilators exert a positive pressure on the airway, which causes inspiration while increasing tidal volume ($V_T$). The inspiratory cycles of these ventilators may vary in volume, pressure, or time. For example, a volume-cycled ventilator—the type used most commonly—delivers a preset volume of air each time, regardless of the amount of lung resistance. A pressure-cycled ventilator generates flow until the machine reaches a preset pressure regardless of the volume delivered or the time required to achieve the pressure. A time-cycled ventilator generates flow for a preset amount of time. A high-frequency ventilator uses high respiratory rates and low $V_T$ to maintain alveolar ventilation.

Negative-pressure ventilators act by creating negative pressure, which pulls the thorax outward and allows air to flow into the lungs. Examples of such ventilators are the iron lung, the cuirass (chest shell), and the body wrap. Negative-pressure ventilators are used mainly to treat neuromuscular disorders, such as Guillain-Barré syndrome, myasthenia gravis, and poliomyelitis.

Other indications for ventilator use include central nervous system disorders, such as cerebral hemorrhage and spinal cord transsection; adult respiratory distress syndrome; pulmonary edema; chronic obstructive pulmonary disease; flail chest; and acute hypoventilation.

## Equipment

Oxygen source • air source that can supply 50 psi • mechanical ventilator • humidifier • ventilator circuit tubing, connectors, and adapters • condensation collection trap • in-line thermometer • gloves • handheld resuscitation bag with reservoir • suction equipment • sterile distilled water • equipment for arterial blood gas (ABG) analysis • optional: oximeter and soft restraints

## Preparation of equipment

In most facilities, respiratory therapists assume responsibility for setting up the ventilator. If necessary, check the manufacturer's instructions for setting it up. In most cases, you'll need to add sterile distilled water to the humidifier and connect the ventilator to the appropriate gas source.

## Implementation

▶ Verify the doctor's order for ventilator support. If the patient isn't already intubated, prepare him for intubation.

▶ When possible, explain the procedure to the patient and his family to help reduce anxiety and fear. Assure the patient and his family that staff members are nearby to provide care.

▶ Perform a complete physical assessment and draw blood for ABG analysis to establish a baseline.

▶ Suction the patient, if necessary.

▶ Plug the ventilator into the electrical outlet and turn it on. Adjust the settings on the ventilator as ordered. (See *Mechanical ventilation glossary.*) Make sure that the ventilator's alarms are set as ordered and that the humidifier is filled with sterile distilled water.

▶ Put on gloves, if you haven't already. Connect the endotracheal tube to the ventilator. Observe for chest expansion, and auscultate for bilateral breath sounds to verify that the patient is being ventilated.

▶ Monitor the patient's ABG values after the initial ventilator setup (usually 20 to 30 minutes), after any changes in ventilator settings, and as the patient's clinical condition indicates to determine whether the patient is being adequately ventilated and to avoid oxygen toxicity. Be prepared to adjust ventilator settings based on ABG analysis.

▶ Check the ventilator tubing frequently for condensation, which can cause resistance to airflow and may also be aspirated by the patient. As needed, drain the condensate into a collection trap or briefly disconnect the patient from the ventilator (ventilating him with a handheld resuscitation bag, if necessary), and empty the water into a receptacle. Don't drain the condensate into the humidifier because the condensate may be contaminated with the patient's secretions.

# Mechanical ventilation glossary

Although a respiratory therapist usually monitors ventilator settings based on the doctor's order, you should understand all of the following terms.

**Assist-control mode:** The assist-control mode allows the ventilator to deliver a preset rate; however, the patient can initiate additional breaths, which trigger the ventilator to deliver the preset tidal volume at positive pressure.

**Continuous positive airway pressure (CPAP):** The CPAP setting prompts the ventilator to deliver positive pressure to the airway throughout the respiratory cycle. It works only on patients who can breathe spontaneously.

**Control mode:** The control mode allows the ventilator to deliver a preset tidal volume at a fixed rate regardless of whether or not the patient is breathing spontaneously.

**Fraction of inspired oxygen ($Fio_2$):** The $Fio_2$ is the amount of oxygen delivered to the patient by the ventilator. The dial or digital display on the ventilator that sets this percentage is labeled by the term oxygen concentration or oxygen percentage.

**I:E ratio:** The I:E ratio compares the duration of inspiration with the duration of expiration. The I:E ratio of normal, spontaneous breathing is 1:2, meaning that expiration is twice as long as inspiration.

**Inspiratory flow rate (IFR):** The inspiratory flow rate IFR denotes the tidal volume delivered within a certain time. Its value can range from 20 to 120 L/minute.

**Minute ventilation or minute volume ($V_E$):** The $V_E$ measurement results from the multiplication of respiratory rate and tidal volume.

**Peak inspiratory pressure (PIP):** Measured by the pressure manometer on the ventilator, the PIP reflects the amount of pressure required to deliver a preset tidal volume.

**Positive end-expiratory pressure (PEEP):** In the PEEP mode, the ventilator is triggered to apply positive pressure at the end of each expiration to increase the area for oxygen exchange by helping to inflate and keep open collapsed alveoli.

**Pressure support ventilation (PSV):** The PSV mode allows the ventilator to apply a preset amount of positive pressure when the patient inspires spontaneously. PSV increases tidal volume while decreasing the patient's breathing workload. This may be used during weaning trials.

**Respiratory rate:** The respiratory rate is the number of breaths per minute delivered by the ventilator; also called frequency.

**Sensitivity setting:** The sensitivity setting determines the amount of effort the patient must exert to trigger the inspiratory cycle.

**Sigh volume:** The sigh volume is a ventilator-delivered breath that is 1½ times as large as the patient's tidal volume.

**Synchronized intermittent mandatory ventilation (SIMV):** The SIMV allows the ventilator to deliver a preset number of breaths at a specific tidal volume. The patient may supplement these mechanical ventilations with his own breaths, in which case the tidal volume and rate are determined by his own inspiratory ability.

**Tidal volume ($V_T$):** $V_T$ refers to the volume of air delivered to the patient with each cycle, usually 12 to 15 cc/kg.

---

▶ Check the in-line thermometer to make sure that the temperature of the air delivered to the patient is close to body temperature.

▶ When monitoring the patient's vital signs, count spontaneous breaths as well as ventilator-delivered breaths.

▶ Change, clean, or dispose of the ventilator tubing and equipment according to your facility's policy to reduce the risk of bacterial contamination. Typically, ventilator tubing should be changed every 48 to 72 hours and sometimes more often.

▶ When ordered, begin to wean the patient from the ventilator. (See *Weaning a patient from the ventilator,* page 334.)

According to the American Association of Critical-Care Nurses' Third National Study Group, weaning from mechanical ventilation is a process consisting of 3 stages: the preweaning stage, the weaning process, and the outcome stage.

# Weaning a patient from the ventilator

Successful weaning depends on the patient's ability to breathe on his own. This means he must have a spontaneous respiratory effort that can keep him ventilated, a stable cardiovascular system, and sufficient respiratory muscle strength and level of consciousness to sustain spontaneous breathing. He also should meet some or all of the following criteria.

## Criteria

▶ Partial pressure of arterial oxygen of 60 mm Hg (50 mm Hg or the ability to maintain baseline levels if he has chronic lung disease) or a fraction of inspired oxygen ($Fio_2$) of 0.4 or less

▶ Partial pressure of arterial carbon dioxide ($Paco_2$) of less than 40 mm Hg (or normal for the patient) or an $Fio_2$ of 0.4 or less if $Paco_2$ is 60 mm Hg or more

▶ Vital capacity of more than 10 ml/kg of body weight

▶ Maximum inspiratory pressure of more than 20 cm $H_2O$

▶ Minute ventilation less than 10 L/minute with a respiratory frequency of less than 30 breaths/minute

▶ Forced expiratory volume in the first second of more than 10 ml/kg of body weight

▶ Ability to double the spontaneous resting minute ventilation

▶ Adequate natural airway or a functioning tracheostomy

▶ Ability to cough and mobilize secretions

▶ Successful withdrawal of any neuromuscular blocker such as pancuronium bromide

▶ Clear or clearing chest X-ray

▶ Absence of infection, acid-base or electrolyte imbalance, hyperglycemia, arrhythmia, renal failure, anemia, fever, or excessive fatigue

## Short-term ventilation

If the patient has received mechanical ventilation for a short time, weaning may be accomplished by progressively decreasing the frequency and tidal volume of the ventilated breaths. Then the patient's endotracheal tube can be converted to a T tube to assess whether his spontaneous respirations are adequate before extubation. If the patient has been mechanically ventilated with 5 cm $H_2O$ or less of positive end-expiratory pressure, the adequacy of his spontaneous breathing can be assessed by using a trial of continuous positive airway pressure on the ventilator.

## Long-term ventilation

If the patient has received mechanical ventilation for a long time, weaning is usually accomplished by switching the ventilator to pressure support ventilation (PSV) with or without intermittent mandatory ventilation (IMV). That way, each of the patient's spontaneous breaths is augmented by the ventilator. As the patient's own respirations improve, IMV and PSV can be decreased.

If the patient doesn't progress satisfactorily using one of these methods, an alternative method of weaning is to disconnect him from the ventilator and place him on a T tube or tracheostomy collar for the ordered amount of time before reconnecting him to the ventilator. The patient then alternates between being on and off the ventilator, increasing the time off the ventilator with each trial.

---

▶ During the preweaning stage, the events leading up to the need for mechanical ventilation are considered and complications that may interfere with weaning are prevented. The health care team determines the patient's readiness for weaning and chooses a strategy and mode of weaning. As the patient stabilizes, he crosses the readiness threshold into the weaning stage.

▶ During the weaning stage, the patient may experience progress and setbacks. Factors related to the patient that may affect weaning during this phase include myocardial function and oxygenation, nutrition, electrolyte balance, ventilatory muscle strength, ventilatory drive and psychological concerns. During the weaning process, assessment criteria that indicate a weaning trial should be stopped include dyspnea, rapid, shallow breathing, facial expression, use of accessory muscles, heart rate, and blood pressure. Facilitative strategies such as biofeedback may also be used during this phase.

▶ The outcome stage includes complete weaning, incomplete weaning where long-term partial or full mechanical ventilatory support may be required, and terminal

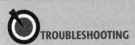

# Responding to ventilator alarms

| Signal | Possible cause | Interventions |
|---|---|---|
| Low-pressure alarm | ▶ Tube disconnected from ventilator | ▶ Reconnect the tube to the ventilator. |
| | ▶ Endotracheal (ET) tube displaced above vocal cords or tracheostomy tube extubated | ▶ Check the tube placement and reposition, if needed. If extubation or displacement has occurred, ventilate the patient manually and call the doctor immediately. |
| | ▶ Leaking tidal volume from low cuff pressure (from an underinflated or ruptured cuff or a leak in the cuff or one-way valve) | ▶ Listen for a whooshing sound around the tube, indicating an air leak. If you hear one, check the cuff pressure. If you can't maintain pressure, call the doctor; he may need to insert a new tube. |
| | ▶ Ventilator malfunction | ▶ Disconnect the patient from the ventilator and ventilate him manually, if necessary. Obtain another ventilator. |
| | ▶ Leak in ventilator circuitry (from loose connection or hole in tubing, loss of temperature-sensitive device, or cracked humidification jar) | ▶ Make sure all connections are intact. Check for holes or leaks in the tubing and replace, if necessary. Check the humidification jar and replace, if cracked. |
| High-pressure alarm | ▶ Increased airway pressure or decreased lung compliance caused by worsening disease | ▶ Auscultate the lungs for evidence of increasing lung consolidation, barotrauma, or wheezing. Call the doctor, if indicated. |
| | ▶ Patient biting on oral ET tube | ▶ Insert a bite block if needed. |
| | ▶ Secretions in airway | ▶ Look for secretions in the airway. To remove them, suction the patient or have him cough. |
| | ▶ Condensate in large-bore tubing | ▶ Check tubing for condensate and remove any fluid. |
| | ▶ Intubation of right mainstem bronchus | ▶ Check tube position. If it has slipped, call the doctor; he may need to reposition it. |
| | ▶ Patient coughing, gagging, or attempting to talk | ▶ If the patient fights the ventilator, the doctor may order a sedative or neuromuscular blocking agent. |
| | ▶ Chest wall resistance | ▶ Reposition the patient to see if doing so improves chest expansion. If repositioning doesn't help, administer the prescribed analgesic. |
| | ▶ Failure of high-pressure relief valve | ▶ Have the faulty equipment replaced. |
| | ▶ Bronchospasm | ▶ Assess the patient for the cause. Report to the doctor and treat the patient, as ordered. |

weaning in which natural death may occur (also called withdrawal of life support).

## Special considerations

▶ Provide emotional support to the patient during all phases of mechanical ventilation to reduce his anxiety and promote successful treatment. Even if the patient is unresponsive, continue to explain all procedures and treatments to him.

▶ Make sure that the ventilator alarms are on at all times. These alarms alert the nursing staff to potentially hazardous conditions and changes in patient status. If an alarm sounds and the problem can't be identified easily, disconnect the patient from the ventilator and use a handheld resuscitation bag to ventilate him. (See *Responding to ventilator alarms*.)

▶ Unless contraindicated, turn the patient from side to side every 1 to 2 hours to facilitate lung expansion and removal of secretions. Perform active or passive range-of-motion exercises for all extremities to reduce the hazards of immobility. If the patient's condition permits, position him upright at regular intervals to increase lung expansion. When moving the patient or the ventilator tubing, be careful to prevent condensation in the tubing from flowing into the lungs because aspiration of this contaminated moisture can cause infection. Provide care for the patient's artificial airway as needed.

▶ Assess the patient's peripheral circulation and monitor his urine output for signs of decreased cardiac output. Watch for signs of fluid volume excess or dehydration.

▶ Place the call light within the patient's reach and establish a method of communication such as a communication board because intubation and mechanical ventilation impair the patient's ability to speak. An artificial airway may help the patient to speak by allowing air to pass through his vocal cords.

▶ Administer a sedative or neuromuscular blocking agent, as ordered, to relax the patient or eliminate spontaneous breathing efforts that can interfere with the ventilator's action. Remember that the patient receiving a neuromuscular blocking drug requires close observation because of his inability to breathe or communicate as well as adequate pain relief or sedation.

▶ If the patient is receiving a neuromuscular blocking agent, make sure that he also receives a sedative. Neuromuscular blocking agents cause paralysis without altering the patient's level of consciousness. Reassure the patient and his family that the paralysis is temporary. Also, make sure that emergency equipment is readily available in case the ventilator malfunctions or the patient is extubated accidentally. Continue to explain all procedures to the patient and take additional steps to ensure his safety, such as raising the side rails of his bed while turning him and covering and lubricating his eyes.

▶ Ensure that the patient gets adequate rest and sleep because fatigue can delay weaning from the ventilator. Provide subdued lighting, safely muffle equipment noises, and restrict staff access to the area to promote quiet during rest periods.

▶ When weaning the patient, continue to observe for signs of hypoxia. Schedule weaning to fit comfortably and realistically with the patient's daily regimen. Avoid scheduling sessions after meals, baths, or lengthy therapeutic or diagnostic procedures. Have the patient help you set up the schedule to give him some sense of control over a frightening procedure. As the patient's tolerance for weaning increases, help him sit up out of bed to improve his breathing and sense of well-being. Suggest diversionary activities to take his mind off breathing.

## Home care
If the patient will be discharged on a ventilator, evaluate the family's or the caregiver's ability and motivation to provide such care. Well before discharge, develop a teaching plan that will address the patient's needs. For example, teaching should include information about ventilator care and settings, artificial airway care, suctioning, respiratory therapy, communication, nutrition, therapeutic exercise, the signs and symptoms of infection, and ways to troubleshoot minor equipment malfunctions.

Also, evaluate the patient's need for adaptive equipment, such as a hospital bed, wheelchair or walker with a ventilator tray, patient lift, and bedside commode. Determine whether the patient needs to travel; if so, select appropriate portable and backup equipment.

Before discharge, have the patient's caregiver demonstrate his ability to use the equipment. At discharge, contact a durable medical equipment vendor and a home health nurse to follow up with the patient. Also, refer the patient to community resources, if available.

## Complications
Mechanical ventilation can cause tension pneumothorax, decreased cardiac output, oxygen toxicity, fluid volume excess caused by humidification, infection, and such GI complications as distention or bleeding from stress ulcers.

## Documentation
▶ Document the date and time of initiation of mechanical ventilation.

▶ Record the type of ventilator used, and note its settings.

▶ Document the patient's response to mechanical ventilation, including vital signs, breath sounds, use of accessory muscles, intake and output, and weight.

▶ Note any complications and nursing actions taken.

▶ Record all pertinent laboratory data, including ABG analysis results and oxygen saturation levels.

▶ During weaning, record the date and time of each session, the weaning method, and baseline and subsequent vital signs, oxygen saturation levels, and ABG values. Again, record the patient's subjective and objective responses, including level of consciousness, respiratory effort, arrhythmia, skin color, and need for suctioning.

▶ Document all complications and nursing actions taken.

▶ If the patient was receiving pressure support ventilation (PSV) or using a T-piece or tracheostomy collar, note the duration of spontaneous breathing and the patient's ability to maintain the weaning schedule.

▶ If using intermittent mandatory ventilation, with or without PSV, record the control breath rate, the time of each breath reduction, and the rate of spontaneous respirations.

## REFERENCES

Agency for Healthcare Research and Quality. *Criteria for Weaning from Mechanical Ventilation.* Evidence Report/Technology Assessment: Number 23. AHRQ Publication No. 00-E028, June 2000. *www.ahrq.gov/clinic/epcsums/mechsumm.htm*

Ahrens, T., et al. "End-Tidal Carbon Dioxide Measurements as a Prognostic Indicator of Outcome of Cardiac Arrest," *American Journal of Critical Care* 10(6):391-98, November 2001.

Henneman, E.A. "Liberating Patients from Mechanical Ventilation: A Team Approach," *Critical Care Nurse* 21(3):25, 27-33, June 2001.

Tasota, F.J., and Dobbin, K. "Weaning Your Patient from Mechanical Ventilation," *Nursing2000* 30(10):41-46, October 2000.

Woodruff, D.W. "How to Ward off Complications of Mechanical Ventilation," *Nursing99* 29(11):34-39, November 1999.

# Mixed venous oxygen saturation monitoring

Mixed venous oxygen saturation ($S\bar{v}O_2$) monitoring uses a fiber-optic thermodilution pulmonary artery (PA) catheter to continuously monitor oxygen delivery to tissues and oxygen consumption by tissues. It allows rapid detection of impaired oxygen delivery, as from decreased cardiac output, hemoglobin level, or arterial oxygen saturation. It also helps evaluate a patient's response to drug therapy, endotracheal tube suctioning, ventilator setting changes, positive end-expiratory pressure, and fraction of inspired oxygen. $S\bar{v}O_2$ usually ranges from 60% to 80%; the normal value is 75%.

## Equipment

Fiber-optic PA catheter ● co-oximeter ● optical module and cable ● gloves

### Preparation of equipment

Review the manufacturer's instructions for assembly and use of the fiber-optic PA catheter. Connect the optical module and cable to the monitor. Next, peel back the wrapping covering the catheter just enough to uncover the fiber-optic connector. Attach the fiber-optic connector to the optical module while allowing the rest of the catheter to remain in its sterile wrapping. Calibrate the fiber-optic catheter by following the manufacturer's instructions.

To prepare for the rest of the procedure, follow instructions for pulmonary catheter insertion. (See *$S\bar{v}O_2$ monitoring equipment,* page 338.)

## Implementation

▶ Wash your hands and put on gloves.

▶ Explain the procedure to the patient to allay his fears and promote cooperation.

▶ Assist with the insertion of the fiber-optic catheter just as you would for a PA catheter.

▶ After the catheter is inserted, confirm that the light intensity tracing on the graphic printout is within normal range to ensure correct positioning and function of the catheter.

▶ Observe the digital readout and record the $S\bar{v}O_2$ on graph paper. Repeat readings at least once each hour to monitor and document trends.

# S̄vo₂ monitoring equipment

The mixed venous oxygen saturation (S̄vo₂) monitoring system consists of a flow-directed pulmonary artery (PA) catheter with fiber-optic filaments, an optical module, and a co-oximeter. The co-oximeter displays a continuous digital S̄vo₂ value; the strip recorder prints a permanent record.

Catheter insertion follows the same technique as with any thermodilution flow-directed PA catheter. The distal lumen connects to an external PA pressure monitoring system; the proximal or central venous pressure lumen connects to another monitoring system or to a continuous-flow administration unit; and the optical module connects to the co-oximeter unit.

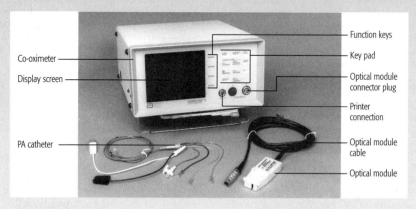

- Function keys
- Key pad
- Optical module connector plug
- Printer connection
- Optical module cable
- Optical module

Co-oximeter
Display screen
PA catheter

**NORMAL S̄vo₂ WAVEFORM**

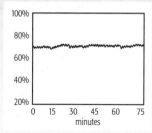

**S̄vo₂ WITH PATIENT ACTIVITIES**

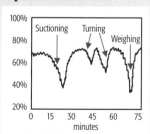

**S̄vo₂ WITH PEEP AND Fɪo₂ CHANGES**

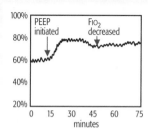

❱ Set the machine alarms 10% above and 10% below the patient's current S$\bar{s}vO_2$ reading.

### Recalibrating the monitor

❱ Draw a mixed venous blood sample from the distal port of the PA catheter. Send it to the laboratory for analysis to compare the laboratory's $\bar{s}vO_2$ reading with that of the fiber-optic catheter.

❱ If the catheter values and the laboratory values differ by more than 4%, follow the manufacturer's instructions to enter the $\bar{s}vO_2$ value obtained by the laboratory into the co-oximeter.

❱ Recalibrate the monitor every 24 hours or whenever the catheter has been disconnected from the optical module.

### Special considerations

❱ If the patient's $\bar{s}vO_2$ drops below 60% or varies by more than 10% for 3 minutes or longer, reassess the patient. If the $\bar{s}vO_2$ doesn't return to the baseline value after nursing interventions, notify the doctor. A decreasing $\bar{s}vO_2$ or a value less than 60% indicates impaired oxygen delivery, as occurs in hemorrhage, hypoxia, shock, arrhythmia, or suctioning. $\bar{s}vO_2$ may also decrease as a result of increased oxygen demand from hyperthermia, shivering, or seizures, for example.

❱ If the intensity of the tracing is low, ensure that all connections between the catheter and co-oximeter are secure and that the catheter is patent and not kinked.

❱ If the tracing is damped or erratic, try to aspirate blood from the catheter to check for patency. If you can't aspirate blood, notify the doctor so that he can replace the catheter. Also, check the PA waveform to determine whether the catheter has wedged. If the catheter has wedged, try to flush the line. Also, turn the patient from side to side and instruct him to cough. If the catheter remains wedged, notify the doctor immediately.

❱ If the tracing shows a high intensity, the catheter may be pressing against a vessel wall. Flush the line. If the tracing doesn't return to normal, notify the doctor so he can reposition the catheter.

### Complications

Thrombosis can result from local irritation by the catheter; however, a heparin flush helps prevent this complication. Thromboembolism also can occur if a thrombus breaks off and lodges in the circulatory system. Monitor the patient for signs and symptoms of infection, such as redness or drainage, at the catheter site.

### Documentation

❱ Document the $\bar{s}vO_2$ value on a flowchart and attach a tracing, as ordered.

❱ Note any significant changes in the patient's status and the results of any interventions. For comparison, note the $\bar{s}vO_2$ as measured by the fiber-optic catheter whenever a blood sample is obtained for laboratory analysis of $\bar{s}vO_2$.

### REFERENCES

Iacobelli, L., et al. "Oxygen Saturation Monitoring," *Minerva Anestesiology* 68(5): 488-91, May 2002.

Turnaoglu, S., et al. "Clinical Applicability of the Substitution of Mixed Venous Oxygen Saturation with Central Venous Oxygen Saturation," *Journal of Cardiothoracic and Vascular Anesthesia* 15(5):574-79, October 2001.

# Nasopharyngeal airway insertion and care

Insertion of a nasopharyngeal airway—soft rubber or latex uncuffed catheter—establishes or maintains a patent airway. This airway is the typical choice for patients who have had recent oral surgery or facial trauma and for patients with loose, cracked, or avulsed teeth. It's also used to protect the nasal mucosa from injury when the patient needs frequent nasotracheal suctioning.

The airway follows the curvature of the nasopharynx, passing through the nose and extending from the nostril to the posterior pharynx. The bevel-shaped pharyngeal end of the airway facilitates insertion, and its funnel-shaped nasal end helps prevent slippage.

Insertion of a nasopharyngeal airway is preferred when an oropharyngeal airway is contraindicated or fails to maintain a patent airway. A nasopharyngeal airway is contraindicated if the patient is receiving anticoagulant therapy or has a hemorrhagic disorder, sepsis, or pathologic nasopharyngeal deformity.

# Inserting a nasopharyngeal airway

First, hold the airway beside the patient's face to make sure it's the proper size (as shown below). It should be slightly smaller than the patient's nostril diameter and slightly longer than the distance from the tip of his nose to his earlobe.

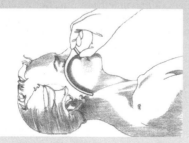

To insert the airway, hyperextend the patient's neck (unless contraindicated). Then push up the tip of his nose and pass the airway into his nostril (as shown below). Avoid pushing against any resistance to prevent tissue trauma and airway kinking.

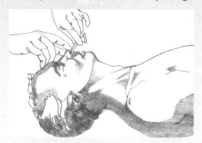

To check for correct airway placement, first close the patient's mouth. Then place your finger over the tube's opening to detect air exchange. Also, depress the patient's tongue with a tongue blade and look for the airway tip behind the uvula

## Equipment
*For insertion*
Nasopharyngeal airway of proper size • tongue blade • water-soluble lubricant • gloves • suction equipment

*For cleaning*
Hydrogen peroxide • water • basin • optional: pipe cleaner

## Preparation of equipment
Measure the diameter of the patient's nostril and the distance from the tip of his nose to his earlobe. Select an airway of slightly smaller diameter than the nostril and of slightly longer length (1″ [2.5 cm]) than measured. The sizes for this type of airway are labeled according to their internal diameter.

The recommended size for a large adult is 8 to 9 mm; for a medium adult, 7 to 8 mm; and for a small adult, 6 to 7 mm. Lubricate the distal half of the airway's surface with a water-soluble lubricant to prevent traumatic injury during insertion.

## Implementation
▶ Put on gloves.
▶ In nonemergency situations, explain the procedure to the patient.
▶ Properly insert the airway. (See *Inserting a nasopharyngeal airway.*)
▶ After the airway is inserted, check it regularly to detect dislodgment or obstruction.
▶ When the patient's natural airway is patent, remove the airway in one smooth motion. If the airway sticks, apply lubricant around the nasal end of the tube and around the nostril; then gently rotate the airway until it's free.

## Special considerations
▶ When you insert the airway, remember to use a chin-lift or jaw-thrust technique to anteriorly displace the patient's mandible. Immediately after insertion, assess the patient's respirations. If absent or inadequate, initiate artificial positive-pressure ventilation with a mouth-to-mask technique, a handheld resuscitation bag, or an oxygen-powered breathing device.
▶ If the patient coughs or gags, the tube may be too long. If so, remove the airway and insert a shorter one.
▶ At least once every 8 hours, remove the airway to check nasal mucous membranes for irritation or ulceration.
▶ Clean the airway by placing it in a basin and rinsing it with hydrogen peroxide and then with water. If secretions remain, use a pipe cleaner to remove them. Reinsert the clean airway into the other nostril (if it's patent) to avoid skin breakdown.

## Complications
Sinus infection may result from obstruction of sinus drainage. Insertion of the air-

way may injure the nasal mucosa and cause bleeding and possibly aspiration of blood into the trachea. Suction as necessary to remove secretions or blood. If the tube is too long, it may enter the esophagus and cause gastric distention and hypoventilation during artificial ventilation. Although semiconscious patients usually tolerate nasopharyngeal airways better than conscious patients, they may still experience laryngospasm and vomiting.

## Documentation

▶ Record the date and time of the airway's insertion.
▶ Document size, cleaning, and removal of the airway.
▶ Record shifts from one nostril to the other.
▶ Note the condition of the mucous membranes.
▶ Document suctioning.
▶ Record any complications and nursing action taken.
▶ Document the patient's reaction to the procedure.

### REFERENCES

American Heart Association in Collaboration with the International Liaison Committee on Resuscitation. "Guidelines 2000 for Cardiopulmonary Resuscitation and Emergency Cardiovascular Care," *Circulation* 102(8 Suppl):I1-384, August 2000.

Edward, D., et al. *Bedside Critical Care Manual*. Philadelphia: Lippincott Williams & Wilkins, 2001.

Rubin, B.K. "Physiology of Airway Mucus Clearance," *Respiratory Care* 47(7):761-68, July 2002.

# Oronasopharyngeal suction

Oronasopharyngeal suction removes secretions from the pharynx by a suction catheter inserted through the mouth or nostril. Used to maintain a patent airway, this procedure helps the patient who can't clear his airway effectively with coughing and expectoration, such as the unconscious or severely debilitated patient. The procedure should be done as often as necessary, depending on the patient's condition.

Because the catheter may inadvertently slip into the lower airway or esophagus, oronasopharyngeal suction is an aseptic procedure that requires sterile equipment. However, clean technique may be used for a tonsil tip suction device. In fact, an alert patient can use a tonsil tip suction device himself to remove secretions.

Nasopharyngeal suctioning should be used with caution in patients who have nasopharyngeal bleeding or spinal fluid leakage into the nasopharyngeal area, in trauma patients, in patients who are receiving anticoagulant therapy, and in those who have blood dyscrasias because these conditions increase the risk of bleeding.

## Equipment

Wall suction or portable suction apparatus ● collection container ● connecting tubing ● water-soluble lubricant ● normal saline solution ● disposable sterile container ● sterile suction catheter (a #12 or #14 French catheter for an adult, #8 or #10 French catheter for a child, or pediatric feeding tube for an infant) ● sterile gloves ● clean gloves ● nasopharyngeal or oropharyngeal airway (optional for frequent suctioning) ● overbed table ● waterproof trash bag ● soap, water, and 70% alcohol for cleaning catheters ● optional: tongue blade and tonsil tip suction device

A commercially prepared kit contains a sterile catheter, disposable container, and sterile gloves.

### Preparation of equipment

Before beginning, check your facility's policy to determine whether a doctor's order is required for oropharyngeal suctioning. Also review the patient's blood gas and oxygen saturation values, and check vital signs. Evaluate the patient's ability to cough and deep-breathe to determine his ability to move secretions up the tracheobronchial tree. Check his history for a deviated septum, nasal polyps, nasal obstruction, traumatic injury, epistaxis, or mucosal swelling.

If no contraindications exist, gather and place the suction equipment on the patient's overbed table or bedside stand. Position the table or stand on your preferred side of the bed to facilitate suctioning. Attach the collection bottle to the suctioning unit, and attach the connecting tubing to it. Date and open the bottle of normal saline solution. Open the waterproof trash bag.

## Tips on airway clearance

Deep breathing and coughing are vital for removing secretions from the lungs. Other techniques used to help clear the airways include diaphragmatic breathing and forced expiration. Here is how to teach these techniques to your patients.

### Diaphragmatic breathing
First, tell the patient to lie in a supine position, with his head elevated 15 to 20 degrees on a pillow. Tell him to place one hand on his abdomen and then inhale so that he can feel his abdomen rise. Explain that this is known as "breathing with the diaphragm."

Next, instruct the patient to exhale slowly through his nose – or, better yet, through pursed lips – while letting his abdomen collapse. Explain that this action decreases his respiratory rate and increases his tidal volume.

Suggest that the patient perform this exercise for 30 minutes several times a day. After he becomes accustomed to the position and has learned to breathe using his diaphragm, he may apply abdominal weights of 8.8 to 11 lb (4 to 5 kg). The weights enhance the movement of the diaphragm toward the head during expiration.

To enhance the effectiveness of exercise, the patient may also manually compress the lower costal margins, perform straight leg lifts, and coordinate the breathing technique with a physical activity such as walking.

### Forced expiration
Explain to the patient that forced expiration helps clear secretions while causing less traumatic injury than does a cough. To perform the technique, tell the patient to forcefully expire without closing his glottis, starting with a mid to low lung volume. Tell him to follow this expiration with a period of diaphragmatic breathing and relaxation.

Inform the patient that if his secretions are in the central airways, he may have to use a more forceful expiration or a cough to clear them.

## Implementation
▶ Explain the procedure to the patient even if he's unresponsive. Inform him that suctioning may stimulate transient coughing or gagging, but tell him that coughing helps to mobilize secretions. If he has been suctioned before, just summarize the reasons for the procedure. Reassure him throughout the procedure to minimize anxiety and fear, which can increase oxygen consumption. Also ask which nostril is more patent.
▶ Wash your hands.
▶ Place the patient in semi-Fowler's or high Fowler's position, if tolerated, to promote lung expansion and effective coughing.
▶ Turn on the suction from the wall or portable unit, and set the pressure according to your facility's policy. The pressure is usually set between 80 and 120 mm Hg; higher pressures cause excessive trauma without enhancing secretion removal. Occlude the end of the connecting tubing to check suction pressure.
▶ Using strict sterile technique, open the suction catheter kit or the packages containing the sterile catheter, disposable container, and gloves. Put on the gloves; con-

sider your dominant hand sterile and your nondominant hand nonsterile. Using your nondominant hand, pour the normal saline solution into the sterile container.
▶ With your nondominant hand, place a small amount of water-soluble lubricant on the sterile area. The lubricant is used to facilitate passage of the catheter during nasopharyngeal suctioning.
▶ Pick up the catheter with your dominant (sterile) hand, and attach it to the connecting tubing. Use your nondominant hand to control the suction valve while your dominant hand manipulates the catheter.
▶ Instruct the patient to cough and breathe slowly and deeply several times before beginning suction. Coughing helps loosen secretions and may decrease the amount of suctioning necessary, while deep breathing helps minimize or prevent hypoxia. (See *Tips on airway clearance.*)

### For nasal insertion
▶ Raise the tip of the patient's nose with your nondominant hand to straighten the passageway and facilitate insertion of the catheter. Without applying suction, gently insert the suction catheter into the patient's

nares. Roll the catheter between your fingers to help it advance through the turbinates. Continue to advance the catheter approximately 5″ to 6″ (13 to 15 cm) until you reach the pool of secretions or the patient begins to cough.

### For oral insertion

▶ Without applying suction, gently insert the catheter into the patient's mouth. Advance it 3″ to 4″ (7.5 to 10 cm) along the side of the patient's mouth until you reach the pool of secretions or the patient begins to cough. Suction both sides of the patient's mouth and pharyngeal area.

### For suctioning

▶ Using intermittent suction, withdraw the catheter from either the mouth or the nose with a continuous rotating motion to minimize invagination of the mucosa into the catheter's tip and side ports. Apply suction for only 10 to 15 seconds at a time to minimize tissue trauma.

▶ Between passes, wrap the catheter around your dominant hand to prevent contamination.

▶ If secretions are thick, clear the lumen of the catheter by dipping it in normal saline solution and applying suction.

▶ Repeat the procedure until gurgling or bubbling sounds stop and respirations are quiet.

▶ After completing suctioning, pull your sterile glove off over the coiled catheter, and discard it and the nonsterile glove along with the container of water.

▶ Flush the connecting tubing with normal saline solution.

▶ Replace the used items so they're ready for the next suctioning and wash your hands.

### Special considerations

▶ If the patient has no history of nasal problems, alternate suctioning between nostrils to minimize traumatic injury. If repeated oronasopharyngeal suctioning is required, the use of a nasopharyngeal or oropharyngeal airway will help with catheter insertion, reduce traumatic injury, and promote a patent airway. To facilitate catheter insertion for oropharyngeal suctioning, depress the patient's tongue with a tongue blade, or ask another nurse to do so. This helps you to visualize the back of the throat and also prevents the patient from biting the catheter.

▶ If the patient has excessive oral secretions, consider using a tonsil tip catheter because this allows the patient to remove oral secretions independently.

▶ Let the patient rest after suctioning while you continue to observe him. The frequency and duration of suctioning depends on the patient's tolerance for the procedure and on any complications. If a patient has borderline oxygenation, hyperoxygenation prior to suctioning me be needed.

### Home care

Oronasopharyngeal suctioning may be performed in the home using a portable suction machine. Under these circumstances, suctioning is a clean rather than a sterile procedure. Properly cleaned catheters can be reused, putting less financial strain on patients.

Catheters should be cleaned by first washing them in soapy water and then boiling them for 10 minutes or soaking them in 70% alcohol for 3 to 5 minutes. The catheters should then be rinsed with normal saline solution or tap water.

Whether the patient requires disposable or reusable suction equipment, you should make sure that he and his caregivers have received proper teaching and support.

### Complications

Increased dyspnea caused by hypoxia and anxiety may result from this procedure. Hypoxia can result because oxygen from the oronasopharynx is removed with the secretions. The amount of oxygen removed varies, depending upon the duration of the suctioning, suction flow and pressure, the size of the catheter in relation to the size of the patient's airway, and his physical condition.

In addition, bloody aspirate can result from prolonged or traumatic suctioning. Water-soluble lubricant can help to minimize traumatic injury.

### Documentation

▶ Record the date, time, reason for suctioning, and technique used

▶ Document amount, color, consistency, and odor (if any) of the secretions

▶ Note the patient's respiratory status before and after the procedure, any complications and the nursing action taken, and the patient's tolerance for the procedure.

**REFERENCES**

American Association for Respiratory Care. "AARC Clinical Practice Guideline: Suctioning of the Patient in the Home," *Respiratory Care* 44(1):99-104, January 1999.

"Tracheal Suctioning of Adults with an Artificial Airway," *Best Practice* 4(4):1-6, 2000.

# Oropharyngeal airway insertion and care

An oropharyngeal airway, a curved rubber or plastic device, is inserted into the mouth to the posterior pharynx to establish or maintain a patent airway. In an unconscious patient, the tongue usually obstructs the posterior pharynx. The oropharyngeal airway conforms to the curvature of the palate, removing the obstruction and allowing air to pass around and through the tube. It also facilitates oropharyngeal suctioning. The oropharyngeal airway is intended for short-term use, as in the postanesthesia or postictal stage. It may be left in place longer as an airway adjunct to prevent the orally intubated patient from biting the endotracheal tube.

The oropharyngeal airway isn't the airway of choice for the patient with loose or avulsed teeth or recent oral surgery. Inserting this airway in the conscious or semiconscious patient may stimulate vomiting and laryngospasm; therefore, you'll usually insert the airway only in the unconscious patient.

## Equipment

*For inserting*
Oral airway of appropriate size ●tongue blade ●padded tongue blade ●gloves ●optional: suction equipment, handheld resuscitation bag or oxygen-powered breathing device

*For cleaning*
Hydrogen peroxide ●water ●basin ●optional: pipe cleaner

*For reflex testing*
Cotton-tipped applicator

## Preparation of equipment

Select an airway of appropriate size for your patient; an oversized airway can obstruct breathing by depressing the epiglottis into the laryngeal opening. Usually, you'll select a small size (size 1 or 2) for an infant or child, a medium size (size 4 or 5) for the average adult, and a large size (size 6) for the large adult. Be sure to confirm the correct size of the airway by placing the airway flange beside the patient's cheek, parallel to his front teeth. If the airway is the right size, the airway curve should reach to the angle of the jaw.

## Implementation

▶ Explain the procedure to the patient even though he may not appear to be alert. Provide privacy and put on gloves to prevent contact with body fluids. If the patient is wearing dentures, remove them so they don't cause further airway obstruction.

▶ Suction the patient, if necessary.

▶ Place the patient in the supine position with his neck hyperextended if this isn't contraindicated.

▶ Insert the airway using the cross-finger or tongue blade technique. (See *Inserting an oral airway*.)

▶ Auscultate the lungs to ensure adequate ventilation.

▶ After the airway is inserted, position the patient on his side to decrease the risk of aspiration of vomitus.

▶ Perform mouth care every 2 to 4 hours as needed. Begin by holding the patient's jaws open with a padded tongue blade and gently removing the airway. Place the airway in a basin, and rinse it with hydrogen peroxide and then water. If secretions remain, use a pipe cleaner to remove them. Complete standard mouth care and reinsert the airway.

▶ While the airway is removed for mouth care, observe the mouth's mucous membranes because tissue irritation or ulceration can result from prolonged airway use.

▶ Frequently check the position of the airway to ensure correct placement.

▶ When the patient regains consciousness and is able to swallow, remove the airway by pulling it outward and downward, following the mouth's natural curvature. After the airway is removed, test the patient's cough and gag reflexes to ensure that removal of the airway wasn't premature and that the patient can maintain his own airway.

▶ To test for the gag reflex, use a cotton-tipped applicator to touch both sides of the posterior pharynx. To test for the cough reflex, gently touch the posterior oropharynx with the cotton-tipped applicator.

## Special considerations

▶ Clear breath sounds on auscultation indicate that the airway is the proper size and in the correct position.

▶ Avoid taping the airway in place because untaping it could delay airway removal, thus increasing the patient's risk of aspiration.

▶ Evaluate the patient's behavior to provide the cue for airway removal. The patient is likely to gag or cough as he becomes more alert, indicating that he no longer needs the airway.

## Complications

Tooth damage or loss, tissue damage, and bleeding may result from insertion. If the airway is too long, it may press the epiglottis against the entrance of the larynx, producing complete airway obstruction. If the airway isn't inserted properly, it may push the tongue posteriorly, aggravating the problem of upper airway obstruction. To prevent traumatic injury, make sure that the patient's lips and tongue aren't between his teeth and the airway.

Immediately after inserting the airway, check for respirations. If respirations are absent or inadequate, initiate artificial positive pressure ventilation by using a mouth-to-mask technique, a handheld resuscitation bag, or an oxygen-powered breathing device.

## Documentation

▶ Record the date and time of the airway's insertion.

▶ Note the size of the airway.

▶ Document removal and cleaning of the airway.

▶ Note the condition of mucous membranes.

▶ Record any suctioning, adverse reactions, and the nursing action taken.

▶ Document the patient's tolerance of the procedure.

## REFERENCES

American Heart Association in Collaboration with the International Liaison Committee on Resuscitation. "Guidelines 2000 for Cardiopulmonary Resuscitation and Emergency Cardiovascular Care," *Circulation* 102(8 Suppl):I1-384, August 2000.

Edwards, D., et al. *Bedside Critical Care Manual*. Philadelphia: Lippincott Williams & Wilkins, 2001.

# Inserting an oral airway

Unless this position is contraindicated, hyperextend the patient's head (as shown below) before using either the cross-finger or tongue blade insertion method.

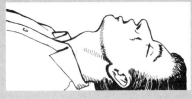

To insert an oral airway using the cross-finger method, place your thumb on the patient's lower teeth and your index finger on his upper teeth. Gently open his mouth by pushing his teeth apart (as shown below).

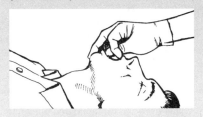

Insert the airway upside down to avoid pushing the tongue toward the pharynx, and slide it over the tongue toward the back of the mouth. Rotate the airway as it approaches the posterior wall of the pharynx so that it points downward (as shown below).

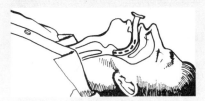

To use the tongue blade technique, open the patient's mouth and depress his tongue with the blade. Guide the airway over the back of the tongue as you did for the cross-finger technique.

# Oxygen administration

A patient will need oxygen therapy when hypoxemia results from a respiratory or cardiac emergency or an increase in metabolic function.

In a respiratory emergency, oxygen administration enables the patient to reduce his ventilatory effort. When conditions such as atelectasis or adult respiratory distress syndrome impair diffusion, or when lung volumes are decreased from alveolar hypoventilation, this procedure boosts alveolar oxygen levels.

In a cardiac emergency, oxygen therapy helps meet the increased myocardial workload as the heart tries to compensate for hypoxemia. Oxygen administration is particularly important for a patient whose myocardium is already compromised, perhaps from a myocardial infarction or cardiac arrhythmia.

When metabolic demand is high (in cases of massive trauma, burns, or high fever, for instance) oxygen administration supplies the body with enough oxygen to meet its cellular needs. This procedure also increases oxygenation in the patient with a reduced blood oxygen-carrying capacity, perhaps from carbon monoxide poisoning or sickle cell crisis.

The adequacy of oxygen therapy is determined by arterial blood gas (ABG) analysis, oximetry monitoring, and clinical examinations. The patient's disease, physical condition, and age will help determine the most appropriate method of administration.

## Equipment

The equipment needed depends on the type of delivery system ordered. (See *Guide to oxygen delivery systems.*)

Equipment generally includes selections from the following list: oxygen source (wall unit, cylinder, liquid tank, or concentrator) ● flowmeter ● adapter, if using a wall unit, or a pressure-reduction gauge, if using a cylinder ● sterile humidity bottle and adapters ● sterile distilled water ● OXYGEN PRECAUTION sign ● appropriate oxygen delivery system (a nasal cannula, simple mask, partial rebreather mask, or nonrebreather mask for low-flow and variable oxygen concentrations, a Venturi mask, aerosol mask, T tube, tracheostomy collar, tent, or oxygen hood for high-flow and specific oxygen concentrations) ● small-diameter and large-diameter connection tubing ● flashlight (for nasal cannula) ● water-soluble lubricant ● gauze pads and tape (for oxygen masks) ● jet adapter for Venturi mask (if adding humidity) ● optional: oxygen analyzer

### Preparation of equipment

Although a respiratory therapist typically is responsible for setting up, maintaining, and managing the equipment, you'll need a working knowledge of the oxygen system being used.

Check the oxygen outlet port to verify flow. Pinch the tubing near the prongs to ensure that an audible alarm will sound if the oxygen flow stops.

## Implementation

▶ Assess the patient's condition. In an emergency situation, verify that he has an open airway before administering oxygen.
▶ Explain the procedure to the patient, and let him know why he needs oxygen to ensure his cooperation.
▶ Check the patient's room to make sure it's safe for oxygen administration. Whenever possible, replace electrical devices with nonelectric ones.

**ALERT!** If the patient is a child and is in an oxygen tent, remove all toys that may produce a spark. Oxygen supports combustion, and the smallest spark can cause a fire.

▶ Place an OXYGEN PRECAUTION sign over the patient's bed and on the door to his room.
▶ Help place the oxygen delivery device on the patient. Make sure it fits properly and is stable.
▶ Monitor the patient's response to oxygen therapy. Check his ABG values during initial adjustments of oxygen flow. When the patient is stabilized, you may use pulse oximetry instead. Check the patient frequently for signs of hypoxia, such as decreased level of consciousness, increased heart rate, arrhythmias, restlessness, perspiration, dyspnea, use of accessory muscles, yawning or flared nostrils, cyanosis, and cool, clammy skin.
▶ Observe the patient's skin integrity to prevent skin breakdown on pressure points from the oxygen delivery device. Wipe moisture or perspiration from the patient's face and from the mask as needed.
▶ If the patient will be receiving oxygen at a concentration above 60% for more than

# Guide to oxygen delivery systems

Patients may receive oxygen through one of several administration systems. Each has its own benefits, drawbacks, and indications for use. The advantages and disadvantages of each system are compared here.

## Nasal cannula

Oxygen is delivered through plastic cannulas in the patient's nostrils.

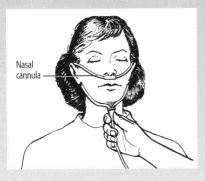

Nasal cannula

### *Advantages*

Safe and simple; comfortable and easily tolerated; nasal prongs can be shaped to fit any face; effective for low oxygen concentrations; allows movement, eating, and talking; inexpensive and disposable.

### *Disadvantages*

Can't deliver concentrations higher than 40%; can't be used in complete nasal obstruction; may cause headaches or dry mucous membranes if flow rate exceeds 6 L/minute; can dislodge easily.

### *Administration guidelines*

Ensure the patency of the patient's nostrils with a flashlight. If patent, hook the cannula tubing behind the patient's ears and under the chin. Slide the adjuster upward under the chin to secure the tubing. If using an elastic strap to secure the cannula, position it over the ears and around the back of the head. Avoid applying it too tightly, which can result in excess pressure on facial structures as well as cannula occlusion. With a nasal cannula, oral breathers achieve the same oxygen delivery as nasal breathers.

## Simple mask

Oxygen flows through an entry port at the bottom of the mask and exits through large holes on the sides of the mask.

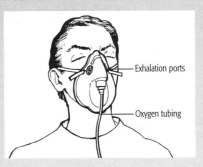

Exhalation ports

Oxygen tubing

### *Advantages*

Can deliver concentrations of 40% to 60%.

### *Disadvantages*

Hot and confining; may irritate patient's skin; tight seal, which may cause discomfort, is required for higher oxygen concentration; interferes with talking and eating; impractical for long-term therapy because of imprecision.

### *Administration guidelines*

Select the mask size that offers the best fit. Place the mask over the patient's nose, mouth, and chin, and mold the flexible metal edge to the bridge of the nose. Adjust the elastic band around the head to hold the mask firmly but comfortably over the cheeks, chin, and bridge of the nose. For elderly or cachectic patients with sunken cheeks, tape gauze pads to the mask over the cheek area to try to create an airtight seal. Without this seal, room air dilutes the oxygen, preventing delivery of the prescribed concentration. A minimum of 5 L/minute is required in all masks to flush expired carbon dioxide from the mask so that the patient doesn't rebreathe it.

*(continued)*

24 hours, watch carefully for signs of oxygen toxicity. Remind the patient to cough and deep-breathe frequently to prevent atelectasis. Also, to prevent the development of serious lung damage, measure ABG values repeatedly to determine whether high oxygen concentrations are still necessary.

# Guide to oxygen delivery systems *(continued)*

### Partial rebreather mask

The patient inspires oxygen from a reservoir bag along with atmospheric air and oxygen from the mask. The first third of exhaled tidal volume enters the bag; the rest exits the mask. Because air entering the reservoir bag comes from the trachea and bronchi, where no gas exchange occurs, the patient rebreathes the oxygenated air he just exhaled.

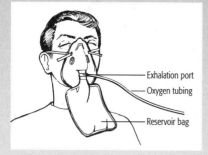

Exhalation port
Oxygen tubing
Reservoir bag

### *Advantages*

Effectively delivers concentrations of 40% to 60%; openings in the mask allow patient to inhale room air if oxygen source fails.

### *Disadvantages*

Tight seal required for accurate oxygen concentration may cause discomfort; interferes with eating and talking; hot and confining; may irritate skin; bag may twist or kink; impractical for long-term therapy.

### *Administration guidelines*

Follow the procedures listed for the simple mask. If the reservoir bag collapses more than slightly during inspiration, raise the flow rate until you see only a slight deflation. Marked or complete deflation indicates insufficient oxygen flow, which could result in carbon dioxide accumulation in the mask and bag. Keep the reservoir bag from twisting or kinking. Ensure free expansion by making sure the bag lies outside the patient's gown and bedcovers.

### Nonrebreather mask

On inhalation, the one-way inspiratory valve opens, directing oxygen from a reservoir bag into the mask. On exhalation, gas exits the mask through the one-way expiratory valves and enters the atmosphere. The patient breathes air only from the bag.

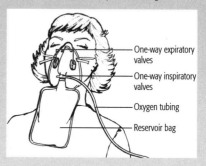

One-way expiratory valves
One-way inspiratory valves
Oxygen tubing
Reservoir bag

### *Advantages*

Delivers the highest possible oxygen concentration (60% to 90%) short of intubation and mechanical ventilation; effective for short-term therapy; doesn't dry mucous membranes; can be converted to a partial rebreather mask, if necessary, by removing the one-way valve.

### *Disadvantages*

Requires a tight seal, which may be difficult to maintain and may cause discomfort; may irritate the patient's skin; interferes with talking and eating; impractical for long-term therapy.

### *Administration guidelines*

Follow procedures listed for the simple mask. Make sure that the mask fits very snugly and that the one-way valves are secure and functioning. Because the mask excludes room air, a valve malfunction could cause carbon dioxide buildup and suffocate an unconscious patient. If the reservoir bag collapses more than slightly during inspiration, raise the flow rate until you see only a slight deflation. Marked or complete deflation indicates an insufficient flow rate. Keep the reservoir bag from twisting or kinking. Ensure free expansion by making sure the bag lies outside the patient's gown and bedcovers.

## Special considerations

**ALERT!** Never administer oxygen by nasal cannula at more than 2 L/minute to a patient with chronic lung disease unless you have a specific order to do so. That is because some patients with chronic lung disease become dependent on a state of hypercapnia and hy-

# Guide to oxygen delivery systems *(continued)*

### CPAP mask

This system allows the spontaneously breathing patient to receive continuous positive airway pressure (CPAP) with or without an artificial airway.

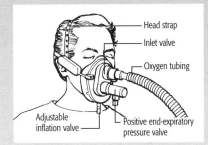

Head strap

Inlet valve

Oxygen tubing

Adjustable inflation valve

Positive end-expiratory pressure valve

#### Advantages

Noninvasively improves arterial oxygenation by increasing functional residual capacity; allows the patient to avoid intubation; allows the patient to talk and cough without interrupting positive pressure.

#### Disadvantages

Requires a tight fit, which may cause discomfort; interferes with eating and talking; heightened risk of aspiration if the patient vomits; increased risk of pneumothorax, diminished cardiac output, and gastric distention; contraindicated in patients with chronic obstructive pulmonary disease, bullous lung disease, low cardiac output, or tension pneumothorax.

#### Administration guidelines

Place one strap behind the patient's head and the other strap over his head to ensure a snug fit. Attach one latex strap to the connector prong on one side of the mask. Then use one hand to position the mask on the patient's face while using the other hand to connect the strap to the other side of the mask. After the mask is applied, assess the patient's respiratory, circulatory, and GI function every hour. Watch for signs of pneumothorax, decreased cardiac output, a drop in blood pressure, and gastric distention.

### Transtracheal oxygen

The patient receives oxygen through a catheter inserted into the base of his neck in a simple outpatient procedure.

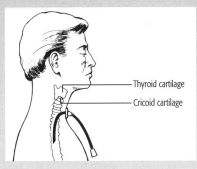

Thyroid cartilage

Cricoid cartilage

#### Advantages

Supplies oxygen to the lungs throughout the respiratory cycle; provides continuous oxygen without hindering mobility; doesn't interfere with eating or talking; doesn't dry mucous membranes; catheter can easily be concealed by a shirt or scarf.

#### Disadvantages

Not suitable for use in patients at risk for bleeding or those with severe bronchospasm, uncompensated respiratory acidosis, pleural herniation into the base of the neck, or high corticosteroid dosages.

#### Administration guidelines

After insertion, obtain a chest X-ray to confirm placement. Monitor the patient for bleeding, respiratory distress, pneumothorax, pain, coughing, or hoarseness. Don't use the catheter for about 1 week following insertion to decrease the risk of subcutaneous emphysema.

*(continued)*

poxia to stimulate their respirations, and supplemental oxygen could cause them to stop breathing. However, long-term oxygen therapy of 12 to 17 hours daily may help patients with chronic lung disease sleep better, survive longer, and experience a reduced incidence of pulmonary hypertension.

# Guide to oxygen delivery systems *(continued)*

### Venturi mask

The mask is connected to a Venturi device, which mixes a specific volume of air and oxygen.

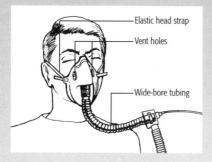

- Elastic head strap
- Vent holes
- Wide-bore tubing

#### *Advantages*

Delivers highly accurate oxygen concentration despite the patient's respiratory pattern because the same amount of air is always entrained; dilute jets can be changed or dial turned to change oxygen concentration; doesn't dry mucous membranes; humidity or aerosol can be added.

#### *Disadvantages*

Confining and may irritate skin; oxygen concentration may be altered if mask fits loosely, tubing kinks, oxygen intake ports become blocked, flow is insufficient, or patient is hyperpneic; interferes with eating and talking; condensate may collect and drip on the patient if humidification is used.

#### *Administration guidelines*

Make sure that the oxygen flow rate is set at the amount specified on each mask and that the Venturi valve is set for the desired fraction of inspired oxygen.

### Aerosols

A face mask, hood, tent, or tracheostomy tube or collar is connected to wide-bore tubing that receives aerosolized oxygen from a jet nebulizer. The jet nebulizer, which is attached near the oxygen source, adjusts air entrainment in a manner similar to the Venturi device.

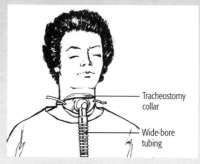

- Tracheostomy collar
- Wide-bore tubing

#### *Advantages*

Administers high humidity; gas can be heated (when delivered through artificial airway) or cooled (when delivered through a tent).

#### *Disadvantages*

Condensate collected in the tracheostomy collar or T tube may drain into the tracheostomy; the weight of the T tube can put stress on the tracheostomy tube.

#### *Administration guidelines*

Guidelines vary with the type of nebulizer used: ultrasonic, large-volume, small-volume, and in-line types. When using a high-output nebulizer, watch for signs of overhydration, pulmonary edema, crackles, and electrolyte imbalance.

---

▶ When monitoring a patient's response to a change in oxygen flow, check the pulse oximetry monitor or measure ABG values 20 to 30 minutes after adjusting the flow. In the interim, monitor the patient closely for any adverse response to the change in oxygen flow.

## Home care

Before discharging a patient who will receive oxygen therapy at home, make sure you're familiar with the types of oxygen therapy, the kinds of services that are available, and the service schedules offered by local home suppliers. Together with the doctor and the patient, choose the device that is best-suited to the patient. (See *Types of home oxygen therapy.*)

If the patient will be receiving transtracheal oxygen therapy, teach him how to properly clean and care for the catheter. Advise him to keep the skin surrounding the insertion site clean and dry to prevent infection.

No matter which device the patient uses, you'll need to evaluate his and his family

## Types of home oxygen therapy

Oxygen therapy can be administered at home using an oxygen tank, an oxygen concentrator, or liquid oxygen.

### Oxygen tank

Commonly used for patients who need oxygen on a standby basis or who need a ventilator at home, the oxygen tank has several disadvantages, including its cumbersome design and the need for frequent refills. Because oxygen is stored under high pressure, the oxygen tank also poses a potential hazard.

### Oxygen concentrator

The oxygen concentrator extracts oxygen molecules from room air. It can be used for low oxygen flow (less than 4 L/minute) and doesn't need to be refilled with oxygen. However, because the oxygen concentrator runs on electricity, it won't function during a power failure.

### Liquid oxygen

This option is commonly used by patients who are oxygen-dependent but still mobile. The liquid oxygen system includes a large liquid reservoir for home use. When the patient wants to leave the house, he fills a portable unit worn over the shoulder; this supplies oxygen for up to several hours, depending on the liter flow.

---

members' ability and motivation to administer oxygen therapy at home. Make sure they understand the reason the patient is receiving oxygen and the safety issues involved in oxygen administration. Teach them how to properly use and clean the equipment and supplies.

If the patient will be discharged with oxygen for the first time, make sure his health insurance covers home oxygen. If it doesn't, find out what criteria he must meet to obtain coverage. Without a third-party payer, he may not be able to afford home oxygen therapy.

### Documentation
▶ Record the date and time of oxygen administration.
▶ Note the type of delivery device used.
▶ Record the oxygen flow rate.
▶ Document the patient's vital signs, skin color, respiratory effort, and breath sounds.
▶ Document the patient's response before and after initiation of therapy.
▶ Note any patient or family teaching provided.

### REFERENCES
American Association for Respiratory Care. "AARC Clinical Practice Guidelines: Oxygen Therapy in the Acute Care Hospital," *Respiratory Care* 36(12):1410-13, December 1991. (Reviewed 2000.)
Wright, J., and White, J. "Continuous Positive Airway Pressure for Obstructive Sleep Apnea," *Cochrane Database of Systematic Reviews* 2(2):CD001106, 2000.

## Prone positioning

Prone positioning is a therapeutic maneuver to improve oxygenation and pulmonary mechanics in patients with acute lung injury or acute respiratory distress syndrome (ARDS). Also known as proning; prone positioning involves physically turning a patient face down from his or her back (supine position). This positioning improves oxygenation in patients by shifting blood flow to regions of the lung that are less severely injured and better aerated.

The criteria for prone positioning frequently include:
▶ Acute onset of respiratory signs and symptoms
▶ Hypoxemia, specifically a partial pressure of arterial oxygen/fraction of inspired oxygen ($PaO_2/FIO_2$) ratio of 300 or less for acute lung injury and a $PaO_2/FIO_2$ ratio of 200 or less for ARDS
▶ Radiological evidence of diffuse bilateral pulmonary infiltrates
▶ No evidence of left atrial hypertension.

The physical challenges of proning have been a traditional barrier to its use. However, equipment innovations such as a lightweight, cushioned frame that straps to the front of the patient before turning, has helped to minimize the risks associated with moving patients and maintaining them in the prone position for several hours at a time.

With the appropriate equipment, proning may also facilitate better movement of the diaphragm by allowing the abdomen to expand more fully. It's usually performed for 6 or more hours a day, for as long as 10 days, until the requirement for a high concentration of inspired oxygen resolves. Patients who respond to the prone position by an increase in the $PaO_2/FIO_2$ ratio of more than 20 or 20% within 2 hours of the patient being turned from supine to prone are classified as responders to prone positioning.

**■■ EVIDENCE BASE** Aside from early intervention, factors predictive of patients' responses are not consistent among studies, and patients' initial responses are not always predictive of their subsequent responses. Patients with extrapulmonary ARDS (such as ARDS due to multiple trauma) appear to respond consistently to prone positioning.

**■■ EVIDENCE BASE** Although research has demonstrated improved oxygenation with proning, It's unclear whether survival rate is increased.

Prone positioning is indicated to support mechanically ventilated patients with ARDS, who require high concentrations of inspired oxygen. It also corrects severe hypoxemia and maintains adequate oxygenation ($PaO_2$ greater than 60%) in patients with acute lung injury, while avoiding ventilator-induced lung injury. Prone positioning improves systemic oxygenation in patients with acute lung injury or ARDS.

It's contraindicated in patients whose heads cannot be supported in a face-down position, or those who are unable to tolerate a head down position. Hemodynamically unstable patients (systolic blood pressure less than 90 mm Hg) despite aggressive fluid resuscitation and vasopressors shouldn't be placed in the prone position. It's also contraindicated in patients who are extremely obese (typically, more than 300 lb), with cerebral hypertension unresponsive to therapy, unstable bone fractures, left ventricular failure (nonpulmonary respiratory failure), and in patients with an active intra-abdominal process.

## Equipment

Vollman Prone Positioner (HillRom) or other prone positioning device

### Preparation of equipment

The positioner is cleaned, according to facility procedure, between positioning turns

and when prone positioning is discontinued.

## Implementation

### Assessing the patient

▶ Assess the patient's hemodynamic status to determine if he will be able to tolerate the prone position.

▶ Assess the patient's mental status prior to prone positioning. Although agitation isn't a contraindication for proning, it must be effectively managed.

▶ Determine whether the patient's size and weight will allow turning him on a generally narrow critical care bed.

▶ If the critical care bed frame is too narrow to allow proning of a patient who weighs more than 300 lb, one option is to move the patient onto a stretcher while supine and then position him back in bed in the prone position.

### Preparing the patient

▶ Explain the purpose and procedure of prone positioning to the patient and his family.

### Before proning

▶ Remove anterior chest wall ECG monitoring leads but make sure the patient's cardiac rate and rhythm can be monitored. These leads will be repositioned onto the patient's back once he is prone.

▶ Provide eye care, if indicated, including lubrication and horizontal taping of eyelids.

▶ Ensure the patient's tongue is inside his mouth; if edematous or protruding, insert a bite block.

▶ Secure the patient's endotracheal tube or tracheotomy tube to prevent dislodgement.

▶ Perform anterior body wound care and dressing changes.

▶ Empty ileostomy or colostomy drainage bags.

**◆ ALERT!** Before a patient is proned, care should be taken to ensure that the endotracheal tube is anchored securely and that all extraneous intravenous catheters and tubing are disconnected. Increased drainage of nasal mucus while patients are prone requires that the endotracheal tube be firmly secured to prevent inadvertent extubation.

▶ Make sure that the brake of the bed is engaged. Attach the surface of the prone positioner to the bed frame, as recommended by the manufacturer.

▶ Position staff appropriately; a minimum of three people is required: one on either side of the bed and one at the head of the bed.

▶ The staff member at the head of the bed is responsible for monitoring the ET tube, mechanical ventilator tubing, and I.V. lines.

▶ Adjust all patient tubing and invasive monitoring lines to prevent dislodgement, kinking, disconnection, or contact with the patient's body during the turning procedure and while the patient remains in the prone position.

**ALERT!** Place all lines inserted in the upper torso over the right or left shoulder, with the exception of chest tubes which are placed at the foot of the bed. All lines inserted in the lower torso are positioned at the foot of the bed.

▶ Turn the patient's face away from the ventilator, placing the endotracheal tubing on the side of the patient's face that is turned away from the ventilator. Loop the remaining tubing above the patient's head. These maneuvers prevent disconnection of the ventilator tubing or kinking of the endotracheal tube during proning.

▶ Place the straps of the prone positioner under the patient's head, chest, and pelvic area.

▶ Attach the proning device to the patient by placing the frame on top of the patient.

▶ Position the nonmovable chest piece, which acts as a marker for the proper device placement, so that it's resting between the patient's clavicles and sixth ribs.

▶ If the patient has a short neck or limited neck range of motion, align the chest piece lower, at the third intercostal space; move both head pieces up to the top of the frame so that only the forehead is supported by the head cushion and the chin is suspended to reduce the risk of skin breakdown.

▶ Adjust the pelvic piece of the device so that it rests ½″ above the iliac crest.

▶ Evaluate the distance between the chest and pelvic pieces to ensure suspension of the abdomen, while preventing bowing of the patient's back.

▶ Adjust the chin and forehead pieces of the device so that facial support is provided in either a face-down or side-lying position without interfering with the endotracheal tube.

▶ Secure the positioning device to the patient by fastening all the soft adjustable straps on one side before tightening them on the opposite side. Once secured, lift the positioner to ensure a secure fit.

**ALERT!** To help ensure a secure fit, look for cushion compression. If the frame isn't tightly secured, shear and friction injuries to the chest and pelvic area may occur.

### Turning the patient

▶ Lower the side rails of the bed, and move the patient to the edge of the bed farthest away from the ventilator by using a draw sheet. The person closest to the patient maintains body contact with the bed at all times, serving as a side rail.

▶ Tuck the straps attached to the steel bar closest to the center of the bed underneath the patient. Then tuck the patient's arm and hand that are resting in the center of the bed under the buttocks. Cross the leg closest to the edge of the bed over the opposite leg at the ankle, which will help with forward motion when the turning process begins.

▶ If the patient's arm can't be straightened to tuck under his buttocks, tuck the arm into the open space between the chest and pelvic pads.

▶ Turn the patient toward the ventilator at a 45-degree angle.

▶ When proning, always turn the patient in the direction of the mechanical ventilator.

▶ The person on the side of the bed with the ventilator grasps the upper steel bar. The person on the other side of the bed grasps the lower steel bar or turning straps of the device.

▶ Lift the patient by the frame into the prone position on the count of three.

▶ Gently move the patient's tucked arm and hand so they are parallel to his body and in a comfortable position.

**ALERT!** To prevent placing stress on the shoulder capsule, take care not to extend the arm position to a 90-degree angle.

▶ Loosen the straps if the patient is clinically stable.

**ALERT!** In the event of an emergency, keep the straps securely fastened in an unstable patient to allow for rapid supine repositioning.

▶ Support the patient's feet with a pillow or towel roll to provide correct flexion while in the prone position.

▶ Pad the patient's elbows to prevent ulnar nerve compression.

▶ Monitor the patient's response to proning through his vital signs, pulse oximetry, and mixed venous oxygen saturation. During the initial proning, arterial blood gases should be obtained within ½ hour of proning and within ½ hour before returning the patient to the supine position.

▶ Reposition the patient's head hourly while in the prone position to prevent facial breakdown. As one person lifts the patient's head, the second person moves the headpieces to provide head support in a different position.

▶ Provide range of motion to arms and legs every 2 hours.

### Returning the patient to the supine position

▶ Securely fasten positioning device straps.

▶ Position the patient on the edge of the bed closest to the ventilator.

▶ Adjust all patient tubing and monitoring lines to prevent dislodgement.

▶ Straighten the patient's arms and rest them on either side of his head. Cross the leg closest to the edge of the bed over the opposite leg.

▶ Using the steel bars of the device, turn the patient to a 45-degree angle away from the ventilator, and then roll him to the supine position.

▶ Position the patient's arms parallel to his body.

▶ Unfasten the positioning device, and remove it from the patient.

## Complications

Potential complications of prone positioning include: inadvertent endotracheal extubation; airway obstruction; decreased oxygen saturation; difficulty coordinating the mechanical ventilator; apical atelectasis; obstructed chest tube; pressure injuries on the weight-bearing parts of the body, including the knees and chest; hemodynamic instability; dislodgement of central venous access; transient dysrhythmias; reversible dependent edema of the face (forehead, eyelids, conjunctiva, lips, and tongue) and anterior chest wall; contractures, enteral feeding intolerance; aspiration of enteral feeding when repositioned supine; and corneal ulceration.

◆ **ALERT!** Critically ill patients with active intra-abdominal processes, regardless of position, are at risk for sepsis and septic shock.

## Special considerations

▶ A doctor's order is usually required before proning critically ill patients.

▶ Proning requires special training and established guidelines to ensure patient safety.

▶ Not all ARDS patients respond favorably to prone positioning, and the benefit of proning sometimes decreases over time.

▶ Patients may require increased sedation during proning.

▶ Proning schedule is generally determined by the patient's ability to maintain improvements in $PaO_2$ while in the prone position.

▶ Use capnography, if possible, to verify correct endotracheal tube placement during proning.

▶ Based on the literature on proning and prevention of pressure injuries, a safe suggestion for repositioning frequency is between 4 and 6 hours.

▶ Proning is discontinued when the patient no longer demonstrates improved oxygenation with the position change.

◆ **ALERT!** It's strongly recommended that lateral rotation therapy be used in conjunction with prone positioning.

## Documentation

▶ Document the patient's response to therapy.

▶ Document the patient's ability to tolerate the turning procedure.

▶ Record the length of time the patient has been in the position.

▶ Document the positioning schedule.

▶ Record monitoring and complications during proning.

▶ Document interventions.

### REFERENCES

Blackburn S, et al. "Neonatal Thermal Care, Part III: The Effect of Infant Position and Temperature Probe Placement," *Neonatal Network* 20(3):25-30, April 2001.

Dalton, H.J. "There and Back Again: Does Prone Positioning have any Value in Respiratory Failure?" *Critical Care Medicine* 30(7):1658, July 2002.

Watanabe, I., et al. "Beneficial Effect of a Prone Position for Patients with Hypoxemia After Transthoracic Esophagectomy," *Critical Care Medicine* 30(8):1799-802, August 2002.

## Pulse and ear oximetry

Performed intermittently or continuously, oximetry is a relatively simple procedure used to monitor arterial oxygen saturation noninvasively. Pulse oximeters usually denote arterial oxygen saturation values with the symbol $SpO_2$, whereas invasively measured arterial oxygen saturation values are denoted by the symbol $SaO_2$. (See *How oximetry works.*)

In this procedure, two diodes send red and infrared light through a pulsating arterial vascular bed, like the one in the fingertip. A photodetector slipped over the finger measures the transmitted light as it passes through the vascular bed, detects the relative amount of color absorbed by arterial blood, and calculates the exact mixed venous oxygen saturation without interference from surrounding venous blood, skin, connective tissue, or bone. Ear oximetry works by monitoring the transmission of light waves through the vascular bed of a patient's earlobe. Results will be inaccurate if the patient's earlobe is poorly perfused, as from a low cardiac output.

### Equipment

Oximeter ● finger or ear pro ● alcohol pad ● nail polish remover, if necessary

### Preparation of equipment

Review the manufacturer's instructions for assembly of the oximeter.

### Implementation

▶ Explain the procedure to the patient.

### For pulse oximetry

▶ Select a finger for the test. Although the index finger is commonly used, a smaller finger may be selected if the patient's fingers are too large for the equipment. Make sure the patient isn't wearing false fingernails, and remove any nail polish from the

### How oximetry works

The pulse oximeter allows noninvasive monitoring of a patient's arterial oxygen saturation ($SaO_2$) levels by measuring the absorption (amplitude) of light waves as they pass through areas of the body that are highly perfused by arterial blood. Oximetry also monitors pulse rate and amplitude.

Light-emitting diodes in a transducer (photodetector) attached to the patient's body (shown below on the index finger) send red and infrared light beams through tissue. The photodetector records the relative amount of each color absorbed by arterial blood and transmits the data to a monitor, which displays the information with each heartbeat. If the $SaO_2$ level or pulse rate varies from preset limits, the monitor triggers visual and audible alarms.

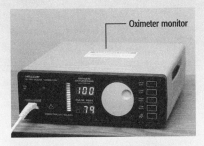

Oximeter monitor

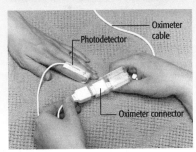

Oximeter cable
Photodetector
Oximeter connector

test finger. Place the transducer (photodetector) probe over the patient's finger so that light beams and sensors oppose each other. If the patient has long fingernails, position the probe perpendicular to the finger, if possible, or clip the fingernail. Always position the patient's hand at heart level to eliminate venous pulsations and to promote accurate readings.

◆ **ALERT!** If you're testing a neonate or a small infant, wrap the probe

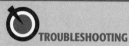

TROUBLESHOOTING

# Diagnosing pulse oximeter problems

To maintain a continuous display of arterial oxygen saturation levels, you'll need to keep the monitoring site clean and dry. Make sure the skin doesn't become irritated from adhesives used to keep disposable probes in place. You may need to change the site if this happens. Disposable probes that irritate the skin also can be replaced by nondisposable models that don't need tape.

Another common problem with pulse oximeters is the failure of the devices to obtain a signal. Your first reaction if this happens should be to check the patient's vital signs. If they're sufficient to produce a signal, check for the following problems.

### Poor connection

See if the sensors are properly aligned. Make sure that wires are intact and securely fastened and that the pulse oximeter is plugged into a power source.

### Inadequate or intermittent blood flow to site

Check the patient's pulse rate and capillary refill time, and take corrective action if blood flow to the site is decreased. This may mean loosening restraints, removing tight-fitting clothes, taking off a blood pressure cuff, or checking arterial and I.V. lines. If none of these interventions works, you may need to find an alternate site. Finding a site with proper circulation may also prove challenging when a patient is receiving vasoconstrictive drugs.

### Equipment malfunctions

Remove the pulse oximeter from the patient, set the alarm limits at 85% and 100%, and try the instrument on yourself or another healthy person. This will tell you if the equipment is working correctly.

---

around the foot so that light beams and detectors oppose each other. For a large infant, use a probe that fits on the great toe and secure the probe to the foot.
▶ Turn on the power switch. If the device is working properly, a beep will sound, a display will light momentarily, and the

pulse searchlight will flash. The $SpO_2$ and pulse rate displays will show stationary zeros. After four to six heartbeats, the $SpO_2$ and pulse rate displays will supply information with each beat, and the pulse amplitude indicator will begin tracking the pulse.

### For ear oximetry
▶ Using an alcohol pad, massage the patient's earlobe for 10 to 20 seconds. Mild erythema indicates adequate vascularization. Following the manufacturer's instructions, attach the ear probe to the patient's earlobe or pinna. Use the ear probe stabilizer for prolonged or exercise testing. Be sure to establish good contact on the ear; an unstable probe may set off the low-perfusion alarm. After the probe has been attached for a few seconds, a saturation reading and pulse waveform will appear on the oximeter's screen.
▶ Leave the ear probe in place for 3 or more minutes until readings stabilize at the highest point, or take three separate readings and average them. Make sure you revascularize the patient's earlobe each time.
▶ After the procedure, remove the probe, turn off and unplug the unit, and clean the probe by gently rubbing it with an alcohol sponge.

## Special considerations
▶ If oximetry has been performed properly, readings are typically accurate. However, certain factors may interfere with accuracy. For example, an elevated bilirubin level may falsely lower $SpO_2$ readings, whereas elevated carboxyhemoglobin or methemoglobin levels, such as occur in heavy smokers and urban dwellers, can cause a falsely elevated $SpO_2$ reading.
▶ If light is a problem, cover the probes; if patient movement is a problem, move the probe or select a different probe; and if ear pigment is a problem, reposition the probe, revascularize the site, or use a finger probe. (See *Diagnosing pulse oximeter problems.*)
▶ Certain intravascular substances, such as lipid emulsions and dyes, can also prevent accurate readings. Other factors that may interfere with accurate results include excessive light (for example, from phototherapy, surgical lamps, direct sunlight, and excessive ambient lighting), excessive patient

movement, excessive ear pigment, hypothermia, hypotension, and vasoconstriction.
▶ If the patient has compromised circulation in his extremities, you can place a
photodetector across the bridge of his nose.
▶ If SpO$_2$ is used to guide weaning the patient from forced inspiratory oxygen, obtain arterial blood gas analysis occasionally
to correlate SpO$_2$ readings with SaO$_2$ levels.
▶ If an automatic blood pressure cuff is
used on the same extremity that is used for
measuring SpO$_2$, the cuff will interfere
with SpO$_2$ readings during inflation.
▶ Normal SpO$_2$ levels for ear and pulse
oximetry are 95% to 100% for adults and
93.8% to 100% by 1 hour after birth for
healthy, full-term neonates. Lower levels
may indicate hypoxemia that warrants intervention. For such patients, follow your
facility's policy or the doctor's orders,
which may include increasing oxygen therapy. If SaO$_2$ levels decrease suddenly, you
may need to resuscitate the patient immediately. Notify the doctor of any significant
change in the patient's condition.

### Documentation
▶ Document the procedure, including:
date, time, procedure type, oximetric measurement, and any action taken.
▶ Record reading on appropriate flowcharts, if indicated.

**EVIDENCE BASE** If you detect a discrepancy between SpO$_2$ and SaO$_2$
values and the patient's clinical appearance, look for possible causes before you
report the results. If troubleshooting measures, such as choosing an alternate monitoring site or changing the probe, don't
reduce the discrepancy, the American
Association for Respiratory Care pulse
oximetry guidelines recommend that you
don't document the SpO$_2$ value. Rather,
document the corrective actions you performed and the SaO$_2$ value obtained by
the arterial blood gas analysis. The acceptable amount of discrepancy varies
with the patient condition and the
oximetry device being used. Always exercise sound clinical judgment.

### REFERENCES
Child Health Corporation of America's Coop-
erative Pulse Oximetry FORUM. "The FO-
RUM Offers Recommendations on Best
Practices in Pediatric Pulse Oximetry,"
*AARC Times* 24(4):36-38, 40-44, April
2000.
Duarte, A.G., and Bidani, A. "Monitoring
Patients with ARDS, Part 2: Pulmonary
Oxygen Uptake," *Journal of Critical Illness*
16(1):38-46, January 2001.
Joint Commission for Accreditation of Health-
care Organizations (2001, February 28).
"Standards Clarification: Physician's Order
to Perform Pulse Oximetry." Available:
*www.jcaho.org/standards_frm.html*
Tate, J., and Tasota, F.J. "Using Pulse Oxime-
try," *Nursing2000* 30(9):30, September
2000.
Vines, D.L., et al. "Current Respiratory Care,
Part 1: Oxygen Therapy, Oximetry,
Bronchial Hygiene," *Journal of Critical Illness* 15(9):507-10, 513-15, September 2000.

## Sputum collection

Secreted by mucous membranes lining the
bronchioles, bronchi, and trachea, sputum
helps protect the respiratory tract from infection. When expelled from the respiratory tract, sputum carries saliva, nasal and sinus secretions, dead cells, and normal oral
bacteria from the respiratory tract. Sputum
specimens may be cultured for identification of respiratory pathogens.
   The usual method of sputum specimen
collection, expectoration, may require ultrasonic nebulization, hydration, or chest
percussion and postural drainage. Less
common methods include tracheal suctioning and, rarely, bronchoscopy. Tracheal
suctioning is contraindicated within 1 hour
of eating and in patients with esophageal
varices, nausea, facial or basilar skull fractures, laryngospasm, or bronchospasm. It
should be performed cautiously in patients
with heart disease because it may precipitate arrhythmias.

### Equipment
*For expectoration*
Sterile specimen container with tight-fitting cap ● gloves ● label ● laboratory request form ● aerosol (such as 10% sodium
chloride, propylene glycol, acetylcysteine,
or sterile or distilled water), if ordered

# Attaching a specimen trap to a suction catheter

Wearing gloves, push the suction tubing onto the male adapter of the in-line trap.

Insert the suction catheter into the rubber tubing of the trap.

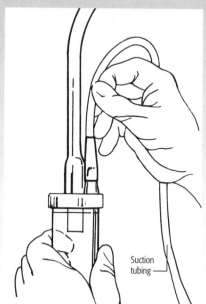

Suction tubing

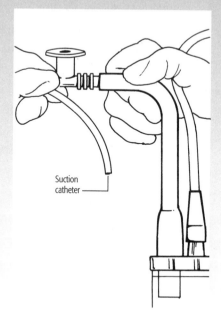

Suction catheter

---

*For tracheal suctioning*
#12 to #14 French sterile suction catheter ● water-soluble lubricant ● label ● laboratory request form ● sterile gloves ● mask ● goggles ● sterile in-line specimen trap (Lukens trap) ● normal saline solution ● portable suction machine ● if wall suction is unavailable, oxygen therapy equipment

Commercial suction kits have all equipment except the suction machine and an in-line specimen container.

### Preparation of equipment
Equipment and preparation depend on the method of collection. Gather the appropriate equipment for the task.

## Implementation
▶ Tell the patient that you'll collect a specimen of sputum (not saliva) and explain the procedure to promote cooperation. If possible, collect the specimen early in the morning, before breakfast, to obtain an overnight accumulation of secretions.

### Collection by expectoration
▶ Instruct the patient to sit in a chair or at the edge of the bed. If he can't sit up, place him in high Fowler's position.
▶ Ask the patient to rinse his mouth with water to reduce specimen contamination. (Avoid mouthwash or toothpaste because they may affect the mobility of organisms in the sputum sample.) Then tell him to cough deeply and expectorate directly into the specimen container. Ask him to produce at least 15 ml of sputum, if possible.
▶ Put on gloves.
▶ Cap the container and, if necessary, clean its exterior. Remove and discard your gloves, and wash your hands thoroughly. Label the container with the patient's name and room number, doctor's name, date and time of collection, and initial diagnosis. Also, include on the laboratory request form whether the patient was febrile or taking antibiotics and whether sputum was induced (because such specimens commonly appear watery and may resemble

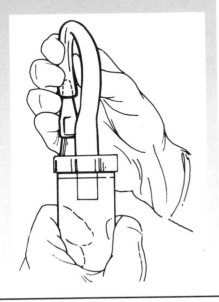

After suctioning, disconnect the in-line trap from the suction tubing and catheter. To seal the container, connect the rubber tubing to the male adapter of the trap.

saliva). Send the specimen to the laboratory immediately.

## Collection by tracheal suctioning

▶ If the patient can't produce an adequate specimen by coughing, prepare to suction him to obtain the specimen. Explain the suctioning procedure to him and tell him that he may cough, gag, or feel short of breath during the procedure.

▶ Check the suction equipment to make sure it's functioning properly. Then place the patient in high Fowler's or semi-Fowler's position.

▶ Administer oxygen to the patient before beginning the procedure.

▶ Wash your hands thoroughly.

▶ Position a mask and goggles over your face.

▶ Put on sterile gloves. Consider one hand sterile and the other hand clean to prevent cross-contamination.

▶ Connect the suction tubing to the male adapter of the in-line specimen trap. At-

tach the sterile suction catheter to the rubber tubing of the trap. (See *Attaching a specimen trap to a suction catheter.*)

▶ Tell the patient to tilt his head back slightly. Then lubricate the catheter with normal saline solution and/or water-soluble lubricant and gently pass it through the patient's nostril without suction.

▶ When the catheter reaches the larynx, the patient will cough. As he does, quickly advance the catheter into the trachea. Tell him to take several deep breaths through his mouth to ease insertion.

▶ To obtain the specimen, apply suction for 5 to 10 seconds but never longer than 15 seconds because prolonged suction can cause hypoxia. If the procedure must be repeated, let the patient rest for four to six breaths. When collection is completed, discontinue the suction, gently remove the catheter, and administer oxygen.

▶ Detach the catheter from the in-line trap, gather it up in your dominant hand, and pull the glove cuff inside out and down around the used catheter to enclose it for disposal. Remove and discard the other glove and your mask and goggles.

▶ Detach the trap from the tubing connected to the suction machine. Seal the trap tightly by connecting the rubber tubing to the male adapter of the trap. Examine the specimen to make sure it's actually sputum, not saliva. Label the trap's container as an expectorated specimen and send it to the laboratory immediately with a completed laboratory request form.

▶ Offer the patient a glass of water or mouthwash.

## Special considerations

▶ If you can't obtain a sputum specimen through tracheal suctioning, perform chest percussion to loosen and mobilize secretions, and position the patient for optimal drainage. After 20 to 30 minutes, repeat the tracheal suctioning procedure.

▶ Before sending the specimen to the laboratory, examine it to make sure it's actually sputum, not saliva, because saliva will produce inaccurate test results.

▶ Because expectorated sputum is contaminated by normal mouth flora, tracheal suctioning provides a more reliable specimen for diagnosis.

▶ If the patient becomes hypoxic or cyanotic during suctioning, remove the catheter immediately and administer oxygen.

▶ If the patient has asthma or chronic bronchitis, watch for aggravated bronchospasms with the use of more than a 10% concentration of sodium chloride or acetylcysteine in an aerosol. If he's suspected of having tuberculosis, don't use more than 20% propylene glycol with water when inducing a sputum specimen because a higher concentration inhibits growth of the pathogen and causes erroneous test results. If propylene glycol isn't available, use 10% to 20% acetylcysteine with water or sodium chloride.

## Complications

Patients with cardiac disease may develop arrhythmias during the procedure as a result of coughing, especially when the specimen is obtained by suctioning. Other potential complications include tracheal trauma or bleeding, vomiting, aspiration, and hypoxemia.

## Documentation

▶ Record the collection method used.
▶ Note time and date of collection.
▶ Document how the patient tolerated the procedure.
▶ Document color and consistency of the specimen, and its proper disposition.

### REFERENCES

Bartoli, M.L., et al. "Quality Evaluation of Samples Obtained by Spontaneous or Induced Sputum: Comparison Between Two Methods of Processing and Relationship with Clinical and Functional Findings," *Journal of Asthma* 39(6):479-86, September 2002.

Ewig, S., et al. "Applying Sputum as a Diagnostic Tool in Pneumonia: Limited Yield, Minimal Impact on Treatment Decisions," *Chest* 121(5):1486-92, May 2002.

# Thoracentesis

Thoracentesis involves the aspiration of fluid or air from the pleural space. It relieves lung tissue compression and respiratory distress by removing accumulated air or fluid that results from injury or conditions such as tuberculosis or cancer. It also provides a specimen of pleural fluid or tissue for bacteriologic or cytolic analysis and allows for introduction of chemotherapeutic agents or other medications into the pleural space. Thoracentesis is contraindicated in patients with bleeding disorders.

## Equipment

Most facilities use a prepackaged thoracentesis tray that typically includes: sterile gloves ● sterile drapes ● 70% isopropyl alcohol or povidone-iodine solution ● 1% or 2% lidocaine ● 5-ml syringe with 21G and 25G needles for anesthetic injection ● 17G thoracentesis needle for aspiration ● 50-ml syringe ● three-way stopcock and tubing ● sterile specimen containers ● sterile hemostat ● sterile 4" × 4" gauze pads.

You'll also need adhesive tape ● sphygmomanometer ● gloves ● stethoscope ● laboratory request slips ● drainage bottles ● optional: Teflon catheter, shaving supplies, biopsy needle, prescribed sedative with 3-ml syringe and 21G needle, and drainage bottles (if the doctor expects a large amount of drainage).

### Preparation of equipment

Assemble all equipment at the patient's bedside or in the treatment area. Check the expiration date on each sterile package and inspect for tears. Prepare the necessary laboratory request form. Be sure to list current antibiotic therapy on the laboratory forms because this will be considered in analyzing the specimens. Make sure the patient has signed an appropriate consent form. Note any drug allergies, especially to the local anesthetic. Have the patient's chest X-rays available.

## Implementation

▶ Explain the procedure to the patient. Inform him that he may feel some discomfort and a sensation of pressure during the needle insertion. Provide privacy and emotional support. Wash your hands.
▶ Obtain baseline vital signs and assess respiratory function.
▶ Administer the prescribed sedative as ordered.
▶ Position the patient. Make sure he's firmly supported and comfortable. Although the choice of position varies, you'll usually seat the patient on the edge of the bed with his legs supported and his head and folded arms resting on a pillow on the overbed table. Or have him straddle a chair backward and rest his head and folded arms on the back of the chair. If the patient is unable to sit, turn him on the unaffected side

with the arm of the affected side raised above his head. Elevate the head of the bed 30 to 45 degrees if such elevation isn't contraindicated. Proper positioning stretches the chest or back and allows easier access to the intercostal spaces.

▶ Remind the patient not to cough, breathe deeply, or move suddenly during the procedure to avoid puncture of the visceral pleura or lung. If the patient coughs, the doctor will briefly halt the procedure and withdraw the needle slightly to prevent puncture.

▶ Expose the patient's entire chest or back, as appropriate.

▶ Shave the aspiration site as ordered.

▶ Wash your hands again before touching the sterile equipment. Then, using sterile technique, open the thoracentesis tray and assist the doctor as necessary in disinfecting the site.

▶ If an ampule of local anesthetic isn't included in the sterile tray and a multidose vial of local anesthetic is to be used, assist the doctor by wiping the rubber stopper with an alcohol pad and holding the inverted vial while the doctor withdraws the anesthetic solution.

▶ After draping the patient and injecting the anesthetic, the doctor attaches a three-way stopcock with tubing to the aspirating needle and turns the stopcock to prevent air from entering the pleural space through the needle.

▶ Attach the other end of the tubing to the drainage bottle.

▶ The doctor then inserts the needle into the pleural space and attaches a 50-ml syringe to the needle's stopcock. A hemostat may be used to hold the needle in place and prevent pleural tear or lung puncture. As an alternative, the doctor may introduce a Teflon catheter into the needle, remove the needle, and attach a stopcock and syringe or drainage tubing to the catheter to reduce the risk of pleural puncture by the needle.

▶ Support the patient verbally throughout the procedure and keep him informed of each step. Assess him for signs of anxiety and provide reassurance as necessary.

▶ Check vital signs regularly during the procedure. Continually observe the patient for such signs of distress as pallor, vertigo, faintness, weak and rapid pulse, decreased blood pressure, dyspnea, tachypnea, diaphoresis, chest pain, blood-tinged mucus,

and excessive coughing. Alert the doctor if such signs develop because they may indicate complications, such as hypovolemic shock and tension pneumothorax.

▶ Put on gloves and assist the doctor as necessary in specimen collection, fluid drainage, and dressing the site.

▶ After the doctor withdraws the needle or catheter, apply pressure to the puncture site using a sterile 4″ × 4″ gauze pad. Then apply a new sterile gauze pad and secure it with tape.

▶ Place the patient in a comfortable position, take his vital signs, and assess his respiratory status.

▶ Label the specimens properly and send them to the laboratory.

▶ Discard disposable equipment. Clean nondisposable items and return them for sterilization.

▶ Check the patient's vital signs and the dressing for drainage every 15 minutes for 1 hour. Continue to assess the patient's vital signs and respiratory status as indicated by his condition.

## Special considerations

▶ To prevent pulmonary edema and hypovolemic shock after thoracentesis, fluid is removed slowly, and no more than 1,000 ml of fluid is removed during the first 30 minutes. Removing the fluid increases the negative intrapleural pressure, which can lead to edema if the lung doesn't reexpand to fill the space.

▶ Pleuritic or shoulder pain may indicate pleural irritation by the needle point.

▶ A chest X-ray is usually ordered after the procedure to detect pneumothorax and evaluate the results of the procedure.

## Complications

Pneumothorax (possibly leading to mediastinal shift and requiring chest tube insertion) can occur if the needle punctures the lung and allows air to enter the pleural cavity. Pyogenic infection can result from contamination during the procedure. Other potential difficulties include pain, cough, anxiety, dry taps, and subcutaneous hematoma.

## Documentation

▶ Record the date and time of thoracentesis.

▶ Document the location of the puncture site.

▶ Record the volume and description (color, viscosity, odor) of the fluid withdrawn.
▶ Note specimens sent to the laboratory.
▶ Record vital signs and respiratory assessment before, during, and after the procedure.
▶ Document any postprocedural tests such as a chest X-ray.
▶ Document complications and the nursing action taken.
▶ Record the patient's reaction to the procedure.

### REFERENCES

Chen, K.Y., et al. "Pneumothorax in the ICU: Patient Outcomes and Prognostic Factors," *Chest* 122(2):678-83, August 2002.
Rubio, E.R., et al. "Thoracoscopic Management of Pleural Effusions in Kaposi's Sarcoma: A Rapid and Effective Alternative for Diagnosis and Treatment," *Southern Medical Journal* 95(8):919-21, August 2002.

# Tracheal cuff-pressure measurement

An endotracheal (ET) or tracheostomy cuff provides a closed system for mechanical ventilation, allowing a desired tidal volume to be delivered to the patient's lungs. To function properly, the cuff must exert enough pressure on the tracheal wall to seal the airway without compromising the blood supply to the tracheal mucosa.

The ideal pressure (known as minimal occlusive volume) is the lowest amount needed to seal the airway. Many authorities recommend maintaining a cuff pressure lower than venous perfusion pressure, usually 16 to 24 cm $H_2O$. (More than 24 cm $H_2O$ may exceed venous perfusion pressure.) Actual cuff pressure will vary with each patient, however.

## Equipment

10-ml syringe • three-way stopcock • cuff pressure manometer • stethoscope • suction equipment • gloves

### Preparation of equipment

Assemble all equipment at the patient's bedside. If measuring with a blood pressure manometer, attach the syringe to one stopcock port; then attach the tubing from the manometer to another port of the stopcock. Turn off the stopcock port where

you'll be connecting the pilot balloon cuff so that air can't escape from the cuff. Use the syringe to instill air into the manometer tubing until the pressure reading reaches 10 mm Hg. This will prevent sudden cuff deflation when you open the stopcock to the cuff and the manometer.

## Implementation

▶ Explain the procedure to the patient. Put on gloves and suction the ET or tracheostomy tube and the patient's oropharynx to remove accumulated secretions above the cuff. Then attach the cuff pressure manometer to the pilot balloon port.
▶ Place the diaphragm of the stethoscope over the trachea and listen for an air leak (as shown below). Keep in mind that a smooth, hollow sound indicates a sealed airway; a loud, gurgling sound indicates an air leak.

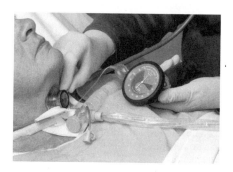

▶ If you don't hear an air leak, press the red button under the dial of the cuff pressure manometer to slowly release air from the balloon on the tracheal tube (as shown below). Auscultate for an air leak.

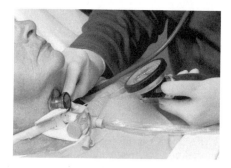

▶ As soon as you hear an air leak, release the red button and gently squeeze the handle of the cuff pressure manometer to inflate the cuff (as shown below). Continue to add air to the cuff until you no longer hear an air leak.

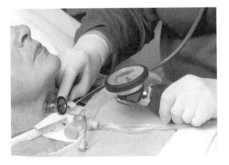

▶ When the air leak ceases, read the dial on the cuff pressure manometer (as shown below). This is the minimal pressure required to effectively occlude the trachea around the tracheal tube. In many cases, this pressure will fall within the green area (16 to 24 cm $H_2O$) on the manometer dial.

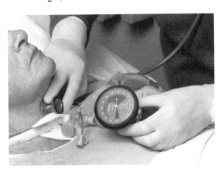

▶ Disconnect the cuff pressure manometer from the pilot balloon port. Document the pressure value.

### Special considerations
▶ Measure cuff pressure at least every 8 hours to avoid overinflation.
▶ Keep in mind that some patients require less pressure, whereas others — for example, those with tracheal malacia (an abnormal softening of the tracheal tissue) — require more pressure. Maintaining the cuff pressure at the lowest possible level will minimize cuff-related problems.
▶ When measuring cuff pressure, keep the connection between the measuring device and the pilot balloon port tight to avoid an air leak that could compromise cuff pressure. If you're using a stopcock, don't leave

the manometer in the OFF position because air will leak from the cuff if the syringe accidentally comes off. Also note the volume of air needed to inflate the cuff. A gradual increase in this volume indicates tracheal dilation or erosion. A sudden increase in volume indicates rupture of the cuff and requires immediate reintubation if the patient is being ventilated.

### Complications
Aspiration of upper airway secretions, underventilation, or coughing spasms may occur if a leak is created during cuff pressure measurement.

### Documentation
▶ After cuff pressure measurement, record the date and time of the procedure, cuff pressure, total amount of air in the cuff after the procedure, any complications and the nursing action taken.
▶ Document the patient's tolerance of the procedure.

### REFERENCES
Schreiber, D. "Trach Care at Home," *RN* 64(7):43-46, July 2001.
Serra, A. "Tracheostomy Care," *Nursing Standard* 14(42):45-52, 54-55, July 2000.
"Standards of Practice: Care of the Patient with a Tracheostomy." *www.cc.nih.gov/ nursing/trach.html*
Tamburri, L.M. "Care of the Patient with a Tracheostomy," *Orthopaedic Nursing* 19(2):49-60, March-April 2000.

# Tracheal suction

Tracheal suction involves the removal of secretions from the trachea or bronchi by means of a catheter inserted through the mouth or nose, a tracheal stoma, a tracheostomy tube, or an endotracheal (ET) tube. In addition to removing secretions, tracheal suctioning also stimulates the cough reflex. This procedure helps maintain a patent airway to promote optimal exchange of oxygen and carbon dioxide and to prevent pneumonia that results from pooling of secretions. Performed as frequently as the patient's condition warrants, tracheal suction calls for strict aseptic technique.

## Equipment

Oxygen source (wall or portable unit and handheld resuscitation bag with a mask, 15-mm adapter, or a positive end-expiratory pressure [PEEP] valve, if indicated) • wall or portable suction apparatus • collection container • connecting tube • goggles • mask • suction catheter kit, or a sterile suction catheter • one sterile glove • one clean glove • disposable sterile solution container • 1-L bottle of sterile water or normal saline solution • sterile water-soluble lubricant (for nasal insertion) • syringe for deflating cuff of ET or tracheostomy tube • waterproof trash bag • optional: sterile towel

### Preparation of equipment

Choose a suction catheter of appropriate size. The diameter should be no larger than half the inside diameter of the tracheostomy or ET tube to minimize hypoxia during suctioning. (A #12 or #14 French catheter may be used for an 8-mm or larger tube.) Place the suction apparatus on the patient's overbed table or bedside stand. Position the table or stand on your preferred side of the bed to facilitate suctioning.

Attach the collection container to the suction unit and the connecting tube to the collection container. Label and date the normal saline solution or sterile water. Open the waterproof trash bag.

## Implementation

▶ Before suctioning, determine whether your facility requires a doctor's order and obtain one, if necessary.
▶ Assess the patient's vital signs, breath sounds, and general appearance to establish a baseline for comparison after suctioning. Review the patient's arterial blood gas values and oxygen saturation levels if they're available. Evaluate the patient's ability to cough and deep-breathe because this will help move secretions up the tracheobronchial tree. If you'll be performing nasotracheal suctioning, check the patient's history for a deviated septum, nasal polyps, nasal obstruction, nasal trauma, epistaxis, or mucosal swelling.
▶ Wash your hands. Explain the procedure to the patient even if he's unresponsive. Tell him that suctioning usually causes transient coughing or gagging but that coughing is helpful for removal of secretions. If the patient has been suctioned previously, summarize the reasons for suctioning. Continue to reassure the patient throughout the procedure to minimize anxiety, promote relaxation, and decrease oxygen demand.
▶ Unless contraindicated, place the patient in semi-Fowler's or high Fowler's position to promote lung expansion and productive coughing.
▶ Remove the top from the normal saline solution or water bottle.
▶ Open the package containing the sterile solution container.
▶ Using sterile technique, open the suction catheter kit and put on the gloves. If using individual supplies, open the suction catheter and the gloves, placing the nonsterile glove on your nondominant hand and then the sterile glove on your dominant hand.
▶ Using your nondominant (nonsterile) hand, pour the normal saline solution or sterile water into the solution container.
▶ Place a small amount of water-soluble lubricant on the sterile area. Lubricant may be used to facilitate passage of the catheter during nasotracheal suctioning.
▶ Place a sterile towel over the patient's chest, if desired, to provide an additional sterile area.
▶ Using your dominant (sterile) hand, remove the catheter from its wrapper. Keep it coiled so it can't touch a nonsterile object. Using your other hand to manipulate the connecting tubing, attach the catheter to the tubing (as shown below).

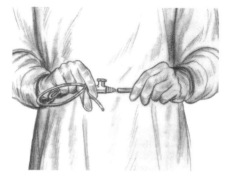

▶ Using your nondominant hand, set the suction pressure according to facility policy. Typically, pressure may be set between 80 and 120 mm Hg. Higher pressures don't enhance secretion removal and may cause traumatic injury. Occlude the suction port

to assess suction pressure (as shown below).

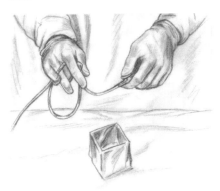

▶ Dip the catheter tip in the saline solution to lubricate the outside of the catheter and reduce tissue trauma during insertion.
▶ With the catheter tip in the sterile solution, occlude the control valve with the thumb of your nondominant hand. Suction a small amount of solution through the catheter (as shown below) to lubricate the inside of the catheter, thus facilitating passage of secretions through it.

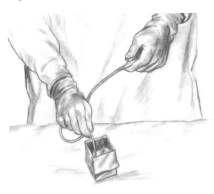

▶ For nasal insertion of the catheter, lubricate the tip of the catheter with the sterile, water-soluble lubricant to reduce tissue trauma during insertion.
▶ If the patient isn't intubated or is intubated but isn't receiving supplemental oxygen or aerosol, instruct him to take three to six deep breaths to help minimize or prevent hypoxia during suctioning.
▶ If the patient isn't intubated but is receiving oxygen, evaluate his need for preoxygenation. If indicated, instruct him to take three to six deep breaths while using his supplemental oxygen. (If needed, the patient may continue to receive supplemental oxygen during suctioning by leaving his nasal cannula in one nostril or by keeping the oxygen mask over his mouth.)
▶ If the patient is being mechanically ventilated, preoxygenate him using either a handheld resuscitation bag or the sigh mode on the ventilator. To use the resuscitation bag, set the oxygen flow meter at 15 L/minute, disconnect the patient from the ventilator, and deliver three to six breaths with the resuscitation bag (as shown below).

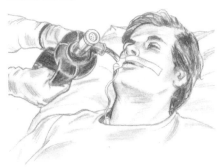

▶ If the patient is being maintained on PEEP, use a resuscitation bag with a PEEP valve.
▶ To preoxygenate using the ventilator, first adjust the fraction of inspired oxygen ($FIO_2$) and tidal volume according to facility policy and patient need. Then, either use the sigh mode or manually deliver three to six breaths. If you have an assistant for the procedure, the assistant can manage the patient's oxygen needs while you perform the suctioning.

### Nasotracheal insertion in a nonintubated patient
▶ Disconnect the oxygen from the patient, if applicable.
▶ Using your nondominant hand, raise the tip of the patient's nose to straighten the passageway and facilitate insertion of the catheter.
▶ Insert the catheter into the patient's nostril while gently rolling it between your fingers to help it advance through the turbinates.
▶ As the patient inhales, quickly advance the catheter as far as possible. To avoid oxygen loss and tissue trauma, don't apply suction during insertion.

‣ If the patient coughs as the catheter passes through the larynx, briefly hold the catheter still and then resume advancement when the patient inhales.

### Insertion in an intubated patient
‣ If you're using a closed system, see *Closed tracheal suctioning.*
‣ Using your nonsterile hand, disconnect the patient from the ventilator.
‣ Using your sterile hand, gently insert the suction catheter into the artificial airway (as shown below). Advance the catheter, without applying suction, until you meet resistance. If the patient coughs, pause briefly and then resume advancement.

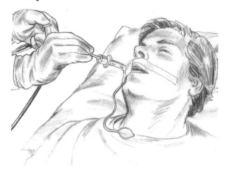

### Suctioning the patient
‣ After inserting the catheter, apply suction intermittently by removing and replacing the thumb of your nondominant hand over the control valve. Simultaneously use your dominant hand to withdraw the catheter as you roll it between your thumb and forefinger. This rotating motion prevents the catheter from pulling tissue into the tube as it exits, thus avoiding tissue trauma. Never suction more than 10 seconds at a time to prevent hypoxia.
‣ If the patient is intubated, use your nondominant hand to stabilize the tip of the ET tube as you withdraw the catheter to prevent mucous membrane irritation or accidental extubation.
‣ If applicable, resume oxygen delivery by reconnecting the source of oxygen or ventilation and hyperoxygenating the patient's lungs before continuing to prevent or relieve hypoxia.
‣ Observe the patient and allow him to rest for a few minutes before the next suctioning. The timing of each suctioning and the length of each rest period depend on his tolerance of the procedure and the absence of complications. To enhance secretion removal, encourage the patient to cough between suctioning attempts.
‣ Observe the secretions. If they're thick, clear the catheter periodically by dipping the tip in the saline solution and applying suction. Normally, sputum is watery and tends to be sticky. Tenacious or thick sputum usually indicates dehydration. Watch for color variations. White or translucent color is normal; yellow indicates pus; green indicates retained secretions or *Pseudomonas* infection; brown usually indicates old blood; red indicates fresh blood; and a "red currant jelly" appearance indicates *Klebsiella* infection. When sputum contains blood, note whether it's streaked or well mixed. Also indicate how often blood appeared. If the patient's heart rate and rhythm are being monitored, observe for arrhythmias. If they occur, stop suctioning and ventilate the patient.
‣ Patients who can't mobilize secretions effectively may need to perform tracheal suctioning after discharge. (See *Tracheal suctioning at home,* page 368.)

### After suctioning
‣ After suctioning, hyperoxygenate the patient being maintained on a ventilator with the handheld resuscitation bag or by using the ventilator's sigh mode, as described earlier.
‣ Readjust the $FIO_2$ and, for ventilated patients, the tidal volume to the ordered settings.
‣ After suctioning the lower airway, assess the patient's need for upper airway suctioning. If the cuff of the ET or tracheostomy tube is inflated, suction the upper airway before deflating the cuff with a syringe. Always change the catheter and sterile glove before resuctioning the lower airway to avoid introducing microorganisms into the lower airway.
‣ Discard the gloves and catheter in the waterproof trash bag. Clear the connecting tubing by aspirating the remaining saline solution or water. Discard and replace suction equipment and supplies according to your facility's policy. Wash your hands.
‣ Auscultate the lungs bilaterally and take vital signs, if indicated, to assess the procedure's effectiveness.

# Closed tracheal suctioning

The closed tracheal suction system can ease removal of secretions and reduce patient complications. Consisting of a sterile suction catheter in a clear plastic sleeve, the system permits the patient to remain connected to the ventilator during suctioning.

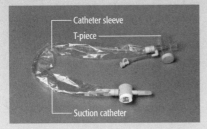

Catheter sleeve
T-piece
Suction catheter

As a result, the patient can maintain the tidal volume, oxygen concentration, and positive end-expiratory pressure delivered by the ventilator while being suctioned. In turn, this reduces the occurrence of suction-induced hypoxemia.

Another advantage of this system is a reduced risk of infection, even when the same catheter is used many times. The caregiver doesn't need to touch the catheter and the ventilator circuit remains closed.

## Implementation

To perform the procedure, gather a closed suction control valve, a T-piece to connect the artificial airway to the ventilator breathing circuit, and a catheter sleeve that encloses the catheter and has connections at each end for the control valve and the T-piece. Then follow these steps:

▶ Remove the closed suction system from its wrapping. Attach the control valve to the connecting tubing.

▶ Depress the thumb suction control valve, and keep it depressed while setting the suction pressure to the desired level.

▶ Connect the T-piece to the ventilator breathing circuit, making sure that the irrigation port is closed;

then connect the T-piece to the patient's endotracheal or tracheostomy tube (as shown below).

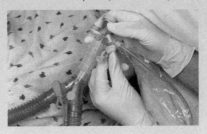

▶ With one hand keeping the T-piece parallel to the patient's chin, use the thumb and index finger of the other hand to advance the catheter through the tube and into the patient's tracheobronchial tree (as shown below).

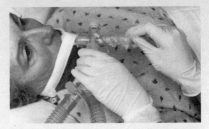

▶ It may be necessary to gently retract the catheter sleeve as you advance the catheter.

▶ While continuing to hold the T-piece and control valve, apply intermittent suction and withdraw the catheter until it reaches its fully extended length in the sleeve. Repeat the procedure as necessary.

▶ After you've finished suctioning, flush the catheter by maintaining suction while slowly introducing normal saline solution or sterile water into the irrigation port.

▶ Place the thumb control valve in the off position.

▶ Dispose of and replace the suction equipment and supplies according to your facility's policy.

▶ Change the closed suction system every 24 hours to minimize the risk of infection.

## Special considerations

▶ Raising the patient's nose into the sniffing position helps align the larynx and pharynx and may facilitate passing the catheter during nasotracheal suctioning. If the patient's condition permits, have an assistant extend the patient's head and neck above his shoulders. The patient's lower

jaw may need to be moved up and forward. If the patient is responsive, ask him to stick out his tongue so he won't be able to swallow the catheter during insertion.

▶ During suctioning, the catheter typically is advanced as far as the mainstem bronchi. However, because of tracheobronchial anatomy, the catheter tends to

# Tracheal suctioning at home

If a patient can't mobilize secretions effectively by coughing, he may have to perform tracheal suctioning at home using either clean or sterile technique. The patient usually uses clean technique, which consists of thorough hand washing and possibly wearing a clean glove. However, a patient with poor hand-washing technique, recurrent respiratory infections, or a compromised immune system or a patient who has had recent surgery may need to use sterile technique.

### Clean technique

Because the cost of disposable catheters can be prohibitive, the patient may reuse the disposable catheter, but the practice remains controversial. If the catheter has thick secretions adhering to it, the patient may clean it with Control III, a quaternary compound.

An alternative to disposable catheters is to use nondisposable, red rubber catheters. However, these catheters contain latex, so use with caution. Consult your facility's policy regarding the care and cleaning of suction catheters in the home setting. Some protocols recommend soaking such catheters in soapy water and then placing them in boiling water for 10 minutes or, alternately, soaking them in 70% alcohol for 3 to 5 minutes and then rinsing in normal saline solution.

### Supplies needed

Obviously, the supplies needed will vary with the technique used. If the patient will be using clean technique, he'll need suction catheter kits (or clean gloves, suction catheters, and basin) and distilled water. If he'll be using sterile technique, everything will need to be sterile: the suction catheters, gloves, basin, and water (or normal saline solution).

The type of suction machine necessary will depend on the patient's needs. You'll need to evaluate the amount of suction the machine provides, how easy it is to clean, how much it costs, the volume of the collection bottles, and whether the machine has an overflow safety device to prevent secretions from entering the compressor. You'll also need to determine whether the patient needs a machine that operates on batteries and, if so, how long the batteries will last and whether and how they can be recharged.

### Nursing goals

Before discharge, the patient and his family should demonstrate the suctioning procedure. They also need to recognize the indications for suctioning, the signs and symptoms of infection, the importance of adequate hydration, and when to use adjunct therapy, such as aerosol therapy, chest physiotherapy, oxygen therapy, or a handheld resuscitation bag. At discharge, arrange for a home health care provider and a durable medical equipment vendor to follow up with the patient.

---

enter the right mainstem bronchi instead of the left. Using an angled catheter (such as a coudé) may help you guide the catheter into the left mainstem bronchus. Rotating the patient's head to the right seems to have a limited effect.

▶ Don't allow the collection container on the suction machine to become more than three-quarters full to keep from damaging the machine.

## Complications

Because oxygen is removed along with secretions, the patient may experience hypoxemia and dyspnea. Anxiety may alter respiratory patterns. Cardiac arrhythmias can result from hypoxia and stimulation of the vagus nerve in the tracheobronchial tree. Tracheal or bronchial trauma can result from traumatic or prolonged suctioning.

Patients with compromised cardiovascular or pulmonary status are at risk for hypoxemia, arrhythmias, hypertension, or hypotension. Patients with a history of nasopharyngeal bleeding, those who are taking anticoagulants, those who have undergone a tracheostomy recently, and those who have a blood dyscrasia are at increased risk for bleeding as a result of suctioning. Use caution when suctioning patients who have increased intracranial pressure because suction may increase pressure further.

If the patient experiences laryngospasm or bronchospasm (rare complications) during suctioning, discuss with the patient's doctor the use of bronchodilators or lidocaine to reduce the risk of this complication.

## Documentation
▶ Record the date and time of the procedure.
▶ Document the technique used.
▶ Note the reason for suctioning.
▶ Note the amount, color, consistency, and odor (if any) of the secretions.
▶ Note complications and the nursing action taken.
▶ Record any pertinent data regarding the patient's subjective response to the procedure.

### REFERENCES
American Association for Respiratory Care. "AARC Clinical Practice Guideline: Suctioning of the Patient in the Home," *Respiratory Care* 44(1):99-104, January 1999.
"As-needed In-line Suction Catheter Changes Were as Safe as and Less Expensive than Daily Scheduled Catheter Changes during Mechanical Ventilation," *Evidence-Based Nursing* 1(3):82, July 1998.
Paul-Allen, J., and Ostrow, C.L. "Survey of Nursing Practices with Closed-System Suctioning," *American Journal of Critical Care* 9(1):9-17, January 2000.
"Tracheal Suctioning of Adults with an Artificial Airway," *Best Practice* 4(4):1-6, 2000.

## Tracheostomy care

Whether a tracheotomy is performed in an emergency situation or after careful preparation, as a permanent measure or as temporary therapy, tracheostomy care has identical goals: to ensure airway patency by keeping the tube free from mucus buildup, to maintain mucous membrane and skin integrity, to prevent infection, and to provide psychological support.

The patient may have one of three types of tracheostomy tube: uncuffed, cuffed, or fenestrated. Tube selection depends on the patient's condition and the doctor's preference.

An *uncuffed* tube, which may be plastic or metal, allows air to flow freely around the tracheostomy tube and through the larynx, reducing the risk of tracheal damage. A *cuffed* tube, made of plastic, is disposable. The cuff and the tube won't separate accidentally inside the trachea because the cuff is bonded to the tube. Also, it doesn't require periodic deflating to lower pressure because cuff pressure is low and evenly distributed against the tracheal wall. Although cuffed tubes may cost more than other tubes, they reduce the risk of tracheal damage. A plastic *fenestrated* tube permits speech through the upper airway when the external opening is capped and the cuff is deflated. It also allows easy removal of the inner cannula for cleaning. However, a fenestrated tube may become occluded.

Whichever tube is used, tracheostomy care should be performed using aseptic technique until the stoma has healed to prevent infection. For recently performed tracheotomies, use sterile gloves for all manipulations at the tracheostomy site. When the stoma has healed, clean gloves may be substituted for sterile ones.

## Equipment
*For aseptic stoma and outer-cannula care*
Waterproof trash bag ● two sterile solution containers ● normal saline solution ● hydrogen peroxide ● sterile cotton-tipped applicators ● sterile 4″ × 4″ gauze pads ● sterile gloves ● prepackaged sterile tracheostomy dressing (or 4″ × 4″ gauze pad) ● equipment and supplies for suctioning and for mouth care ● water-soluble lubricant or topical antibiotic cream ● materials as needed for cuff procedures and for changing tracheostomy ties (see below)

*For aseptic inner-cannula care*
All of the preceding equipment plus a prepackaged commercial tracheostomy-care set, or sterile forceps ● sterile nylon brush ● sterile 6″ (15 cm) pipe cleaners ● clean gloves ● a third sterile solution container ● disposable temporary inner cannula (for a patient on a ventilator)

*For changing tracheostomy ties*
30″ (76-cm) length of tracheostomy twill tape ● bandage scissors ● sterile gloves ● hemostat

*For emergency tracheostomy tube replacement*
Sterile tracheal dilator or sterile hemostat ● sterile obturator that fits the tracheostomy tube in use ● extra sterile tracheostomy tube and obturator in appropriate size ● suction equipment and supplies

(Keep these supplies in full view in the patient's room at all times for easy access in case of emergency. Consider taping an emergency sterile tracheostomy tube in a sterile wrapper to the head of the bed for easy access in an emergency.)

*For cuff procedures*
5- or 10-ml syringe • padded hemostat • stethoscope

### Preparation of equipment
Wash your hands and assemble all equipment and supplies in the patient's room. Check the expiration date on each sterile package and inspect the package for tears. Open the waterproof trash bag and place it next to you so that you can avoid reaching across the sterile field or the patient's stoma when discarding soiled items.

Establish a sterile field near the patient's bed (usually on the overbed table) and place equipment and supplies on it. Pour normal saline solution, hydrogen peroxide, or a mixture of equal parts of both solutions into one of the sterile solution containers; then pour normal saline solution into the second sterile container for rinsing. For inner-cannula care, you may use a third sterile solution container to hold the gauze pads and cotton-tipped applicators saturated with cleaning solution. If you'll be replacing the disposable inner cannula, open the package containing the new inner cannula while maintaining sterile technique. Obtain or prepare new tracheostomy ties, if indicated.

### Implementation
▶ Assess the patient's condition to determine his need for care.
▶ Explain the procedure to the patient even if he's unresponsive. Provide privacy.
▶ Place the patient in semi-Fowler's position (unless it's contraindicated) to decrease abdominal pressure on the diaphragm and promote lung expansion.
▶ Remove any humidification or ventilation device.
▶ Using sterile technique, suction the entire length of the tracheostomy tube to clear the airway of any secretions that may hinder oxygenation.
▶ Reconnect the patient to the humidifier or ventilator, if necessary.

### Cleaning a stoma and outer cannula
▶ Put on sterile gloves if you aren't already wearing them.
▶ With your dominant hand, saturate a sterile gauze pad with the cleaning solution. Squeeze out the excess liquid to prevent accidental aspiration. Wipe the patient's neck under the tracheostomy tube flanges and twill tapes.
▶ Saturate a second pad and wipe until the skin around the tracheostomy is cleaned. Use more pads or cotton-tipped applicators to clean the stoma site and the tube's flanges. Wipe only once with each pad and then discard it to prevent contamination of a clean area with a soiled pad.
▶ Rinse debris and peroxide (if used) with one or more sterile 4″ × 4″ gauze pads dampened in normal saline solution. Dry the area thoroughly with additional sterile gauze pads; then apply a new sterile tracheostomy dressing.
▶ Remove and discard your gloves.

### Cleaning a nondisposable inner cannula
▶ Put on sterile gloves.
▶ Using your nondominant hand, remove and discard the patient's tracheostomy dressing. Then, with the same hand, disconnect the ventilator or humidification device and unlock the tracheostomy tube's inner cannula by rotating it counterclockwise. Place the inner cannula in the container of hydrogen peroxide.
▶ Working quickly, use your dominant hand to scrub the cannula with the sterile nylon brush. If the brush doesn't slide easily into the cannula, use a sterile pipe cleaner.
▶ Immerse the cannula in the container of normal saline solution and agitate it for about 10 seconds to rinse it thoroughly.
▶ Inspect the cannula for cleanliness. Repeat the cleaning process, if necessary. If it's clean, tap it gently against the inside edge of the sterile container to remove excess liquid and prevent aspiration. Don't dry the outer surface because a thin film of moisture acts as a lubricant during insertion.
▶ Reinsert the inner cannula into the patient's tracheostomy tube. Lock it in place and then gently pull on it to make sure it's positioned securely. Reconnect the mechanical ventilator. Apply a new sterile tracheostomy dressing.

▶ If the patient can't tolerate being disconnected from the ventilator for the time it takes to clean the inner cannula, replace the existing inner cannula with a clean one and reattach the mechanical ventilator. Then clean the cannula just removed from the patient and store it in a sterile container for the change.

### Caring for a disposable inner cannula
▶ Put on clean gloves.
▶ Using your dominant hand, remove the patient's inner cannula. After evaluating the secretions in the cannula, discard it properly.
▶ Pick up the new inner cannula, touching only the outer locking portion. Insert the cannula into the tracheostomy and, following the manufacturer's instructions, lock it securely.

### Changing tracheostomy ties
▶ Obtain assistance from another nurse or a respiratory therapist because of the risk of accidental tube expulsion during this procedure. Patient movement or coughing can dislodge the tube.
▶ Wash your hands thoroughly and put on sterile gloves if you aren't already wearing them.
▶ If you aren't using commercially packaged tracheostomy ties, prepare new ties from a 30″ (76-cm) length of twill tape by folding one end back 1″ (2.5 cm) on itself. Then, with the bandage scissors, cut a ½″ (1.5-cm) slit down the center of the tape from the folded edge.
▶ Prepare the other end of the tape the same way.
▶ Hold both ends together and, using scissors, cut the resulting circle of tape so that one piece is approximately 10″ (25.5 cm) long and the other is about 20″ (51 cm) long.
▶ Help the patient into semi-Fowler's position if possible.
▶ After your assistant puts on gloves, instruct her to hold the tracheostomy tube in place to prevent its expulsion during replacement of the ties. If you must perform the procedure without assistance, fasten the clean ties in place before removing the old ties to prevent tube expulsion.
▶ With the assistant's gloved fingers holding the tracheostomy tube in place, cut the soiled tracheostomy ties with the bandage scissors or untie them and discard the ties.

Be careful not to cut the tube of the pilot balloon.
▶ Thread the slit end of one new tie a short distance through the eye of one tracheostomy tube flange from the underside; use the hemostat, if needed, to pull the tie through. Then thread the other end of the tie completely through the slit end and pull it taut so it loops firmly through the flange. This avoids knots that can cause throat discomfort, tissue irritation, pressure, and necrosis at the patient's throat.
▶ Fasten the second tie to the opposite flange in the same manner.
▶ Instruct the patient to flex his neck while you bring the ties around to the side and tie them together with a square knot. Flexion produces the same neck circumference as coughing and helps prevent an overly tight tie. Instruct your assistant to place one finger under the tapes as you tie them to ensure that they're tight enough to avoid slippage but loose enough to prevent choking or jugular vein constriction. Placing the closure on the side allows easy access and prevents pressure necrosis at the back of the neck when the patient is recumbent.
▶ After securing the ties, cut off the excess tape with the scissors and instruct your assistant to release the tracheostomy tube.
▶ Make sure the patient is comfortable and can reach the call button easily.
▶ Check tracheostomy-tie tension often on patients with traumatic injury, radical neck dissection, or cardiac failure because neck diameter can increase from swelling and cause constriction; also check neonatal or restless patients frequently because ties can loosen and cause tube dislodgment.

### Concluding tracheostomy care
▶ Replace any humidification device.
▶ Provide mouth care as needed because the oral cavity can become dry and malodorous or develop sores from encrusted secretions.
▶ Observe soiled dressings and any suctioned secretions for amount, color, consistency, and odor.
▶ Properly clean or dispose of all equipment, supplies, solutions, and trash according to policy.
▶ Take off and discard your gloves.
▶ Make sure that the patient is comfortable and that he can easily reach the call button.
▶ Make sure all necessary supplies are readily available at the bedside.

▶ Repeat the procedure at least once every 8 hours or as needed. Change the dressing as often as necessary regardless of whether you also perform the entire cleaning procedure, because a wet dressing with exudate or secretions predisposes the patient to skin excoriation, breakdown, and infection.

### Deflating and inflating a tracheostomy cuff
▶ Read the cuff manufacturer's instructions because cuff types and procedures vary widely.
▶ Assess the patient's condition, explain the procedure to him, and reassure him. Wash your hands thoroughly.
▶ Help the patient into semi-Fowler's position, if possible, or place him in a supine position so secretions above the cuff site will be pushed up into his mouth if he's receiving positive-pressure ventilation.
▶ Suction the oropharyngeal cavity to prevent pooled secretions from descending into the trachea after cuff deflation.
▶ Release the padded hemostat clamping the cuff inflation tubing, if a hemostat is present.
▶ Insert a 5- or 10-ml syringe into the cuff pilot balloon and very slowly withdraw all air from the cuff. Leave the syringe attached to the tubing for later reinflation of the cuff. Slow deflation allows positive lung pressure to push secretions upward from the bronchi. Cuff deflation may also stimulate the patient's cough reflex, producing additional secretions.
▶ Remove any ventilation device. Suction the lower airway through any existing tube to remove all secretions. Then reconnect the patient to the ventilation device.
▶ Maintain cuff deflation for the prescribed time. Observe the patient for adequate ventilation, and suction as necessary. If the patient has difficulty breathing, reinflate the cuff immediately by depressing the syringe plunger very slowly. Use a stethoscope to listen over the trachea for the air leak, then inject the least amount of air needed to achieve an adequate tracheal seal.
▶ When inflating the cuff, you may use the minimal-leak technique or the minimal occlusive volume technique to help gauge the proper inflation point.
▶ If you're inflating the cuff using cuff pressure measurement, be careful not to exceed 25 mm Hg. If pressure exceeds 25 mm Hg, notify the doctor because you may need to change to a larger size tube, use higher inflation pressures, or permit a larger air leak. Recommended cuff pressure is about 18 mm Hg.
▶ After you've inflated the cuff, if the tubing doesn't have a one-way valve at the end, clamp the inflation line with a padded hemostat (to protect the tubing) and remove the syringe.
▶ Check for a minimal-leak cuff seal. You shouldn't feel air coming from the patient's mouth, nose, or tracheostomy site, and a conscious patient shouldn't be able to speak.
▶ Be alert for air leaks from the cuff itself. Suspect a leak if injection of air fails to inflate the cuff or increase cuff pressure, if you're unable to inject the amount of air you withdrew, if the patient can speak, if ventilation fails to maintain adequate respiratory movement with pressures or volumes previously considered adequate, or if air escapes during the ventilator's inspiratory cycle.
▶ Note the exact amount of air used to inflate the cuff to detect tracheal malacia if more air is consistently needed.
▶ Make sure the patient is comfortable and can easily reach the call button and communication aids.
▶ Properly clean or dispose of all equipment, supplies, and trash according to facility policy.
▶ Replenish any used supplies and make sure all necessary emergency supplies are at the bedside.

### Special considerations
▶ Keep appropriate equipment at the patient's bedside for immediate use in an emergency.
▶ Consult the doctor about first-aid measures you can use for your tracheostomy patient should an emergency occur. Follow facility policy regarding procedure if a tracheostomy tube is expelled or if the outer cannula becomes blocked. If the patient's breathing is obstructed, for example, when the tube is blocked with mucus that can't be removed by suctioning or by withdrawing the inner cannula, call the appropriate code and provide manual resuscitation with a handheld resuscitation bag or reconnect the patient to the ventilator. Don't remove the tracheostomy tube entirely because this may allow the airway to close completely. Use extreme caution when at-

tempting to reinsert an expelled tracheostomy tube because of the risk of tracheal trauma, perforation, compression, and asphyxiation. Reassure the patient until the doctor arrives (usually a minute or less in this type of code or emergency).

▶ Refrain from changing tracheostomy ties unnecessarily during the immediate postoperative period before the stoma track is well formed (usually 4 days) to avoid accidental dislodgment and expulsion of the tube. Unless secretions or drainage is a problem, ties can be changed once per day.

▶ Refrain from changing a single-cannula tracheostomy tube or the outer cannula of a double-cannula tube. Because of the risk of tracheal complications, the doctor usually changes the cannula, with the frequency of change depending on the patient's condition.

▶ If the patient's neck or stoma is excoriated or infected, apply a water-soluble lubricant or topical antibiotic cream as ordered. Remember not to use a powder or an oil-based substance on or around a stoma because aspiration can cause infection and abscess.

▶ Replace all equipment, including solutions, regularly according to policy to reduce the risk of nosocomial infections.

## Home care

If the patient is being discharged with a tracheostomy, start self-care teaching as soon as he's receptive. Teach the patient how to change and clean the tube. If he's being discharged with suction equipment (a few patients are), make sure he and his family feel knowledgeable and comfortable about using this equipment.

## Complications

The following complications can occur within the first 48 hours after tracheostomy tube insertion: hemorrhage at the operative site, causing drowning; bleeding or edema in tracheal tissue, causing airway obstruction; aspiration of secretions; introduction of air into the pleural cavity, causing pneumothorax; hypoxia or acidosis, triggering cardiac arrest; and introduction of air into surrounding tissues, causing subcutaneous emphysema.

Secretions collecting under dressings and twill tape can encourage skin excoriation and infection. Hardened mucus or a slipped cuff can occlude the cannula opening and obstruct the airway. Tube displacement can stimulate the cough reflex if the tip rests on the carina, or it can cause blood vessel erosion and hemorrhage. Just the presence of the tube or cuff pressure can produce tracheal erosion and necrosis.

## Documentation

▶ Record the date and time of the procedure and type of procedure.

▶ Document amount, consistency, color, and odor of secretions; stoma and skin condition; the patient's respiratory status; change of the tracheostomy tube by the doctor; the duration of any cuff deflation; the amount of any cuff inflation; and cuff pressure readings and specific body position.

▶ Note any complications and the nursing action taken.

▶ Document patient or family teaching and their comprehension and progress.

▶ Document the patient's tolerance of the treatment.

### REFERENCES

National Institutes of Health, Clinical Center Nursing Department (1999, September 21). "Standards of Practice: Care of the Patient with a Tracheostomy." Available: *www.cc.nih.gov/nursing/trach.html*

Schreiber, D. "Trach Care at Home," *RN* 64(7): 43-46, July 2001.

Serra, A. "Tracheostomy Care," *Nursing Standard* 14(42):45-52,54-55, July 2000.

Tamburri, L.M. "Care of the Patient with a Tracheostomy," *Orthopaedic Nursing* 19(2):49-60, March-April 2000.

# 7

# Neurologic care

APPROPRIATE SUPPORTIVE CARE REQUIRES THAT YOU ASSESS AND DOCUMENT NEUROLOGIC vital signs. At the same time, you must also assess other systems for complications arising from neurologic dysfunction.

Make sure to assess neurologic vital signs, especially the patient's orientation level. The patient with neurologic impairment may experience changes in perception that range from confusion to psychosis. Unaddressed, such disorientation further impairs the patient's ability to participate in recovery. Recognizing this will help you to intervene appropriately.

Respiratory assessment is an important part of an overall neurologic assessment. This is because patients with neurologic damage, especially those with traumatic brain or spinal cord injury, are at considerable risk for respiratory complications. These injuries may depress the respiratory control center and paralyze the muscles used for breathing. As a result, brain tissue, which is especially sensitive to blood oxygen levels, can quickly be damaged by inadequate oxygenation.

Patients with neurologic impairment may experience ineffective cerebral perfusion and increased intracranial pressure. They may also experience neurologic impairment caused by a seizure disorder or a spinal cord injury.

# Protocols

## Managing the patient experiencing ineffective cerebral perfusion

### Purpose
To rapidly identify signs of altered cerebral perfusion, and take necessary steps to limit neurologic deficit related to the altered perfusion

### Collaborative level
Interdependent

### Expected patient outcomes
▶ The patient will preserve cerebral function.
▶ The patient will improve neurologic deficit.
▶ The patient will maintain stable vital signs and adequate blood pressure.
▶ The patient will remain free from injury.
▶ The patient will maintain a patent airway with adequate ventilation.

### Definition of terms
▶ *Stroke:* Broad term used to signify the acute onset of a neurologic deficit resulting from the disruption of the blood supply to the brain. Stroke can be ischemic or hemorrhagic. Ischemic stroke is classified as either thrombotic or embolic. Hemorrhagic stroke refers to bleeding in the intracranial spaces or into the brain itself.
▶ *Transient ischemic event (TIA):* Temporary loss or decrease in blood flow to the brain resulting in transient focal symptoms. Duration of symptoms is usually less than 1 hour.
▶ *Subarachnoid hemorrhage:* Bleeding into the subarachnoid space, most commonly the result of an aneurysm rupture; can also be the result of trauma.
▶ *Intracerebral hemorrhage:* Bleeding into the brain tissue, usually the result of hypertension.

### Indications
Treatment
▶ Acute ischemic stroke
▶ TIA
▶ Intracerebral hemorrhage
▶ Subarachnoid hemorrhage

## Prevention
▶ Aspiration pneumonia
▶ Malnutrition
▶ Skin breakdown
▶ Infection
▶ Recurrent stroke
▶ Deep vein thrombosis (DVT) and pulmonary embolus
▶ Seizure

## Assessment guidance
### Signs and symptoms
#### Middle cerebral artery (most common)
▶ Contralateral hemiparesis of the face, arm, and leg
▶ Homonymous hemianopsia
▶ Aphasia (left hemisphere involvement)
▶ Sensory impairment in the same area as hemiplegia

#### Anterior cerebral artery
▶ Impaired gait
▶ Contralateral hemiparesis of foot or leg
▶ Abulia
▶ Flat affect

#### Posterior cerebral artery
▶ Homonymous hemianopsia
▶ Memory deficits
▶ Perseveration
▶ Visual field deficits

#### Cerebellar stroke
▶ Nausea
▶ Vomiting
▶ Incoordination
▶ Dizziness

#### Level of consciousness
▶ Unusually not affected in ischemic stroke
▶ Commonly depressed with hemorrhage
▶ Headache (more common with hemorrhage)
▶ Hypertension

### Diagnostic studies
#### Laboratory tests
▶ Complete blood count
▶ Prothrombin time and partial thromboplastin time
▶ Chemistry

#### Imaging tests
▶ Computed tomography (CT) scan
▶ Magnetic resonance imaging

▶ Angiography identifies vessel abnormalities; used primarily with subarachnoid hemorrhage
▶ Echocardiogram

#### Other
▶ Carotid Doppler
▶ EEG

## Nursing interventions
### Early care
▶ Ensure that the patient's airway is patent.
▶ Administer supplemental oxygen as ordered.
▶ Take a baseline neurologic assessment.
▶ Evaluate the patient for thrombolytic therapy (presentation within 3 hours of onset of symptoms), and identify any contraindication to thrombolytic therapy.
▶ Obtain a CT scan immediately to rule out hemorrhage.
▶ Monitor the patient for a neurologic deficit; neurologic assessment is needed at a minimum of every 2 hours for 24 hours.
▶ Monitor the patient's blood pressure, and maintain within 10% of baseline; don't aggressively lower in ischemic infarct.
▶ Prepare the patient for urgent craniotomy, if indicated.

### Continuing care
▶ Complete diagnostic studies to determine etiology.
▶ Increase the patient's activity as soon as he's hemodynamically stable.
▶ Assist the patient with an exercise program.
▶ Encourage the patient to participate in activities of daily living.
▶ Institute a bowel program.
▶ Remove the indwelling urinary catheter as soon as possible, and institute a bladder training program, if necessary, to maintain continence.
▶ Maintain an adequate fluid balance.
▶ Monitor the patient for signs of increased intracranial pressure (ICP).
▶ Assess the patient for signs of dysphagia.
▶ Maintain the patient's diet as recommended.
▶ Institute postoperative craniotomy care.

### Recovery care
▶ Assess the patient's self-care capabilities in conjunction with therapies.
▶ Make appropriate referrals.

▶ Obtain the necessary durable medical equipment.
▶ Plan for the patient's transfer to acute rehabilitation if indicated.

## Patient teaching
▶ Be sure to cover these important points with the patient and family:
−signs and symptoms of decreased perfusion
−emergency response to noted signs and symptoms
−all medication information, which includes dosages reasons for taking and side effects
−home safety measures related to the deficit
−how to reduce risk of recurrent stroke
−risk factors and how to minimize and control
−bowel and bladder elimination program
−nutritional guidelines and feeding techniques
−use of assistive devices
−guidelines for exercise and activity.

## Precautions
▶ If thrombolytics are administered, monitor the patient carefully for signs of hemorrhage.
▶ If hemorrhage is suspected, stop the infusion immediately; consider a neurosurgical consult.
▶ If ischemic stroke involved a large area, monitor the patient carefully for signs of increased ICP in the first 72 hours.
▶ Have the patient ambulate as soon as possible to decrease the risk of DVT.

## Documentation
▶ Document the full baseline neurologic assessment.
▶ Record frequent follow-up assessments.
▶ Document the patient's vital signs.
▶ Record diagnostic study results.
▶ Record nursing interventions.
▶ Document doctor notification and intervention.
▶ Note the patient's response to treatment.
▶ Document patient teaching.

## Related procedures
▶ Arterial pressure monitoring
▶ Endotracheal intubation
▶ Endotracheal tube care
▶ Feeding tube insertion and removal
▶ Indwelling catheter care and removal
▶ Manual ventilation
▶ Mechanical ventilation
▶ Nasopharyngeal airway insertion and care
▶ Oropharyngeal airway insertion and care
▶ Passive range-of-motion exercises
▶ Physical assessment
▶ Sequential compression therapy
▶ Transcranial Doppler monitoring

## REFERENCES
*Diseases,* 2nd ed. Professional Guide Series. Springhouse, Pa.: Lippincott Williams & Wilkins, 2002.
Weinberger, J. *Contemporary Diagnosis and Management of Stroke.* Newtown, Pa.: Handbooks in Healthcare, 2000.

## ORGANIZATIONS
American Heart Association: *www.strokeassociation.org*
National Institute of Neurologic Disease: *www.ninds.nih.gov/stroke*
National Stroke Association: *www.stroke.org*
*Stroke:* A Journal of the American Heart Association: *www.stroke.ahajournals.org*

# Managing the patient with increased intracranial pressure

## Purpose
To identify and rapidly treat patients with increased intracranial pressure

## Collaborative level
Interdependent

## Expected patient outcomes
▶ The patient will maintain neurologic function.
▶ The patient will maintain adequate ventilation.
▶ The patient will maintain adequate cerebral perfusion pressure.
▶ The patient won't experience herniation syndrome.

## Definition of terms
▶ *Intracranial pressure (ICP):* Pressure normally exerted by the cerebral spinal fluid in the intracranial cavity as it circulates around the brain and spinal cord. Normal pressure is 0 to 15 mm Hg.

▶ *Cerebral perfusion pressure (CPP):* Blood pressure gradient used to estimate adequacy of cerebral circulation. Calculated as mean arterial pressure (MAP).

▶ *Mass effect:* Shifting of brain structures, resulting from pressure caused by cerebral edema or a space-occupying lesion; can lead to herniation of brain tissue.

▶ *Cushing triad:* Elevation in blood pressure with widened blood pressure and bradycardia. Very late sign of increased ICP indicating herniation.

## Indications
### Treatment
**Increased ICP**
*Conditions that increase brain volume*
▶ Tumor
▶ Abscess
▶ Cerebral edema

*Conditions that increase blood volume*
▶ Hematomas and hemorrhages
▶ Obstruction to venous outflow
▶ Hyperemia
▶ Hypercapnia

*Conditions that increase cerebrospinal fluid*
▶ Increased production of cerebrospinal fluid (CSF)
▶ Decreased absorption of CSF
▶ Obstruction to flow of CSF

### Prevention
▶ Herniation syndromes
▶ Respiratory failure
▶ Skin breakdown
▶ Infection
▶ GI bleeding

## Assessment guidance
### Early signs and symptoms
▶ Change in level of consciousness (LOC), which is the single most important indicator of early increase in ICP
▶ Ipsilateral pupil dilation, decreased response to light
▶ Motor weakness
▶ Dysfunction of extraocular movement
▶ Headache
▶ Seizure, if from space-occupying lesion

### Later signs and symptoms
▶ Further deterioration in LOC to coma
▶ Hemiplegia to decorticate-decerebrate posturing

▶ Worsening headache
▶ Impaired brainstem reflexes
▶ Changes in vital signs (Cushing triad, which is a very late sign)
▶ Vomiting (more common in children)

### Diagnostic studies
**Imaging tests**
▶ CT scan
▶ Magnetic resonance imaging

## Nursing interventions
▶ Maintain a patent airway.
▶ Prevent hypoxia and hypercarbia.
▶ Keep suctioning to a minimum (less than 15 seconds); always preoxygenate the patient.
▶ Monitor the patient's ICP in response to interventions.
▶ Perform frequent neurologic assessments.
▶ Maintain adequate blood pressure to ensure CPP greater than 70 mm Hg.
▶ Maintain the patient's head in the neutral position.
▶ Maintain normothermia.
▶ Avoid severe hip flexion.
▶ Perform passive range-of-motion exercises.
▶ Maintain euvolemia; monitor intake and output carefully.
▶ Maintain ICP monitoring system according to facility policy.
▶ Plan nursing activities to allow for rest periods to decrease pressure spikes.
▶ Maintain seizure precautions.
▶ Institute DVT prophylaxis, as appropriate.
▶ Administer stool softeners and osmotic diuretics.
▶ Sedate the patient to decrease restlessness or agitation.
▶ Monitor electrolyte level.
▶ Monitor urine and osmolarities when using diuretic therapy.
▶ Prepare the patient for cranial surgery as indicated.
▶ Provide postoperative cranial care.
▶ Assess family coping mechanisms, and refer the patient to social services as needed.
▶ Offer emotional support.

## Patient teaching
▶ Explain to the patient and family the reason for the patient's increased ICP.
▶ Explain all procedures and interventions.
▶ Discuss the patient's need for rehabilitation.
▶ Explain all studies being done.
▶ Provide information on support groups and community resources.

## Precautions
▶ Infection is a common complication of ICP monitoring; monitor carefully for signs and symptoms.
▶ Seizure and hyperthermia increase ICP and will make the condition worse.

## Documentation
▶ Record ICP.
▶ Document vital signs, blood pressure with MAP, CPP, and temperature.
▶ Record neurologic assessment.
▶ Document nursing interventions, medications given, and the patient's response.
▶ Record doctor notification and intervention.

## Related procedures
▶ Arterial pressure monitoring
▶ Central venous line insertion and removal
▶ Central venous pressure monitoring
▶ Cerebral blood flow monitoring
▶ Cerebrospinal fluid drainage
▶ Endotracheal intubation
▶ Endotracheal tube care
▶ Feeding tube insertion and removal
▶ I.V. bolus injection
▶ Indwelling catheter care and removal
▶ Intracranial pressure monitoring
▶ Manual ventilation
▶ Mechanical ventilation
▶ Nasopharyngeal airway insertion and care
▶ Oropharyngeal airway insertion and care
▶ Passive range-of-motion exercises
▶ Physical assessment
▶ Postoperative care
▶ Preoperative care
▶ Sequential compression therapy

### REFERENCES
*Diseases,* 2nd ed. *Professional Guide Series.* Springhouse, Pa.: Lippincott Williams & Wilkins, 2002.

Lower, J. "Facing Neuro Assessment Fearlessly," *Nursing* 32(2):58-64, February 2002.
March, K. "Intracranial Pressure Monitoring and Assessing Intracranial Compliance in Brain Injury," *Critical Care Nursing Clinics of North America* 12(4):429-36, December 2000.

# Managing the patient with seizure disorder

## Purpose
To prevent physical injury and ensure patient safety; to accurately observe and report seizure characteristics, physical findings, and assessment

## Collaborative level
Interdependent

## Expected patient outcomes
▶ The patient will remain free from injury.
▶ The patient will avoid aspiration.

## Definition of terms
▶ *Palilalia:* Involuntary repetition of a syllable or phrase.
▶ *Impaired consciousness:* The inability to respond normally to exogenous stimuli because of altered awareness or responsiveness.
▶ *Responsiveness:* The ability of the patient to carry out simple commands or willed movement.
▶ *Awareness:* The patient's contact with events during a particular period in terms of question and recall.
▶ *Status epilepticus:* A condition in which epileptic seizures continue or are repeated without regaining consciousness for 30 minutes or more.
▶ *Aura:* A subjective sensation or objective finding preceding a seizure.

## Indications
Treatment
▶ New-onset seizure disorder
▶ Known seizure disorder

Prevention
▶ Respiratory arrest
▶ Oral trauma
▶ Head trauma
▶ Stress fractures
▶ Aspiration pneumonia
▶ Postictal pulmonary edema

▶ Status epilepticus
▶ Hypotension
▶ Cardiac arrhythmias
▶ Metabolic abnormalities
▶ Hypoglycemia
▶ Hyperthermia
▶ Rhabdomyolysis
▶ Renal failure
▶ Cerebral edema

## Assessment guidance
### Signs and symptoms
#### Auras
▶ Somatosensory: Numbness, tingling, weak electric shock or sense of movement
▶ Visual: Flashes of light or colors, visual illusions, or hallucinations
▶ Auditory: Humming, buzzing, or hissing
▶ Olfactory and gustatory: Unpleasant odors and tastes
▶ Autonomic: Epigastric sensations, flushing, pallor, sweating, pupil dilation, and diaphoresis
▶ Dysphasic: Speech arrest, vocalization, and palilalia
▶ Dysmnesic: Distortion of memory, dreamy state, flashback, and sense of deja vu
▶ Cognitive: Distortions of time sense and sensations of unreality
▶ Affective: Fear, pleasure, displeasure, rage, anger, irritability, elation, and eroticism

#### Seizures
*Simple partial seizure*
▶ No impairment of awareness
▶ Motor: Clonus, jerking, increased tone
▶ Versive: Conjugate eye movements and turning of head to side
▶ Postural: Asymmetric dystonic posturing
▶ Aphasic: Speech arrest or disruption while conscious

*Complex partial seizure*
▶ Impairment of awareness
▶ Automatism phenomenon: Alimentary chewing movements, increased salivation or borborygmus
▶ Mimetic: Face movements resulting in expressions of fear, bewilderment, discomfort, laughing, or crying
▶ Gestural: Repetitive movements of hands and fingers or sexual gestures
▶ Staring
▶ May be preceded by simple partial seizure, with or without postictal confusion

*Absence seizure*
▶ Staring, motionless distant appearance
▶ Suppression of mental function, complete abolition of awareness, responsiveness, and memory
▶ No postictal period

*Myoclonic seizure*
▶ Sudden, brief, shocklike contractions that may be generalized or confined to one area or muscle group
▶ No loss of consciousness

*Tonic seizure*
▶ Impairment of consciousness
▶ Sudden-onset increased tone in extensor muscles, leading to fall
▶ Brief periods of apnea or high-pitched cry
▶ More prevalent during sleep
▶ Last seconds to 1 minute
*Atonic seizure*
▶ Sudden loss of muscle tone, with patient dropping to the ground
▶ Impaired consciousness during fall only

*Clonic seizure*
▶ Loss or impairment of consciousness
▶ Brief generalized tonic spasm and then bilateral jerks

*Tonic-clonic seizure*
▶ Unconsciousness; may be preceded by simple or complex partial seizure
▶ Tonic contraction of muscles with loss of postural control
▶ Cry caused by contraction of respiratory muscles forcing exhalation
▶ Generalized contraction of all muscles in all four extremities
▶ Possible fecal and urinary incontinence
▶ Possible tongue biting

### Diagnostic studies
#### Laboratory tests
▶ Serum chemistry panel including glucose, sodium, calcium, magnesium, and blood urea nitrogen to rule out metabolic cause
▶ CBC to rule out infection as cause
▶ Toxic screen (if alcohol or drug abuse or withdrawal is suspected)

#### Imaging tests
▶ MRI scan
▶ CT scan
▶ Positron emission tomography scan

### Other
▶ Lumbar puncture, if malignancy or infection is cause of seizure
▶ EEG (4-hour sleep-deprived) to confirm presence of abnormal electrical activity, providing information about the type of seizure disorder and location of seizure focus
▶ Pulse oximetry or arterial blood gas (ABG) analysis, if hypoxia is suspected as the cause

## Nursing interventions
▶ Ensure a patent airway.
▶ Make the patient as comfortable as possible.
▶ Remove harmful objects from around the patient.
▶ Protect the patient's head and body from injury.
▶ Loosen tight clothing and eyeglasses.
▶ After a seizure, place the patient in recovery position (lateral decubitus) to prevent aspiration and promote drainage.
▶ An oral airway may be inserted after a seizure during unconsciousness to maintain the airway and assist in draining secretions to prevent aspiration.
▶ Examine the patient for signs of injury.
▶ Monitor the patient's vital signs.
▶ Remain with the patient throughout the seizure.
▶ Insert or maintain an I.V. line with normal saline solution.
▶ Notify the doctor.
▶ Draw chemistry panel, CBC, toxicology, and antiepileptic levels.
▶ Draw blood for ABG analysis.
▶ Obtain pulse oximetry.
▶ Give supplemental oxygen.
▶ Note time of onset and duration, patient activity at time of onset, sequence of events, sensory phenomena, motor activity, postural tone, laterality of movements, incontinence, tongue biting, alteration of consciousness, automatisms, tonic movements, clonic movements, pupillary, skin or respiratory changes, and patient response after seizure.
▶ Assess precipitating factors, such as anxiety, sleep deprivation, fever, menstrual cycle, alcohol, hyperventilation, flickering lights, or television.
▶ Offer comfort and reassurance after the seizure.
▶ Allow the patient to express and deal with fear, anxiety, and grief.

## Patient teaching
▶ Evaluate the patient's knowledge of seizures and treatments.
▶ Teach the patient and his family the importance of complying with the prescribed drug regimen, concerns for adverse effects, and the need for follow-up care.
▶ Advise the patient on the importance of wearing a medical identification bracelet.
▶ Teach the patient when antiepileptic drug levels are ordered to have blood drawn before taking his morning dose of medication.
▶ Teach the caregiver ways to keep the patient safe.
▶ Teach the patient and his family the importance of the patient wearing a helmet when bike riding, avoiding contact sports, and never swimming alone.
▶ Teach the patient and his family about seizure triggers.
▶ Teach the patient and his family the importance of keeping a seizure diary.
▶ Teach the patient and his family that bathroom doors should always open out.
▶ Explain driving restrictions and loss of license per each state protocol.
▶ Refer the patient and his family to support groups.
▶ Give the patient the phone number for the Epilepsy Foundation of America.

## Precautions
▶ Never force anything between the patient's teeth during a seizure.
▶ Don't move the patient during a seizure.

## Documentation
▶ Document the seizure on the patient's medical record, including the time of onset and duration, the patient's activity at the time of onset, sequence of events, and sensory phenomena.
▶ Record the patient's motor activity, postural tone, and laterality of movements.
▶ Note any incontinence, tongue biting, alteration of consciousness, automatisms, and tonic or clonic movements.
▶ Document the patient's pupillary, skin, or respiratory changes.
▶ Note patient response following seizure.
▶ Document vital signs, including an electrocardiogram if possible.

## Related procedures
▶ Arterial puncture for blood gas analysis
▶ Cardiac monitoring

▶ Cardiopulmonary resuscitation
▶ I.V. bolus injection
▶ Neurologic assessment
▶ Oxygen administration
▶ Physical assessment
▶ Prone positioning
▶ Pulse and ear oximetry
▶ Rectal suppositories and ointments
▶ Seizure precautions
▶ Venipuncture

**REFERENCES**
Brown, T., and Holmes, G. *Handbook of Epilepsy,* 2nd ed. Philadelphia: Lippincott Williams & Wilkins, 2000.
Kammerman, S., and Wasserman, L. "Seizure Disorders: Part 1. Classification and Diagnosis." *Western Journal of Medicine* 175(2): 99-103, August 2001.
Kammerman, S., and Wasserman, L. "Seizure Disorders Part 2. Treatment." *Western Journal of Medicine* 175(3):184-88, September 2001.
Sirven, J., and Malamut, B. *Clinical Neurology of the Older Adult.* Philadelphia: Lippincott Williams & Wilkins, 2002.

**ORGANIZATIONS**
Epilepsy Foundation of America: *www.efa.org*
National Institute of Neurological Disorders and Stroke: *www.ninds.nih.gov*

# Managing the patient with spinal cord injury

## Purpose
To rapidly treat and stabilize the patient with a compromised spinal cord injury

## Collaborative level
Interdependent

## Expected patient outcomes
▶ The patient will maintain a patent airway.
▶ The patient will maintain hemodynamic stability.
▶ The patient will preserve or improve neurologic function.
▶ The patient will optimize his functional outcome.
▶ The patient will help prevent complications.

## Definition of terms
▶ *Complete spinal cord injury:* Total loss of motor and sensory function below the level of the lesion, usually causing irreversible damage.
▶ *Incomplete spinal cord injury:* Preservation of some degree of motor or sensory loss below the level of the lesion, indicating some sparing of tract. Has better prognosis than complete spinal cord injury.
▶ *Quadriplegia:* Paralysis of all four extremities, caused by an injury above T1.
▶ *Paraplegia:* Paralysis of the lower extremities, caused by injury to the thoracic, lumbar, sacral, or coccygeal area of the spine.
▶ *Spinal shock:* Areflexia with flaccid paralysis, usually occurring immediately after the injury and lasting days to months; the return of reflex activity signals resolution of spinal shock.
▶ *Autonomic dysreflexia:* Vasomotor response to noxious stimuli, most commonly bowel or bladder dysfunction, occurring below the level of the injury; usually in patients with an injury above T6.

## Indications
Treatment
▶ Spinal cord dysfunction related to acute trauma
▶ Spinal cord dysfunction related to tumor or vascular compromise

Prevention
▶ Respiratory failure
▶ Bradycardia
▶ Hypotension
▶ DVT
▶ GI bleeding
▶ Skin breakdown
▶ Infection
▶ Depression

## Assessment guidance
*Acute emergency room*
▶ Airway, breathing, and circulation
▶ Motor and sensory examination to identify neurologic level of injury
▶ Vital signs indicating spinal shock: bradycardia and hypotension
▶ Associated injuries identified and treated
▶ Acute trauma history compared with evidence of compressive lesion or vascular compromise

*Continuing acute care*
▶ Ongoing motor and sensory examination
▶ Signs of dysautonomia: severe sudden onset of headache, hypertension, flushing

## Diagnostic studies
### Imaging tests
▶ Lumbar spine X-ray
▶ CT scan
▶ MRI

## Nursing interventions
▶ Maintain a patent airway; use a nasal airway if indicated.
▶ Monitor vital capacity and tidal volume.
▶ Assess the patient's use of accessory muscles and diaphragm for breathing.
▶ Perform chest percussion and assisted cough.
▶ Administer methylprednisolone therapy.
▶ Maintain endotracheal tube and ventilator.
▶ Perform oral care every 2 hours while the patient is intubated.
▶ Maintain adequate blood pressure; treat spinal shock if clinical signs of shock are present.
▶ Maintain immobilization device as indicated (hard collar, halo, cervical traction).
▶ Assess the patient for changes in neurologic level with any change in position early in injury.
▶ Prepare the patient for stabilization surgery as indicated.
▶ Perform passive range-of-motion exercises.
▶ Monitor intake and output carefully; hypervolemia occurs easily in spinal shock.
▶ Maintain the ICP monitoring system per facility policy.
▶ Institute DVT prophylaxis as appropriate.
▶ Begin bowel program.
▶ Maintain adequate nutrition; enteral feeding is preferable.
▶ Perform skin care to prevent loss of skin integrity.
▶ Prevent urinary tract infections.
▶ Prevent renal calculi by maintaining adequate fluid intake.
▶ Institute rehabilitation therapies as soon as hemodynamic stability is established.
▶ Assess the patient's and family's coping mechanisms; refer them to social services as needed.
▶ Offer emotional support.

## Patient teaching
▶ Explain all procedures and interventions.
▶ Explain all treatment options.
▶ Instruct the patient about quad-assisted cough.
▶ If the patient is discharged in a halo vest, teach pin site care and recognition of adequate traction.
▶ Explain signs and symptoms of autonomic dysreflexia, with actions to take.
▶ Explain how to maintain skin integrity.
▶ Teach the patient how to maintain bowel and bladder function.
▶ Teach the need for rehabilitation.
▶ Instruct the patient in range-of-motion exercises.
▶ Explain all studies being done.
▶ Provide the patient with information on support groups and community resources.

## Precautions
▶ Watch for signs and symptoms of infection, a common complication of increased ICP.
▶ Prevent seizures and hyperthermia, which will increase ICP and make the condition worse.

## Documentation
▶ Record vital signs and intake and output.
▶ Document motor and sensory assessment.
▶ Note vital capacity and tidal volume.
▶ Document traction weight, pin site condition, alignment, and halo-vest condition.
▶ Record nursing interventions, response to interventions, medications given, and doctor notification and intervention.

## Related procedures
▶ Arterial pressure monitoring
▶ Central venous line insertion and removal
▶ Central venous pressure monitoring
▶ Cervical collar application
▶ Endotracheal intubation
▶ Endotracheal tube care
▶ Feeding tube insertion and removal
▶ Halo-vest traction
▶ I.V. bolus injection
▶ Indwelling catheter care and removal
▶ Manual ventilation
▶ Mechanical ventilation
▶ Nasopharyngeal airway insertion and care
▶ Oropharyngeal airway insertion and care
▶ Passive range-of-motion exercises

▶ Physical assessment
▶ Postoperative care
▶ Preoperative care
▶ Pressure ulcer care
▶ Sequential compression therapy
▶ Skull tongs care

## REFERENCES

Alspach, J.G., ed. American Association of Critical Care Nurses. Core Curriculum for Critical Care Nursing, 5th ed. Philadelphia: W.B. Saunders Company, 1998.

*Diseases,* 2nd ed. *Professional Guide Series.* Springhouse, Pa.: Lippincott Williams & Wilkins, 2002.

## ORGANIZATIONS

National Spinal Cord Injury Association: *www.spinalcord.org*
American Association of Neurological Surgeons: *www.neurosurgery.org*
National Institute of Neurological Diseases and Stroke: *www.ninds.nih.gov*
Paralyzed Veterans of America: *www.pva.org*

# Procedures

# Cerebral blood flow monitoring

Traditionally, caregivers have estimated cerebral blood flow (CBF) in neurologically compromised patients by calculating cerebral perfusion pressure. However, modern technology permits continuous regional blood flow monitoring at the bedside.

A sensor placed on the cerebral cortex calculates CBF in the capillary bed by thermal diffusion. Thermistors within the sensor detect the temperature differential between two metallic plates—one heated, one neutral. This differential is inversely proportional to CBF: As the differential decreases, CBF increases, and vice versa. This monitoring technique reveals important information about the effects of interventions on CBF. It also yields continuous real-time values for CBF, which are essential in conditions in which compromised blood flow may put the patient at risk for complications, such as ischemia and infarction.

CBF monitoring is indicated whenever CBF alterations are anticipated. It's used most commonly in patients with subarachnoid hemorrhage (in which a vasospasm may restrict blood flow), trauma associated with high ICP, or vascular tumors.

## Equipment

CBF monitoring requires a special sensor that attaches to a computer data system or to a small analog monitor that operates on a battery for patient transport.

*For care of site*
Sterile 4″ × 4″ gauze pads ● clean gloves ● sterile gloves ● povidone-iodine solution or ointment ● adhesive tape

*For removing sensor*
Sterile suture removal tray ● 1″ adhesive tape ● sterile 4″ × 4″ gauze pads ● clean gloves ● sterile gloves ● suture material

## Preparation of equipment

Make sure that the patient or a family member is fully informed about the procedures involved in CBF monitoring and obtain a consent form. If the patient will need CBF monitoring after surgery, advise him that a sensor will be in place for about 3 days. Tell the patient that the insertion site will be covered with a dry, sterile dressing. Mention that the sensor may be removed at the bedside.

### Setting up the sensor monitor

Depending on the type of system you're using, you may need to verify that a battery has been inserted in the monitor to allow CBF monitoring during patient transport to the intensive care unit.

# Inserting a CBF sensor

Typically, the surgeon inserts a cerebral blood flow (CBF) sensor during a craniotomy. He tunnels the sensor toward the craniotomy site and then carefully inserts the metallic plates of the thermistor to make sure that they continuously contact the surface of the cerebral cortex. After closing the dura and replacing the bone flap, he closes the scalp.

**INSERTION SITE**

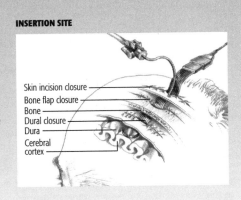

Skin incision closure
Bone flap closure
Bone
Dural closure
Dura
Cerebral cortex

**SENSOR**

The sensor measures CBF by means of thermistors housed inside it. The thermistors consist of two metallic plates—one heated and one neutral. The sensor detects the temperature difference between the two plates. This difference is inversely proportional to CBF. As CBF increases, the temperature difference decreases, and vice versa.

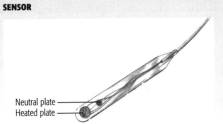

Neutral plate
Heated plate

First, assemble the following equipment at the bedside: a monitor and a sensor cable with an attached sensor. Attach the distal end of the sensor cable (from the patient's head) to the SENSOR CONNECT port on the monitor. When the sensor cable is securely in place, press the ON key to activate the monitor.

Next, calibrate the system by pressing the CAL key. You should see the red light appear on the CAL button. Ideally, you'll begin by calibrating the sensor to 00.0 by pressing the directional arrows. Readouts of plus or minus 0.1 are also acceptable.

## Implementation

▶ The surgeon typically inserts the sensor in the operating room during or following a craniotomy. (Occasionally, he may insert it through a burr hole.) He implants the sensor far from major blood vessels and verifies that the metallic plates have good contact with the brain surface. (See *Inserting a CBF sensor.*)

▶ Press the RUN key to display the CBF reading. Observe the monitor's digital display and document the baseline value.

▶ Record the CBF hourly. Be sure to watch for trends and correlate values with the patient's clinical status. Be aware that stimulation or activity may cause a 10% increase or decrease in CBF. If you detect a 20% increase or decrease, suspect poor contact between the sensor and the cerebral cortex.

◆ **ALERT!** In the patient with a head injury, cerebral perfusion pressure shouldn't fall below 70 mm Hg. If the patient's cerebral perfusion pressure falls below 70 mm Hg, the blood flow to his brain may be inadequate.

### Caring for the insertion site

▶ Wash your hands. Put on clean gloves, and remove the dressing from the sensor insertion site.

▶ Observe the site for CSF leakage, a potential complication. Then remove and discard your gloves.

▶ Next, put on sterile gloves. Using aseptic technique, clean the insertion site with a gauze pad soaked in povidone-iodine solution. Clean the site, starting at the center and working outward in a circular pattern.

▶ Using a new gauze pad soaked with povidone-iodine solution, clean the exposed part of the sensor from the insertion site to the end of the sensor. Apply povidone-iodine ointment to the insertion site if your facility's policy permits.

▶ Next, place sterile 4″ × 4″ gauze pads over the insertion site to completely cover it. Tape all edges securely to create an occlusive dressing.

### Removing the sensor

▶ In most cases, the CBF sensor remains in place for about 3 days when used for postoperative monitoring.

▶ Explain the procedure to the patient; then wash your hands. Put on clean gloves, remove the dressing, and dispose of the gloves and dressing properly.

▶ Open the suture removal tray and the package of suture material. The surgeon removes the anchoring sutures and then gently removes the sensor from the insertion site.

▶ After the surgeon closes the wound with stitches, put on sterile gloves, apply a folded gauze pad to the site, and tape it in place. Observe the condition of the site, including any leakage.

### Special considerations

▶ CBF fluctuates with the brain's metabolic demands, ranging from 60 to 90 ml/100 g/minute normally. However, the patient's neurologic condition dictates the acceptable range. For instance, in a patient in a coma, CBF may be half the normal value; in a patient in a barbiturate-induced coma with burst suppression on the EEG, CBF may be as low as 10 ml/100 g/minute. Vasospasm secondary to subarachnoid hemorrhage may result in CBF below 40 ml/100 g/minute. In an awake patient, CBF above 90 ml/100 g/minute may indicate hyperemia.

▶ If you suspect poor contact between the sensor and the cerebral cortex, turn the patient toward the side of the sensor or gently wiggle the catheter back and forth (using a sterile-gloved hand). To determine whether these maneuvers have improved contact

between the sensor and the cortex, observe the CBF value on the monitor as you perform them.

▶ If your patient has low CBF but no neurologic signs that indicate ischemia, suspect a fluid layer (a small hematoma) between the sensor and the cortex.

▶ As with ICP monitoring, CBF monitoring may lead to infection. Administer prophylactic antibiotics as ordered and maintain a sterile dressing around the insertion site. CSF leakage, another potential complication, may occur at the sensor insertion site. To prevent leakage, the surgeon usually places an additional suture at the site.

▶ To reduce the risk of infection, change the dressing at the insertion site daily.

### Documentation

▶ Document cleaning of the site, appearance of the site, and dressing changes.

▶ After sensor removal, document any leakage from the site.

### REFERENCES

Barker, E. *Neuroscience Nursing.* St. Louis: Mosby–Year Book, Inc., 1994.

Gupta, A.K. "Monitoring the Injured Brain in the Intensive Care Unit," *Journal of Postgraduate Medicine* 48(3):218-25, July-September 2002.

Hickey, J.V. *The Clinical Practice of Neurological and Neurosurgical Nursing,* 5th ed. Philadelphia: Lippincott Williams & Wilkins, 2003.

# Cerebrospinal fluid drainage

Cerebrospinal fluid drainage aims to reduce CSF pressure to the desired level and then to maintain it at that level. Fluid can be withdrawn from the lateral ventricle (ventriculostomy) or the lumbar subarachnoid space, depending on the indication and the desired outcome. Ventricular drainage is used to reduce increased ICP, whereas lumbar drainage is used to aid healing of the dura mater. External CSF drainage is used most commonly to manage increased ICP and to facilitate spinal or cerebral dural healing after traumatic injury or surgery. In either case, CSF is drained by a catheter or a ventriculostomy tube in a sterile, closed drainage collection system.

Other therapeutic uses include ICP monitoring via the ventriculostomy; direct instillation of medications, contrast media, or air for diagnostic radiology; and aspiration of CSF for laboratory analysis.

To place the ventricular drain, the doctor inserts a ventricular catheter through a burr hole in the patient's skull. Usually, this is done in the operating room, with the patient receiving a general anesthetic but it may also be performed at the bedside in the intensive care unit or the emergency department. To place the lumbar subarachnoid drain, the doctor may administer a local spinal anesthetic at bedside or in the operating room. (See *CSF drainage using a ventricular drain.*)

## Equipment

Overbed table ● sterile gloves ● sterile cotton-tipped applicators ● povidone-iodine solution ● alcohol pads ● sterile fenestrated drape ● 3-ml syringe for local anesthetic ● 25G ¾″ needle for injecting anesthetic ● local anesthetic (usually 1% lidocaine) ● 18G or 20G sterile spinal needle or Tuohy needle ● #5 French whistle-tip catheter or ventriculostomy tube ● external drainage set (includes drainage tubing and sterile collection bag) ● suture material ● 4″ × 4″ dressings ● paper tape ● lamp or another light source ● I.V. pole ● ventriculostomy tray ● twist drill ● optional: pain medication (such as an analgesic), and an anti-infective agent (such as an antibiotic)

### Preparation of equipment

Open all equipment using sterile technique. Check all packaging for breaks in seals and for expiration dates. After the doctor places the catheter, connect it to the external drainage system tubing. Secure connection points with tape or a connector. Place the collection system, including drip chamber and collection bag, on an I.V. pole.

## Implementation

▶ Explain the procedure to the patient and family. Make sure the patient or a responsible family member signs a consent form and document according to policy.
▶ Wash your hands thoroughly.
▶ Perform a baseline neurologic assessment, including vital signs, to help detect alterations or signs of deterioration.

---

# CSF drainage using a ventricular drain

Cerebrospinal fluid (CSF) drainage aims to control intracranial pressure (ICP) during treatment for traumatic injury or other conditions that cause an increase in ICP. A commonly used procedures is described below.

### Ventricular drain

For a ventricular drain, the doctor makes a burr hole in the patient's skull and inserts the catheter into the ventricle. The distal end of the catheter is connected to a closed drainage system.

**CLOSED DRAINAGE SYSTEM**

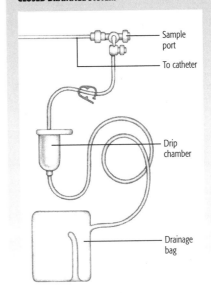

Sample port

To catheter

Drip chamber

Drainage bag

---

### Inserting a ventricular drain
▶ Place the patient in the supine position.
▶ Place the equipment tray on the overbed table and unwrap the tray.
▶ Adjust the height of the bed so that the doctor can perform the procedure comfortably.
▶ Illuminate the area of the catheter insertion site.
▶ Shave the patient's hair at the area of the insertion site.

▶ The doctor will clean the insertion site and administer a local anesthetic. He'll put on sterile gloves and drape the insertion site.

▶ To insert the drain, the doctor will request a ventriculostomy tray with a twist drill. After completing the ventriculostomy, he'll connect the drainage system and suture the catheter in place. He'll then cover the insertion site with a sterile dressing.

### Inserting a lumbar subarachnoid drain

▶ Position the patient in a side-lying position with his chin tucked to his chest and knees drawn up to his abdomen, as for a lumbar puncture. Urge him to remain as still as possible during the procedure. He may also be positioned sitting up at the bedsie leaning forward over a bedside table.

▶ To insert the drain, the doctor attaches a Tuohy needle (or spinal needle) to the whistle-tip catheter. After the doctor removes the needle, he connects the drainage system, sutures or tapes the catheter securely in place, and covers it with a sterile dressing.

### Monitoring CSF drainage

▶ Maintain a continuous hourly output of CSF by raising or lowering the drainage system drip chamber. To maintain CSF outflow, the drip chamber should be slightly lower than or at the level of the lumbar drain insertion site. Sometimes you may need to carefully raise or lower the drip chamber to increase or decrease CSF flow. For ventricular drains, ensure that the flow chamber of the ICP monitoring setup remains positioned as ordered.

▶ With ventricular drains, also monitor the drainage and correlate the drainge amounts to changes in ICP readings.

▶ To drain CSF as ordered, put on gloves, and then turn the main stopcock on to drainage. This allows CSF to collect in the graduated flow chamber. Document the time and the amount of CSF obtained. Then turn the stopcock off to drainage. To drain the CSF from this chamber into the drainage bag, release the clamp below the flow chamber. Never empty the drainage bag. Instead, replace it when full using sterile technique.

▶ Check the dressing frequently for drainage, which could indicate CSF leakage.

▶ Check the tubing for patency by watching the CSF drops in the drip chamber or by lowering the height of the drip chamber and watching for flow of CSF.

▶ Observe the CSF for color, clarity, amount, blood, and sediment. CSF specimens for laboratory analysis should be obtained from the collection port attached to the tubing, not from the collection bag.

▶ Change the collection bag when it's full or every 24 hours according to your facility's policy.

## Special considerations

▶ Maintaining a continual hourly output of CSF is essential to prevent overdrainage or underdrainage. Underdrainage or lack of CSF may reflect kinked tubing, catheter displacement, or a drip chamber placed higher than the catheter insertion site. Overdrainage can occur if the drip chamber is placed too far below the catheter insertion site.

▶ For patients with a ventriculostomy, raising or lowering the head of the bed can affect the CSF flow rate. When changing the patient's position, reposition the drip chamber.

▶ Patients with lumbar drains are usually kept in a flat position especially if the drain is placed for spinal dural tear.

▶ Patients may experience a chronic headache during continuous CSF drainage. Reassure the patient that this isn't unusual; administer analgesics as appropriate but be aware that this may also indicate overdrainage (headache, tachycardia, diaphoresis and nausea).

## Complications

Symptoms of excessive CSF drainage include headache, tachycardia, diaphoresis, and nausea. Acute overdrainage may result in collapsed ventricles (more common with ventricular drains), tonsillar herniation, and medullary compression (with lumbar drains if ICP is increased).

◆ **ALERT!** If drainage accumulates too rapidly, clamp the system and notify the doctor immediately. Then perform a complete neurologic assessment on the patient. This constitutes a potential neurosurgical emergency.

Cessation of drainage may indicate clot formation. If you can't quickly identify the cause of the obstruction, notify the doctor.

If drainage is blocked, the patient may develop signs of increased ICP, more commonly with a verntricular drain.

Infection may cause meningitis. To prevent this, administer antibiotics as ordered and maintain a sterile closed system with dry sterile dressings over the site.

## Documentation

▶ Record the time and date of the insertion procedure and the patient's response.
▶ Record routine vital signs and neurologic assessment findings at least every 4 hours.
▶ Document the color, clarity, and amount of CSF at least every 8 hours.
▶ Record hourly and 24-hour CSF output and describe the condition of the dressing.

### REFERENCES

Hickey, J.V. *The Clinical Practice of Neurological and Neurosurgical Nursing,* 5th ed. Philadelphia: Lippincott Williams & Wilkins, 2002.

Montgomery, K.L. "SOP: Care of the Patient with Lumbar Subarachnoid Drainage System." NIH Clinical Center Nursing Dept. Revised March 1998. *www.cc.nih.gov/ nursing/lumsubdr.htm*

# Halo-vest traction

Halo-vest traction immobilizes the head and neck after traumatic injury to the cervical vertebrae — the most common of all spinal injuries. This procedure, which can prevent further injury to the spinal cord, is performed by an orthopedic surgeon or a neurosurgeon, with nursing assistance, in the emergency department, a specially equipped room, or in the operating room after surgical reduction of vertebral injuries. The halo-vest traction device consists of a metal ring that fits over the patient's head and metal bars that connect the ring to a plastic vest that distributes the weight of the entire apparatus around the chest. (See *Comparing halo-vest traction devices,* page 390.)

When in place, halo-vest traction allows the patient greater mobility than traction with skull tongs. It also carries less risk of infection because it doesn't require skin incisions and drill holes to position skull pins.

## Equipment

Halo-vest traction unit ● halo ring ● cervical collar or sandbags (if needed) ● plastic vest, board or padded headrest ● tape measure ● halo ring conversion chart ● scissors and razor ● 4″ × 4″ gauze pads ● povidone-iodine solution ● sterile gloves ● Allen wrench ● four positioning pins ● multiple-dose vial of 1% lidocaine (with or without epinephrine) ● alcohol pads ● 3-ml syringe ● 25G needles ● five sterile skull pins (one more than needed) ● torque screwdriver ● sheepskin liners ● cotton-tipped applicators ● ordered cleaning solution ● medicated powder or cornstarch ● sterile water or normal saline solution ● optional: hair dryer and pain medication (such as an analgesic)

Most facilities supply packaged halo-vest traction units that include software (such as jacket and sheepskin liners), hardware (such as halo, head pins, upright bars, and screws), and tools (such as torque screwdriver, two conventional wrenches, Allen wrench, and screws and bolts). These units don't include sterile gloves, povidone-iodine solution, sterile drapes, cervical collars, or equipment for local anesthetic injection.

### Preparation of equipment

Obtain a halo-vest traction unit with halo rings and plastic vests in several sizes. Vest sizes are based on chest circumference measured at the xyphoid process. However, coat size for a male or bra size for a female may be substituted. Check the expiration date of the prepackaged tray and check the outside covering for damage to ensure the sterility of the contents. Then assemble the equipment at the patient's bedside.

## Implementation

▶ Check the support that was applied to the patient's neck on the way to the hospital. If necessary, apply the cervical collar immediately or immobilize the head and neck with sandbags. Keep the cervical collar or sandbags in place until the halo is applied. This support will then be carefully removed to facilitate application of the vest. Because the patient is likely to be frightened, try to reassure him.
▶ Remove the headboard and any furniture at the head of the bed to provide ample

# Comparing halo-vest traction devices

| Type | Description | Advantages |
|------|-------------|------------|
| Low profile (standard)<br>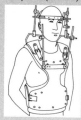 | ▶ Traction and compression are produced by threaded support rods on either side of the halo ring.<br>▶ Flexion and extension are obtained by moving the swivel arm to an anterior or posterior position, depending on the location of the skull pins. | ▶ Immobilizes cervical spine fractures while allowing the patient mobility<br>▶ Facilitates surgery of the cervical spine and permits flexion and extension<br>▶ Allows airway intubation without losing skeletal traction<br>▶ Facilitates necessary alignment by an adjustment at the junction of the threaded support rods and horizontal frame |
| Mark II<br>(type of low profile)<br>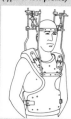 | ▶ Traction and compression are produced by threaded support rods on either side of the halo ring.<br>▶ Flexion and extension are obtained by swivel clamps, which allow the bars to intersect and hold at any angle. | ▶ Enables the doctor to assemble the metal framework more quickly<br>▶ Allows unobstructed access for anteroposterior and lateral X-rays of the cervical spine<br>▶ Allows the patient to wear his usual clothing because uprights are shaped closer to the body |
| Mark III<br>(update of Mark II)<br>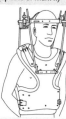 | ▶ Traction and compression are produced by threaded support rods on either side of the halo ring.<br>▶ Flexion and extension are accommodated by a serrated split articulation coupling attached to the halo ring, which can be adjusted in 4-degree increments. | ▶ Simplifies application while promoting patient comfort<br>▶ Eliminates shoulder pressure and discomfort by using a flexible padded strap instead of the vest's solid plastic shoulder<br>▶ Accommodates the tall patient with modified hardware and shorter uprights and allows unobstructed access for medial and lateral X-rays |
| Trippi-Wells tongs<br>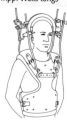 | ▶ Traction is produced by four pins that compress the skull.<br>▶ Flexion and extension are obtained by adjusting the midline vertical plate. | ▶ Applies tensile force to the neck or spine while allowing the patient mobility<br>▶ Makes it possible to change from mobile to stationary traction without interrupting traction<br>▶ Adjusts to three planes for mobile and stationary traction<br>▶ Allows unobstructed access for medial and lateral X-rays |

working space. Then carefully place the patient's head on a board or on a padded headrest that extends beyond the edge of the bed.

♦ **ALERT!** Never put the patient's head on a pillow before applying the halo, to avoid further injury to the spinal cord.

▶ Elevate the bed to a working level that gives the doctor easy access to the front and back of the halo unit.

▶ Stand at the head of the bed and see if the patient's chin lines up with his midsternum, indicating proper alignment. If ordered, support the patient's head in your hands and gently rotate the neck into alignment without flexing or extending it.

### Assisting with halo application

▶ Ask another nurse to help you with the procedure.

▶ Explain the procedure to the patient, wash your hands, and provide privacy.

▶ Have the assisting nurse hold the patient's head and neck stable while the doctor removes the cervical collar or sandbags. Maintain this support until the halo is secure while you assist with pin insertion.

▶ The doctor measures the patient's head with a tape measure and refers to the halo ring conversion chart to determine the correct ring size. (The ring should clear the head by ⅝" [1.6 cm] and fit ½" [1.3 cm] above the bridge of the nose.)

▶ The doctor selects four pin sites: ½" above the lateral one-third of each eyebrow and ½" above the top of each ear in the occipital area. He also takes into account the degree and type of correction needed to provide proper cervical alignment.

▶ Trim and shave the hair at the pin sites with scissors or a razor to facilitate subsequent care and help prevent infection. Put on gloves. Then use 4" × 4" gauze pads soaked in povidone-iodine solution to clean the sites.

▶ Open the halo-vest unit using sterile technique to avoid contamination. The doctor puts on the sterile gloves and removes the halo and the Allen wrench. He then places the halo over the patient's head and inserts the four positioning pins to hold the halo in place temporarily.

▶ Help the doctor prepare the anesthetic. First, clean the injection port of the multiple-dose vial of lidocaine with the alcohol pad. Then invert the vial so the doctor can insert a 25G needle attached to the 3-ml syringe and withdraw the anesthetic.

▶ The doctor injects the anesthetic at the four pin sites. He may change needles on the syringe after each injection.

▶ The doctor removes four of the five skull pins from the sterile setup and firmly screws in each pin at a 90-degree angle to the skull. When the pins are in place, he removes the positioning pins. He then tightens the skull pins with the torque screwdriver.

### Applying the vest

▶ After the doctor measures the patient's chest and abdomen, he selects a vest of appropriate size.

▶ Place the sheepskin liners inside the front and back of the vest to make it more comfortable and help prevent pressure ulcers.

▶ Help the doctor carefully raise the patient while the other nurse supports the head and neck. Slide the back of the vest under the patient and gently lay him down. The doctor then fastens the front of the vest on the patient's chest using Velcro straps.

▶ The doctor attaches the metal bars to the halo and vest and tightens each bolt in turn to avoid tightening any single bolt completely, causing maladjusted tension. When halo-vest traction is in place, X-rays should be taken immediately to check the depth of the skull pins and verify proper alignment.

### Caring for the patient

▶ Take routine and neurologic vital signs at least every 2 hours for 24 hours (preferably every hour for 48 hours) and then every 4 hours until stable.

♦ **ALERT!** Notify the doctor immediately if you observe any decrease in motor function or any decreased sensation; these changes in baseline findings could indicate spinal cord trauma.

▶ Put on gloves. Gently clean the pin sites every 4 hours with cotton-tipped applicators dipped in cleaning solution. Rinse the sites with sterile water or normal saline solution to remove any excess cleaning solution. Then clean the pin sites with povidone-iodine solution or other ordered solution. Meticulous pin-site care prevents infection and removes debris that might block drainage and lead to abscess formation. Watch for signs of infection—a loose pin, swelling or redness, purulent drainage, pain at the site—and notify the doctor if these signs develop.

▶ The doctor retightens the skull pins with the torque screwdriver 24 and 48 hours after the halo is applied. If the patient complains of a headache after the pins are tightened, obtain an order for an analgesic. If pain occurs with jaw movement, notify the doctor because this may indicate that pins have slipped onto the thin temporal plate.

▶ Examine the halo-vest unit every shift to make sure that everything is secure and that the patient's head is centered within the halo. If the vest fits correctly, you should be able to insert one or two fingers under the jacket at the shoulder and chest when the patient is lying in a supine position.

▶ Wash the patient's chest and back daily. First, place the patient on his back. Loosen the bottom Velcro straps so you can get to the chest and back. Then, reaching under the vest, wash and dry the skin. Check for tender, reddened areas or pressure spots that may develop into ulcers. If necessary, use a hair dryer to dry damp sheepskin because moisture predisposes the skin to pressure ulcer formation. Lightly dust the skin with medicated powder or cornstarch to prevent itching. If itching persists, check to see if the patient is allergic to sheepskin and if any drug he's taking might cause a skin rash. If your facility's policy allows, change the vest lining as necessary.

▶ Turn the patient on his side (less than 45 degrees) to wash his back. Then close the vest.

▶ Be careful not to put any stress on the apparatus, which could knock it out of alignment and lead to subluxation of the cervical spine.

## Special considerations

✦ **ALERT!** Keep two conventional wrenches available at all times. In case of cardiac arrest, use them to remove the distal anterior bolts. Pull the two upright bars outward. Unfasten the Velcro straps and remove the front of the vest. Use the sturdy back of the vest as a board for cardiopulmonary resuscitation (CPR). Many vests now have a hinged front to raise the vest plate for CPR. Be sure ypou know the type of vest the pa-

tient has. To prevent subluxating the cervical injury, start CPR with the jaw thrust maneuver, which avoids hyperextension of the neck. Pull the patient's mandible forward while maintaining proper head and neck alignment. This pulls the tongue forward to open the airway.

▶ Never lift the patient up by the vertical bars. This could strain or tear the skin at the pin sites or misalign the traction.

▶ To prevent falls, walk with the ambulatory patient. Remember, he'll have trouble seeing objects at or near his feet, and the weight of the halo-vest unit (about 10 lb [4.5 kg]) may throw him off balance. If the patient is in a wheelchair, lower the leg rests to prevent the chair from tipping backward.

▶ Because the vest limits chest expansion, routinely assess pulmonary function, especially in a patient with pulmonary disease.

## Home care

Teach the patient to turn slowly—in small increments—to avoid losing his balance. Remind him to avoid bending forward because the extra weight of the halo apparatus could cause him to fall. Teach him to bend at the knees rather than the waist.

Have a physical therapist teach the patient how to use assistive devices to extend his reach and to help him put on socks and shoes. Suggest that he wear shirts that button in front and that are larger than usual to accommodate the halo-vest.

Most important, teach the patient about pin-site care, shampooing, and hair care.

## Complications

Manipulating the patient's neck during application of halo-vest traction may cause subluxation of the spinal cord, or it could push a bone fragment into the spinal cord, possibly compressing the cord and causing paralysis below the break.

Inaccurate positioning of the skull pins can lead to a puncture of the skull and dura mater, causing a loss of CSF and a serious central nervous system infection. Nonsterile technique during application of the halo or inadequate pin-site care can also lead to infection at the pin sites. Pressure ulcers can develop if the vest fits poorly or chafes the skin.

## Documentation

▶ Record the date and time that the halo-vest traction was applied.

▶ Note the length of the procedure and the patient's response.

▶ After application, record routine and neurologic vital signs.

▶ Document pin-site care and note any signs of infection.

### REFERENCES

Chen, H.J., et al. "One-stage Posterior Decompression and Fusion Using a Luque Rod for Occipito-Cervical Instability and Neural Compression," *Spinal Cord* 39(2):101-108, February 2001.

Papagelopoulos, P.J., et al. "Halo Pin Intracranial Penetration and Epidural Abscess in a Patient with a Previous Cranioplasty: Case Report and Review of the Literature," *Spine* 26(19):E463-67, October 2001.

# Intracranial pressure monitoring

Intracranial pressure monitoring measures pressure exerted by the brain, blood, and CSF against the inside of the skull. Indications for monitoring ICP include head trauma with bleeding or edema, overproduction or insufficient absorption of CSF, cerebral hemorrhage, and space-occupying brain lesions. ICP monitoring can detect elevated ICP early, before clinical danger signs develop. Prompt intervention can then help avert or diminish neurologic damage caused by cerebral hypoxia and shifts of brain mass.

The four basic ICP monitoring systems are intraventricular catheter, subarachnoid bolt, epidural sensor, and intraparenchymal pressure monitoring. (See *Understanding ICP monitoring systems*, pages 394 and 395.)

Regardless of which system is used, the procedure is typically performed by a neurosurgeon in the operating room, emergency department, or intensive care unit.

Insertion of an ICP monitoring device requires sterile technique to reduce the risk of central nervous system (CNS) infection. Setting up equipment for the monitoring systems also requires strict asepsis.

## Equipment

Monitoring unit and transducers ● 16 to 20 sterile 4″ × 4″ gauze pads ● linen-saver pads ● shave preparation tray or hair scissors ● sterile drapes ● povidone-iodine solution ● sterile gown ● surgical mask ● sterile gloves ● head dressing supplies (including two rolls of 4″ elastic gauze dressing, one roll of 4″ roller gauze, and adhesive tape) ● optional: suction apparatus, I.V. pole, and yardstick

### Preparation of equipment

Monitoring units and setup protocols are varied and complex and differ among health care facilities. Check your facility's guidelines for your particular unit.

Various types of preassembled ICP monitoring units are also available, each with its own setup protocols. These units are designed to reduce the risk of infection by eliminating the need for multiple stopcocks, manometers, and transducer dome assemblies. Some facilities use units that have miniaturized transducers rather than transducer domes.

## Implementation

▶ Explain the procedure to the patient or his family. Make sure the patient or a responsible family member has signed a consent form.

▶ Determine whether the patient is allergic to iodine preparations.

▶ Provide privacy if the procedure is being done in an open emergency department or intensive care unit. Wash your hands.

▶ Obtain baseline routine and neurologic vital signs to aid in prompt detection of decompensation during the procedure.

▶ Place the patient in the supine position and elevate the head of the bed 30 degrees (or as ordered). Document the number of bed crank rotations, or hang a yardstick on an I.V. pole and mark the exact elevation.

▶ Place linen-saver pads under the patient's head. Shave or clip his hair at the insertion site, as indicated by the doctor, to decrease the risk of infection. Carefully fold and remove the linen-saver pads to avoid spilling loose hair onto the bed. Drape the patient with sterile drapes. Then scrub the insertion site for 2 minutes with povidone-iodine solution.

▶ The doctor puts on the sterile gown, mask, and sterile gloves. He then opens the interior wrap of the sterile supply tray and

# Understanding ICP monitoring systems

Intracranial pressure (ICP) can be monitored using one of four systems.

### Intraventricular catheter monitoring

In intraventricular catheter monitoring, which monitors ICP directly, the doctor inserts a small polyethylene or silicone rubber catheter into the lateral ventricle through a burr hole.

Although this method measures ICP most accurately, it carries the greatest risk of infection. This is the only type of ICP monitoring that allows evaluation of brain compliance and drainage of significant amounts of cerebrospinal fluid (CSF).

Contraindications usually include stenotic cerebral ventricles, cerebral aneurysms in the path of catheter placement, and suspected vascular lesions.

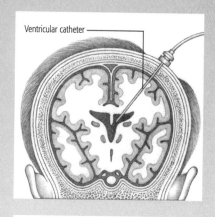

Ventricular catheter

### Subarachnoid bolt monitoring

Subarachnoid bolt monitoring involves insertion of a special bolt into the subarachnoid space through a twist-drill burr hole that's positioned in the front of the skull behind the hairline.

Placing the bolt is easier than placing an intraventricular catheter, especially if a computed tomography scan reveals that the cerebrum has shifted or the ventricles have collapsed. This type of ICP monitoring also carries less risk of infection and parenchymal damage because the bolt doesn't penetrate the cerebrum.

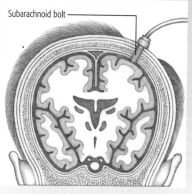

Subarachnoid bolt

### Epidural or subdural sensor monitoring

ICP can also be monitored from the epidural or subdural space. For epidural monitoring, a fiber-optic sensor is inserted into the epidural space through a burr hole. This system's main drawback is its questionable accuracy because ICP isn't being measured directly from a CSF-filled space.

For subdural monitoring, a fiber-optic transducer-tipped catheter is tunneled through a burr hole, and its tip is placed on brain tissue under the dura mater. The main drawback to this method is its inability to drain CSF.

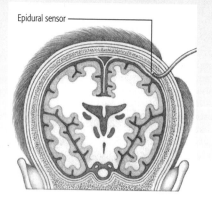

Epidural sensor

## Understanding ICP monitoring systems *(continued)*

### Intraparenchymal monitoring

In intraparenchymal monitoring, the doctor inserts a catheter through a small subarachnoid bolt and, after puncturing the dura, advances the catheter a few centimeters into the brain's white matter. There is no need to balance or calibrate the equipment after insertion.

Although this method doesn't provide direct access to CSF, measurements are accurate because brain tissue pressures correlate well with ventricular pressures. Intraparenchymal monitoring may be used to obtain ICP measurements in patients with compressed or dislocated ventricles.

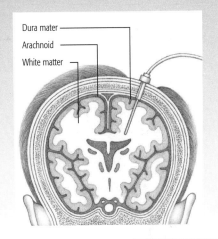

Dura mater
Arachnoid
White matter

proceeds with insertion of the catheter or bolt.

▶ To facilitate placement of the device, hold the patient's head in your hands or attach a long strip of 4″ roller gauze to one side rail, and bring it across the patient's forehead to the opposite rail. Reassure the conscious patient to help ease his anxiety. Talk to him frequently to assess his level of consciousness (LOC) and detect signs of deterioration. Watch for cardiac arrhythmias and abnormal respiratory patterns.

▶ After insertion, put on sterile gloves and apply povidone-iodine solution and a sterile dressing to the site. If not done by the doctor, connect the catheter to the appropriate monitoring device, depending on the system used. (See *Setting up a ventriculostomy ICP monitoring system,* page 396.)

▶ If the doctor has set up a ventriculostomy drainage system, attach the drip chamber to the headboard or bedside I.V. pole as ordered.

■◆ **ALERT!** Positioning the drip chamber too high may raise ICP; positioning it too low may cause excessive CSF drainage.

▶ Inspect the insertion site at least every 24 hours (or according to facility policy) for redness, swelling, and drainage. Clean the site, reapply povidone-iodine solution, and apply a  dry sterile dressing.

▶ Assess the patient's clinical status and take routine and neurologic vital signs every hourly or as ordered. Make sure you've obtained orders for pressure parameters from the doctor.

▶ Calculate cerebral perfusion pressure (CPP) hourly; use the equation:
CPP = MAP − ICP (MAP refers to mean arterial pressure).

▶ Observe digital ICP readings and waves. Remember, the trend of readings is more significant than any single reading. (See *Interpreting ICP waveforms,* pages 397 and 398.) If you observe continually elevated ICP readings, note how long they're sustained. If they last several minutes, notify the doctor immediately. Finally, record and describe any CSF drainage.

### Special considerations

■◆ **ALERT!** In infants, ICP monitoring can be performed without penetrating the scalp. In this external method, a photoelectric transducer with a pressure-sensitive membrane is taped to the anterior fontanel. The transducer responds to pressure at the site and transmits readings to a bedside monitor and recording system. The external method is restricted to infants because pressure readings can be obtained only at fontanels, the incompletely ossified areas of the skull.

# Setting up a ventriculostomy ICP monitoring system

To set up a ventriculostomy intracranial pressure (ICP) monitoring system, follow these steps, using strict aseptic technique:

▶ Begin by opening a sterile towel. On the sterile field, place a 20-ml luer-lock syringe, an 18G needle, a 250-ml bag filled with normal saline solution (with outer wrapper removed), and a disposable transducer.
▶ Put on sterile gloves and gown and fill the 20-ml syringe with normal saline solution from the I.V. bag.
▶ Remove the injection cap from the patient line and attach the syringe. Turn the system stopcock off to the short end of the patient line and flush through to the drip chamber (as shown below). Allow a few drops to flow through the flow chamber (the manometer), the tubing, and the one-way valve into the drainage bag. (Fill the tubing and the manometer slowly to minimize air bubbles. If air bubbles surface, make sure to force them from the system.)

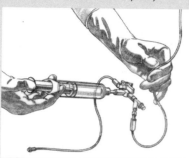

▶ Attach the manometer to the I.V. pole at the head of the bed.
▶ Slide the drip chamber onto the manometer and align the chamber to the zero point (as shown below).

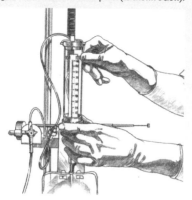

▶ Next, connect the transducer to the monitor.
▶ Put on a new pair of sterile gloves.
▶ Keeping one hand sterile, turn the patient stopcock off to the patient.
▶ Align the zero point with the center line of the patient's head, level with the middle of the ear (as shown below).

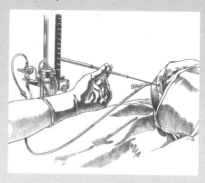

▶ Lower the flow chamber to zero and turn the stopcock off to the dead-end cap. With a clean hand, balance the system according to monitor guidelines.
▶ Turn the system stopcock off to drainage and raise the flow chamber to the ordered height (as shown below).

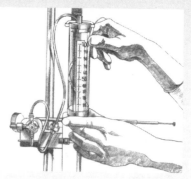

▶ Return the stopcock to the ordered position and observe the monitor for the return of ICP patterns.

# Interpreting ICP waveforms

Three waveforms—A, B, and C—are used to monitor intracranial pressure (ICP). A waves are an ominous sign of intracranial decompensation and poor compliance. B waves correlate with changes in respiration, and C waves correlate with changes in arterial pressure.

### Normal waveform

A normal ICP waveform typically shows a steep upward systolic slope followed by a downward diastolic slope with a dicrotic notch. In most cases, this waveform occurs continuously and indicates an ICP between 0 and 15 mm Hg—normal pressure.

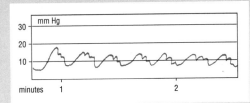

### A waves

The most clinically significant ICP waveforms are A waves, which may reach elevations of 50 to 100 mm Hg, persist for 5 to 20 minutes, then drop sharply, signaling exhaustion of the brain's compliance mechanisms. A waves may come and go, spiking from temporary rises in thoracic pressure or from a condition that increas-

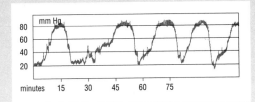

es ICP beyond the brain's compliance limits. Activities, such as sustained coughing or straining during defecation, can cause temporary elevations in thoracic pressure.

### B waves

B waves, which appear sharp and rhythmic with a sawtooth pattern, occur every 1½ to 2 minutes and may reach elevations of 50 mm Hg. The clinical significance of B waves isn't clear, but the waves correlate with respiratory changes and may occur more frequently with decreasing compensation. Because B

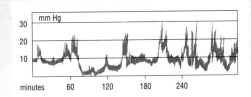

waves sometimes precede A waves, notify the doctor if B waves occur frequently.

### C waves

Like B waves, C waves are rapid and rhythmic, but they aren't as sharp. Clinically insignificant, they may fluctuate with respirations or systemic blood pressure changes.

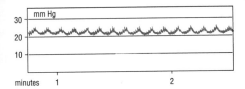

*(continued)*

▶ Osmotic diuretic agents, such as mannitol, reduce cerebral edema by shrinking intracranial contents. Given by I.V. drip or bolus, mannitol draws water from tissues into plasma; it doesn't cross the blood-brain barrier. Monitor serum electrolyte levels and osmolality readings closely because the patient may become dehydrated

## Interpreting ICP waveforms *(continued)*

### Waveform showing equipment problem

A waveform such as the one shown at right signals a problem with the transducer or monitor. Check for line obstruction and determine whether the transducer needs rebalancing

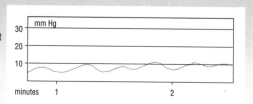

very quickly. Be aware that a rebound increase in ICP may occur. (See *Nursing management of increased ICP.*) To avoid rebound increased ICP, 50 ml of albumin may be given with the mannitol bolus. Note, however, that you'll see a residual rise in ICP before it decreases. If your patient has heart failure or severe renal dysfunction, monitor for problems in adapting to the increased intravascular volumes.

▶ Monitor intake and output carefully to maintain normovolume to ensure adequate MAP. This will assure good CSF pressure.

▶ Although their use is controversial, steroids may be used to lower elevated ICP by reducing sodium and water concentration in the brain. They're usually given with antacids and famotidine or ranitidine because they may produce peptic ulcers. Observe for possible GI bleeding. Also monitor blood glucose levels because steroids may cause hyperglycemia.

▶ A barbiturate-induced coma depresses the reticular activating system and reduces the brain's metabolic demand. Reduced demand for oxygen and energy reduces cerebral blood flow, thereby lowering ICP.

▶ Hyperventilation with oxygen from a handheld resuscitation bag or ventilator helps rid the patient of excess carbon dioxide, thereby constricting cerebral vessels and reducing cerebral blood volume and ICP. However, only normal brain tissues respond because blood vessels in damaged areas have reduced vasoconstrictive ability.

◆ **ALERT!** Because hyperventilation with a handheld resuscitation bag or a ventilator can cause ischemia, it should only be performed in an acute situation to reduce increased increased ICP until other measures can be used.

▶ Before tracheal suctioning, hyperventilate the patient with 100% oxygen as ordered. Apply suction for a maximum of 15 seconds. Avoid inducing hypoxia because this condition greatly increases cerebral blood flow.

▶ Because fever raises brain metabolism, which increases cerebral blood flow, fever reduction (achieved by administering acetaminophen, sponge baths, or a hypothermia blanket) also helps to reduce ICP. However, rebound increases in ICP and brain edema may occur if rapid rewarming takes place after hypothermia or if cooling measures induce shivering.

▶ Withdrawal of CSF through the drainage system reduces CSF volume and thus reduces ICP. Although less commonly used, surgical removal of a skull-bone flap provides room for the swollen brain to expand. If this procedure is performed, keep the site clean and dry to prevent infection and maintain sterile technique when changing the dressing.

## Complications

CNS infection, the most common hazard of ICP monitoring, can result from contamination of the equipment setup or of the insertion site.

◆ **ALERT!** Excessive loss of CSF can result from faulty stopcock placement or a drip chamber that is positioned too low. Such loss can rapidly decompress the cranial contents and damage bridging cortical veins, leading to hematoma formation. Decompression can also lead to rupture of existing hematomas or aneurysms, causing hemorrhage.

Watch for signs of impending or overt decompensation: pupillary dilation (unilat-

# Nursing management of increased ICP

By performing nursing care gently, slowly, and cautiously, you can help manage, or even significantly reduce, increased intracranial pressure (ICP). If possible, urge the patient to participate in his own care. Here are some steps you can take to manage increased ICP:

▶ Plan your care to include rest periods between activities. This allows the patient's ICP to return to baseline, thus avoiding lengthy and cumulative pressure elevations.

▶ Speak to the patient before attempting any procedures, even if he appears comatose. Touch him on an arm or leg first before touching him in a more personal area, such as the face or chest. This is especially important if the patient doesn't know you or if he's confused or sedated.

▶ Suction the patient only when needed to remove secretions and maintain airway patency. Avoid depriving him of oxygen for long periods while suctioning; always hyperventilate the patient with oxygen before and after the procedure. Monitor his heart rate while suctioning. If multiple catheter passes are needed to clear secretions, hyperventilate the patient between them to bring ICP as close to baseline as possible.

▶ To promote venous drainage, keep the patient's head in the midline position, even when he's positioned on his side. Avoid flexing the neck or hip more than 90 degrees, and keep the head of the bed elevated 30 to 45 degrees.

▶ To avoid increasing intrathoracic pressure, which raises ICP, discourage Valsalva's maneuver and isometric muscle contractions. To avoid isometric contractions, distract the patient when giving him painful injections (by asking him to wiggle his toes and by massaging the area before injection to relax the muscle) and have him concentrate on breathing through difficult procedures such as bed-to-stretcher transfers. To keep the patient from holding his breath when moving around in bed, tell him to relax as much as possible during position changes. If necessary, administer a stool softener to help prevent constipation and unnecessary straining during defecation.

▶ If the patient is heavily sedated, monitor his respiratory rate and blood gas levels. Depressed respirations will compromise ventilations and oxygen exchange. Maintaining adequate respiratory rate and volume will help reduce ICP.

▶ If you're in a specialty unit, you may be able to routinely hyperventilate the patient to counter sustained ICP elevations. This procedure is one of the best ways to reduce high ICP at the bedside for short periods. Consult your facility's protocol.

---

eral or bilateral); decreased pupillary response to light; decreasing LOC; rising systolic blood pressure and widening pulse pressure; bradycardia; slowed, irregular respirations; and, in late decompensation, decerebrate posturing.

## Documentation

▶ Record the time and date of the insertion procedure and the patient's response.
▶ Note the insertion site and the type of monitoring system used.
▶ Record ICP digital readings and waveforms and CCP hourly in your notes, in a flowchart, or directly on readout strips, depending on your facility's policy.
▶ Document any factors that may affect ICP (for example, drug administration, stressful procedures, or sleep).
▶ Record routine and neurologic vital signs hourly and describe the patient's clinical status.

▶ Note the amount, character, and frequency of any CSF drainage (for example, "between 6 p.m. and 7 p.m., 15 ml of blood-tinged CSF"). Also record the ICP reading in response to drainage.

## REFERENCES

Hickey, J.V. *The Clinical Practice of Neurological and Neurosurgical Nursing,* 5th ed. Philadelphia: Lippincott Williams & Wilkins, 2003.

Kirkness, C.J., et al. "Intracranial Pressure Waveform Analysis: Clinical and Research Implications," *Journal of Neuroscience Nursing* 32(5):271-77, October 2000.

March, K. "Intracranial Pressure Monitoring and Assessing Intracranial Compliance in Brain Injury," *Critical Care Nursing Clinics of North America* 12(4):429-35, December 2000.

# Lumbar puncture

Lumbar puncture involves the insertion of a sterile needle into the subarachnoid space of the spinal canal, usually between the third and fourth lumbar vertebrae. This procedure is used to detect the presence of blood in CSF, to obtain CSF specimens for laboratory analysis, and to inject dyes or gases for contrast in radiologic studies. It's also used to administer drugs or anesthetics and to relieve ICP by removing CSF.

Performed by a doctor with a nurse assisting, lumbar puncture requires sterile technique and careful patient positioning. This procedure is contraindicated in patients with lumbar deformity, increased ICP or infection at the puncture site.

## Equipment

Overbed table • one or two pairs of sterile gloves for the doctor • sterile gloves for the nurse • povidone-iodine solution • sterile gauze pads • alcohol sponges • sterile fenestrated drape • 3-ml syringe for local anesthetic • 25G ¾″ sterile needle for injecting anesthetic • local anesthetic (usually 1% lidocaine) • 18G or 20G ½″ spinal needle with stylet (22G needle for children) • three-way stopcock • manometer • small adhesive bandage • three sterile collection tubes with stoppers • laboratory request forms • labels • light source such as a gooseneck lamp • optional: patient-care reminder

Disposable lumbar puncture trays contain most of the needed sterile equipment.

### Preparation of equipment

Gather the equipment and take it to the patient's bedside.

## Implementation

▶ Explain the procedure to the patient to ease his anxiety and ensure his cooperation. Make sure a consent form has been signed.
▶ Inform the patient that he may experience headache after lumbar puncture but reassure him that his cooperation during the procedure minimizes such an effect.
▶ Immediately before the procedure, provide privacy and instruct the patient to void.
▶ Wash your hands thoroughly.

# Positioning for lumbar puncture

Have the patient lie on his side at the edge of the bed, with his chin tucked to his chest and his knees drawn up to his abdomen. Make sure the patient's spine is curved and his back is at the edge of the bed (as shown below). This position widens the spaces between the vertebrae, easing needle insertion. The patient can also sit up at the beside leaning forward over the bedside table.

To help the patient maintain this position, place one of your hands behind his neck and the other hand behind his knees and pull gently. Hold the patient firmly in this position throughout the procedure to prevent accidental needle displacement.

### Patient positioning

Typically, the doctor inserts the needle between the third and fourth lumbar vertebrae (as shown below).

**PATIENT POSITIONING**

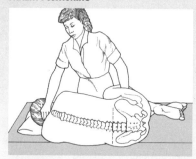

**NEEDLE INSERTION**

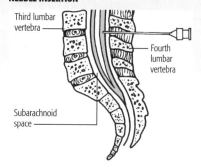

Third lumbar vertebra

Fourth lumbar vertebra

Subarachnoid space

▶ Open the equipment tray on an overbed table, being careful not to contaminate the sterile field when you open the wrapper.

▶ Provide adequate lighting at the puncture site using a gooseneck lamp and adjust the height of the patient's bed to allow the doctor to perform the procedure comfortably.

▶ Position the patient and reemphasize the importance of remaining as still as possible to minimize discomfort and trauma. (See *Positioning for lumbar puncture.*)

▶ The doctor cleans the puncture site with sterile gauze pads soaked in povidone-iodine solution, wiping in a circular motion away from the puncture site; he uses three different pads to prevent contamination of spinal tissues by the body's normal skin flora. Next, he drapes the area with the fenestrated drape to provide a sterile field. (If the doctor uses povidone-iodine pads instead of sterile gauze pads, he may remove his sterile gloves and put on another pair to avoid introducing povidone-iodine into the subarachnoid space with the lumbar puncture needle.)

▶ If no ampule of anesthetic is included on the equipment tray, clean the injection port of a multidose vial of anesthetic with an alcohol pad. Then invert the vial 45 degrees so that the doctor can insert a 25G needle and syringe and withdraw the anesthetic for injection.

▶ Before the doctor injects the anesthetic, tell the patient he'll experience a transient burning sensation and local pain. Ask him to report any other persistent pain or sensations because they may indicate irritation or puncture of a nerve root, requiring repositioning of the needle.

▶ When the doctor inserts the sterile spinal needle into the subarachnoid space between the third and fourth lumbar vertebrae, instruct the patient to remain still and breathe normally. If necessary, hold the patient firmly in position to prevent sudden movement that may displace the needle.

▶ If the lumbar puncture is being performed to administer contrast media for radiologic studies or spinal anesthetic, the doctor injects the dye or anesthetic at this time.

▶ When the needle is in place, the doctor attaches a manometer with a three-way stopcock to the needle hub to read CSF pressure. If ordered, help the patient extend his legs to provide a more accurate pressure reading.

▶ The doctor then detaches the manometer and allows CSF to drain from the needle hub into the collection tubes. When he has collected 2 to 3 ml in each tube, mark the tubes in sequence, insert a stopper to secure them, and label them.

▶ If the doctor suspects an obstruction in the spinal subarachnoid space, he may check for Queckenstedt's sign. After he takes an initial CSF pressure reading, compress the patient's jugular vein for 10 seconds as ordered. This increases ICP and, if no subarachnoid block exists, causes CSF pressure to rise as well. The doctor then takes pressure readings every 10 seconds until the pressure stabilizes.

▶ Put on sterile gloves.

▶ After the doctor collects the specimens and removes the spinal needle, clean the puncture site with povidone-iodine and apply a small adhesive bandage.

▶ Remove and discard gloves.

▶ Send the CSF specimens to the laboratory immediately, with completed laboratory request forms.

## Special considerations

▶ During lumbar puncture, watch closely for signs of adverse reaction: elevated pulse rate, pallor, and clammy skin. Alert the doctor immediately to any significant changes.

▶ The patient may be ordered to lie flat for 2 hours after the procedure. If necessary, place a patient-care reminder on his bed to this effect.

▶ Collected CSF specimens must be sent to the laboratory immediately; they can't be refrigerated for later transport.

## Complications

Headache is the most common adverse effect of lumbar puncture. Others include a reaction to the anesthetic, meningitis, epidural or subdural abscess, bleeding into the spinal canal, CSF leakage through the dural defect remaining after needle withdrawal, local pain caused by nerve root irritation, edema or hematoma at the puncture site, transient difficulty voiding, and fever. The most serious complications of lumbar puncture, although rare, are tonsillar herniation and medullary compression.

## Documentation

▶ Record the initiation and completion times of the procedure.

# Differentiating among seizure types

The hallmark of epilepsy is recurring seizures, which can be classified as partial or generalized. Some patients may be affected by more than one type.

## Partial seizures

Arising from a localized area in the brain, partial seizures cause specific symptoms. In some patients, partial seizure activity may be spread to the entire brain, causing a generalized seizure. Partial seizures include simple partial (jacksonian motor-type and sensory type), complex partial (psychomotor or temporal lobe), and secondarily generalized partial seizures.

## Simple partial jacksonian motor-type seizure

The simple jacksonian motor-type seizure begins as a localized motor seizure, which is characterized by a spread of abnormal activity to adjacent areas of the brain. Typically, the patient experiences a stiffening or jerking in one extremity, accompanied by a tingling sensation in the same area. For example, the seizure may start in the thumb and spread to the entire hand and arm. The patient seldom loses consciousness, although the seizure may secondarily progress to a generalized tonic-clonic seizure.

## Simple partial sensory-type seizure

Perception is distorted in the simple partial sensory-type seizure. Symptoms can include hallucinations, flashing lights, tingling sensations, vertigo, or déjà vu (the feeling of having experienced something before).

## Complex partial seizure

Symptoms of the complex partial seizure are variable, but usually include purposeless behavior. The patient may experience an aura and exhibit overt signs, including a glassy stare, picking at his clothes, aimless wandering, lip smacking or chewing motions, and unintelligible speech. The seizure may last for a few seconds or as long as 20 minutes. Afterward, mental confusion may last for several minutes; as a result, an observer may mistakenly suspect psychosis or intoxication with alcohol or drugs. The patient has no memory of his actions during the seizure.

## Secondarily generalized partial seizure

The secondarily generalized partial seizure can be either simple or complex and can progress to a generalized seizure. An aura may precede the progression. Loss of consciousness occurs immediately or within 1 to 2 minutes of the start of the progression.

## Generalized seizures

As the term suggests, generalized seizures cause a general electrical abnormality within the brain. They include several distinct types.

## Absence (petit mal) seizure

The absence seizure occurs most commonly in children, but it also may affect adults. It usually begins with a brief change in the level of consciousness, indicated by blinking or rolling of the eyes or a blank stare, and slight mouth movements. The patient retains his posture and continues preseizure activity without difficulty. Typically, the seizure lasts 1 to 10 seconds. The impairment is so brief that the patient is sometimes unaware of it. If not properly treated, these seizures can recur as often as 100 times a day. An absence seizure may progress to a generalized tonic-clonic seizure.

## Myoclonic seizure

Also called bilateral massive epileptic monoclonus, the myoclonic seizure is marked by brief, involuntary muscular jerks of the body or extremities, which may occur in a rhythmic manner, and a brief loss of consciousness.

## Generalized tonic-clonic (grand mal) seizure

Typically, the generalized tonic-clonic seizure begins with a loud cry, precipitated by air rushing from the lungs through the vocal cords. The patient falls to the ground, losing consciousness. The body stiffens (tonic phase) and then alternates between episodes of muscle spasm and relaxation (clonic phase).

---

▶ Document the patient's response, administration of drugs, number of specimen tubes collected, time of transport to the laboratory, and color, consistency, and any other characteristics of the collected specimens.

## Differentiating among seizure types *(continued)*

Tongue biting, incontinence, labored breathing, apnea, and subsequent cyanosis may also occur. The seizure stops in 2 to 5 minutes, after abnormal electrical conduction of the neurons is completed. The patient then regains consciousness, but is somewhat confused and may have difficulty talking. If he can talk, he may complain of drowsiness, fatigue, headache, muscle soreness, and arm or leg weakness. He may fall into a deep sleep after the seizure.

### Akinetic seizure
Characterized by a general loss of postural tone and a temporary loss of consciousness, the akinetic seizure occurs in young children. It's sometimes called a "drop attack" because it causes the child to fall.

### REFERENCES
Chadwick, D.R., and Lever, A.M. "The Impact of New Diagnostic Methodologies in the Management of Meningitis in Adults at a Teaching Hospital," *QJM-Monthly Journal of the Association of Physicians* 95(10): 663-70, October 2002.

Mignot, E., et al. "The Role of Cerebrospinal Fluid Hypocretin Measurement in the Diagnosis of Narcolepsy and Other Hypersomnias," *Archives of Neurology* 59(10): 1553-62, October 2002.

# Seizure precautions

Seizures are paroxysmal events associated with abnormal electrical discharges of neurons in the brain. Partial seizures are usually unilateral, involving a localized or focal area of the brain. Generalized seizures involve the entire brain. (See *Differentiating among seizure types.*) When a patient has a generalized seizure, nursing care aims to protect him from injury and prevent serious complications. Appropriate care also includes observation of seizure characteristics to help determine the area of the brain involved.

Patients considered at risk for seizures are those with a history of seizures and those with conditions that predispose them to seizures. These conditions include metabolic abnormalities, such as hypocalcemia, hypoglycemia, and pyridoxine deficiency; brain tumors or other space-occupying lesions; infections, such as meningitis, encephalitis, and brain abscess; traumatic injury, especially if the dura mater was penetrated; ingestion of toxins, such as mercury, lead, or carbon monoxide; genetic abnormalities, such as tuberous sclerosis

and phenylketonuria; perinatal injuries; and cerebrovascular accident. Patients at risk for seizures need precautionary measures to help prevent injury if a seizure occurs. (See *Precautions for generalized seizures,* page 404.)

### Equipment
Oral airway • suction equipment • side rail pads • seizure activity record • additional equipment: I.V. • normal saline solution • oxygen • endotracheal intubation equipment

### Implementation
▶ If you're with a patient when he experiences an aura, help him into bed, raise the side rails, and adjust the bed flat. If he's away from his room, lower him to the floor and place a pillow, blanket, or other soft material under his head to keep it from hitting the floor.
▶ Stay with the patient during the seizure and be ready to intervene if complications such as airway obstruction develop. If necessary, have another staff member obtain the appropriate equipment and notify the doctor of the obstruction.
▶ Provide privacy, if possible.
▶ Depending on your facility's policy, if the patient is in the beginning of the tonic phase of the seizure, you may insert an oral airway into his mouth so that his tongue doesn't block his airway. If an oral airway isn't available, don't try to hold his mouth open or place your hands inside because you may be bitten. After the patient's jaw becomes rigid, don't force the airway into place because you could break his teeth or cause another injury. Some clinicians ad-

# Precautions for generalized seizures

By taking appropriate precautions, you can help protect the patient from injury, aspiration, and airway obstruction should he have a seizure. Plan your precautions using information obtained from the patient's history. What kind of seizure has the patient previously had? Is he aware of exacerbating factors? Sleep deprivation, missed doses of anticonvulsants, and even upper respiratory infections can increase seizure frequency in the patient who has had seizures. Was his previous seizure an acute episode, or did it result from a chronic condition?

### Gather the equipment

Based on answers provided in the patient's history, you can tailor your precautions to his needs. Start by gathering the appropriate equipment, including a hospital bed with full-length side rails, commercial side rail pads or six bath blankets (four for a crib), adhesive tape, an oral airway, and oral or nasal suction equipment.

### Bedside preparations

Now carry out the precautions you think appropriate for the patient. Remember that a patient with preexisting seizures who's being admitted for a change in medication, treatment for an infection, or detoxification may have an increased risk of seizures.

▶ Explain the reasons for the precautions to the patient.

▶ To protect the patient's limbs, head, and feet from injury if he has a seizure while in bed, cover the side rails, headboard, and footboard with side rail pads or bath blankets. If you use blankets, keep them in place with adhesive tape. Keep the side rails raised while the patient is in bed to prevent falls. Keep the bed in a low position to minimize any injuries that may occur if the patient climbs over the rails.

▶ Place an airway at the patient's bedside, or tape it to the wall above the bed according to your facility's protocol. Keep suction equipment nearby in case you need to establish a patent airway. Explain to the patient how the airway will be used.

▶ If the patient has frequent or prolonged seizures, prepare an I.V. heparin lock to facilitate administration of emergency medications.

---

vocate waiting until the seizure subsides before inserting the airway.

▶ Move hard or sharp objects out of the patient's way and loosen his clothing.

▶ Don't forcibly restrain the patient or restrict his movements during the seizure because the force of the patient's movements against restraints could cause muscle strain or even joint dislocation.

▶ Continually assess the patient during the seizure. Observe the earliest symptom, such as head or eye deviation, as well as how the seizure progresses, what form it takes, and how long it lasts. Your description may help determine the seizure's type and cause.

▶ If this is the patient's first seizure, notify the doctor immediately. If the patient has had seizures before, notify the doctor only if the seizure activity is prolonged or if the patient fails to regain consciousness. (See *Understanding status epilepticus.*)

▶ If ordered, establish an I.V. line and infuse normal saline solution at a keep-vein-open rate.

▶ If the seizure is prolonged and the patient becomes hypoxemic, administer oxygen as ordered. Some patients may require endotracheal intubation.

▶ For a patient known to be diabetic, administer 50 ml of dextrose 50% in water by I.V. push as ordered. For a patient known to be an alcoholic, a 100-mg bolus of thiamine may be ordered to stop the seizure.

▶ After the seizure, turn the patient on his side and apply suction, if necessary, to facilitate drainage of secretions and maintain a patent airway. Insert an oral airway, if needed.

▶ Check for injuries.

▶ Reorient and reassure the patient as necessary.

▶ When the patient is comfortable and safe, document what happened during the seizure.

▶ Place side rail pads on the bed in case the patient experiences another seizure.

▶ After the seizure, monitor vital signs and mental status every 15 to 20 minutes for 2 hours.

▶ Ask the patient about his aura and activities preceding the seizure. The type of aura (such as auditory, visual, olfactory, gustatory, or somatic) helps pinpoint the site in the brain where the seizure originated.

### Special considerations
▶ Because a seizure commonly indicates an underlying disorder, such as meningitis or a metabolic or electrolyte imbalance, a complete diagnostic workup will be ordered if the cause of the seizure isn't evident.

### Complications
The patient who experiences a seizure may experience an injury, respiratory difficulty, and decreased mental capability. Common injuries include scrapes and bruises suffered when the patient hits objects during the seizure and traumatic injury to the tongue caused by biting. If you suspect a serious injury, such as a fracture or deep laceration, notify the doctor and arrange for appropriate evaluation and treatment.

Changes in respiratory function may include aspiration, airway obstruction, and hypoxemia. After the seizure, complete a respiratory assessment and notify the doctor if you suspect a problem. Expect most patients to experience a postictal period of decreased mental status lasting 30 minutes to 24 hours. Reassure the patient that this doesn't indicate incipient brain damage.

### Documentation
▶ Document that the patient requires seizure precautions and record all precautions taken.
▶ Record the date and the time the seizure began as well as its duration and any precipitating factors. Identify any sensation that may be considered an aura. If the seizure was preceded by an aura, have the patient describe what he experienced.
▶ Record any involuntary behavior that occurred at the onset, such as lip smacking, chewing movements, or hand and eye movements. Describe where the movement began and the parts of the body involved. Note any progression or pattern to the activity.
▶ Document whether the patient's eyes deviated to one side and whether the pupils changed in size, shape, equality, or reaction to light.

---

## Understanding status epilepticus

A continuous seizure state unless interrupted by emergency interventions, status epilepticus can occur in all seizure types. The most life-threatening example is generalized tonic-clonic status epilepticus, which is a continuous generalized tonic-clonic seizure without intervening return of consciousness.

Status epilepticus, always an emergency, is accompanied by respiratory distress. It can result from abrupt withdrawal of anticonvulsant medications, hypoxic or metabolic encephalopathy, acute head trauma, or septicemia secondary to encephalitis or meningitis.

Emergency treatment of status epilepticus usually consists of diazepam, phenytoin, or phenobarbital; dextrose 50% I.V. (when seizures are secondary to hypoglycemia); and thiamine I.V. (in the presence of chronic alcoholism or withdrawal).

---

▶ Note if the patient's teeth were clenched or open.
▶ Record any incontinence, vomiting, or salivation that occurred during the seizure.
▶ Note the patient's response to the seizure. Was he aware of what happened? Did he fall into a deep sleep after the seizure? Was he upset or ashamed?
▶ Document any medications given, complications experienced during the seizure, and interventions performed.
▶ Record the patient's post-seizure mental status.

### REFERENCES
Brodie, M.J., et al. *Epilepsy, Fast Facts,* 2nd ed. Oxford, England: Health Press Limited, 2001.
Hickey, J.V. *The Clinical Practice of Neurological and Neurosurgical Nursing,* 5th ed. Philadelphia: Lippincott Williams & Wilkins, 2003.

## Skull tongs care

Applying skeletal traction with skull tongs immobilizes the cervical spine after a fracture or dislocation, invasion by tumor or infection, or surgery. Three types of skull

# Types of skull tongs

Skull (or cervical) tongs consist of a stainless steel body with a pin at the end of each arm. Each pin is about ⅛″ (0.3 cm) in diameter and has a sharp tip.

### Crutchfield tongs
The pins are placed about 5″ (12.5 cm) apart in line with the long axis of the cervical spine.

### Gardner-Wells tongs
The pins are farther apart, inserted slightly above the patient's ears.

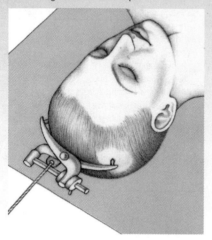

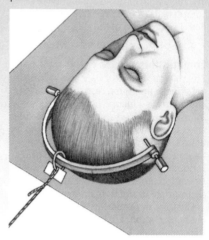

tongs are commonly used: Crutchfield, Gardner-Wells, and Vinke. (See *Types of skull tongs.*)

Crutchfield tongs are applied by incising the skin with a scalpel, drilling a hole in the exposed skull, and inserting the pins on the tongs into the hole. Gardner-Wells tongs and Vinke tongs are applied less invasively. Gardner-Wells tongs have spring-loaded pins attached to the tongs. These pins are advanced gently into the scalp. Then the tongs are tightened to secure the apparatus.

When any tong device is in place, traction is created by extending a rope from the center of the tongs over a pulley and attaching weights to it. With the help of X-ray monitoring, the weights are adjusted to establish reduction, if necessary, and to maintain alignment. Meticulous pin-site care (three times per day to prevent infection) and frequent observation of the traction apparatus to make sure it's working properly are required.

Skull tongs can also be used to reduce a subluxation and restore normal anatomic positioning in cervical degenerative disease.

## Equipment
Three sterile specimen containers ● one bottle each of ordered cleaning solution, normal saline solution, and povidone-iodine solution ● sterile, cotton-tipped applicators ● sandbags or cervical collar (hard or soft) ● fine mesh gauze strips ● 4″ × 4″ gauze pads ● sterile gloves ● sterile basin ● sterile scissors ● hair clippers ● optional: turning frame and antibacterial ointment

### Preparation of equipment
Bring the equipment to the patient's room. Place the sterile specimen containers on the bedside table. Fill one with a small amount of cleaning solution, one with normal saline solution, and one with povidone-iodine solution. Then set out the cotton-tipped applicators. Keep the sandbags or cervical collar handy for emergency immobilization of the head and neck if the pins in the tongs should slip.

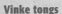

### Vinke tongs
The pins are placed at the parietal bones, near the widest transverse diameter of the skull, about 1" (2.5 cm) above the helix.

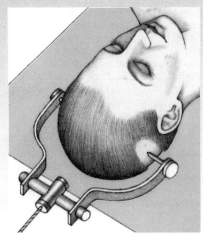

## Implementation
▶ Explain the procedure to the patient and wash your hands. Inform the patient that pin sites usually feel tender for several days after the tongs are applied. Tell him that he'll also feel some muscular discomfort in the injured area.
▶ Before providing care, observe each pin site carefully for signs of infection, such as loose pins, swelling or redness, or purulent drainage. Use hair clippers to trim the patient's hair around the pin sites, when necessary, to facilitate assessment.
▶ Put on gloves and gently wipe each pin site with a cotton-tipped applicator dipped in cleaning solution to loosen and remove crusty drainage. Repeat with a fresh applicator as needed for thorough cleaning. Use a separate applicator for each site to avoid cross-contamination. Next, wipe each site with normal saline solution to remove excess cleaning solution. Finally, wipe with povidone-iodine solution to provide asepsis at the site and prevent infection.
▶ After providing care, discard all pin-site cleaning materials.

▶ If the pin sites are infected, apply a povidone-iodine wrap as ordered. First, obtain strips of fine mesh gauze or cut a 4" × 4" gauze pad into strips (using sterile scissors and wearing sterile gloves). Soak the strips in a sterile basin of povidone-iodine solution or normal saline solution as ordered and squeeze out the excess solution. Wrap one strip securely around each pin site. Leave the strip in place to dry until you provide care again. Removing the dried strip aids in debridement and helps clear the infection.
▶ Check the traction apparatus—rope, weights, and pulleys—at the start of each shift, every 4 hours, and as necessary (for example, after position changes). Make sure the rope hangs freely and that the weights never rest on the floor or become caught under the bed.

## Special considerations
▶ Occasionally, the doctor may prefer an antibacterial ointment for pin-site care instead of povidone-iodine solution. To remove old ointment, wrap a cotton-tipped applicator with a 4" × 4" gauze pad, moisten it with cleaning solution, and gently clean each site. Keep a box of sterile gauze pads handy at the patient's bedside.
▶ Watch for signs and symptoms of loose pins, such as persistent pain or tenderness at pin sites, redness, and drainage. The patient may also report feeling or hearing the pins move.
▶ If you suspect a pin has loosened or slipped, don't turn the patient until the doctor examines the skull tongs and fixes them as needed.
▶ If the pins pull out, immobilize the patient's head and neck with sandbags or apply a cervical collar. Then carefully remove the traction weights. Apply manual traction to the patient's head by placing your hands on each side of the mandible and pulling very gently while maintaining proper alignment. After you stabilize the alignment, have someone send for the doctor immediately. Remain calm and reassure the patient. When traction is reestablished, take neurologic vital signs.

◆◆ **ALERT!** Never add or subtract weights to the traction apparatus without an order from the doctor. Doing so can cause neurologic impairment.
▶ Take neurologic vital signs at the beginning of each shift, every 4 hours, and as

necessary (for example, after turning or transporting the patient). Carefully assess the function of cranial nerves, which may be impaired by pin placement. Note any asymmetry, deviation, or atrophy. Review the patient's chart to determine baseline neurologic vital signs on admission to the facility and immediately after the tongs were applied.

▶ Monitor respirations closely and keep suction equipment handy. Remember, injury to the cervical spine may affect respiration. Be alert for signs of respiratory distress, such as unequal chest expansion and an irregular or altered respiratory rate or pattern.

▶ Patients with skull tongs may be placed on a turning frame to facilitate turning without disrupting vertebral alignment. Establish a turning schedule for the patient (usually a supine position for 2 hours and then a prone position for 1 hour) to help prevent complications of immobility.

▶ Never remove a patient from the bed or turning frame when transporting him to another department.

### Complications

Infection, excessive tractive force, or osteoporosis can cause the skull pins to slip or pull out. Because this interrupts traction, the patient must receive immediate attention to prevent further injury.

### Documentation

▶ Record the date, time, and type of pin-site care and the patient's response to the procedure in your notes.

▶ Document any signs of infection.

▶ Note whether any weights were added or removed.

▶ Record neurologic vital signs, the patient's respiratory status, and the turning schedule on the Kardex.

### REFERENCES

Papagelopoulos, P.J., et al. "Halo Pin Intracranial Penetration and Epidural Abscess in a Patient with a Previous Cranioplasty: Case Report and Review of the Literature," *Spine* 26(19):E463-67, October 2001.

Parney, I.F., et al. "Hepburn and the Development of Skull Tongs for Cervical Spine Traction," *Neurosurgery* 47(6):1430-32, December 2000; discussion 1432-33.

# Transcranial Doppler monitoring

Transcranial Doppler ultrasonography is a noninvasive method of monitoring blood flow in the intracranial vessels, specifically the circle of Willis. This procedure is used in the intensive care unit to monitor patients who have experienced cerebrovascular disorders, such as stroke, head trauma, or subarachnoid hemorrhage. It can help detect intracranial stenosis, vasospasm, and arteriovenous malformations as well as assess collateral pathways. Because it has the advantage of monitoring a continuous waveform, it can be used in intraoperative monitoring of cerebral circulation.

Transcranial Doppler ultrasonography is also used to monitor the effect of ICP changes on the cerebral circulation, to monitor patient response to various medications, and to evaluate carbon dioxide reactivity, which may be impaired or lost from arterial obstruction or trauma. In addition, it has been used to confirm brain death.

The transcranial Doppler unit transmits pulses of high-frequency ultrasound, which are then reflected back to the transducer by the red blood cells moving in the vessel being monitored. This information is then processed by the instrument into an audible signal and a velocity waveform, which is displayed on the monitor. The displayed waveform is actually a moving graph of blood flow velocities with TIME displayed along the horizontal axis, VELOCITY displayed along the vertical axis, and AMPLITUDE represented by various colors or intensities within the waveform. The heart's contractions speed up the movement of blood cells during systole and slow it down during diastole, resulting in a waveform that varies in velocity over the cardiac cycle.

The major benefits of transcranial Doppler monitoring are that it provides instantaneous, real-time information about cerebral blood flow and that it's noninvasive and painless for the patient. Also, the unit itself is portable and easy to use. The major disadvantage is that it relies on the ability of ultrasound waves to penetrate thin areas of the cranium; this is difficult if the patient has thickening of the temporal bone, which increases with age.

The transcranial Doppler unit should always be used with its power set at the lowest level needed to provide an adequate waveform. This procedure requires specialized training to ensure accurate vessel identification and correct interpretation of the signals.

## Equipment
Transcranial Doppler unit • transducer with an attachment system • terry cloth headband • ultrasonic coupling gel • marker

## Implementation
▶ Explain the procedure to the patient and answer any questions he has about the procedure as thoroughly as possible.
▶ Place the patient in the proper position—usually the supine position.
▶ Turn the Doppler unit on and observe as it performs a self-test. The screen should show six parameters: PEAK (CM/S), MEAN (CM/S), DEPTH (M/M), DELTA (%), EMBOLI (AGR), and PIL.
▶ Enter the patient's name and identification number in the appropriate place on the Doppler unit. Depending on the unit you're using, you may need to enter additional information, such as the patient's diagnosis or the doctor's name.
▶ Indicate the vessel that you wish to monitor (usually the right or left middle cerebral artery [MCA]). You'll also need to set the approximate depth of the vessel within the skull (50 mm for the MCA).
▶ Next, use the keypad to increase the power level to 100% to initially locate the signal. You can later decrease the level as needed, depending on the thickness of the patient's skull.
▶ Examine the temporal region of the patient's head, and mentally identify the three windows of the transtemporal access route: posterior, middle, and anterior (as shown below).

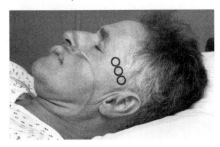

▶ Apply a generous amount of ultrasonic gel at the level of the temporal bone between the tragus of the ear and the end of the eyebrow, and over the area of the three windows.
▶ Next, place the transducer on the posterior window. Angle the transducer slightly in an anterior direction and slowly move it in a narrow circle. This movement is commonly called the "flashlighting" technique. As you hold the transducer at an angle and perform flashlighting, also begin to very slowly move the transducer forward across the temporal area. As you do this, listen for the audible signal with the highest pitch. This sound corresponds to the highest velocity signal, which corresponds to the signal of the vessel you are assessing. You can also use headphones to let you better evaluate the audible signal and provide patient privacy.
▶ After you've located the highest-pitched signal, use a marker to draw a circle around the transducer head on the patient's temple (as shown below). Note the angle of the transducer so that you can duplicate it after the transducer attachment system is in place.

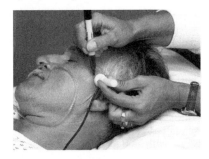

▶ Next, place the transducer system on the patient. To do this, first place the plate of the transducer attachment system over the patient's temporal area; match the circular opening in the plate exactly with the circle drawn on the patient's head. Then, holding the plate in place, encircle the patient's head with the straps attached to the system. Finally, tighten the straps so that the transducer attachment system will stay in place on the patient's head.
▶ Fill the circular opening in the plate with the ultrasonic gel.
▶ Place the transducer in the gel-filled opening in the attachment system plate. Using the plastic screws provided, loosely

# Comparing velocity waveforms

A normal transcranial Doppler signal is usually characterized by mean velocities that fall within the normal reported values. Additional information can be gathered by evaluating the shape of the velocity waveform.

### Effect of significant proximal vessel obstruction

A delayed systolic upstroke can be seen in a waveform when significant proximal vessel obstruction is present.

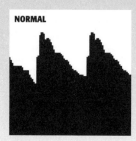

NORMAL

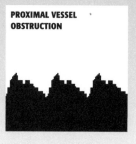

PROXIMAL VESSEL OBSTRUCTION

### Effect of increased cerebrovascular resistance

Changes in cerebrovascular resistance, as occur with increased intracranial pressure, cause a decrease in diastolic flow.

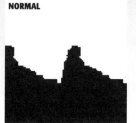

NORMAL

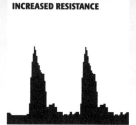

INCREASED RESISTANCE

---

secure the two plates together. This will hold the transducer in place but allow it to rotate for the best angle.

▶ Adjust the position and angle of the transducer until you again hear the highest-pitched audible signal. When you hear this signal, look at the waveform on the monitor screen. You should see a clear waveform with a bright white line (called an envelope) at the upper edge of the waveform. The envelope exactly follows the contours of the waveform itself.

▶ If the envelope doesn't follow the waveform's contours, adjust the GAIN setting. If the signal is wrapping around the screen, use the SCALE key to increase the scale and the BASELINE key to drop the baseline.

▶ When you've determined that you have the strongest, highest-pitched signal and the best waveform, lock the transducer in place by tightening the plastic screws (as shown at right). The tightened plates will

hold the transducer at the angle you've chosen. Disconnect the transducer handle.

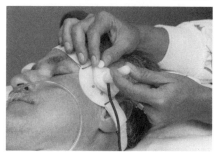

▶ Place a wide terry cloth headband over the transducer attachment system and secure it around the patient's head to provide additional stability for the transducer.

▶ Look at the monitor screen. You should be able to see a waveform and read the numeric values of the peak, mean velocities, and pulsatility index (PI1) above the displayed waveform. The shape of the waveform reveals more information. (See *Comparing velocity waveforms.*)

## Special considerations

▶ Velocity changes in the transcranial Doppler signal correlate with changes in cerebral blood flow. The parameter that most clearly reflects this change is the mean velocity. First, establish a baseline for the mean velocity. Then, as the patient's velocity increases or decreases, the value (%) will change negatively or positively from the baseline.

▶ Emboli appear as high-intensity transients that occur randomly during the cardiac cycle. Emboli make a distinctive "clicking," "chirping," or "plunking" sound. You can set up an emboli counter to count either the total number of emboli aggregates or the number of embolic events per minute.

▶ Various screens can be stored on the system's hard drive and can be recalled or printed.

▶ Before using the transcranial Doppler system, be sure to remove turban head dressings or thick dressings over the test site.

## Documentation

▶ Record the date and the time that the monitoring began and which artery is being monitored.

▶ Document any patient teaching as well as the patient's tolerance of the procedure.

### REFERENCES

"Cerebral Microemboli and Cognitive Impairment." *Journal of Neurological Sciences* 203-204(c):211-14, November 2002.

Gupta, A.K. "Monitoring the Injured Brain in the Intensive Care Unit," *Journal of Postgraduate Medicine,* 48(3):218-25, July-September 2002.

# 8

# Gastrointestinal care

## Protocols 413

## Procedures 419

GASTROINTESTINAL (GI) CONDITIONS AFFECT JUST ABOUT EVERYONE AT ONE TIME OR another. These conditions, so intimately tied to psychological health and stability, range from simple changes in bowel habits to life-threatening disorders that require major surgery and radical lifestyle changes.

Care for the patient with a GI condition also varies widely. For example, the patient with simple constipation may need only brief teaching about diet and exercise. But someone with colorectal cancer may need ongoing nursing care ranging from encouragement and support during the diagnostic workup to meticulous colostomy care during recovery.

A patient having a GI procedure, especially one that's uncomfortable or embarrassing, needs considerable emotional support. Helping him maintain his sense of dignity while eliciting his cooperation requires a skillful blend of compassion and judgment.

# Protocols

## Managing the patient receiving enteral nutrition

### Purpose
To provide nutrition, calories, minerals, and vitamins to meet the metabolic requirements of the patient with a condition that prevents him from doing so on his own

### Collaborative level
Interdependent

### Expected patient outcomes
▶ The patient will receive tube feeding to meet metabolic body requirements.
▶ The patient will receive normal breathing pattern assessment during tube feeding administration.

### Definition of terms
▶ *Enteral nutrition:* Nutrients given via the GI tract when the patient can't swallow, chew, or ingest food but can still absorb nutrients.
▶ *Tube feeding:* Administration of enteral nutrition through a tube inserted into the stomach, duodenum, or jejunum.
▶ *Percutaneous endoscopic gastrostomy:* Tube for feeding that's placed directly in the stomach.
▶ *Jejunostomy tube:* Tube for feeding that's placed directly in the jejunum; commonly used if aspiration has occurred.

### Indications
Treatment
▶ Trouble swallowing or an inability to swallow
▶ Esophageal obstruction
▶ Cancer adjunct therapy
▶ Altered level of consciousness
▶ Head or neck surgery
▶ Facial trauma

Prevention
▶ Malnutrition
▶ Dehydration
▶ Electrolyte imbalances

### Assessment guidance
Signs and symptoms
▶ Trouble swallowing or an inability to swallow
▶ Unconscious or unable to be aroused
▶ Poor understanding of the need for nutrients
▶ Wounds or incisions on the face or neck region
▶ Thinning, lackluster hair
▶ Dry skin or mucous membranes
▶ Poor muscle tone

Diagnostic studies
*Laboratory tests*
▶ Hemoglobin and hematocrit
▶ Albumin
▶ Total protein
▶ Serum iron
▶ Transferrin level

▶ Cholesterol
▶ Lymphocyte count
▶ Mineral and vitamin levels
▶ Electrolyte levels

*Imaging tests*
▶ X-rays for obstructions or other abnormalities and to confirm tube placement after insertion
▶ Swallowing studies to assess swallowing reflex

## Nursing interventions
▶ Determine appropriate weight for the patient's age, sex, and height.
▶ Determine the patient's needed calorie intake.
▶ Monitor intake and output.
▶ Weigh the patient daily.
▶ Assess the patient's oral cavity and assist with oral hygiene as necessary.
▶ Monitor nutrition-influenced laboratory values.
▶ Give enteral feedings.
▶ Provide proper feeding tube care.
▶ Verify tube placement before feeding.
▶ Monitor the patient for residual gastric contents.
▶ Keep head of bed elevated 30 degrees for feedings.
▶ Assess the patient's respiratory system for signs of aspiration.

## Patient teaching
▶ Teach the importance of a well-balanced diet to meet the metabolic demands of daily living.
▶ Tell the patient to weigh himself every day.
▶ Discuss reasons for tube feedings with the patient.
▶ Teach the patient how tube feeding nutrition will assist with nutritional requirements.
▶ Teach the patient feeding tube care and maintenance.
▶ Tell patient how to change tube feeding setup.
▶ Instruct the patient about feeding formula preparation and safety.

## Precautions
▶ Monitor the patient for proper tube feeding placement and functioning and to prevent tube dislodgment.
▶ Ensure proper handling of feeding formula.

▶ Check expiration dates on tube formula.
▶ Monitor the patient for signs of aspiration if a nasogastric (NG) tube is present.
▶ Monitor the patient for changes in bowel habits and adjust formula as appropriate.

## Contraindications
▶ Intestinal obstruction
▶ Severe pancreatitis
▶ Intractable vomiting or diarrhea
▶ Paralytic ileus

## Documentation
▶ Document the patient's intake and output, calorie intake, and weight.
▶ Note the amount and rate of enteral nutrition and how the patient tolerated the feedings.
▶ Document tube care delivered and site observation.
▶ Document that teachings have been completed and note the patient's response.

## Related procedures
▶ Feeding tube insertion and removal
▶ Gastric lavage
▶ Gastrostomy feeding button care
▶ Gavage feeding
▶ Nasoenteric-decompression tube insertion and removal
▶ Nasogastric tube care
▶ Nasogastric tube insertion and removal
▶ Transabdominal tube feedings
▶ Tube feedings

### REFERENCES
Craven, R.F., and Hirnle, C.J. *Fundamentals of Nursing.* Philadelphia: Lippincott Williams & Wilkins, 2000.
Ignatavicius, D.D., and Workman, M.L. *Medical-Surgical Nursing.* Philadelphia: W.B. Saunders Co., 2002.
*Mosby's Medical, Nursing, & Allied Health Dictionary,* 6th ed. St. Louis: Mosby–Year Book, Inc., 2002.
Potter, P.A., and Perry, A.G. *Fundamentals of Nursing.* St. Louis: Mosby–Year Book, Inc., 2001.

# Managing the patient with a bowel diversion

## Purpose
To teach the patient about stoma and pouch care, to prevent or minimize complications

## Collaborative level
Interdependent

## Expected patient outcomes
▶ The patient will preserve positive body image and social contact.
▶ The patient will preserve skin integrity around the stoma site.

## Definition of terms
▶ *Stoma:* An opening created through the body surface; in this case, to drain bowel contents.
▶ *Ileostomy:* Surgically created opening of the ileum onto the abdominal surface, for the emptying of bowel contents.
▶ *Colostomy:* Surgically created opening of the colon onto the abdominal surface, for the emptying of bowel contents.
▶ *Continent ileostomy:* An ileostomy that drains into a created pouch or reservoir in the abdomen. Continence occurs through a one-way nipple valve.
▶ *Colostomy irrigation:* Instillation of fluid into the colon through the stoma, to stimulate bowel evacuation. This procedure establishes a pattern for regular bowel movements.
▶ *Ostomy pouch:* A collection appliance (pouch) to collect fecal contents from incontinent ostomies. Pouches are applied directly to abdominal skin and require a skin barrier for application. Skin barriers are sized according to stoma dimensions.

## Indications
### Treatment
▶ Bowel cancer
▶ Inflammatory bowel disease
▶ Tumors
▶ Severe abdominal trauma or wounds

### Prevention
▶ Bowel rest for severely inflamed bowel

## Assessment guidance
### Signs and symptoms
▶ Abdominal pain
▶ Bowel irregularity or change in bowel characteristics
▶ Vomiting
▶ Nausea
▶ Weight loss
▶ Abdominal tenderness or rigidity
▶ Abdominal mass

## Diagnostic studies
### Laboratory tests
▶ Hemoglobin and hematocrit
▶ Complete blood count (CBC)
▶ Electrolyte levels

### Imaging tests
▶ Abdominal X-ray
▶ Abdominal series
▶ Barium enema
▶ Endoscopy or colonoscopy

## Nursing interventions
▶ Assess the stoma.
▶ Care for, change, and empty the ostomy pouch.
▶ Irrigate the colostomy, if applicable.
▶ Provide emotional support.

## Patient teaching
▶ Teach the importance of a healthy stoma appearance.
▶ Instruct the patient on proper pouch fitting, changing, and emptying.
▶ Teach proper stoma care.
▶ Provide the patient with techniques to prevent odors.
▶ Teach about colostomy irrigation, if applicable.
▶ Tell the patient to avoid foods that cause gas or odors.

## Precautions
▶ Ensure proper pouch fitting to prevent leakage or skin irritation.

## Documentation
▶ Document stoma appearance and pouch contents and characteristics.
▶ Record the pouch-changing regimen, including wafer size and type of equipment used.
▶ Note the irrigation results.
▶ Document the patient's attitude toward appliance.

## Related procedures
▶ Colostomy and ileostomy care
▶ Continent ileostomy care

## REFERENCES
Craven, R.F., and Hirnle, C.J. *Fundamentals of Nursing.* Philadelphia: Lippincott Williams & Wilkins, 2000.
*Mosby's Medical, Nursing, & Allied Health Dictionary,* 6th ed. St. Louis: Mosby–Year Book, Inc., 2002.

Potter, P.A., and Perry, A.G. *Fundamentals of Nursing.* St. Louis: Mosby–Year Book, Inc., 2001.

Smeltzer, S.C., and Bare, B.G. *Brunner & Suddarth's Medical-Surgical Nursing.* Philadelphia: Lippincott Williams & Wilkins, 2000.

## ORGANIZATIONS

American Cancer Society: *www.cancer.org*

Crohn's and Colitis Foundation of America, 368 Park Avenue South, New York, NY 10016-8804

International Association for Enterostomal Therapy, 2081 Business Circle Drive, Suite 290, Irvine, CA 92715

International Foundation for Bowel Dysfunction, Box 17864, Milwaukee, WI 53217

National Foundation for Ileitis and Colitis, 295 Madison Avenue, New York, NY 10017

# Managing the patient with alteration in bowel function

## Purpose
To provide treatment measures to effectively induce a bowel movement and prevent future bowel alterations

## Collaborative level
Interdependent

## Expected patient outcomes
▶ The patient will pass soft, formed stool every 1 to 3 days.
▶ The patient will pass stool without straining.
▶ The patient will identify measures to prevent or treat constipation.

## Definition of terms
▶ *Constipation:* Abnormal infrequency or irregularity of bowel movements, hardening of the stool, or difficulty of stool passage.
▶ *Perceived constipation:* Subjective diagnosis of constipation, in which an individual's bowel pattern isn't consistent with his perceived-as-normal bowel habits. Commonly, laxatives are used and lead to chronic laxative abuse.
▶ *Fecal impaction:* Accumulation of hardened stool that an individual is unable to move. Seeping liquid diarrhea is often a sign because only liquid can pass the obstruction.

## Indications
### Treatment
▶ No bowel movement, accompanied by abdominal distention and discomfort
▶ Straining with attempted bowel evacuation
▶ Passage of hard, dry, minimal-amount stool

### Prevention
▶ History of frequent episodes of constipation
▶ Dependent use of laxatives to induce bowel movements
▶ Prescribed multiple medications that may cause constipation
▶ Limited physical mobility

## Assessment guidance
### Signs and symptoms
▶ No bowel movement for several days
▶ Discomfort in abdominal region
▶ Full feeling with abdominal pressure
▶ Decreased appetite
▶ Needing to strain for a small amount of hard stool
▶ Abdominal distention
▶ Palpable rectal mass
▶ Hard, dry, small-volume stool
▶ Borborygmus
▶ Abdominal area tender to palpate

### Diagnostic studies
*Laboratory tests*
▶ Fecal occult blood test

*Imaging tests*
▶ Barium enema
▶ Sigmoidoscopy

*Other*
▶ Digital rectal examination

## Nursing interventions
▶ Monitor the patient's bowel frequency and habits.
▶ Perform bowel assessment.
▶ Encourage physical activity.
▶ Encourage adequate fluid intake.
▶ Review the patient's current medications.
▶ Provide privacy for defecation.
▶ Monitor the patient for fecal impaction.

## Patient teaching
▶ Teach preventive measures of constipation, such as a high-fiber diet, fluid intake, and physical activity.)

▶ Tell the patient when to seek medical attention.

▶ Instruct the patient to attend to signs of defecation in a timely manner.

▶ Have the patient develop a bowel schedule by using a stimulus for bowel movements.

▶ Teach the patient about the proper use of laxatives and other bowel aids.

## Precautions
▶ Monitor the patient for signs of fecal impaction or obstruction.

## Contraindications
▶ Don't administer an enema if bowel obstruction is suspected.

▶ Don't administer an enema after prostate or rectal surgery.

## Documentation
▶ Record frequency and characteristics of all bowel movements.

▶ Document any aids used for defecation.

▶ Record patient's understanding of bowel habit instructions.

▶ Document abdominal assessment.

▶ Note signs and symptoms of altered bowel functioning.

## Related procedures
▶ Fecal occult blood test
▶ Stool collection

## REFERENCES
Ackley, B.J., and Ladwig, G.B. *Nursing Diagnosis Handbook.* St. Louis: Mosby–Year Book, Inc., 2002.

Ignatavicius, D.D., and Workman, M.L. *Medical-Surgical Nursing.* Philadelphia: W.B. Saunders Co., 2002.

Smeltzer, S.C., and Bare, B.G. *Brunner & Suddarth's Medical-Surgical Nursing.* Philadelphia: Lippincott Williams & Wilkins, 2000.

# Managing the patient with imbalanced nutrition

## Purpose
To provide sufficient nutrients to meet the daily metabolic demands to prevent or minimize complications of malnutrition

## Collaborative level
Interdependent

## Expected patient outcomes
▶ The patient will make progressive weight gain toward desirable goal or weight at appropriate goal.

▶ The patient will understand the need for sufficient calorie intake to balance metabolic demands.

▶ The patient won't develop malnutrition signs or symptoms.

▶ The patient will identify factors that led to imbalanced nutrition.

## Definition of terms
▶ *Malnutrition:* Disorder of nutrition resulting from unbalanced, insufficient dietary intake resulting from impaired absorption or intake.

▶ *Enteral nutrition:* Nutrients given via the GI tract when the patient can't swallow, chew, or ingest food but can still absorb nutrients.

▶ *Parenteral nutrition:* Nutrients given by a route other than the GI tract, usually the I.V. route.

▶ *Tube feeding:* Administration of enteral nutrition through a tube inserted into the stomach, duodenum, or jejunum.

▶ *Partial enteral nutrition:* Nutrients given through fortified supplements.

## Indications
Treatment
▶ Malnutrition
▶ Nothing-by-mouth status or receiving only standard I.V. therapy for more than 7 days
▶ Inability to maintain adequate nutrition through eating
▶ Inability to swallow
▶ Inability to consume nutrients because of critical illness
▶ Malabsorption syndrome
▶ Bowel rest from GI disorders

Prevention
▶ Upcoming GI surgery
▶ Need for increased calorie intake for anticipated healing or recovery

## Assessment guidance
Signs and symptoms
▶ Admitted weight loss
▶ Problems swallowing
▶ Altered taste sensation
▶ Aversion to eating
▶ Abdominal pain
▶ Nausea, vomiting, or diarrhea

▶ Dry skin
▶ Red, dry oral cavity
▶ Confusion
▶ Lackluster hair with possible thinning or loss
▶ Poor muscle tone

### Diagnostic studies
*Laboratory tests*
▶ Hemoglobin and hematocrit
▶ Albumin
▶ Total protein
▶ Serum iron
▶ Transferrin
▶ Cholesterol
▶ Lymphocyte count
▶ Mineral and vitamin levels
▶ Electrolyte levels
▶ Lactose tolerance test
▶ Schilling test

*Imaging tests*
▶ Small intestine biopsy
▶ GI X-rays
▶ Barium enema

## Nursing interventions
▶ Determine appropriate weight for the patient's age, sex, and height.
▶ Assist the patient with goal development for improving nutritional status and weight gain as needed.
▶ Monitor the patient's intake and output.
▶ Weigh the patient daily.
▶ Assess the patient's ability to consume nutrients.
▶ Assist the patient with nutritional intake as needed.
▶ Assess the patient's oral cavity and assist with oral hygiene as necessary.
▶ Make the patient's environment as pleasant as possible for mealtime.
▶ Assist the patient in planning his meal, providing choices that are nutritionally balanced.
▶ Monitor nutrition-influenced laboratory values.
▶ Provide nutritional supplements.
▶ Monitor the patient's enteral or parenteral feedings if applicable.
▶ Provide proper feeding tube care if applicable.

## Patient teaching
▶ Teach the importance of following a well-balanced diet to meet metabolic demands of daily living.
▶ Teach fundamentals of a well-balanced diet.
▶ Instruct the patient to weigh himself every day.
▶ Explain how to set a realistic weight goal and time frame.
▶ Explain the reasons for supplements to the patient.
▶ Teach how tube feeding will assist with nutritional requirements.
▶ Instruct the patient about feeding tube care and maintenance.
▶ Instruct the patient about how to change tube feeding setup.

## Precautions
▶ Monitor the patient for proper tube feeding placement and functioning and prevent dislodgment.
▶ Ensure proper handling of supplements.
▶ Check expiration dates on tube feedings and supplements.
▶ Monitor the patient for signs of aspiration if an NG tube is present.

## Contraindications
Enteral feedings
▶ Intestinal obstruction
▶ Severe pancreatitis
▶ Intractable vomiting or diarrhea
▶ Paralytic ileus

## Documentation
▶ Document intake and output.
▶ Note calorie intake.
▶ Record weight.
▶ Document percentage of meals and supplements taken.
▶ Document the amount and rate of enteral or parenteral nutrition and patient tolerance.
▶ Note tube care delivered and site observation.
▶ Record instructions completed and patient's response.

## Related procedures
▶ Feeding tube insertion and removal
▶ Gastric lavage
▶ Gastrostomy feeding button care
▶ Lipid emulsions
▶ Nasoenteric-decompression tube care

▶ Nasoenteric-decompression tube insertion and removal
▶ Nasogastric tube care
▶ Nasogastric tube insertion and removal
▶ Patient monitoring during parenteral nutrition
▶ Peripheral I.V. line insertion
▶ Peripheral I.V. line maintenance
▶ PICC insertion and removal
▶ Total parenteral nutrition
▶ Transabdominal tube feedings
▶ Tube feedings
▶ Venipuncture

### REFERENCES

Ackley, B.J., and Ladwig, G.B. *Nursing Diagnosis Handbook.* St. Louis: Mosby–Year Book, Inc., 2002.

Ignatavicius, D.D., and Workman, M.L. *Medical-Surgical Nursing.* Philadelphia: W.B. Saunders Co., 2002.

*Mosby's Medical, Nursing, & Allied Health Dictionary,* 6th ed. St. Louis: Mosby–Year Book, Inc., 2002.

Potter, P.A., and Perry, A.G. *Fundamentals of Nursing.* St. Louis: Mosby–Year Book, Inc., 2001.

Smeltzer, S.C., and Bare, B.G. *Brunner & Suddarth's Medical-Surgical Nursing.* Philadelphia: Lippincott Williams & Wilkins, 2000.

# Procedures

## Abdominal paracentesis

A bedside procedure, abdominal paracentesis involves the aspiration of fluid from the peritoneal space through a needle, trocar, or cannula inserted in the abdominal wall. Used to diagnose and treat massive ascites resistant to other therapy, the procedure helps determine the cause of ascites while relieving the pressure created by ascites. It may also precede other procedures, including radiography, peritoneal dialysis, and surgery. With abdominal paracentesis, the health care team can also detect intra-abdominal bleeding after traumatic injury and obtain a peritoneal fluid specimen for laboratory analysis. The procedure must be performed cautiously in pregnant patients and in those with bleeding tendencies or unstable vital signs.

Nursing responsibilities during abdominal paracentesis include preparing the patient, monitoring his condition and providing emotional support during the procedure, assisting the doctor, and obtaining specimens for laboratory analysis.

### Equipment

Tape measure ● sterile gloves ● clean gloves ● gown ● goggles ● linen-saver pads ● four Vacutainer laboratory tubes ● two large glass Vacutainer bottles (1,000 ml or larger) ● dry, sterile pressure dressing ● laboratory request forms ● povidone-iodine solution ● local anesthetic (multidose vial of 1% or 2% lidocaine with epinephrine) ● 4″ × 4″ sterile gauze pads ● sterile paracentesis tray (containing needle, trocar, cannula, three-way stopcock) ● disposable sterile drapes ● marking pen ● 5-ml syringe with 22G or 25G needle ● optional: povidone-iodine ointment, alcohol sponge, 50-ml syringe, suture materials, and salt-poor albumin

### Implementation

▶ Explain the procedure to the patient to ease his anxiety and promote cooperation. Reassure him that he should feel no pain, but that he may feel a stinging sensation from the local anesthetic injection and pressure from the needle or trocar and cannula insertion. He may also sense pressure when the doctor aspirates abdominal fluid.
▶ Make sure to obtain the patient's signed consent form.
▶ Instruct the patient to void before the procedure; or insert an indwelling urinary catheter, if ordered, to minimize the risk of accidental bladder injury from the needle or trocar and cannula insertion.

# Positioning the patient for abdominal paracentesis

Help the patient sit up in bed, or allow him to sit on the side of the bed with additional support for his back and arms.

When the patient takes this position, gravity helps fluid to accumulate in the lower abdominal cavity. The internal abdominal structures provide counterresistance and additional pressure to facilitate fluid flow.

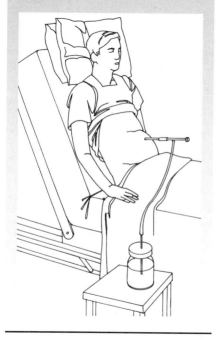

▶ Identify and record baseline values: vital signs, weight, and abdominal girth. (Use the tape measure to gauge the patient's abdominal girth at the umbilical level.) Indicate the abdominal area measured with a felt-tipped marking pen. Baseline data will be used to monitor the patient's status.
▶ Help the patient sit up in bed or in a chair that fully supports his arms and legs so that fluid accumulates in the lower abdomen. Or help him sit on the side of the bed and use pillows to support his back. (See *Positioning the patient for abdominal paracentesis.*)

▶ Expose the patient's abdomen from diaphragm to pubis. Keep the rest of the patient covered to avoid chilling him.
▶ Make the patient as comfortable as possible, and place a linen-saver pad under him for protection from drainage.
▶ Remind the patient to stay as still as possible during the procedure to prevent injury from the needle or trocar and cannula.
▶ Wash your hands. Open the paracentesis tray using aseptic technique to ensure a sterile field. Next, put on gloves before assisting the doctor as he prepares the patient's abdomen with povidone-iodine solution, drapes the operative site with sterile drapes, and administers the local anesthetic.
▶ If the paracentesis tray doesn't contain a sterile ampule of anesthetic, wipe the top of a multidose vial of anesthetic solution with an alcohol sponge, and invert the vial at a 45-degree angle. This will allow the doctor to insert the sterile 5-ml syringe with the 22G or 25G needle and withdraw the anesthetic without touching the nonsterile vial.
▶ Using the scalpel, the doctor may make a small incision before inserting the needle or trocar and cannula (usually 1″ to 2″ [2.5 to 5 cm] below the umbilicus). Listen for a popping sound. This signifies that the needle or trocar has pierced the peritoneum.
▶ Assist the doctor collect specimens in the proper containers. Wear clean gloves, gown, and goggles to protect you from possible body fluid contamination. If the doctor orders substantial drainage, connect the three-way stopcock and tubing to the cannula. Run the other end of the tubing to a large sterile Vacutainer. Or aspirate the fluid with a three-way stopcock and 50-ml syringe.
▶ Gently turn the patient from side to side to enhance drainage, if necessary.
▶ As the fluid drains, monitor the patient's vital signs every 15 minutes. Observe him closely for vertigo, faintness, diaphoresis, pallor, heightened anxiety, tachycardia, dyspnea, and hypotension, especially if more than 1,500 ml of peritoneal fluid was aspirated at one time. This loss may induce a fluid shift and hypovolemic shock.
▶ Immediately report signs of shock to the doctor; he may order you to administer salt-poor albumin I.V. to prevent hypovolemia and a decline in renal function.

▶ When the procedure ends and the doctor removes the needle or trocar and cannula, he may suture the incision. Wearing sterile gloves, apply the dry, sterile pressure dressing and povidone-iodine ointment to the site. Help the patient assume a comfortable position.

▶ Monitor the patient's vital signs and check the dressing for drainage every 15 minutes for 1 hour, every 30 minutes for 2 hours, every hour for 4 hours, and then every 4 hours for 24 hours to detect delayed reactions to the procedure. Make sure to note drainage color, amount, and character.

▶ Label the Vacutainer specimen tubes, and send them to the laboratory with the appropriate laboratory request forms. If the patient is receiving antibiotics, note this on the request form. This information will be considered during the fluid analysis.

▶ Make sure that you remove and dispose of all equipment properly.

## Special considerations

▶ Throughout this procedure, try to help the patient remain still to prevent accidental perforation of abdominal organs.

▶ If the patient shows any signs of hypovolemic shock, reduce the vertical distance between the needle or the trocar and cannula and the drainage collection container to slow the drainage rate. If necessary, stop the drainage.

▶ To prevent fluid shifts and hypovolemia, limit aspirated fluid to between 1,500 and 2,000 ml. If peritoneal fluid doesn't flow easily, try repositioning the patient to facilitate drainage. Also, verify suction in the Vacutainer collection bottle when you connect it to the drainage tubing, and be sure to use macrodrip tubing without a backflow device.

▶ After the procedure, observe for peritoneal fluid leakage. If this develops, notify the doctor. Always maintain daily patient weight and abdominal girth records. Compare these values with the baseline figures to detect recurrent ascites.

## Complications

Removing large amounts of fluid may cause hypotension, oliguria, and hyponatremia. If an excessive amount of fluid (more than 2 L) is removed, ascitic fluid tends to form again, drawing fluid from extracellular tissue throughout the body. Oth-er possible complications include perforation of abdominal organs by the needle or the trocar and cannula, wound infection, and peritonitis.

## Documentation

▶ Record the date and time of the procedure, the puncture site location, and whether the wound was sutured.

▶ Document the amount, color, viscosity, and odor of aspirated fluid in your notes and in the fluid intake and output record.

▶ Record the patient's vital signs, weight, and abdominal girth measurements before and after the procedure.

▶ Note the patient's tolerance of the procedure, vital signs, and any signs and symptoms of complications during the procedure.

▶ Document the number of specimens sent to the laboratory

## REFERENCES

Edward, D., et al. *Bedside Critical Care Manual.* Philadelphia: Lippincott Williams & Wilkins, 2001.

Stephenson, J., and Gilbert, J. "The Development of Clinical Guidelines on Paracentesis for Ascites Related to Malignancy," *Palliative Medicine* 16(3):213-18, May 2002.

# Colostomy and ileostomy care

A patient with an ascending or transverse colostomy or an ileostomy must wear an external pouch to collect emerging fecal matter, which will be watery or pasty. Besides collecting waste matter, the pouch helps to control odor and protect the stoma and peristomal skin. Most disposable pouching systems can be used for 2 to 7 days; some models last even longer.

All pouching systems need to be changed immediately if a leak develops, and every pouch must be emptied when it's one-third to one-half full. The patient with an ileostomy may need to empty his pouch four or five times daily.

Naturally, the best time to change the pouching system is when the bowel is least active, usually between 2 and 4 hours after meals. After a few months, most patients can predict the best changing time.

The selection of a pouching system should take into consideration which sys-

# Comparing ostomy pouching systems

Manufactured in many shapes and sizes, ostomy pouches are fashioned for comfort, safety, and easy application. For example, a disposable closed-end pouch may meet the needs of a patient who irrigates his ostomy, who wants added security, or who wants to discard the pouch after each bowel movement. Another patient may prefer a reusable, drainable pouch. Some commonly available pouches are described below.

### Disposable pouches

The patient who must empty his pouch often (because of diarrhea or a new colostomy or ileostomy) may prefer a one-piece, drainable, disposable pouch with a closure clamp attached to a skin barrier (below left).

These transparent or opaque, odor-proof, plastic pouches come with attached adhesive or karaya seals. Some pouches have microporous adhesive or belt tabs. The bottom opening allows for easy draining. This pouch may be used permanently or temporarily, until stoma size stabilizes.

Also disposable and made of transparent or opaque odor-proof plastic, a one-piece disposable closed-end pouch (below right) may come in a kit with adhesive seal, belt tabs, skin barrier, or carbon filter for gas release. A patient with a regular bowel elimination pattern may choose this style for additional security and confidence.

Also made of transparent or opaque odor-proof plastic, this style comes with belt tabs and usually snaps to the skin barrier with a flange mechanism.

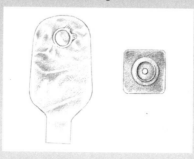

### Reusable pouches

Typically manufactured from sturdy, opaque, hypoallergenic plastic, the reusable pouch comes with a separate custom-made faceplate and O-ring (as shown below). Some pouches have a pressure valve for releasing gas. The device has a 1- to 2-month life span, depending on how frequently the patient empties the pouch.

Reusable equipment may benefit a patient who needs a firm faceplate or who wishes to minimize cost. However, many reusable ostomy pouches aren't odor-proof.

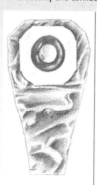
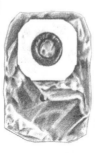

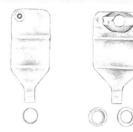

A two-piece disposable drainable pouch with separate skin barrier (top of next column) permits frequent changes and also minimizes skin breakdown.

tem provides the best adhesive seal and skin protection for the individual patient. The type of pouch selected also depends on the stoma's location and structure, availability of supplies, wear time, consistency of effluent, personal preference, and finances.

Pouching systems may be drainable or closed-bottomed, disposable or reusable, adhesive-backed, and one-piece or two-piece. (See *Comparing ostomy pouching systems.*)

## Equipment

Pouching system • stoma measuring guide • stoma paste (if drainage is watery to pasty or stoma secretes excess mucus) • plastic bag • water • washcloth and towel • closure clamp • toilet or bedpan • water or pouch cleaning solution • gloves • facial tissues • optional: ostomy belt, paper tape, mild nonmoisturizing soap, skin shaving equipment, liquid skin sealant, pouch deodorant

## Implementation

Provide privacy and emotional support.

### Fitting the pouch and skin barrier

▶ For a pouch with an attached skin barrier, measure the stoma with the stoma measuring guide. Select the opening size that matches the stoma.

▶ For an adhesive-backed pouch with a separate skin barrier, measure the stoma with the measuring guide and select the opening that matches the stoma. Trace the selected size opening onto the paper back of the skin barrier's adhesive side. Cut out the opening. (If the pouch has precut openings, which can be handy for a round stoma, select an opening that is ⅛" larger than the stoma. If the pouch comes without an opening, cut the hole ⅛" wider than the measured tracing.) The cut-to-fit system works best for an irregularly shaped stoma.

▶ For a two-piece pouching system with flanges, see *Applying a skin barrier and pouch,* page 424.

▶ Avoid fitting the pouch too tightly because the stoma has no pain receptors. A constrictive opening could injure the stoma or skin tissue without the patient feeling warning discomfort. Also avoid cutting the opening too big because this may expose the skin to fecal matter and moisture.

▶ The patient with a descending or sigmoid colostomy who has formed stools and whose ostomy doesn't secrete much mucus may choose to wear only a pouch. In this case, make sure the pouch opening closely matches the stoma size.

▶ Between 6 weeks and 1 year after surgery, the stoma will shrink to its permanent size. At that point, pattern-making

preparations will be unnecessary unless the patient gains weight, has additional surgery, or injures the stoma.

### Applying or changing the pouch

▶ Collect all equipment.

▶ Wash your hands and provide privacy.

▶ Explain the procedure to the patient. As you perform each step, explain what you are doing and why because the patient will eventually perform the procedure himself.

▶ Put on gloves.

▶ Remove and discard the old pouch. Wipe the stoma and peristomal skin gently with a facial tissue.

▶ Carefully wash with mild soap and water and dry the peristomal skin by patting gently. Allow the skin to dry thoroughly. Inspect the peristomal skin and stoma. If necessary, shave surrounding hair (in a direction away from the stoma) to promote a better seal and avoid skin irritation from hair pulling against the adhesive.

▶ If applying a separate skin barrier, peel off the paper backing of the prepared skin barrier, center the barrier over the stoma, and press gently to ensure adhesion.

▶ You may want to outline the stoma on the back of the skin barrier (depending on the product) with a thin ring of stoma paste to provide extra skin protection. (Skip this step if the patient has a sigmoid or descending colostomy, formed stools, and little mucus.)

▶ Remove the paper backing from the adhesive side of the pouching system and center the pouch opening over the stoma. Press gently to secure.

▶ For a pouching system with flanges, align the lip of the pouch flange with the bottom edge of the skin barrier flange. Gently press around the circumference of the pouch flange, beginning at the bottom, until the pouch securely adheres to the barrier flange. (The pouch will click into its secured position.) Holding the barrier against the skin, gently pull on the pouch to confirm the seal between flanges.

▶ Encourage the patient to stay quietly in position for about 5 minutes to improve adherence. The patient's body warmth also helps to improve adherence and soften a rigid skin barrier.

▶ Attach an ostomy belt to further secure the pouch, if desired. (Some pouches have

# Applying a skin barrier and pouch

Fitting a skin barrier and ostomy pouch properly can be done in a few steps. Shown below is a two-piece pouching system with flanges, which is commonly used.

Measure the stoma using a measuring guide.

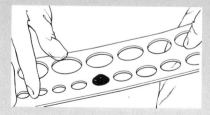

Trace the appropriate circle carefully on the back of the skin barrier.

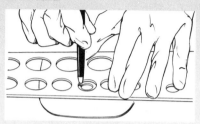

Cut the circular opening in the skin barrier. Bevel the edges to keep them from irritating the patient.

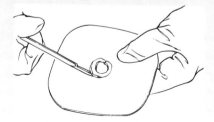

Remove the backing from the skin barrier and moisten it or apply barrier paste as needed along the edge of the circular opening.

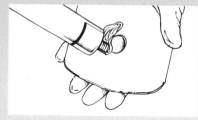

Center the skin barrier over the stoma, adhesive side down, and gently press it to the skin.

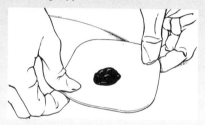

Gently press the pouch opening onto the ring until it snaps into place.

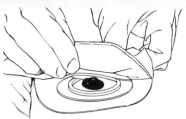

belt loops, and others have plastic adapters for belts.)
▶ Leave a bit of air in the pouch to allow drainage to fall to the bottom.
▶ Apply the closure clamp, if necessary.
▶ If desired, apply paper tape in a picture-frame fashion to the pouch edges for additional security.

## Emptying the pouch
▶ Put on gloves.
▶ Tilt the bottom of the pouch upward and remove the closure clamp.
▶ Turn up a cuff on the lower end of the pouch and allow it to drain into the toilet or bedpan.
▶ Wipe the bottom of the pouch and reapply the closure clamp.

If desired, the bottom portion of the pouch can be rinsed with cool tap water. Don't aim water up near the top of the pouch because this may loosen the seal on the skin.

A two-piece flanged system can also be emptied by unsnapping the pouch. Let the drainage flow into the toilet.

Release flatus through the gas release valve if the pouch has one. Otherwise, release flatus by tilting the pouch bottom upward, releasing the clamp, and expelling the flatus. To release flatus from a flanged system, loosen the seal between the flanges. (Some pouches have gas release valves.)

Never make a pinhole in a pouch to release gas. This destroys the odor-proof seal.

Remove gloves.

## Special considerations

After performing and explaining the procedure to the patient, encourage the patient's increasing involvement in self-care.

Use adhesive solvents and removers only after patch-testing the patient's skin because some products may irritate the skin or produce hypersensitivity reactions. Consider using a liquid skin sealant, if available, to give skin tissue additional protection from drainage and adhesive irritants.

Remove the pouching system if the patient reports burning or itching beneath it or purulent drainage around the stoma. Notify the doctor or therapist of any skin irritation, breakdown, rash, or unusual appearance of the stoma or peristomal area.

Use commercial pouch deodorants, if desired. However, most pouches are odor-free, and odor should only be evident when you empty the pouch or if it leaks. Before discharge, suggest that the patient avoid odor-causing foods, such as fish, eggs, onions, and garlic.

If the patient wears a reusable pouching system, suggest that he obtain two or more systems so that he can wear one while the other dries after cleaning with soap and water or a commercially prepared cleaning solution.

## Complications

Failure to fit the pouch properly over the stoma or improper use of a belt can injure the stoma. Be alert for a possible allergic reaction to adhesives and other ostomy products.

## Documentation

Record the date and time of the pouching system change.

Note the character of drainage, including color, amount, type, and consistency.

Document the appearance of the stoma and the peristomal skin.

Document patient teaching and describe the teaching content.

Record the patient's response to self-care and evaluate his learning progress.

## REFERENCES

Craven, R., and Hirnle, C.J. *Fundamentals of Nursing: Human Health and Function.* 4th ed. Philadelphia: Lippincott Williams & Wilkins, 2002.

# Continent ileostomy care

An alternative to a conventional ileostomy, a continent, or pouch, ileostomy (also called a Kock ileostomy or an ileal pouch) features an internal reservoir fashioned from the terminal ileum. This procedure may be used for a patient who requires proctocolectomy for chronic ulcerative colitis or multiple polyposis. Other patients may have a traditional ileostomy converted to a continent ileostomy. This procedure is contraindicated in Crohn's disease or gross obesity. Patients who need emergency surgery and those who can't care for the pouch are also unlikely to have this procedure.

The length of preoperative hospitalization varies with the patient's condition. Nursing responsibilities include providing bowel preparation, antibiotic therapy, and emotional support. After surgery, nursing responsibilities include ensuring patency of the drainage catheter, assessing GI function, caring for the stoma and peristomal skin, managing pain resulting from surgery and, if necessary, perineal skin care.

Daily patient teaching on pouch intubation and drainage usually begins soon after surgery. Continuous drainage is maintained for about 2 to 6 weeks to allow the suture lines to heal. During this period, a drainage catheter is attached to low intermittent suction. After the suture line heals, the patient learns how to drain the pouch himself.

## Understanding pouch construction

Depending on the patient and related factors during intestinal surgery, the doctor may construct a pouch to collect fecal matter internally. To make such a pouch, the doctor loops about 12" (30 cm) of ileum and sutures the inner sides together.

He opens the loop with a U-shaped cut and seams the inside to create a smooth lining. Then he fashions a nipple or valve between what is becoming the pouch and what will be the stoma. He folds the open ileum over, sews the pouch closed, and fixes the pouch to the abdominal wall.

Because the pouch holds fecal matter in reserve, the patient benefits from not having to change and empty ostomy equipment. Instead, he empties and irrigates the pouch as needed by inserting a catheter through the stoma and into the pouch.

Initially after surgery, the nurse performs this procedure until the patient can do it himself.

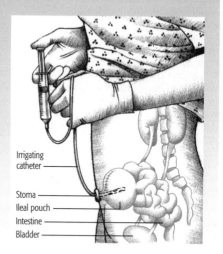

Irrigating catheter —

Stoma —
Ileal pouch —
Intestine —
Bladder —

## Equipment

Leg drainage bag ● bedside drainage bag ● normal saline solution ● 50-ml catheter-tip syringe ● extra continent ileostomy catheter ● 4" × 4" × 1" foam dressing and Montgomery straps ● 20-ml syringe with adapter ● precut drain dressing ● gloves ● water-soluble lubricant ● graduated container ● skin sealant ● optional: commercial catheter securing device

## Implementation

Nursing interventions for a patient undergoing a continent ileostomy range from standard preoperative and postoperative care to pouch care and patient teaching.

### Preoperative care

▶ Reinforce and, if necessary, supplement the doctor's explanation of a continent ileostomy and its implications for the patient. (See *Understanding pouch construction*.)
▶ Assess patient and family attitudes related to the operation and to the forthcoming changes in the patient's body image.
▶ Provide encouragement and support.

### Postoperative care

▶ When the patient returns to his room, attach the drainage catheter emerging from the ileostomy to continuous gravity drainage.
▶ A leg drainage bag may be attached to the patient's thigh during ambulation.
▶ Irrigate the catheter with 30 ml of normal saline solution as ordered and needed to prevent catheter obstruction and allow fluid return by gravity. During the early postoperative period, keep the pouch empty; drainage will be serosanguineous.
▶ Monitor fluid intake and output.
▶ Check the catheter frequently once the patient begins eating solid food to ensure that neither mucus nor undigested food particles block it.
▶ If the patient complains of abdominal cramps, distention, and nausea—symptoms of bowel obstruction—the catheter may be clogged. Gently irrigate with 20 to 30 ml of water or normal saline solution until the catheter drains freely. Then move the catheter slightly or rotate it gently to help clear the obstruction. Finally, try milking the catheter. If these measures fail, notify the doctor.
▶ Check the stoma frequently for color, edema, and bleeding. Normally pink to red, a stoma that turns dark red or blue-red may have a compromised blood supply.
▶ To care for the stoma and peristomal skin, put on gloves. Remove the dressing, gently clean the peristomal area with water

and pat it dry. Use a skin sealant around the stoma to prevent skin irritation.

▶ One way to apply a stoma dressing is to slip a precut drain dressing around the catheter to cover the stoma. Cut a hole slightly larger than the lumen of the catheter in the center of a 4″ × 4″ × 1″ piece of foam. Disconnect the catheter from the drainage bag and insert the distal end of the catheter through the hole in the foam. Slide the foam pad onto the dressing. Secure the foam in place with Montgomery straps. Secure the catheter by wrapping the strap ties around it or by using a commercial catheter securing device. Then reconnect the catheter to the drainage bag. (The surgeon will remove the drainage catheter when he determines that the suture line has healed.)

▶ Assess the peristomal skin for irritation from moisture.

▶ To reduce discomfort from gas pains, encourage the patient to ambulate. Also recommend that he avoid swallowing air (to minimize gas pains) by chewing food well, limiting conversation while eating, and not drinking from a straw.

## Draining the pouch

▶ Provide privacy, explain the procedure to the patient, and wash your hands.

▶ Put on gloves.

▶ Have the patient with a pouch conversion sit on the toilet to help him feel more at ease during the procedure.

▶ Remove the stoma dressing.

▶ Encourage the patient to relax his abdominal muscles to allow the catheter to slide easily into the pouch.

▶ Lubricate the tip of the drainage catheter tip with the water-soluble lubricant and insert it in the stoma. Gently push the catheter downward. (The direction of insertion may vary depending on the patient.)

▶ When the catheter reaches the nipple valve of the internal pouch or reservoir (after about 2″ or 2½″ [5 or 6.5 cm]), you'll feel resistance. Instruct the patient to take a deep breath as you exert gentle pressure on the catheter to insert it through the valve. If this fails, have the patient lie supine and rest for a few minutes. Then, with the patient still supine, try to insert the catheter again.

▶ Gently advance the catheter to the suture marking made by the surgeon.

▶ Let the pouch drain completely. This usually takes 5 to 10 minutes. With thick drainage or a clogged catheter, the process may take 30 minutes.

▶ If the tube clogs, irrigate with 30 ml of water or normal saline using the 50-ml catheter-tip syringe. Also, rotate and milk the tube. If these steps fail, remove, rinse, and reinsert the catheter.

▶ Remove the catheter after completing drainage.

▶ Measure output, subtracting the amount of irrigant used.

▶ Rinse the catheter thoroughly with warm water.

▶ Clean the peristomal area and apply a fresh stoma dressing.

## Predischarge teaching

▶ Make sure the patient can properly intubate and drain the pouch himself.

▶ Provide the patient with appropriate equipment. If the postoperative drainage catheter is still in place, teach the patient how to care for it properly.

▶ Make sure the patient has a pouch-draining schedule and give him appropriate pamphlets or video instructions on pouch care.

▶ Make sure the patient feels comfortable calling the doctor, nurse, or appropriate other caregivers with questions or problems.

▶ Tell the patient where to obtain supplies.

▶ Refer the patient to a local ostomy group.

▶ Provide dietary counseling.

## Special considerations

▶ Never aspirate fluid from the catheter because the resulting negative pressure may damage inflamed tissue.

▶ The first few times you intubate the pouch, the patient may be tense, making insertion difficult. Encourage relaxation. To shorten drainage time, have the patient cough, press gently on his abdomen over the pouch, or suddenly tighten his abdominal muscles and then relax them.

▶ Keep an accurate record of intake and output to ensure fluid and electrolyte balance. The average daily output should be 1,000 ml. Report inadequate or excessive output (more than 1,400 ml daily).

## Complications

Common postoperative complications include obstruction, fistula, pouch perforation, nipple valve dysfunction, abscesses, diarrhea, skin irritation, stenosis of the stoma, and bacterial overgrowth in the pouch.

## Documentation

▶ Record the date, time, and all aspects of preoperative and postoperative care.
▶ Document the condition of the stoma and peristomal skin.
▶ Document diet, medications.
▶ Record intubations.
▶ Document patient teaching and discharge planning.

### REFERENCES

Edward, D., et al. *Bedside Critical Care Manual*. Philadelphia: Lippincott Williams & Wilkins, 2001.
Litle, V.R., et al. "The Continent Ileostomy: Long-term Durability and Patient Satisfaction," *Journal of Gastrointestinal Surgery* 3(6):625-32, November-December 1999.

# Esophageal tube care

Although the doctor inserts an esophageal tube, the nurse cares for the patient during and after intubation. Typically, the patient is in the intensive care unit for close observation and constant care. The environment may help to increase the patient's tolerance for the procedure and may help to control bleeding. Sedatives may be contraindicated, especially for a patient with portal systemic encephalopathy.

Most important, the patient who has an esophageal tube in place to control variceal bleeding (typically from portal hypertension) must be observed closely for esophageal rupture because varices weaken the esophagus. Additionally, possible traumatic injury from intubation or esophageal balloon inflation increases the chance of rupture. Emergency surgery is usually performed if a rupture occurs, but the operation has a low success rate.

## Equipment

Manometer ● two 2-L bottles of normal saline solution ● irrigation set ● water-soluble lubricant ● several cotton-tipped applicators ● mouth-care equipment ● nasopharyngeal suction apparatus ● several #12 French suction catheters ● intake and output record sheets ● gloves ● goggles ●

sedatives ● traction weights or football helmet ● scissors

## Implementation

▶ To ease the patient's anxiety, explain the care that you'll give.
▶ Provide privacy. Wash your hands and put on gloves and goggles.
▶ Monitor the patient's vital signs every 5 minutes to 1 hour as ordered. A change in vital signs may signal complications or recurrent bleeding.
▶ If the patient has a Sengstaken-Blakemore or Minnesota tube, check the pressure gauge on the manometer every 30 to 60 minutes to detect any leaks in the esophageal balloon and to verify the set pressure.
▶ Maintain drainage and suction on gastric and esophageal aspiration ports as ordered. This is important because fluid accumulating in the stomach may cause the patient to regurgitate the tube, and fluid accumulating in the esophagus may lead to vomiting and aspiration.
▶ Irrigate the gastric aspiration port as ordered, using the irrigation set and normal saline solution. Frequent irrigation keeps the tube from clogging. Obstruction in the tube can lead to regurgitation of the tube and vomiting.
▶ To prevent pressure ulcers, clean the patient's nostrils and apply water-soluble lubricant frequently. Use warm water to loosen crusted nasal secretions before applying the lubricant with cotton-tipped applicators.
▶ Provide mouth care often to rid the patient's mouth of foul-tasting matter and to relieve dryness from mouth breathing.
▶ Use #12 French catheters to provide gentle oral suctioning, if necessary, to help remove secretions.
▶ Offer emotional support. Keep the patient as quiet as possible and administer sedatives, if ordered.
▶ A football helmet or traction weights may be used to secure the tube. If used, make sure that the traction weights hang from the foot of the bed at all times. Never rest them on the bed. Instruct housekeepers and other coworkers not to move the weights because reduced traction may change the position of the tube.
▶ Elevate the head of the bed about 25 degrees to ensure countertraction for the weights.

▶ Keep the patient on complete bed rest because exertion, such as coughing or straining, increases intra-abdominal pressure, which may trigger further bleeding.

▶ Keep the patient in semi-Fowler's position to reduce blood flow into the portal system and to prevent reflux into the esophagus.

▶ Monitor intake and output as ordered.

## Special considerations

▶ Observe the patient carefully for esophageal rupture indicated by signs and symptoms of shock, increased respiratory difficulties, and increased bleeding. Tape scissors to the head of the bed so you can cut the tube quickly to deflate the balloons if asphyxia develops. When performing this emergency intervention, hold the tube firmly close to the nostril before cutting.

▶ If using traction, release the tension before deflating any balloons. If weights and pulleys supply traction, remove the weights. If a football helmet supplies traction, untape the esophageal tube from the face guard before deflating the balloons. Deflating the balloon under tension triggers a rapid release of the entire tube from the nose, which may injure mucous membranes, initiate recurrent bleeding, and obstruct the airway.

▶ If the doctor orders an X-ray study to check the tube's position or to view the chest, lift the patient in the direction of the pulley and then place the X-ray film behind his back. Never roll him from side to side because pressure exerted on the tube in this way may shift the tube's position. Similarly, lift the patient to make the bed or to assist him with the bedpan.

## Complications

Esophageal rupture, the most life-threatening complication associated with esophageal balloon tamponade, can occur at any time but is most likely to occur during intubation or inflation of the esophageal balloon. Asphyxia may result if the balloon moves up the esophagus and blocks the airway. Aspiration of pooled esophageal secretions may also complicate this procedure.

## Documentation

▶ Read the manometer hourly and record the esophageal pressures.

▶ Record when the balloons are deflated and by whom.

▶ Document vital signs, the condition of the patient's nostrils, routine care, and any drugs administered.

▶ Record the color, consistency, and amount of gastric returns.

▶ Record any signs and symptoms of complications and the nursing actions taken.

▶ Document gastric port and NG tube irrigations.

▶ Maintain accurate intake and output records.

## REFERENCES

Alvares, J.F., et al. "Tracheal Obstruction After Insertion of a Self-expanding Metal Esophageal Stent: Successful Management with an Endotracheal Tube,.Steroids, and Radiotherapy," *Endoscopy* 34(7):592, July 2002.

Edward, D., et al. *Bedside Critical Care Manual.* Philadelphia: Lippincott Williams & Wilkins, 2001.

# Esophageal tube insertion and removal

Used to control hemorrhage from esophageal or gastric varices, an esophageal tube is inserted nasally or orally and advanced into the esophagus or stomach. Ordinarily, a doctor inserts and removes the tube. In an emergency situation, a nurse may remove it.

Once the tube is in place, a gastric balloon secured at the end of the tube can be inflated and drawn tightly against the cardia of the stomach. The inflated balloon secures the tube and exerts pressure on the cardia. The pressure, in turn, controls the bleeding varices.

Most tubes also contain an esophageal balloon to control esophageal bleeding. (See *Types of esophageal tubes,* page 430.) Usually, gastric or esophageal balloons are deflated after 24 hours. If the balloon remains inflated longer than 24 hours, pressure necrosis may develop and cause further hemorrhage or perforation.

Other procedures to control bleeding include irrigation with tepid or iced saline solution and drug therapy with a vasopressor. Used with the esophageal tube, these procedures provide effective, temporary control of acute variceal hemorrhage.

# Types of esophageal tubes

When working with patients who have an esophageal tube, remember the advantages of the most common types.

### Sengstaken-Blakemore tube

This triple-lumen, double-balloon tube has a gastric aspiration port, which allows you to obtain drainage from below the gastric balloon and to instill medication.

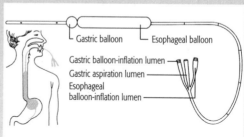

### Linton tube

This triple-lumen, single-balloon tube has a port for gastric aspiration and one for esophageal aspiration as well. Additionally, the Linton tube reduces the risk of esophageal necrosis because it doesn't have an esophageal balloon.

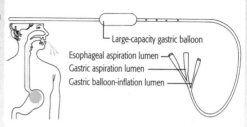

### Minnesota esophagogastric tamponade tube

This esophageal tube has four lumens and two balloons. The device provides pressure-monitoring ports for both balloons without the need for Y-connectors. One port is used for gastric suction; the other for esophageal suction.

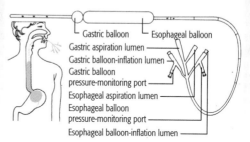

## Equipment

Esophageal tube ● NG tube (if using a Sengstaken-Blakemore tube) ● two suction sources ● basin of ice ● irrigation set ● 2 L of normal saline solution ● two 60-ml syringes ● water-soluble lubricant ● ½" or 1" adhesive tape ● stethoscope ● foam nose guard ● four rubber-shod clamps (two clamps and two plastic plugs for a Minnesota tube) ● anesthetic spray (as ordered) ● traction equipment (football helmet or a basic frame with traction rope, pulleys, and a 1-lb [0.5-kg] weight) ● mercury aneroid manometer ● Y-connector tube (for Sengstaken-Blakemore or Linton tube) ● basin of water ● cup of water with straw ● scissors ● gloves ● gown ● waterproof marking pen ● goggles ● sphygmomanometer

## Preparation of equipment

Keep the traction helmet at the bedside or attach traction equipment to the bed so that either is readily available after tube insertion. Place the suction machines nearby and plug them in. Open the irrigation set and fill the container with normal saline solution. Place all equipment within reach.

Test the balloons on the esophageal tube for air leaks by inflating them and submerging them in the basin of water. If no bubbles appear in the water, the balloons are intact. Remove them from the water and deflate them. Clamp the tube lumens, so that the balloons stay deflated during insertion.

To prepare the Minnesota tube, connect the mercury aneroid manometer to the gastric pressure monitoring port. Note the pressure when the balloon fills with 100, 200, 300, 400, and 500 cc of air.

Check the aspiration lumens for patency and make sure that they're labeled according to their purpose. If they aren't identified, label them carefully with the marking pen.

Chill the tube in a basin of ice. This will stiffen it and facilitate insertion.

## Implementation

▶ Explain the procedure and its purpose to the patient and provide privacy.
▶ Wash your hands and put on gloves, gown, and goggles to protect yourself from splashing blood.
▶ Assist the patient into semi-Fowler's position and turn him slightly toward his left side. This position promotes stomach emptying and helps prevent aspiration.
▶ Explain that the doctor will inspect the patient's nostrils (for patency).
▶ To determine the length of tubing needed, hold the balloon at the patient's xiphoid process and then extend the tube to the patient's ear and forward to his nose. Using a waterproof pen, mark this point on the tubing.
▶ Inform the patient that the doctor will spray his throat (posterior pharynx) and nostril with an anesthetic to minimize discomfort and gagging during intubation.
▶ After lubricating the tip of the tube with water-soluble lubricant to reduce friction and facilitate insertion, the doctor will pass the tube through the more patent nostril. As he does, he'll direct the patient to tilt his chin toward his chest and to swallow when he senses the tip of the tube in the back of his throat. Swallowing helps to advance the tube into the esophagus and prevents intubation of the trachea. (If the doctor introduces the tube orally, he'll direct the patient to swallow immediately.) As the patient swallows, the doctor quickly advances the tube at least ½" (1.3 cm) beyond the previously marked point on the tube.

▶ To confirm tube placement, the doctor will aspirate stomach contents through the gastric port. He'll also auscultate the stomach with a stethoscope as he injects air. After partially inflating the gastric balloon with 50 to 100 cc of air, he'll order an X-ray of the abdomen to confirm correct placement of the balloon. Before fully inflating the balloon, he'll use the 60-ml syringe to irrigate the stomach with normal saline solution and empty the stomach as completely as possible. This helps the patient avoid regurgitating gastric contents when the balloon inflates.
▶ After confirming tube placement, the doctor will fully inflate the gastric balloon (250 to 500 cc of air for a Sengstaken-Blakemore tube; 700 to 800 cc of air for a Linton tube) and clamp the tube using rubber-shod clamps. If he's using a Minnesota tube, he'll connect the pressure-monitoring port for the gastric balloon lumen to the mercury manometer and then inflate the balloon in 100-cc increments until it fills with up to 500 cc of air. As he introduces the air, he'll monitor the intragastric balloon pressure to make sure the balloon stays inflated. Then he'll clamp the ports. For the Sengstaken-Blakemore or Minnesota tube, the doctor will gently pull on the tube until he feels resistance, which indicates that the gastric balloon is inflated and exerting pressure on the cardia of the stomach. When he senses that the balloon is engaged, he'll place the foam nose guard around the area where the tube emerges from the nostril.
▶ Be ready to tape the nose guard in place around the tube. This helps to minimize pressure on the nostril from the traction and decreases the risk of necrosis.
▶ With the nose guard secured, traction can be applied to the tube with a traction rope and a 1-lb (0.5-kg) weight, or the tube can be pulled gently and taped secure

# Securing an esophageal tube

To reduce the risk of the gastric balloon's slipping down or away from the cardia of the stomach, secure an esophageal tube to a football helmet. Tape the tube to the face guard, as shown, and fasten the chin strap.

To remove the tube quickly, unfasten the chin strap and pull the helmet slightly forward. Cut the tape and the gastric balloon and esophageal balloon lumens. Be sure to hold onto the tube near the patient's nostril.

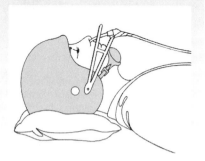

tightly to the face guard of a football helmet. (See *Securing an esophageal tube*.)
▶ With pulley-and-weight traction, lower the head of the bed to about 25 degrees to produce countertraction.
▶ Lavage the stomach through the gastric aspiration lumen with normal saline solution (iced or tepid) until the return fluid is clear. The vasoconstriction thus achieved stops the hemorrhage; the lavage empties the stomach. Any blood detected later in the gastric aspirate indicates that bleeding remains uncontrolled.
▶ Attach one of the suction sources to the gastric aspiration lumen. This empties the stomach, helps prevent nausea and possible vomiting, and allows continuous observation of the gastric contents for blood.
▶ If the doctor inserted a Sengstaken-Blakemore or a Minnesota tube, he'll inflate the esophageal balloon as he inflates the gastric balloon to compress the esophageal varices and control bleeding.

To do this with a Sengstaken-Blakemore tube, attach the Y-connector tube to the esophageal lumen. Then attach a sphygmomanometer inflation bulb to one end of the

Y-connector and the manometer to the other end. Inflate the esophageal balloon until the pressure gauge ranges between 30 and 40 mm Hg and clamp the tube.

To do this with a Minnesota tube, attach the mercury manometer directly to the esophageal pressure-monitoring outlet. Then, using the 60-ml syringe and pushing the air slowly into the esophageal balloon port, inflate the balloon until the pressure gauge ranges from 35 to 45 mm Hg.
▶ Check the balloon pressure every 2 hours.
▶ Set up esophageal suction to prevent accumulation of secretions that may cause vomiting and pulmonary aspiration. This is important because swallowed secretions can't pass into the stomach if the patient has an inflated esophageal balloon in place. If the patient has a Linton or a Minnesota tube, attach the suction source to the esophageal aspiration port. If the patient has a Sengstaken-Blakemore tube, advance an NG tube through the other nostril into the esophagus to the point where the esophageal balloon begins and attach the suction source as ordered.

## Removing the tube
▶ The doctor will deflate the esophageal balloon by aspirating the air with a syringe. (He may order the esophageal balloon to be deflated at 5-mm Hg increments every 30 minutes for several hours.) Then if bleeding doesn't recur, he'll remove the traction from the gastric tube and deflate the gastric balloon (also by aspiration). The gastric balloon is always deflated just before removing the tube to prevent the balloon from riding up into the esophagus or pharynx and obstructing the airway or, possibly, causing asphyxia or rupture.
▶ After disconnecting all suction tubes, the doctor will gently remove the esophageal tube. If he feels resistance, he'll aspirate the balloons again. (To remove a Minnesota tube, he'll grasp it near the patient's nostril and cut across all four lumens approximately 3″ [7.5 cm] below that point. This ensures deflation of all balloons.)
▶ After the tube has been removed, assist the patient with mouth care.

## Special considerations
▶ If the patient appears cyanotic or if other signs of airway obstruction develop during tube placement, remove the tube immedi-

ately because it may have entered the trachea instead of the esophagus. After intubation, keep scissors taped to the head of the bed. If respiratory distress occurs, cut across all lumens while holding the tube at the nares and remove the tube quickly. Unless contraindicated, the patient can sip water through a straw during intubation to facilitate tube advancement.

▶ Keep in mind that the intraesophageal balloon pressure varies with respirations and esophageal contractions. Baseline pressure is the important pressure.

▶ The balloon on the Linton tube should stay inflated no longer than 24 hours because necrosis of the cardia may result. Usually, the doctor removes the tube only after a trial period (lasting at least 12 hours) with the esophageal balloon deflated or with the gastric balloon tension released from the cardia to check for rebleeding. In some facilities, the doctor may deflate the esophageal balloon for 5 to 10 minutes every hour to temporarily relieve pressure on the esophageal mucosa.

## Complications
Erosion and perforation of the esophagus and gastric mucosa may result from the tension placed on these areas by the balloons during traction. Esophageal rupture may result if the gastric balloon accidentally inflates in the esophagus. Acute airway occlusion may result if the balloon dislodges and moves upward into the trachea. Other erosions, nasal tissue necrosis, and aspiration of oral secretions may also complicate the patient's condition.

## Documentation
▶ Record the date and time of insertion and removal, the type of tube used, and the name of the doctor who performed the procedure.

▶ Document the intraesophageal balloon pressure (for Sengstaken-Blakemore and Minnesota tubes), intragastric balloon pressure (for Minnesota tube), or amount of air injected (for Sengstaken-Blakemore and Linton tubes).

▶ Record the amount of fluid used for gastric irrigation and the color, consistency, and amount of gastric returns, before and after lavage.

## REFERENCES
Alvares, J.F., et al. "Tracheal Obstruction After Insertion of a Self-expanding Metal Esophageal Stent: Successful Management with an Endotracheal Tube, Steroids, and Radiotherapy," *Endoscopy* 34(7):592, July 2002.

Edward, D., et al. *Bedside Critical Care Manual.* Philadelphia: Lippincott Williams & Wilkins, 2001.

# Fecal occult blood test

Fecal occult blood tests are valuable for determining the presence of occult blood (hidden GI bleeding) and for distinguishing between true melena and melena-like stools. Certain medications, such as iron supplements and bismuth compounds, can darken stools so that they resemble melena.

Two common occult blood screening tests are Hematest (an orthotolidine reagent tablet) and the Hemoccult slide (filter paper impregnated with guaiac). Both tests produce a blue reaction in a fecal smear if occult blood loss exceeds 5 ml in 24 hours. A newer test, ColoCARE, requires no fecal smear.

Occult blood tests are particularly important for early detection of colorectal cancer because 80% of patients with this disorder test positive. However, a single positive test result doesn't necessarily confirm GI bleeding or indicate colorectal cancer. To confirm a positive result, the test must be repeated at least three times while the patient follows a meatless, high-residue diet. Even then, a confirmed positive test doesn't necessarily indicate colorectal cancer. It does indicate the need for further diagnostic studies because GI bleeding can result from many causes other than cancer, such as ulcers and diverticula. These tests are easily performed on collected specimens or smears from a digital rectal examination.

## Equipment
Test kit ● gloves ● glass or porcelain plate ● tongue blade or other wooden applicator

## Implementation
▶ Put on gloves and collect a stool specimen.

# Home tests for fecal occult blood

Most fecal occult blood tests require the patient to collect a specimen of his stool and smear some of it on a slide. In contrast, some new tests don't require the patient to handle stool, making the procedure safer and simpler. One example is a test called ColoCARE.

If the patient will be performing the ColoCARE test at home, tell him to avoid red meat and vitamin C supplements for 2 days before the test. He should check with his doctor about discontinuing any medications before the test. Some drugs that may interfere with test results are aspirin, indomethacin, corticosteroids, phenylbutazone, reserpine, dietary supplements, anticancer drugs, and anticoagulants.

Tell the patient to flush the toilet twice just before performing the test to remove any toilet-cleaning chemicals from the tank. Tell him to defecate into the toilet, but to throw no toilet paper into the bowl. Within 5 minutes, he should remove the test pad from its pouch and float it printed side up on the surface of the water. Tell him to watch the pad for 15 to 30 seconds for any evidence of blue or green color changes and have him record the result on the reply card.

Emphasize that he should perform this test with three consecutive bowel movements and then send the completed card to his doctor. However, he should call his doctor immediately if he notes a positive color change in the first test.

## Hematest reagent tablet test

▶ Use a wooden applicator to smear a bit of the stool specimen on the filter paper supplied with the test kit. Or, after performing a digital rectal examination, wipe the finger you used for the examination on a square of the filter paper.
▶ Place the filter paper with the stool smear on a glass plate.
▶ Remove a reagent tablet from the bottle and immediately replace the cap tightly. Then place the tablet in the center of the stool smear on the filter paper.
▶ Add one drop of water to the tablet and allow it to soak in for 5 to 10 seconds. Add a second drop, letting it run from the tablet onto the specimen and filter paper. If nec-

essary, tap the plate gently to dislodge any water from the top of the tablet.
▶ After 2 minutes, the filter paper will turn blue if the test is positive. Don't read the color that appears on the tablet itself or that develops on the filter paper after the 2-minute period.
▶ Note the results and discard the filter paper.
▶ Remove and discard your gloves and wash your hands thoroughly.

## Hemoccult slide test

▶ Open the flap on the slide packet and use a wooden applicator to apply a thin smear of the stool specimen to the guaiac-impregnated filter paper exposed in box A. Or, after performing a digital rectal examination, wipe the finger you used for the examination on a square of the filter paper.
▶ Apply a second smear from another part of the specimen to the filter paper exposed in box B because some parts of the specimen may not contain blood.
▶ Allow the specimens to dry for 3 to 5 minutes.
▶ Open the flap on the reverse side of the slide package and place 2 drops of Hemoccult developing solution on the paper over each smear. A blue reaction will appear in 30 to 60 seconds if the test is positive.
▶ Record the results and discard the slide package.
▶ Remove and discard your gloves and wash your hands thoroughly.

## Special considerations

▶ Make sure stool specimens aren't contaminated with urine, soap solution, or toilet tissue and test them as soon as possible after collection.
▶ Test samples from several portions of the same specimen because occult blood from the upper GI tract isn't always evenly dispersed throughout the formed stool; likewise, blood from colorectal bleeding may occur mostly on the outer stool surface.
▶ Check the condition of the reagent tablets and note their expiration date. Use only fresh tablets and discard outdated ones. Protect Hematest tablets from moisture, heat, and light.
▶ If repeat testing is necessary after a positive screening test, explain the test to the patient. Instruct him to maintain a high-fiber diet and to refrain from eating red meat, poultry, fish, turnips, and horserad-

ish for 48 to 72 hours before the test as well as throughout the collection period because these substances may alter test results.

▶ As ordered, have the patient discontinue the use of iron preparations, bromides, iodides, rauwolfia derivatives, indomethacin, colchicine, salicylates, potassium, phenylbutazone, oxyphenbutazone, bismuth compounds, steroids, and ascorbic acid for 48 to 72 hours before the test and during it to ensure accurate test results and avoid possible bleeding, which some of these compounds may cause.

### Home care

If the patient will be using the Hemoccult slide packet at home, advise him to complete the label on the slide packet before specimen collection. If he'll be using a ColoCARE test packet, inform him that this test is a preliminary screen for occult blood in his stool. Tell him that he won't have to obtain a stool specimen to perform the test but that he should follow your instructions carefully. (See *Home tests for fecal occult blood*.)

### Documentation

▶ Record the time and date of the test, the result, and any unusual characteristics of the stool tested.
▶ Document positive results to the doctor.

### REFERENCES

Little, J., et al. "Asymptomatic Colorectal Neoplasia and Fecal Characteristics: A Case-control Study of Subjects Participating in the Nottingham Fecal Occult Blood Screening Trial," *Diseases of the Colon and Rectum* 45(9):1233-41, September 2002.

Seeff, L.C., et al. "Are We Doing Enough To Screen for Colorectal Cancer? Findings from the 1999 Behavioral Risk Factor Surveillance System," *Journal of Family Practice* 51(9):761-66, September 2002.

# Feeding tube insertion and removal

Inserting a feeding tube nasally or orally into the stomach or duodenum allows a patient who can't or won't eat to receive nourishment. The feeding tube also permits administration of supplemental feedings to a patient who has very high nutritional requirements, such as an unconscious patient or one with extensive burns. Typically, a feeding tube is inserted by a nurse as ordered. The preferred feeding tube route is nasal, but the oral route may be used for patients with such conditions as a deviated septum or a head or nose injury.

The doctor may order duodenal feeding when the patient can't tolerate gastric feeding or when he expects gastric feeding to produce aspiration. Absence of bowel sounds or possible intestinal obstruction contraindicates using a feeding tube.

Feeding tubes differ somewhat from standard NG tubes. Made of silicone, rubber, or polyurethane, feeding tubes have small diameters and great flexibility. This reduces oropharyngeal irritation, necrosis from pressure on the tracheoesophageal wall, distal esophageal irritation, and discomfort from swallowing. To facilitate passage, some feeding tubes are weighted with tungsten, and some need a guide wire to keep them from curling in the back of the throat.

These small-bore tubes usually have radiopaque markings and a water-activated coating, which provides a lubricated surface.

### Equipment

*For insertion*
Feeding tube (#6 to #18 French, with or without guide) ● linen-saver pad ● gloves ● hypoallergenic tape ● water-soluble lubricant ● cotton-tipped applicators ● skin preparation (such as compound benzoin tincture) ● facial tissues ● penlight ● small cup of water with straw, or ice chips ● emesis basin ● 60-ml syringe ● stethoscope ● water

*During use*
Mouthwash or normal saline solution ● toothbrush

*For removal*
Linen-saver pad ● tube clamp ● bulb syringe

#### Preparation of equipment

Have the proper size tube available. Usually, the doctor orders the smallest-bore tube that will allow free passage of the liquid feeding formula. Read the instructions on the tubing package carefully because tube characteristics vary according to manufacturer. (For example, some tubes have marks at the appropriate lengths for gastric, duodenal, and jejunal insertion.)

Examine the tube to make sure it's free from defects, such as cracks or rough or sharp edges. Next, run water through the tube. This checks for patency, activates the coating, and facilitates removal of the guide.

## Implementation
▶ Explain the procedure to the patient and show him the tube so that he knows what to expect and can cooperate more fully.
▶ Provide privacy. Wash your hands and put on gloves.
▶ Assist the patient into semi-Fowler's or high Fowler's position.
▶ Place a linen-saver pad across the patient's chest to protect him from spills.
▶ To determine the tube length needed to reach the stomach, first extend the distal end of the tube from the tip of the patient's nose to his earlobe. Coil this portion of the tube around your fingers so the end will remain curved until you insert it. Then extend the uncoiled portion from the earlobe to the xiphoid process. Use a small piece of hypoallergenic tape to mark the total length of the two portions.

### Inserting the tube nasally
▶ Using a penlight, assess nasal patency. Inspect nasal passages for a deviated septum, polyps, or other obstructions. Occlude one nostril, then the other, to determine which has the better airflow. Assess the patient's history of nasal injury or surgery.
▶ Lubricate the curved tip of the tube (and the feeding tube guide, if appropriate) with a small amount of water-soluble lubricant to ease insertion and prevent tissue injury.
▶ Ask the patient to hold the emesis basin and facial tissues in case he needs them.
▶ To advance the tube, insert the curved, lubricated tip into the more patent nostril and direct it along the nasal passage toward the ear on the same side. When it passes the nasopharyngeal junction, turn the tube 180 degrees to aim it downward into the esophagus. Tell the patient to lower his chin to his chest to close the trachea. Then give him a small cup of water with a straw, or ice chips. Direct him to sip the water or suck on the ice and swallow frequently. This will ease the tube's passage. Advance the tube as he swallows.

### Inserting the tube orally
▶ Have the patient lower his chin to close his trachea and ask him to open his mouth.
▶ Place the tip of the tube at the back of the patient's tongue, give water, and instruct the patient to swallow as above. Remind him to avoid clamping his teeth down on the tube. Advance the tube as he swallows.

### Positioning the tube
▶ Keep passing the tube until the tape marking the appropriate length reaches the patient's nostril or lips.
▶ To check tube placement, attach the syringe filled with 10 cc of air to the end of the tube. Gently inject the air into the tube as you auscultate the patient's abdomen with the stethoscope about 3″ (7.5 cm) below the sternum. Listen for a whooshing sound, which signals that the tube has reached its target in the stomach. If the tube remains coiled in the esophagus, you'll feel resistance when you inject the air, or the patient may belch.
▶ If you hear a whooshing sound, gently try to aspirate gastric secretions. Successful aspiration confirms correct tube placement. If no gastric secretions return, the tube may be in the esophagus. You'll need to advance the tube or reinsert it before proceeding.
▶ After confirming proper tube placement, remove the tape marking the tube length.
▶ Tape the tube to the patient's nose and remove the guide wire. *Note:* In some cases, X-rays may be ordered to verify tube placement.
▶ To advance the tube to the duodenum, especially a tungsten-weighted tube, position the patient on his right side. This lets gravity assist tube passage through the pylorus. Move the tube forward 2″ to 3″ (5 to 7.5 cm) hourly until X-ray studies confirm duodenal placement. (An X-ray must confirm placement before feeding begins because duodenal feeding can cause nausea and vomiting if accidentally delivered to the stomach.)
▶ Apply a skin preparation to the patient's cheek before securing the tube with tape. This helps the tube adhere to the skin and also prevents irritation.
▶ Tape the tube securely to the patient's cheek to avoid excessive pressure on his nostrils.

## Removing the tube
▶ Protect the patient's chest with a linen-saver pad.
▶ Flush the tube with air, clamp or pinch it to prevent fluid aspiration during withdrawal, and withdraw it gently but quickly.
▶ Promptly cover and discard the used tube.

## Special considerations
▶ Flush the feeding tube every 8 hours with up to 60 ml of normal saline solution or water to maintain patency. Retape the tube at least daily and as needed. Alternate taping the tube toward the inner and outer side of the nose to avoid constant pressure on the same nasal area. Inspect the skin for redness and breakdown.
▶ Provide nasal hygiene daily using the cotton-tipped applicators and water-soluble lubricant to remove crusted secretions. Also help the patient brush his teeth, gums, and tongue with mouthwash or saline solution at least twice daily.
▶ If the patient can't swallow the feeding tube, use a guide to aid insertion.
▶ Precise feeding-tube placement is especially important because small-bore feeding tubes may slide into the trachea without causing immediate signs of respiratory distress, such as coughing, choking, gasping, or cyanosis. However, the patient will usually cough if the tube enters the larynx. To make sure that the tube clears the larynx, ask the patient to speak. If he can't, the tube is in the larynx. Withdraw the tube at once and reinsert.
▶ When aspirating gastric contents to check tube placement, pull gently on the syringe plunger to prevent trauma to the stomach lining or bowel. If you meet resistance during aspiration, stop the procedure because resistance may result simply from the tube lying against the stomach wall. If the tube coils above the stomach, you won't be able to aspirate stomach contents. To rectify this, change the patient's position or withdraw the tube a few inches, readvance it, and try to aspirate again. If the tube was inserted with a guide wire, don't use the guide wire to reposition the tube. The doctor may do so, using fluoroscopic guidance.

## Home care
If your patient will use a feeding tube at home, make appropriate home care nursing referrals and teach the patient and caregivers how to use and care for a feeding tube. Teach them how to obtain equipment, insert and remove the tube, prepare and store feeding formula, and solve problems with tube position and patency.

## Complications
Prolonged intubation may lead to skin erosion at the nostril, sinusitis, esophagitis, esophagotracheal fistula, gastric ulceration, and pulmonary and oral infection.

## Documentation
▶ For tube insertion, record the date, time, tube type and size, insertion site, area of placement, and confirmation of proper placement.
▶ Record the name of the person performing the procedure.
▶ For tube removal, record the date and time.
▶ Document the patient's tolerance of the procedure.

### REFERENCES
Bowers, S. "All About Tubes: Your Guide to Enteral Feeding Devices," *Nursing2000* 30(12):41-47, December 2000.
Craven, R., and Hirnle, C.J. *Fundamentals of Nursing: Human Health and Function,* 4th ed. Philadelphia: Lippincott Williams & Wilkins, 2002.
Guenter, P., and Silkroski, M. *Tube Feeding: Practical Guidelines and Nursing Protocols.* Gaithersburg, Md.: Aspen Pubs., Inc., 2001.
Stone, S.J., et al. "Bedside Placement of Postpyloric Feeding Tubes," *AACN Clinical Issues* 11(4):517-30, November 2000.

# Gastric lavage

After poisoning or a drug overdose, especially in patients who have central nervous system depression or an inadequate gag reflex, gastric lavage flushes the stomach and removes ingested substances through a gastric lavage tube. The procedure is also used to empty the stomach in preparation for endoscopic examination. For patients with gastric or esophageal bleeding, lavage with tepid or iced water or normal saline solution may be used to stop bleeding. However, some controversy exists over the effec-

## Is iced lavage effective?

Some experts question the effectiveness of using an iced irrigant for gastric lavage to treat GI bleeding. Here's why.

Iced irrigating solutions stimulate the vagus nerve, which triggers increased hydrochloric acid secretion. In turn, this stimulates gastric motility, which can irritate the bleeding site.

Some doctors prefer using unchilled normal saline solution (which may prevent rapid electrolyte loss) or even water if the patient must avoid sodium. They point out that no research exists to support the use of iced irrigant to stop acute GI bleeding.

---

tiveness of iced lavage for this purpose. (See *Is iced lavage effective?*)

Gastric lavage can be continuous or intermittent. Typically, this procedure is done in the emergency department or intensive care unit by a doctor, gastroenterologist, or nurse; a wide-bore lavage tube is almost always inserted by a gastroenterologist.

Gastric lavage is contraindicated after ingestion of a corrosive substance (such as lye, petroleum distillates, ammonia, alkalis, or mineral acids) because the lavage tube may perforate the already compromised esophagus.

Correct lavage tube placement is essential for patient safety because accidental misplacement (in the lungs, for example) followed by lavage can be fatal. Other complications of gastric lavage include bradyarrhythmias and aspiration of gastric fluids.

### Equipment
Lavage setup (two graduated containers for drainage, three pieces of large-lumen rubber tubing, Y-connector, and a clamp or hemostat) ● 2 to 3 L of normal saline solution, tap water, or appropriate antidote as ordered ● I.V. pole ● basin of ice, if ordered ● Ewald tube or any large-lumen gastric tube, typically #36 to #40 French (see *Using wide-bore gastric tubes*) ● water-soluble lubricant or anesthetic ointment ● stethoscope ● ½" hypoallergenic tape ● 50-ml bulb or catheter-tip syringe ● gloves ● face shield ● linen-saver pad or towel ●

Yankauer or tonsil-tip suction device ● suction apparatus ● labeled specimen container ● laboratory request form ● norepinephrine ● optional: patient restraints and charcoal tablets

A prepackaged, syringe-type irrigation kit may be used for intermittent lavage. For poisoning or a drug overdose, however, the continuous lavage setup may be more appropriate to use because it's a faster and more effective means of diluting and removing the harmful substance.

### Preparation of equipment
Set up the lavage equipment. (See *Preparing for gastric lavage,* page 440.) If iced lavage is ordered, chill the desired irrigant (water or normal saline solution) in a basin of ice. Lubricate the end of the lavage tube with the water-soluble lubricant or anesthetic ointment.

❖ **ALERT!** Correct lavage tube placement is essential for patient safety because accidental misplacement (in the lungs, for example) followed by lavage can be fatal.

### Implementation
◗ Explain the procedure to the patient, provide privacy, and wash your hands.
◗ Put on gloves and a face shield.
◗ Drape the towel or linen-saver pad over the patient's chest to protect him from spills.
◗ The doctor inserts the lavage tube nasally and advances it slowly and gently because forceful insertion may injure tissues and cause epistaxis. He checks the tube's placement by injecting about 30 cc of air into the tube with the bulb syringe and then auscultating the patient's abdomen with a stethoscope. If the tube is in place, he'll hear the sound of air entering the stomach.
◗ Because the patient may vomit when the lavage tube reaches the posterior pharynx during insertion, be prepared to suction the airway immediately with either a Yankauer or a tonsil-tip suction device.
◗ When the lavage tube passes the posterior pharynx, help the patient into Trendelenburg's position and turn him toward his left side in a three-quarter prone posture. This position minimizes passage of gastric contents into the duodenum and may prevent the patient from aspirating vomitus.
◗ After securing the lavage tube nasally or orally with tape and making sure the irrig-

ant inflow tube on the lavage setup is clamped, connect the unattached end of this tube to the lavage tube. Allow the stomach contents to empty into the drainage container before instilling any irrigant. This confirms proper tube placement and decreases the risk of overfilling the stomach with irrigant and inducing vomiting. If you're using a syringe irrigation set, aspirate stomach contents with a 50-ml bulb or catheter-tip syringe before instilling the irrigant.

▶ When you confirm proper tube placement, begin gastric lavage by instilling about 250 ml of irrigant to assess the patient's tolerance and prevent vomiting. If you're using a syringe, instill about 50 ml of solution at a time until you've instilled between 250 and 500 ml.

▶ Clamp the inflow tube and unclamp the outflow tube to allow the irrigant to flow out. If you're using the syringe irrigation kit, aspirate the irrigant with the syringe and empty it into a calibrated container. Measure the outflow amount to make sure that it equals at least the amount of irrigant you instilled. This prevents accidental stomach distention and vomiting. If the drainage amount falls significantly short of the instilled amount, reposition the tube until sufficient solution flows out. Gently massage the abdomen over the stomach to promote outflow.

▶ Repeat the inflow-outflow cycle until returned fluids appear clear. This signals that the stomach no longer holds harmful substances or that bleeding has stopped.

▶ Assess the patient's vital signs, urine output, and level of consciousness (LOC) every 15 minutes. Notify the doctor of any changes.

▶ If ordered, remove the lavage tube.

### Special considerations

▶ To control GI bleeding, the doctor may order continuous irrigation of the stomach with an irrigant and a vasoconstrictor, such as norepinephrine. After the stomach absorbs norepinephrine, the portal system delivers the drug directly to the liver, where it's metabolized. This prevents the drug from circulating systemically and initiating a hypertensive response. Or the doctor may direct you to clamp the outflow tube for a prescribed period after instilling the irrigant and the vasoconstrictive med-

# Using wide-bore gastric tubes

If you need to deliver a large volume of fluid rapidly through a gastric tube (when irrigating the stomach of a patient with profuse gastric bleeding or poisoning, for example), a wide-bore gastric tube usually serves best. Typically inserted orally, these tubes remain in place only long enough to complete the lavage and evacuate stomach contents.

### Ewald tube

In an emergency, using this single-lumen tube with several openings at the distal end allows you to aspirate large amounts of gastric contents quickly.

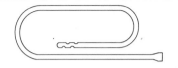

### Levacuator tube

This tube has two lumens. Use the larger lumen for evacuating gastric contents; the smaller, for instilling an irrigant.

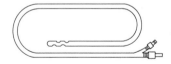

### Edlich tube

This single-lumen tube has four openings near the closed distal tip. A funnel or syringe may be connected at the proximal end. Like the Ewald tube, the Edlich tube allows you to withdraw large quantities of gastric contents quickly.

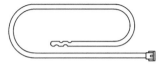

ication and before withdrawing it. This allows the mucosa time to absorb the drug.

▶ Never leave a patient alone during gastric lavage. Observe continuously for any changes in LOC and monitor vital signs fre-

# Preparing for gastric lavage

Prepare the lavage setup as follows:
▶ Connect one of the three pieces of large-lumen tubing to the irrigant container.
▶ Insert the stem of the Y-connector in the other end of the tubing.
▶ Connect the remaining two pieces of tubing to the free ends of the Y-connector.
▶ Place the unattached end of one of the tubes into one of the drainage containers. (Later, you'll connect the other piece of tubing to the patient's gastric tube.)
▶ Clamp the tube leading to the irrigant.
▶ Suspend the entire setup from the I.V. pole, hanging the irrigant container at the highest level.

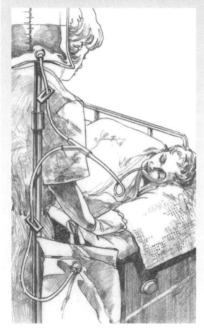

quently because the natural vagal response to intubation can depress the patient's heart rate.
▶ If you need to restrain the patient, secure restraints on the same side of the bed or stretcher so you can free them quickly without moving to the other side of the bed.

▶ Remember also to keep tracheal suctioning equipment nearby and watch closely for airway obstruction caused by vomiting or excess oral secretions. Throughout gastric lavage, you may need to suction the oral cavity frequently to ensure an open airway and prevent aspiration. For the same reasons, and if he doesn't exhibit an adequate gag reflex, the patient may require an endotracheal tube before the procedure.
▶ When aspirating the stomach for ingested poisons or drugs, save the contents in a labeled container to send to the laboratory for analysis, along with a laboratory request form. If ordered, after lavage to remove poisons or drugs, mix charcoal tablets with the irrigant (water or normal saline solution) and administer the mixture through the NG tube. The charcoal will absorb any remaining toxic substances. The tube may be clamped temporarily, allowed to drain via gravity, attached to intermittent suction, or removed.
▶ When performing gastric lavage to stop bleeding, keep precise intake and output records to determine the amount of bleeding. When large volumes of fluid are instilled and withdrawn, serum electrolyte and arterial blood gas levels may be measured during or at the end of lavage.

## Complications

Vomiting and subsequent aspiration, the most common complication of gastric lavage, occur more commonly in a groggy patient. Bradyarrhythmias also may occur. After iced lavage especially, the patient's body temperature may drop, thereby triggering cardiac arrhythmias.

## Documentation

▶ Record the date and time of lavage, size and type of NG tube used, volume and type of irrigant, and amount of drained gastric contents.
▶ Document information on the intake and output record sheet; include your observations, including the color and consistency of drainage.
▶ Document precisely the patient's vital signs and LOC, any drugs instilled through the tube, and the time the tube was removed.
▶ Document how the patient tolerated the procedure.

## REFERENCES

Blazys, D. "Tips on Gastric Lavage," *Journal of Emergency Nursing* 25(3):200, June 1999.

Blazys, D. "Use of Lavage in Treating Overdose," *Journal of Emergency Nursing* 26(4): 394-98, August 2000.

Clegg, T., and Hope, K. "The First Line Response for People Who Self-poison: Exploring the Options for Gut Decontamination," *Journal of Advanced Nursing* 30(6): 1360-67, December 1999.

Craven, R., and Hirnle, C.J. *Fundamentals of Nursing: Human Health and Function,* 4th ed. Philadelphia: Lippincott Williams & Wilkins, 2002.

Vale, J.A. The American Academy of Toxicology. Position Statement: Gastric Lavage. *www.clintox.org/Pos_Statements/Gastric_Lavage.html*

# Gastrostomy feeding button care

A gastrostomy feeding button serves as an alternative feeding device for an ambulatory patient who is receiving long-term enteral feedings. Approved by the Food and Drug Administration for 6-month implantation, feeding buttons can be used to replace gastrostomy tubes, if necessary.

The feeding button has a mushroom dome at one end and two wing tabs and a flexible safety plug at the other. When inserted into an established stoma, the button lies almost flush with the skin, with only the top of the safety plug visible.

The button can usually be inserted into a stoma in less than 15 minutes. In addition to its cosmetic appeal, the device is easily maintained, reduces skin irritation and breakdown, and is less likely to become dislodged or to migrate than an ordinary feeding tube. A one-way, antireflux valve mounted just inside the mushroom dome prevents accidental leakage of gastric contents. The device usually requires replacement after 3 to 4 months, typically because the antireflux valve wears out.

## Equipment

Gastrostomy feeding button of the correct size (all three sizes, if the correct one isn't known) ● obturator ● water-soluble lubricant ● gloves ● feeding accessories, including adapter, feeding catheter, food syringe or bag, and formula ● catheter clamp ● cleaning equipment, including water, a syringe, cotton-tipped applicator, pipe cleaner, and mild soap or povidone-iodine solution ● optional: I.V. pole and pump to provide continuous infusion over several hours

## Implementation

▶ Explain the insertion, reinsertion, and feeding procedure to the patient. Tell him the doctor will perform the initial insertion.

▶ Wash your hands and put on gloves. (See *How to reinsert a gastrostomy feeding button,* page 442.)

▶ Attach the adapter and feeding catheter to the syringe or feeding bag. Clamp the catheter and fill the syringe or bag and catheter with formula. Refill the syringe before it's empty. These steps prevent air from entering the stomach and distending the abdomen.

▶ Open the safety plug and attach the adapter and feeding catheter to the button. Elevate the syringe or feeding bag above stomach level and gravity-feed the formula for 15 to 30 minutes, varying the height as needed to alter the flow rate. Use a pump for continuous infusion or for feedings lasting several hours.

▶ After the feeding, flush the button with 10 ml of water and clean the inside of the feeding catheter with a cotton-tipped applicator and water to preserve patency and to dislodge formula or food particles. Then lower the syringe or bag below stomach level to allow burping. Remove the adapter and feeding catheter. The antireflux valve should prevent gastric reflux. Then snap the safety plug into place to keep the lumen clean and prevent leakage if the antireflux valve fails. If the patient feels nauseated or vomits after the feeding, vent the button with the adapter and feeding catheter to control emesis.

▶ Wash the catheter and syringe or feeding bag in warm soapy water and rinse thoroughly. Clean the catheter and adapter with a pipe cleaner. Rinse well before using for the next feeding. Soak the equipment once per week according to the manufacturer's recommendations.

# How to reinsert a gastrostomy feeding button

If your patient's gastrostomy feeding button pops out (with coughing, for instance), you or he will need to reinsert the device. Here are some steps to follow

### Prepare the equipment
Collect the feeding button, an obturator, and a water-soluble lubricant. If the button will be reinserted, wash it with soap and water and rinse it thoroughly.

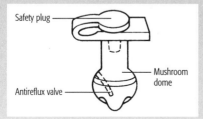

### Insert the button
▶ Check the depth of the patient's stoma to make sure you have the correct size feeding button. Then clean around the stoma.
▶ Lubricate the obturator with a water-soluble lubricant and distend the button several times to ensure the antireflux valve's patency within the button.
▶ Lubricate the mushroom dome and the stoma. Gently push the button through the stoma into the stomach.

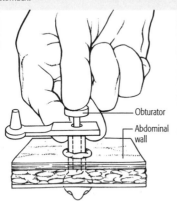

▶ Remove the obturator by gently rotating it as you withdraw it, to keep the antireflux valve from adhering to it. If the valve sticks, gently push the obturator back into the button until the valve closes.
▶ After removing the obturator, make sure the valve is closed. Then close the flexible safety plug, which should be relatively flush with the skin surface.

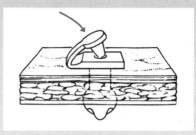

▶ If you need to administer a feeding right away, open the safety plug and attach the feeding adapter and feeding tube. Deliver the feeding as ordered.

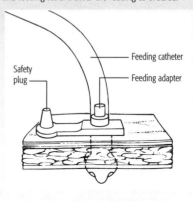

## Special considerations
▶ If the button pops out while feeding, reinsert it, estimate the formula already delivered, and resume feeding.
▶ Once daily, clean the peristomal skin with mild soap and water or povidone-iodine and let the skin air-dry for 20 minutes to avoid skin irritation. Also, clean the site whenever spillage from the feeding bag occurs.

## Home care

Before discharge, make sure the patient can insert and care for the gastrostomy feeding button. If necessary, teach him or a family member how to reinsert the button by first practicing on a model. Offer written instructions and answer his questions on obtaining replacement supplies.

## Documentation

▶ Record the feeding time and duration, amount and type of feeding formula used, and the patient's tolerance of the procedure.
▶ Document intake and output records as necessary. Note the appearance of the stoma and surrounding skin.

### REFERENCES

Craven, R., and Hirnle, C.J. *Fundamentals of Nursing: Human Health and Function,* 4th ed. Philadelphia: Lippincott Williams & Wilkins, 2002.
Guenter, P., and Silkroski, M. *Tube Feeding: Practical Guidelines and Nursing Protocols.* Gaithersburg, Md.: Aspen Pubs., Inc., 2001.

# Nasoenteric-decompression tube care

The patient with a nasoenteric-decompression tube needs special care and continuous monitoring to ensure tube patency, to maintain suction and bowel decompression, and to detect such complications as fluid-electrolyte imbalances related to aspiration of intestinal contents. Precise intake and output records are an integral part of the patient's care. Frequent mouth and nose care is also essential to provide comfort and to prevent skin breakdown. Last, a patient with a nasoenteric-decompression tube will need encouragement and support during insertion and removal of the tube and while the tube is in place.

## Equipment

Suction apparatus with intermittent suction capability (stationary or portable unit) • container of water • intake and output record sheets • mouthwash and water mixture • sponge tipped swabs • water-soluble lubricant or petroleum jelly • cotton-tipped applicators • safety pin • tape or rubber band • disposable irrigation set • irrigant •

labels for tube lumens • optional: throat comfort measures, such as gargle, viscous lidocaine, throat lozenges, ice collar, sour hard candy, or gum

### Preparation of equipment

Assemble the suction apparatus and set up the suction unit. If indicated, test the unit by turning it on and placing the end of the suction tubing in a container of water. If the tubing draws in water, the unit works.

## Implementation

▶ Explain to the patient and his family the purpose of the procedure. Answer questions clearly and thoroughly to ease anxiety and enhance cooperation.
▶ After tube insertion, have the patient lie quietly on his right side for about 2 hours to promote the tube's passage. After the tube advances past the pylorus, the tube can be advanced 2″ (5 cm) per hour as ordered.
▶ After the tube advances to the desired position, coil the excess external tubing and secure it to the patient's gown or bed linens with a safety pin attached to tape or a rubber band looped around it. This prevents kinks in the tubing, which would interrupt suction. When in the desired location, the tube may be taped to the patient's face.
▶ Maintain slack in the tubing so the patient can move comfortably and safely in bed. Show him how far he can move without dislodging the tube.
▶ After securing the tube, connect it to the tubing on the suction machine to begin decompression.
▶ Check the suction machine at least every 2 hours to confirm proper functioning and to ensure tube patency and bowel decompression. Excessive negative pressure may draw the mucosa into the tube openings, impair the suction's effectiveness, and injure the mucosa. By using intermittent suction, you may avoid these problems. To check functioning in an intermittent suction unit, look for drainage in the connecting tube and dripping into the collecting container. Empty the container every 8 hours and measure the contents.
▶ After decompression and before extubation, as ordered, provide a clear-to-full liquid diet to assess bowel function.
▶ Record intake and output accurately to monitor fluid balance. If you irrigate the

## Clearing a nasoenteric-decompression tube obstruction

If the patient's nasoenteric-decompression tube appears to be obstructed, notify the doctor right away. He may order measures such as these to restore patency quickly and efficiently.

▶ First, disconnect the tube from the suction source and irrigate with normal saline solution. Use gravity flow to help clear the obstruction unless ordered otherwise.

▶ If irrigation doesn't reestablish patency, the tube may be obstructed by its position against the gastric mucosa. To rectify this, tug slightly on the tube to move it away from the mucosa.

▶ If gentle tugging doesn't restore patency, the tube may be kinked and may need additional manipulation. Before proceeding, however, take the following precautions:

– Never reposition or irrigate a nasoenteric-decompression tube (without a doctor's order) in a patient who has had GI surgery.

– Avoid manipulating a tube in a patient who had the tube inserted during surgery. To do so may disturb new sutures.

– Don't try to reposition a tube in a patient who was difficult to intubate (because of an esophageal stricture, for example).

---

tube, its length may prohibit aspiration of the irrigant, so record the amount of instilled irrigant as "intake." Typically, normal saline solution supersedes water as the preferred irrigant because water, which is hypotonic, may increase electrolyte loss through osmotic action, especially if you irrigate the tube often.

▶ Observe the patient for signs and symptoms of disorders related to suctioning and intubation. Signs and symptoms of dehydration, a fluid-volume deficit, or a fluid-electrolyte imbalance include dry skin and mucous membranes, decreased urine output, lethargy, exhaustion, and fever.

▶ Watch for signs and symptoms of pneumonia related to the patient's inability to clear his pharynx or cough effectively with a tube in place. Be alert for fever, chest pain, tachypnea or labored breathing, and

diminished breath sounds over the affected area.

▶ Observe drainage characteristics: color, amount, consistency, odor, and any unusual changes.

▶ Provide mouth care frequently (at least every 4 hours) to increase the patient's comfort and promote a healthy oral cavity. If the tube remains in place for several days, mouth-breathing will leave the lips, tongue, and other tissues dry and cracked.

▶ Encourage the patient to brush his teeth or rinse his mouth with the mouthwash and water mixture.

▶ Lubricate the patient's lips with either wet sponge tipped swabs or petroleum jelly applied with a cotton-tipped applicator.

▶ At least every 4 hours, gently clean and lubricate the patient's external nostrils with either petroleum jelly or water-soluble lubricant on a cotton-tipped applicator to prevent skin breakdown.

▶ Watch for peristalsis to resume, signaled by bowel sounds, passage of flatus, decreased abdominal distention and possibly, a spontaneous bowel movement. These signs may require tube removal.

### Special considerations

▶ For a Miller-Abbott tube, clamp the lumen leading to the mercury balloon and label it DO NOT TOUCH. Label the other lumen SUCTION. Marking the tube may prevent accidentally instilling irrigant into the wrong lumen.

▶ If the suction machine works improperly, replace it immediately. If the machine works properly but no drainage accumulates in the collection container, suspect an obstruction in the tube.

▶ As ordered, irrigate the tube with the irrigation set to clear the obstruction. (See *Clearing a nasoenteric-decompression tube obstruction.*)

▶ If your patient is ambulatory and his tube connects to a portable suction unit, he may move short distances while connected to the unit. Or, if feasible and ordered, the tube can be disconnected and clamped briefly while he moves around.

▶ If the tubing irritates the patient's throat or makes him hoarse, offer relief with mouthwash, gargles, viscous lidocaine, throat lozenges, an ice collar, sour hard candy, or gum as appropriate.

▶ If the tip of the balloon falls below the ileocecal valve (confirmed by X-ray), the tube can't be removed nasally. It has to be advanced and removed through the anus.
▶ If the balloon at the end of the tube protrudes from the anus, notify the doctor. Most likely, the tube can be disconnected from suction, the proximal end severed, and the remaining tube removed gradually through the anus either manually or by peristalsis.

## Complications

In addition to fluid-volume deficit, electrolyte imbalance, and pneumonia, potential complications include mercury poisoning (from a ruptured mercury-filled balloon) and intussusception of the bowel (from the weight of the mercury in the balloon).

## Documentation

▶ Record the frequency and type of mouth and nose care provided. Describe the therapeutic effect, if any.
▶ Document the amount, color, consistency, and odor of the drainage obtained each time you empty the collection container.
▶ Record the amount of drainage on the intake and output sheet.
▶ Always document the amount of any irrigant or other fluid introduced through the tube or taken orally by the patient.
▶ If the suction machine malfunctions, note the length of time it wasn't functioning and the nursing action taken.
▶ Document the amount and character of any vomitus.
▶ Record the patient's tolerance of the tube's insertion and removal.

### REFERENCES

Hoffmann, S., et al. "Nasogastric Tube Versus Gastrostomy Tube for Gastric Decompression in Abdominal Surgery: A Prospective, Randomized Trial Comparing Patients' Tube-related Inconvenience," *Langenbecks Archives of Surgery* 386(6):402-409, November 2001.
Lee, S.S., et al. "Endoscopically Placed Nasogastrojejunal Feeding Tubes: A Safe Route for Enteral Nutrition in Patients with Hepatic Encephalopathy," *American Surgeon* 68(2):196-200, February 2002.

# Nasoenteric-decompression tube insertion and removal

The nasoenteric-decompression tube is inserted nasally and advanced beyond the stomach into the intestinal tract. It's used to aspirate intestinal contents for analysis and to treat intestinal obstruction. The tube may also help to prevent abdominal distention after GI surgery. A doctor usually inserts or removes a nasoenteric-decompression tube; sometimes, however, a nurse removes it.

A balloon or rubber bag at one end of the tube holds mercury (or air or water) to stimulate peristalsis and facilitate the tube's passage through the pylorus and into the intestinal tract. (See *Common types of nasoenteric-decompression tubes,* page 446.)

## Equipment

Sterile 10-ml syringe ● 21G needle ● nasoenteric-decompression tube ● container of water ● 5 to 10 ml of mercury or water, as ordered ● suction-decompression equipment ● gloves ● towel or linen-saver pad ● water-soluble lubricant ● 4″ × 4″ gauze pad ● ½″ hypoallergenic tape ● bulb syringe or 60-ml catheter-tip syringe ● rubber band ● safety pin ● clamp ● specimen container ● basin of ice or warm water ● penlight ● waterproof marking pen ● glass of water with straw ● optional: ice chips and local anesthetic

### Preparation of equipment

Stiffen a flaccid tube by chilling it in a basin of ice to facilitate insertion. To make a stiff tube flexible, dip it into warm water.

Check the tube's balloon for leaks. If you're using a Cantor or Harris tube, inject 10 cc of air into the balloon with a 10-ml syringe and 21G needle. If you're using a Miller-Abbott or Dennis tube, attach a 10-ml syringe to the distal balloon port. Immerse the balloon in a container of water and watch for air bubbles. Bubble-free water means that the balloon is free of leaks. Then remove the balloon from the water. Mercury, air, or water is added to the balloon either before or after insertion of the tube, depending on the type of tube used. Follow the manufacturer's recommendations.

# Common types of nasoenteric-decompression tubes

The type of nasoenteric-decompression tube chosen will depend on the size of the patient and his nostrils, the estimated duration of intubation, and the reason for the procedure. For example, to remove viscous material from the patient's intestinal tract, the doctor may select a tube with a wide bore and a single lumen.

Whichever tube you use, you'll need to provide good mouth care and check the patient's nostrils often for signs of irritation. If you see signs of irritation, retape the tube so that it doesn't cause tension and then lubricate the nostril. Or check with the doctor to see if the tube can be inserted through the other nostril.

Most tubes are impregnated with a radiopaque mark so that placement can easily be confirmed by X-ray or other imaging technique. The most commonly used nasoenteric-decompression tubes are shown below.

### Cantor tube

The Cantor tube is a 10' (3-m) long, single-lumen tube with a balloon that can hold mercury at its distal tip. The tube may be used to relieve bowel obstructions and to aspirate intestinal contents.

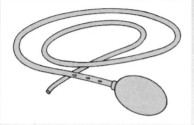

### Miller-Abbott tube

The Miller-Abbott tube is a 10' long tube with two lumens: one for inflating the distal balloon with air and one for instilling mercury or water. Also used for bowel obstruction, the tube allows aspiration of intestinal contents.

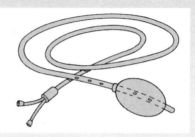

### Harris tube

Measuring only 6' (1.8 m) long, the Harris tube is a single-lumen tube that also ends with a balloon that holds mercury. Used primarily for treating a bowel obstruction, the tube allows lavage of the intestinal tract, usually with a Y-tube attached.

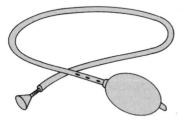

### Dennis tube

The Dennis tube is a 10' long, three-lumen sump tube and is used to decompress the intestinal tract before or after GI surgery. Each lumen is marked to denote its use: irrigation, drainage, and balloon inflation.

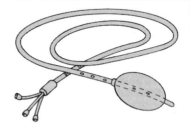

Set up suction-decompression equipment, if ordered, and make sure it works properly.

## Implementation

▶ Explain the procedure to the patient, forewarning him that he may experience some discomfort. Provide privacy and adequate lighting. Wash your hands and put on gloves.

▶ Position the patient as the doctor specifies, usually in semi-Fowler's or high Fowler's position. You may also need to help the patient hold his neck in a hyper-extended position.

▶ Protect the patient's chest with a linen-saver pad or towel.

▶ Agree with the patient on a signal that can be used to stop the insertion briefly, if necessary.

### Assisting with insertion

▶ The doctor assesses the patency of the patient's nostrils. To evaluate which nostril has better airflow in a conscious patient, he holds one nostril closed and then the other as the patient breathes. In an unconscious patient, he examines each nostril with a penlight to check for polyps, a deviated septum, or other obstruction.

▶ To decide how far the tube must be inserted to reach the stomach, the doctor places the tube's distal end at the tip of the patient's nose and then extends the tube to the earlobe and down to the xiphoid process. He either marks the tube with a waterproof marking pen or holds it at this point.

▶ The doctor applies water-soluble lubricant to the first few inches of the tube to reduce friction and tissue trauma and to facilitate insertion.

▶ If the balloon already contains mercury or water, the doctor holds it so the fluid runs to the bottom. Then he pinches the balloon closed to retain the fluid as the insertion begins.

▶ Tell the patient to breathe through his mouth or to pant as the balloon enters his nostril. After the balloon begins its descent, the doctor releases his grip on it, allowing the weight of the fluid to pull the tube into the nasopharynx. When the tube reaches the nasopharynx, the doctor instructs the patient to lower his chin and to swallow. In some cases, the patient may sip water through a straw to facilitate swallowing as the tube advances, but not after the tube reaches the trachea. This prevents injury from aspiration. The doctor continues to advance the tube slowly to prevent it from curling or kinking in the stomach.

▶ To confirm the tube's passage into the stomach, the doctor aspirates stomach contents with a bulb syringe.

▶ When the doctor confirms proper placement of a Miller-Abbott tube, he injects the appropriate amount of mercury (commonly between 2 and 5 ml) into the balloon lumen.

▶ To keep the tube out of the patient's eyes and to help avoid undue skin irritation, fold a 4″ × 4″ gauze pad in half and tape it to the patient's forehead with the fold directed toward the patient's nose. The doctor can slide the tube through this sling, leaving enough slack for the tube to advance.

▶ Position the patient as directed to help advance the tube. He'll typically lie on his right side until the tube clears the pylorus (about 2 hours). The doctor will confirm passage by X-ray.

▶ After the tube clears the pylorus, the doctor may direct you to advance it 2″ to 3″ (5 to 7.5 cm) every hour and to reposition the patient until the premeasured mark reaches the patient's nostril. Gravity and peristalsis will help advance the tube. (Notify the doctor if you can't advance the tube.)

▶ Keep the remaining premeasured length of tube well lubricated to ease passage and prevent irritation.

▶ Don't tape the tube while it advances to the premeasured mark unless the doctor asks you to do so.

▶ After the tube progresses the necessary distance, the doctor will order an X-ray to confirm tube positioning. When the tube is in place, secure the external tubing with tape to help prevent further progression.

▶ Loop a rubber band around the tube and pin the rubber band to the patient's gown with a safety pin.

▶ If ordered, attach the tube to intermittent suction.

### Removing the tube

▶ Assist the patient into semi-Fowler's or high Fowler's position. Drape a linen-saver pad or towel across the patient's chest.

▶ Wash your hands and put on gloves.

▶ Clamp the tube and disconnect it from the suction. This prevents the patient from aspirating any gastric contents that leak from the tube during withdrawal.

▶ If your patient has a double-lumen Miller-Abbott tube or a triple-lumen Dennis tube, attach a 10-ml syringe to the balloon port and withdraw the mercury. Place the mercury in a specimen container and follow your facility's protocol for safe disposal. (If you're working with a single-lumen Cantor or Harris tube, you'll with-

draw the mercury after you remove the tube.)
▶ Slowly withdraw between 6″ and 8″ (15 and 20.5 cm) of the tube. Wait 10 minutes and withdraw another 6″ to 8″. Wait another 10 minutes. Continue this procedure until the tube reaches the patient's esophagus (with about 18″ [45.5 cm] of the tube remaining inside the patient). At this point, you can gently withdraw the tube completely with the mercury in the balloon.

## Special considerations
▶ For a double- or triple-lumen tube, note which lumen accommodates balloon inflation and which accommodates drainage.
▶ An alternative method for removing a single-lumen tube is to withdraw it gently into the pharynx. Ask the patient to open his mouth. Then grasp the tube and mercury balloon and gently pull them outside of the patient's mouth. Remove mercury from the bag with a needle and syringe. Then pull the tube and empty balloon through the patient's nose. Never forcibly remove a tube if you meet resistance. Notify the doctor instead.
▶ Apply a local anesthetic, if ordered, to the nostril or the back of the throat to dull sensations and the gag reflex for intubation. Letting the patient gargle with a liquid anesthetic or hold ice chips in his mouth for a few minutes serves the same purpose.
▶ Mercury can be disposed of only by a licensed hazardous-waste disposal company. Put the container of mercury into a plastic bag, and send it to the appropriate department for disposal, according to your facility's policy.

## Complications
Nasoenteric-decompression tubes may cause reflux esophagitis, nasal or oral inflammation, and nasal, laryngeal, or esophageal ulceration.

## Documentation
▶ Record the date and time the nasoenteric-decompression tube was inserted and by whom.
▶ Record the patient's tolerance of the procedure.
▶ Document the type of tube used; the suction type and amount; and the color, amount, and consistency of drainage.

▶ Note the date, time, and name of the person removing the tube and the patient's tolerance of the removal procedure.

### REFERENCES
Hoffmann, S., et al. "Nasogastric Tube Versus Gastrostomy Tube for Gastric Decompression in Abdominal Surgery: A Prospective, Randomized Trial Comparing Patients' Tube-related Inconvenience," *Langenbecks Archives of Surgery* 386(6):402-409, November 2001.
Lee, S.S., et al. "Endoscopically Placed Nasogastrojejunal Feeding Tubes: A Safe Route for Enteral Nutrition in Patients with Hepatic Encephalopathy," *American Surgeon* 68(2):196-200, February 2002.

# Nasogastric tube care

Providing effective NG tube care requires meticulous monitoring of the patient and the equipment. Monitoring the patient involves checking drainage from the NG tube and assessing GI function. Monitoring the equipment involves verifying correct tube placement and irrigating the tube to ensure patency and to prevent mucosal damage.

Specific care measures vary only slightly for the most commonly used NG tubes: the single-lumen Levin tube and the double-lumen Salem sump tube.

## Equipment
Irrigant (usually normal saline solution) • irrigant container • 60-ml catheter-tip syringe • bulb syringe • suction equipment • sponge-tipped swabs or toothbrush and toothpaste • petroleum jelly • ½″ or 1″ hypoallergenic tape • water-soluble lubricant • gloves • stethoscope • linen-saver pad • optional: emesis basin

### Preparation of equipment
Make sure the suction equipment works properly. (See *Common gastric suction devices.*) When using a Salem sump tube with suction, connect the larger, primary lumen (for drainage and suction) to the suction equipment and select the appropriate setting as ordered (usually low constant suction). If the doctor doesn't specify the setting, follow the manufacturer's directions. A Levin tube usually calls for intermittent low suction.

# Common gastric suction devices

Various suction devices are available for applying negative pressure to nasogastric (NG) and other drainage tubes. Two common types are shown here.

### Portable suction machine

In the portable suction machine, a vacuum created intermittently by an electric pump draws gastric contents up the NG tube and into the collecting bottle.

### Stationary suction machine

A stationary wall-unit apparatus can provide intermittent or continuous suction. On-off switches and variable power settings let you set and adjust the suction force on either machine.

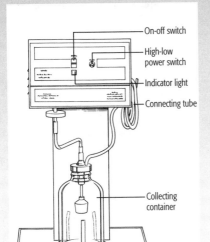

- On-off switch
- High-low power switch
- Indicator light
- Connecting tube
- Collecting container

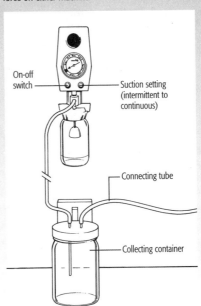

- On-off switch
- Suction setting (intermittent to continuous)
- Connecting tube
- Collecting container

## Implementation

▶ Explain the procedure and provide privacy.

▶ Wash your hands and put on gloves.

### Irrigating an NG tube

▶ Review the irrigation schedule (usually every 4 hours), if the doctor orders this procedure.

▶ Inject 10 cc of air and auscultate the epigastric area with a stethoscope and aspirate stomach contents to check correct positioning in the stomach and to prevent the patient from aspirating the irrigant.

▶ Measure the amount of irrigant in the bulb syringe or in the 60-ml catheter-tip syringe (usually 10 to 20 ml) to maintain an accurate intake and output record.

▶ When using suction with a Salem sump tube or a Levin tube, unclamp and disconnect the tube from the suction equipment while holding it over a linen-saver pad or an emesis basin to collect any drainage.

▶ Slowly instill the irrigant into the NG tube. (When irrigating the Salem sump tube, you may instill small amounts of solution into the vent lumen without interrupting suction; however, you should instill greater amounts into the larger, primary lumen.)

▶ Gently aspirate the solution with the bulb syringe or 60-ml catheter-tip syringe or connect the tube to the suction equipment as ordered. Gentle aspiration prevents excessive pressure on a suture line and on delicate gastric mucosa. Report any bleeding.

▶ Reconnect the tube to suction after completing irrigation.

### Instilling a solution through an NG tube

▶ If the doctor orders instillation, inject the solution, and don't aspirate it. Note the amount of instilled solution as "intake" on the intake and output record.

▶ Reattach the tube to suction as ordered.

▶ After attaching the Salem sump tube's primary lumen to suction, instill 10 to 20 cc of air into the vent lumen to verify patency. Listen for a soft hiss in the vent. If you don't hear this sound, suspect a clogged tube; recheck patency by instilling 10 ml of normal saline solution and 10 to 20 cc of air in the vent.

### Monitoring patient comfort and condition

▶ Provide mouth care once a shift or as needed. Depending on the patient's condition, use sponge-tipped swabs to clean his teeth or assist him to brush them with toothbrush and toothpaste. Coat the patient's lips with petroleum jelly to prevent dryness from mouth breathing.

▶ Change the tape securing the tube as needed or at least daily. Clean the skin, apply fresh tape, and dab water-soluble lubricant on the nostrils as needed.

▶ Regularly check the tape that secures the tube because sweat and nasal secretions may loosen the tape.

▶ Assess bowel sounds regularly (every 4 to 8 hours) to verify GI function.

▶ Measure the drainage amount and update the intake and output record every 8 hours. Be alert for electrolyte imbalances with excessive gastric output.

▶ Inspect gastric drainage and note its color, consistency, odor, and amount. Normal gastric secretions have no color or appear yellow-green from bile and have a mucoid consistency. Immediately report any drainage with a coffee-bean color; this may indicate bleeding. If you suspect that the drainage contains blood, use a screening test (such as Hematest) for occult blood according to your facility's policy.

### Special considerations

▶ Irrigate the NG tube with 30 ml of irrigant before and after instilling medication. Wait for about 30 minutes, or as ordered, after instillation, before reconnecting the suction equipment to allow sufficient time for the medication to be absorbed.

▶ When no drainage appears, check the suction equipment for proper function. Then, holding the NG tube over a linen-saver pad or an emesis basin, separate the tube and the suction source. Check the suction equipment by placing the suction tubing in an irrigant container. If the apparatus draws the water, check the NG tube for proper function. Note the amount of water drawn into the suction container on the intake and output record.

▶ A dysfunctional NG tube may be clogged or incorrectly positioned. Attempt to irrigate the tube, reposition the patient, or rotate and reposition the tube. However, if the tube was inserted during surgery, avoid this maneuver to ensure that the movement doesn't interfere with gastric or esophageal sutures. Notify the doctor.

▶ If you can ambulate the patient and interrupt suction, disconnect the NG tube from the suction equipment. Clamp the tube to prevent stomach contents from draining out of the tube.

▶ If the patient has a Salem sump tube, watch for gastric reflux in the vent lumen when pressure in the stomach exceeds atmospheric pressure. This problem may result from a clogged primary lumen or from a suction system that is set up improperly. Assess the suction equipment for proper functioning. Then irrigate the NG tube and instill 30 cc of air into the vent tube to maintain patency. Don't attempt to stop reflux by clamping the vent tube. Unless contraindicated, elevate the patient's torso more than 30 degrees, and keep the vent tube above his midline to prevent a siphoning effect.

### Complications

Epigastric pain and vomiting may result from a clogged or improperly placed tube. Any NG tube—the Levin tube in particular—may move and aggravate esophagitis, ulcers, or esophageal varices, causing hemorrhage. Perforation may result from aggressive intubation. Dehydration and electrolyte imbalances may result from removing body fluids and electrolytes by suctioning. Pain, swelling, and salivary dysfunction may signal parotitis, which occurs in dehydrated, debilitated patients. Intubation can cause nasal skin breakdown and discomfort and increased mucous secretions. Aspiration pneumonia may result from gastric reflux. Vigorous suction may damage the gastric mucosa and cause significant bleeding, possibly interfering with endoscopic assessment and diagnosis.

## Documentation
▶ Regularly record tube placement confirmation (usually every 4 to 8 hours).
▶ Document precisely fluid intake and output, including the instilled irrigant.
▶ Document the irrigation schedule and note the actual time of each irrigation.
▶ Record drainage color, consistency, odor, and amount.
▶ Note tape change times and condition of the nares.

### REFERENCES
Craven, R., and Hirnle, C.J. *Fundamentals of Nursing: Human Health and Function,* 4th ed. Philadelphia: Lippincott Williams & Wilkins, 2002.

Guenter, P., and Silkroski, M. *Tube Feeding: Practical Guidelines and Nursing Protocols.* Gaithersburg, Md.: Aspen Pubs., Inc., 2001.

# Nasogastric tube insertion and removal

Usually inserted to decompress the stomach, an NG tube can prevent vomiting after major surgery. An NG tube is typically in place for 48 to 72 hours after surgery, by which time peristalsis usually resumes. It may remain in place for shorter or longer periods, however, depending on its use.

The NG tube has other diagnostic and therapeutic applications, especially in assessing and treating upper GI bleeding, collecting gastric contents for analysis, performing gastric lavage, aspirating gastric secretions, and administering medications and nutrients.

Inserting an NG tube requires close observation of the patient and verification of proper placement. Removing the tube requires careful handling to prevent injury or aspiration. The tube must be inserted with extra care in pregnant patients and in those with an increased risk of complications. For example, the doctor will order an NG tube for a patient with aortic aneurysm, myocardial infarction, gastric hemorrhage, or esophageal varices only if he believes that the benefits outweigh the risks of intubation.

Most NG tubes have a radiopaque marker or strip at the distal end so that the tube's position can be verified by X-ray studies. If the position can't be confirmed, the doctor may order fluoroscopy to verify placement.

The most common NG tubes are the Levin tube, which has one lumen, and the Salem sump tube, which has two lumens, one for suction and drainage and a smaller one for ventilation. Air flows through the vent lumen continuously. This protects the delicate gastric mucosa by preventing a vacuum from forming should the tube adhere to the stomach lining. The Moss tube, which has a triple lumen, is usually inserted during surgery. (See *Types of NG tubes,* page 452.)

## Equipment
*For inserting an NG tube*
Tube (usually #12, #14, #16, or #18 French for a normal adult) • towel or linen-saver pad • facial tissues • emesis basin • penlight • 1″ or 2″ hypoallergenic tape • gloves • water-soluble lubricant • cup or glass of water with straw (if appropriate) • stethoscope • tongue blade • catheter-tip or bulb syringe or irrigation set • safety pin • ordered suction equipment • optional: metal clamp, ice, alcohol pad, warm water, large basin or plastic container, and rubber band

*For removing an NG tube*
Stethoscope • gloves • catheter-tip syringe • normal saline solution • towel or linen-saver pad • adhesive remover • optional: clamp

### Preparation of equipment
Inspect the NG tube for defects, such as rough edges or partially closed lumens. Then check the tube's patency by flushing it with water. To ease insertion, increase a stiff tube's flexibility by coiling it around your gloved fingers for a few seconds or by

## Types of NG tubes

The doctor will choose the type and diameter of nasogastric (NG) tube that best suits the patient's needs, including lavage, aspiration, enteral therapy, or stomach decompression. Choices may include the Levin and Salem sump tubes.

### Levin tube

The Levin tube is a rubber or plastic tube with a single lumen, a length of 42″ to 50″ (106.5 to 127 cm), and holes at the tip and along the side.

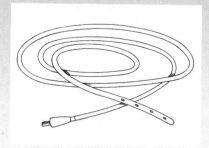

### Salem sump tube

The Salem sump tube is a double-lumen tube made of clear plastic and has a blue sump port (pigtail) that allows atmospheric air to enter the patient's stomach. Thus, the tube floats freely and doesn't adhere to or damage gastric mucosa. The larger port of this 48″ (121.9-cm) tube serves as the main suction conduit. The tube has openings at 45, 55, 65, and 75 cm as well as a radiopaque line to verify placement.

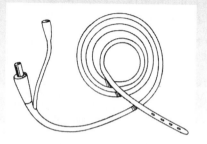

dipping it into warm water. Stiffen a limp rubber tube by briefly chilling it in ice.

## Implementation

▶ Whether you're inserting or removing an NG tube, provide privacy, wash your hands, and put on gloves before inserting the tube. Check the doctor's order to determine the type of tube that should be inserted.

### Inserting an NG tube

▶ Explain the procedure to the patient to ease anxiety and promote cooperation. Inform her that she may experience some nasal discomfort, that she may gag, and that her eyes may water. Emphasize that swallowing will ease the tube's advancement.

▶ Agree on a signal that the patient can use if she wants you to stop briefly during the procedure.

▶ Gather and prepare all necessary equipment.

▶ Help the patient into high Fowler's position unless contraindicated.

▶ Stand at the patient's right side if you're right-handed or at her left side if you're left-handed to ease insertion.

▶ Drape the towel or linen-saver pad over the patient's chest to protect her gown and bed linens from spills.

▶ Have the patient gently blow her nose to clear her nostrils.

▶ Place the facial tissues and emesis basin well within the patient's reach.

▶ Help the patient face forward with her neck in a neutral position.

▶ To determine how long the NG tube must be to reach the stomach, hold the end of the tube at the tip of the patient's nose. Extend the tube to the patient's earlobe and then down to the xiphoid process (as shown below).

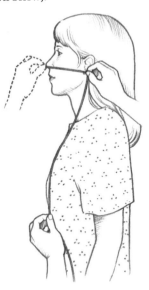

▶ Mark this distance on the tubing with the tape. (Average measurements for an adult range from 22″ to 26″ [56 to 66 cm].) It may be necessary to add 2″ (5 cm) to this measurement in tall individuals to ensure entry into the stomach.
▶ To determine which nostril will allow easier access, use a penlight and inspect for a deviated septum or other abnormalities. Ask the patient if she ever had nasal surgery or a nasal injury. Assess airflow in both nostrils by occluding one nostril at a time while the patient breathes through her nose. Choose the nostril with the better airflow.
▶ Lubricate the first 3″ (7.6 cm) of the tube with a water-soluble gel to minimize injury to the nasal passages. Using a water-soluble lubricant prevents lipoid pneumonia, which may result from aspiration of an oil-based lubricant or from accidental slippage of the tube into the trachea.
▶ Instruct the patient to hold her head straight and upright.
▶ Grasp the tube with the end pointing downward, curve it, if necessary, and carefully insert it into the more patent nostril (as shown below).

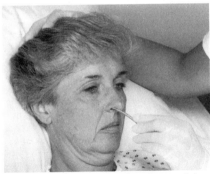

▶ Aim the tube downward and toward the ear closer to the chosen nostril. Advance it slowly to avoid pressure on the turbinates and resultant pain and bleeding.
▶ When the tube reaches the nasopharynx, you'll feel resistance. Instruct the patient to lower her head slightly to close the trachea and open the esophagus. Then rotate the tube 180 degrees toward the opposite nostril to redirect it so that the tube won't enter the patient's mouth.
▶ Unless contraindicated, offer the patient a cup or glass of water with a straw. Direct her to sip and swallow as you slowly advance the tube (as shown below). This helps the tube pass to the esophagus. (If you aren't using water, ask the patient to swallow.)

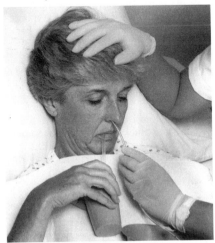

## Ensuring proper tube placement

▶ Use a tongue blade and penlight to examine the patient's mouth and throat for signs of a coiled section of tubing (especially in an unconscious patient). Coiling indicates an obstruction.

▶ Keep an emesis basin and facial tissues readily available for the patient.

▶ As you carefully advance the tube and the patient swallows, watch for respiratory distress signs, which may mean the tube is in the bronchus and must be removed immediately.

▶ Stop advancing the tube when the tape mark reaches the patient's nostril.

▶ Attach a catheter-tip or bulb syringe to the tube and try to aspirate stomach contents (as shown below). If you don't obtain stomach contents, position the patient on her left side to move the contents into the stomach's greater curvature, and aspirate again.

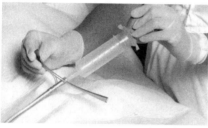

![Alert icon] **ALERT!** When confirming tube placement, never place the tube's end in a container of water. If the tube should be mispositioned in the trachea, the patient may aspirate water. Also, water without bubbles doesn't confirm proper placement. Instead, the tube may be coiled in the trachea or the esophagus.

▶ If you still can't aspirate stomach contents, advance the tube 1″ to 2″ (2.5 to 5 cm). Then inject 10 cc of air into the tube. At the same time, auscultate for air sounds with your stethoscope placed over the epigastric region. You should hear a whooshing sound if the tube is patent and properly positioned in the stomach.

▶ If these tests don't confirm proper tube placement, you'll need X-ray verification.

▶ Secure the NG tube to the patient's nose with hypoallergenic tape or another designated tube holder (as shown above right). If the patient's skin is oily, wipe the bridge of the nose with an alcohol pad and allow to dry. You will need about 4″ (10 cm) of 1″

tape. Split one end of the tape up the center about 1½″ (3.8 cm). Make tabs on the split ends (by folding sticky sides together). Stick the uncut tape end on the patient's nose so that the split in the tape starts about ½″ (1.3 cm) to 1½″ from the tip of her nose. Crisscross the tabbed ends around the tube. Then apply another piece of tape over the bridge of the nose to secure the tube.

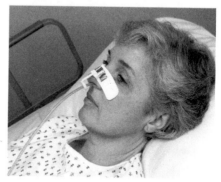

▶ Alternatively, stabilize the tube with a prepackaged product that secures and cushions it at the nose.

▶ To reduce discomfort from the weight of the tube, tie a slipknot around the tube with a rubber band, and then secure the rubber band to the patient's gown with a safety pin, or wrap another piece of tape around the end of the tube and leave a tab. Then fasten the tape tab to the patient's gown.

▶ Attach the tube to suction equipment, if ordered, and set the designated suction pressure.

▶ Provide frequent nose and mouth care while the tube is in place.

## Removing an NG tube

▶ Explain the procedure to the patient, informing her that it may cause some nasal discomfort and sneezing or gagging.

▶ Assess bowel function by auscultating for peristalsis or flatus.

▶ Help the patient into semi-Fowler's position. Then drape a towel or linen-saver pad across her chest to protect her gown and bed linens from spills.

▶ Wash your hands and put on gloves.

▶ Using a catheter-tip syringe, flush the tube with 10 ml of normal saline solution to ensure that the tube doesn't contain stomach contents that could irritate tissues during tube removal.

▶ Untape the tube from the patient's nose and then unpin it from her gown.

▶ Clamp the tube by folding it in your hand.

▶ Ask the patient to hold her breath to close the epiglottis. Then withdraw the tube gently and steadily. (When the distal end of the tube reaches the nasopharynx, you can pull it quickly.)

▶ When possible, immediately cover and remove the tube because its sight and odor may nauseate the patient.

▶ Assist the patient with thorough mouth care, and clean the tape residue from her nose with adhesive remover.

▶ For the next 48 hours, monitor the patient for signs of GI dysfunction, including nausea, vomiting, abdominal distention, and food intolerance. GI dysfunction may necessitate reinsertion of the tube.

### Special considerations

▶ A helpful device for calculating the correct tube length is Ross-Hanson tape. Place the narrow end of this measuring tape at the tip of the patient's nose. Again, extend the tape to the patient's earlobe and down to the tip of the xiphoid process. Mark this distance on the edge of the tape labeled "nose to ear to xiphoid." The corresponding measurement on the opposite edge of the tape is the proper insertion length.

▶ If the patient has a deviated septum or other nasal condition that prevents nasal insertion, pass the tube orally after removing any dentures, if necessary. Sliding the tube over the tongue, proceed as you would for nasal insertion.

▶ When using the oral route, remember to coil the end of the tube around your hand. This helps curve and direct the tube downward at the pharynx.

▶ If your patient is unconscious, tilt her chin toward her chest to close the trachea. Then advance the tube between respirations to ensure that it doesn't enter the trachea.

▶ While advancing the tube in an unconscious patient (or in a patient who can't swallow), stroke the patient's neck to encourage the swallowing reflex and facilitate passage down the esophagus.

▶ While advancing the tube, observe for signs that it has entered the trachea, such as choking or breathing difficulties in a

---

## Using an NG tube at home

If the patient will need to have a nasogastric (NG) tube in place at home – for example, for short-term feeding or gastric decompression – find out who will insert the tube. If the patient will have a home care nurse, identify her and, if possible, tell the patient when to expect her.

If the patient or a family member will perform the procedure, you'll need to provide additional instruction and supervision. Use the following checklist to prepare your teaching topics:

▶ how and where to obtain equipment needed for home intubation

▶ how to insert the tube

▶ how to verify tube placement by aspirating stomach contents

▶ how to correct tube misplacement

▶ how to prepare formula for tube feeding

▶ how to store formula, if appropriate

▶ how to administer formula through the tube

▶ how to remove and dispose of an NG tube

▶ how to clean and store a reusable NG tube

▶ how to use the NG tube for gastric decompression, if appropriate

▶ how to set up and operate suctioning equipment

▶ how to troubleshoot suctioning equipment

▶ how to perform mouth care and other hygienic procedures.

---

conscious patient and cyanosis in an unconscious patient or a patient without a cough reflex. If these signs occur, remove the tube immediately. Allow the patient time to rest; then try to reinsert the tube.

▶ After tube placement, vomiting suggests tubal obstruction or incorrect position. Assess immediately to determine the cause.

### Home care

An NG tube may be inserted or removed at home. Indications for insertion include gastric decompression and short-term feeding. A home care nurse or the patient may insert the tube, deliver the feeding, and remove the tube. (See *Using an NG tube at home*.)

## Complications

Potential complications of prolonged intubation with an NG tube include skin erosion at the nostril, sinusitis, esophagitis, esophagotracheal fistula, gastric ulceration, and pulmonary and oral infection. Additional complications that may result from suction include electrolyte imbalances and dehydration.

## Documentation

▶ Record the type and size of the NG tube and the date, time, and route of insertion.
▶ Document the type and amount of suction, if used.
▶ Record the drainage, including the amount, color, character, consistency, and odor.
▶ Document the patient's tolerance of the procedure.
▶ Record the date and time the tube is removed.
▶ Document the color, consistency, and amount of gastric drainage.
▶ Note the patient's tolerance of the removal procedure.

### REFERENCES

Craven, R., and Hirnle, C.J. *Fundamentals of Nursing: Human Health and Function,* 4th ed. Philadelphia: Lippincott Williams & Wilkins, 2002.
Guenter, P., and Silkroski, M. *Tube Feeding: Practical Guidelines and Nursing Protocols.* Gaithersburg, Md.: Aspen Pubs., Inc., 2001.

# Rectal tube insertion and removal

Whether GI hypomotility simply slows the normal release of gas and feces or results in paralytic ileus, inserting a rectal tube may relieve the discomfort of distention and flatus. Decreased motility may result from various medical or surgical conditions, certain medications (such as atropine sulfate), or even swallowed air. Conditions that contraindicate using a rectal tube include recent rectal or prostatic surgery, recent myocardial infarction, and diseases of the rectal mucosa.

## Equipment

Stethoscope ● linen-saver pads ● drape ● water-soluble lubricant ● commercial kit or #22 to #32 French rectal tube of soft rubber or plastic container (such as an emesis basin, a plastic bag, or a water bottle with vent) ● tape ● gloves ● linens

## Implementation

▶ Bring all equipment to the patient's bedside, provide privacy, and wash your hands.
▶ Explain the procedure and encourage the patient to relax.
▶ Check for abdominal distention. Using the stethoscope, auscultate for bowel sounds.
▶ Place the linen-saver pads under the patient's buttocks to absorb any drainage that may leak from the tube.
▶ Position the patient in the left-lateral Sims' position to facilitate rectal tube insertion.
▶ Put on gloves.
▶ Drape the patient's exposed buttocks.
▶ Lubricate the rectal tube tip with water-soluble lubricant to ease insertion and prevent rectal irritation.
▶ Lift the patient's right buttock to expose the anus.
▶ Insert the rectal tube tip into the anus, advancing the tube 2″ to 4″ (5 to 10 cm) into the rectum. Direct the tube toward the umbilicus along the anatomic course of the large intestine.
▶ As you insert the tube, tell the patient to breathe slowly and deeply, or suggest that he bear down as he would for a bowel movement to relax the anal sphincter and ease insertion.
▶ Using tape, secure the rectal tube to the buttocks. Then attach the tube to the container to collect possible leakage.
▶ Remove the tube after 15 to 20 minutes. If the patient reports continued discomfort or if gas wasn't expelled, you can repeat the procedure in 2 or 3 hours, if ordered.
▶ Clean the patient and replace soiled linens and the linen-saver pad. Make sure the patient feels as comfortable as possible. Again, check for abdominal distention and listen for bowel sounds.
▶ If you'll reuse the equipment, clean it and store it in the bedside cabinet; otherwise discard the tube.

## Special considerations

▶ Inform the patient about each step and reassure him throughout the procedure to encourage cooperation and promote relaxation.

▶ Fastening a plastic bag (like a balloon) to the external end of the tube lets you observe gas expulsion. Leaving a rectal tube in place indefinitely does little to promote peristalsis, can reduce sphincter responsiveness, and may lead to permanent sphincter damage or pressure necrosis of the mucosa.

▶ Repeat insertion periodically to stimulate GI activity. If the tube fails to relieve distention, notify the doctor.

## Documentation

▶ Record the date and time you insert the tube.

▶ Document the amount, color, and consistency of any evacuated matter.

▶ Record the patient's abdomen on percussion: hard, distended, soft, or drumlike.

▶ Note bowel sounds before and after insertion.

### REFERENCES

Edward, D., et al. *Bedside Critical Care Manual.* Philadelphia: Lippincott Williams & Wilkins, 2001.

Kanehira, E., et al. "Early Clinical Results of Endorectal Surgery Using a Newly Designed Rectal Tube with a Side Window," *Surgical Endoscopy* 16(1):14-17, January 2002.

# Stool collection

Stool specimens are collected to determine the presence of blood, ova and parasites, bile, fat, pathogens, or such substances as ingested drugs. Gross examination of stool characteristics, such as color, consistency, and odor, can reveal such conditions as GI bleeding and steatorrhea.

Stool specimens are collected randomly or for specific periods such as 72 hours. Because stool specimens can't be obtained on demand, proper collection requires careful instructions to the patient to ensure an uncontaminated specimen.

## Equipment

Specimen container with lid ● gloves ● two tongue blades ● paper towel ● bedpan or portable commode ● two patient-care re-

minders (for timed specimens) ● laboratory request form ● optional: enema

## Implementation

▶ Explain the procedure to the patient and to the family members, if possible, to ensure their cooperation and prevent inadvertent disposal of timed stool specimens.

### Collecting a random specimen

▶ Tell the patient to notify you when he has the urge to defecate. Have him defecate into a clean, dry bedpan or commode. Instruct him not to contaminate the specimen with urine or toilet tissue because urine inhibits fecal bacterial growth and toilet tissue contains bismuth, which interferes with test results.

▶ Put on gloves.

▶ Using a tongue blade, transfer the most representative stool specimen from the bedpan to the container and cap the container. If the patient passes blood, mucus, or pus with the stool, include this with the specimen.

▶ Wrap the tongue blade in a paper towel and discard it. Remove and discard your gloves and wash your hands thoroughly to prevent cross-contamination.

### Collecting a timed specimen

▶ Place a patient-care reminder stating SAVE ALL STOOLS over the patient's bed, in his bathroom, and in the utility room.

▶ After putting on gloves, collect the first specimen, and include this in the total specimen.

▶ Obtain the timed specimen as you would a random specimen, but remember to transfer all stools to the specimen container.

▶ If a stool specimen must be obtained with an enema, use only tap water or normal saline solution.

▶ As ordered, send each specimen to the laboratory immediately with a laboratory request form or, if permitted, refrigerate the specimens collected during the test period and send them when collection is complete. Remove and discard gloves.

▶ Make sure the patient is comfortable after the procedure and that he has the opportunity to thoroughly clean his hands and perianal area. Perineal care may be necessary for some patients.

### Special considerations

▶ Never place a stool specimen in a refrigerator that contains food or medication to prevent contamination.
▶ Notify the doctor if the stool specimen looks unusual.

### Home care

If the patient is to collect a specimen at home, instruct him to collect it in a clean container with a tight-fitting lid, wrap the container in a brown paper bag, and keep it in the refrigerator (separate from any food items) until it can be transported.

### Documentation

▶ Record the time of the specimen collection and transport to the laboratory.
▶ Note stool color, odor, and consistency, and any unusual characteristics.
▶ Document whether the patient had difficulty passing the stool.

### REFERENCES

Edward, D., et al. *Bedside Critical Care Manual*. Philadelphia: Lippincott Williams & Wilkins, 2001.
Yucesoy, M., et al. "Detection of Toxin Production in *Clostridium difficile* Strains by Three Different Methods," *Clinical Microbiology and Infection* 8(7):413-18, July 2002.

# Transabdominal tube feedings

To access the stomach, duodenum, or jejunum, the doctor may place a tube through the patient's abdominal wall. This procedure may be done surgically or percutaneously.

A gastrostomy or jejunostomy tube is usually inserted during intra-abdominal surgery. The tube may be used for feeding during the immediate postoperative period or it may provide long-term enteral access, depending on the type of surgery. Typically, the doctor will suture the tube in place to prevent gastric contents from leaking.

In contrast, a percutaneous endoscopic gastrostomy (PEG) or a percutaneous endoscopic jejunostomy (PEJ) tube can be inserted endoscopically without the need for laparotomy or general anesthesia. Typically, the insertion is done in the endoscopy suite or at the patient's bedside. A PEG or

PEJ tube may be used for nutrition, drainage, and decompression. Contraindications to endoscopic placement include obstruction (such as an esophageal stricture or duodenal blockage), previous gastric surgery, morbid obesity, and ascites. These conditions would necessitate surgical placement.

With either type of tube placement, feedings may begin after 24 hours (or when peristalsis resumes).

After a time, the tube may need replacement, and the doctor may recommend a similar tube, such as an indwelling urinary catheter or a mushroom catheter, or a gastrostomy button—a skin-level feeding tube.

### Equipment

*For feeding*
Feeding formula ● 120 ml of water ● large-bulb or catheter-tip syringe ● 4″ × 4″ gauze pads ● soap ● skin protectant ● hypoallergenic tape ● gravity-drip administration bags ● mouthwash ● toothpaste or mild salt solution ● gloves ● stethoscope ● optional: enteral infusion pump

*For decompression*
Suction apparatus with tubing and straight drainage collection set

### Preparation of equipment

Always check the expiration date on commercially prepared feeding formulas. If the formula has been prepared by the dietitian or pharmacist, check the preparation time and date. Discard any opened formula that is more than 1 day old.

Commercially prepared administration sets and enteral pumps allow continuous formula administration. Place the desired amount of formula into the gavage container and purge air from the tubing. To avoid contamination, hang only a 4- to 6-hour supply of formula at a time.

### Implementation

▶ Provide privacy and wash your hands.
▶ Explain the procedure to the patient. Tell him, for example, that feedings usually start at a slow rate and increase as tolerated. After he tolerates continuous feedings, he may progress to intermittent feedings as ordered.

▶ Assess for bowel sounds before feeding and Monitor patient for abdominal distention.

▶ Ask the patient to sit, or assist him into semi-Fowler's position, for the entire feeding. This helps to prevent esophageal reflux and pulmonary aspiration of the formula. For an intermittent feeding, have him maintain this position throughout the feeding and for 30 minutes to 1 hour afterward.

▶ Put on gloves. Before starting the feeding, measure residual gastric contents. Attach the syringe to the feeding tube and aspirate. If the contents measure more than twice the amount infused, hold the feeding and recheck in 1 hour. If residual contents still remain too high, notify the doctor. Chances are the formula isn't being absorbed properly. Keep in mind that residual contents will be minimal with PEJ tube feedings.

▶ Allow 30 ml of water to flow into the feeding tube to establish patency.

▶ Be sure to administer formula at room temperature. Cold formula may cause cramping.

### Intermittent feedings

▶ Allow gravity to help the formula flow over 30 to 45 minutes. Faster infusions may cause bloating, cramps, or diarrhea.

▶ Begin intermittent feeding with a low volume (200 ml) daily. According to the patient's tolerance, increase the volume per feeding as needed to reach the desired calorie intake.

▶ When the feeding finishes, flush the feeding tube with 30 to 60 ml of water. This maintains patency and provides hydration.

▶ Cap the tube to prevent leakage.

▶ Rinse the feeding administration set thoroughly with hot water to avoid contaminating subsequent feedings. Allow it to dry between feedings.

### Continuous feedings

▶ Measure residual gastric contents every 4 hours.

▶ To administer the feeding with a pump, set up the equipment according to the manufacturer's guidelines, and fill the feeding bag. To administer the feeding by gravity, fill the container with formula and purge air from the tubing.

▶ Monitor the gravity drip rate or pump infusion rate frequently to ensure accurate delivery of formula.

▶ Flush the feeding tube with 30 to 60 ml of water every 4 hours to maintain patency and to provide hydration.

▶ Monitor intake and output to anticipate and detect fluid or electrolyte imbalances.

### Decompression

▶ To decompress the stomach, connect the PEG port to the suction device with tubing or straight gravity drainage tubing. Jejunostomy feeding may be given simultaneously via the PEJ port of the dual-lumen tube.

### Tube exit site care

▶ Provide daily skin care.

▶ Gently remove the dressing by hand. Never cut away the dressing over the catheter because you might cut the tube or the sutures holding the tube in place.

▶ At least daily and as needed, clean the skin around the tube's exit site using a 4″ × 4″ gauze pad soaked in the prescribed cleaning solution. When healed, wash the skin around the exit site daily with soap. Rinse the area with water and pat dry. Apply skin protectant, if necessary.

▶ Anchor a gastrostomy or jejunostomy tube to the skin with hypoallergenic tape to prevent peristaltic migration of the tube. This also prevents tension on the suture anchoring the tube in place.

▶ Coil the tube, if necessary, and tape it to the abdomen to prevent pulling and contamination of the tube. PEG and PEJ tubes have toggle-bolt-like internal and external bumpers that make tape anchors unnecessary. (See *Caring for a PEG or PEJ site,* page 460.)

## Special considerations

▶ If the patient vomits or complains of nausea, feeling too full, or regurgitation, stop the feeding immediately and assess his condition. Flush the feeding tube and attempt to restart the feeding in 1 hour (measure residual gastric contents first). You may have to decrease the volume or rate of feedings. If the patient develops dumping syndrome, which includes nausea, vomiting, cramps, pallor, and diarrhea, the feedings may have been given too quickly.

▶ Provide oral hygiene frequently. Brush all surfaces of the teeth, gums, and tongue

# Caring for a PEG or PEJ site

The exit site of a percutaneous endoscopic gastrostomy (PEG) or percutaneous endoscopic jejunostomy (PEJ) tube requires routine observation and care. Follow these care guidelines:

▶ Change the dressing daily while the tube is in place.

▶ After removing the dressing, carefully slide the tube's outer bumper away from the skin (as shown below) about ½″ (1.5 cm).

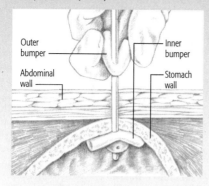

Outer bumper — Inner bumper

Abdominal wall — Stomach wall

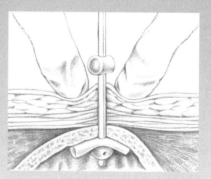

▶ Examine the skin around the tube. Look for redness and other signs of infection or erosion.

▶ Gently depress the skin surrounding the tube and inspect for drainage (as shown above right). Expect minimal wound drainage initially after implantation. This should subside in about 1 week.

▶ Inspect the tube for wear and tear. (A tube that wears out will need replacement.)

▶ Clean the site with the prescribed cleaning solution. Then apply povidone-iodine ointment over the exit site according to your facility's guidelines.

▶ Rotate the outer bumper 90 degrees (to avoid repeating the same tension on the same skin area), and slide the outer bumper back over the exit site.

▶ If leakage appears at the PEG tube site, or if the patient risks dislodging the tube, apply a sterile gauze dressing over the site. Don't put sterile gauze underneath the outer bumper. Loosening the anchor this way allows the feeding tube free play, which could lead to wound abscess.

▶ Write the date and time of the dressing change on the tape.

---

at least twice daily using mouthwash, toothpaste, or a mild salt solution.

▶ You can administer most tablets and pills through the tube by crushing them and diluting as necessary. (However, don't crush enteric-coated or sustained-release drugs, which lose their effectiveness when crushed.) Medications should be in liquid form for administration.

▶ Control diarrhea resulting from dumping syndrome by using continuous pump or gravity-drip infusions, diluting the feeding formula, or adding antidiarrheal medications.

### Home care

Instruct the patient and family members or other caregivers in all aspects of enteral feedings, including tube maintenance and site care. Specify signs and symptoms to

report to the doctor, define emergency situations and review actions to take.

When the tube needs replacement, advise the patient that the doctor may insert a replacement gastrostomy button or a latex, indwelling, or mushroom catheter after removing the initial feeding tube. The procedure may be done in the doctor's office or your facility's endoscopy suite.

As the patient's tolerance of tube feeding improves, he may wish to try syringe feedings rather than intermittent feedings. If appropriate, teach him how to feed himself by the syringe method. (See *Teaching the patient about syringe feeding.*)

### Complications

Common complications related to transabdominal tubes include GI or other systemic problems, mechanical malfunction, and

# Teaching the patient about syringe feeding

If the patient plans to feed himself by syringe when he returns home, you'll need to teach him how to do this before he's discharged. Here are some points to emphasize.

### Initial instructions
First, show the patient how to clamp the feeding tube, remove the syringe's bulb or plunger, and place the tip of the syringe into the feeding tube (as shown below). Then tell him to instill between 30 and 60 ml of water into the feeding tube to make sure it stays open and patent.

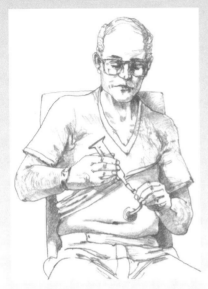

Next, tell him to pour the feeding solution into the syringe and begin the feeding (as shown above right). As the solution flows into the stomach, show him how to tilt the syringe to allow air bubbles to escape. Describe the discomfort that air bubbles may cause.

### Tips for free flow
When about one-fourth of the feeding solution remains, direct the patient to refill the syringe.

Caution him to avoid letting the syringe empty completely. Doing so may result in abdominal cramping and gas.

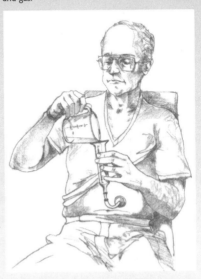

Show the patient how to increase and decrease the solution's flow rate by raising or lowering the syringe. Explain that he may need to dilute a thick solution to promote free flow.

### Finishing up
Inform the patient that the feeding infusion process should take at least 15 minutes. If the process takes less than 15 minutes, dumping syndrome may result.

Show the patient the steps needed to finish the feeding, including how to flush the tube with water, clamp the tube, and clean the equipment for later use. If he's using disposable gear, urge him to discard it properly. Review how to store unused feeding solution as appropriate.

---

metabolic disturbances. Cramping, nausea, vomiting, bloating, and diarrhea may be related to medication; rapid infusion rate; formula contamination, osmolarity, or temperature (too cold or too warm); fat malabsorption; or intestinal atrophy from malnutrition. Constipation may result from inadequate hydration or insufficient exercise.

Systemic problems may be caused by pulmonary aspiration, infection at the tube exit site, or contaminated formula. Proper positioning during feeding, verification of tube placement, meticulous skin care, and aseptic formula preparation are ways to prevent these complications.

Typical mechanical problems include tube dislodgment, obstruction, or impairment. For example, a PEG or PEJ tube may migrate if the external bumper loosens. Occlusion may result from incompletely crushed and liquefied medication particles or inadequate tube flushing. Further, the tube may rupture or crack from age, drying, or frequent manipulation.

Monitor the patient for vitamin and mineral deficiencies, glucose tolerance, and fluid and electrolyte imbalances, which may follow bouts of diarrhea or constipation.

## Documentation

◗ On the intake and output record, document the date, time, and amount of each feeding and the water volume instilled.
◗ Separately maintain total volumes for nutrients and water, to allow calculation of nutrient intake.
◗ Document the type of formula, the infusion method and rate.
◗ Document the amount of residual gastric contents.
◗ Record complications and abdominal assessment findings.
◗ Record the patient's tolerance of the procedure and formula.
◗ Note patient-teaching topics covered and the patient's progress in self-care.

### REFERENCES

Bowers, S. "All About Tubes: Your Guide to Enteral Feeding Devices," *Nursing2000* 30(12):41-47, December 2000.
Craven, R., and Hirnle, C.J. *Fundamentals of Nursing: Human Health and Function,* 4th ed. Philadelphia: Lippincott Williams & Wilkins, 2002.
Guenter, P., and Silkroski, M. *Tube Feeding: Practical Guidelines and Nursing Protocols.* Gaithersburg, Md.: Aspen Pubs., Inc., 2001.
Stone, S.J., et al. "Bedside Placement of Postpyloric Feeding Tubes," *AACN Clinical Issues* 11(4):517-30, November 2000.

# Tube feedings

Tube feeding involves delivery of a liquid feeding formula directly to the stomach (known as gastric gavage), duodenum, or jejunum. Gastric gavage typically is indicated for a patient who can't eat normally because of dysphagia or oral or esophageal obstruction or injury. Gastric feedings also may be given to an unconscious or intubated patient or to a patient recovering from GI tract surgery who can't ingest food orally.

Duodenal or jejunal feedings decrease the risk of aspiration because the formula bypasses the pylorus. Jejunal feedings result in reduced pancreatic stimulation; thus, the patient may require an elemental diet.

Patients usually receive gastric feedings on an intermittent schedule. For duodenal or jejunal feedings, however, most patients seem to better tolerate a continuous slow drip.

Liquid nutrient solutions come in various formulas for administration through an NG tube, small-bore feeding tube, gastrostomy or jejunostomy tube, percutaneous endoscopic gastrostomy or jejunostomy tube, or gastrostomy feeding button. Tube feeding is contraindicated in patients who have no bowel sounds or a suspected intestinal obstruction.

## Equipment
*For gastric feedings*
Feeding formula ● graduated container ● 120 ml of water ● gavage bag with tubing and flow regulator clamp ● towel or linen-saver pad ● 60-ml syringe ● stethoscope ● optional: infusion controller and tubing set (for continuous administration), adapter to connect gavage tubing to feeding tube

*For duodenal or jejunal feedings*
Feeding formula ● enteral administration set containing a gavage container, drip chamber, roller clamp or flow regulator, and tube connector ● I.V. pole ● 60-ml syringe with adapter tip ● water ● optional: pump administration set (for an enteral infusion pump), Y-connector

*For nasal and oral care*
Cotton-tipped applicators ● water-soluble lubricant ● sponge-tipped swabs ● petroleum jelly

A bulb syringe or large catheter-tip syringe may be substituted for a gavage bag after the patient demonstrates tolerance for a gravity drip infusion. The doctor may order an infusion pump to ensure accurate delivery of the prescribed formula.

## Preparation of equipment

Make sure to refrigerate formulas prepared in the dietary department or pharmacy. Refrigerate commercial formulas only after opening them. Check the date on all formula containers. Discard expired commercial formula. Use powdered formula within 24 hours of mixing. Always shake the container well to mix the solution thoroughly.

Allow the formula to warm to room temperature before administration. Cold formula can increase the chance of diarrhea. Never warm it over direct heat or in a microwave because heat may curdle the formula or change its chemical composition. Also, hot formula may injure the patient.

Pour 60 ml of water into the graduated container. After closing the flow clamp on the administration set, pour the appropriate amount of formula into the gavage bag. Hang no more than a 4- to 6-hour supply at one time to prevent bacterial growth.

Open the flow clamp on the administration set to remove air from the lines. This keeps air from entering the patient's stomach and causing distention and discomfort.

## Implementation

▶ Provide privacy and wash your hands.
▶ Inform the patient that he'll receive nourishment through the tube and explain the procedure to him. If possible, give him a schedule of subsequent feedings.
▶ If the patient has a nasal or oral tube, cover his chest with a towel or linen-saver pad to protect him and the bed linens from spills.
▶ Assess the patient's abdomen for bowel sounds and distention.

## Delivering a gastric feeding

▶ Elevate the bed to semi-Fowler's or high Fowler's position to prevent aspiration by gastroesophageal reflux and to promote digestion.
▶ Check placement of the feeding tube to be sure it hasn't slipped out since the last feeding.

**⚠ ALERT!** Never give a tube feeding until you're sure the tube is properly positioned in the patient's stomach. Administering a feeding through a mis-placed tube can cause formula to enter the patient's lungs.

▶ To check tube patency and position, remove the cap or plug from the feeding tube and use the syringe to inject 5 to 10 cc of air through the tube. At the same time, auscultate the patient's stomach with the stethoscope. Listen for a whooshing sound to confirm tube positioning in the stomach. Also aspirate stomach contents to confirm tube patency and placement.
▶ To assess gastric emptying, aspirate and measure residual gastric contents. Hold feedings if residual volume is greater then the predetermined amount specified in the doctor's order (usually 50 to 100 ml). Reinstill any aspirate obtained.
▶ Connect the gavage bag tubing to the feeding tube. Depending on the type of tube used, you may need to use an adapter to connect the two.
▶ If you're using a bulb or catheter-tip syringe, remove the bulb or plunger and attach the syringe to the pinched-off feeding tube to prevent excess air from entering the patient's stomach, causing distention. If you're using an infusion controller, thread the tube from the formula container through the controller according to the manufacturer's directions. Blue food dye can be added to the feeding to quickly identify aspiration. Purge the tubing of air and attach it to the feeding tube.
▶ Open the regulator clamp on the gavage bag tubing and adjust the flow rate appropriately. When using a bulb syringe, fill the syringe with formula and release the feeding tube to allow formula to flow through it. The height at which you hold the syringe will determine the flow rate. When the syringe is three-quarters empty, pour more formula into it.
▶ To prevent air from entering the tube and the patient's stomach, never allow the syringe to empty completely. If you're using an infusion controller, set the flow rate according to the manufacturer's directions. Always administer a tube feeding slowly—typically 200 to 350 ml over 15 to 30 minutes, depending on the patient's tolerance and the doctor's order—to prevent sudden stomach distention, which can cause nausea, vomiting, cramps, or diarrhea.
▶ After administering the appropriate amount of formula, flush the tubing by adding about 60 ml of water to the gavage

bag or bulb syringe, or manually flush it using a barrel syringe. This maintains the tube's patency by removing excess formula, which could occlude the tube.

▶ If you're administering a continuous feeding, flush the feeding tube every 4 hours to help prevent tube occlusion. Monitor gastric emptying every 4 hours.

▶ To discontinue gastric feeding (depending on the equipment you're using), close the regulator clamp on the gavage bag tubing, disconnect the syringe from the feeding tube, or turn off the infusion controller.

▶ Cover the end of the feeding tube with its plug or cap to prevent leakage and contamination of the tube.

▶ Leave the patient in semi-Fowler's or high Fowler's position for at least 30 minutes.

▶ Rinse all reusable equipment with warm water. Dry it and store it in a convenient place for the next feeding. Change equipment every 24 hours or according to your facility's policy.

### Delivering a duodenal or jejunal feeding

▶ Elevate the head of the bed and place the patient in low Fowler's position.

▶ Open the enteral administration set and hang the gavage container on the I.V. pole.

▶ If you're using a nasoduodenal tube, measure its length to check tube placement. Remember that you may not get any residual when you aspirate the tube.

▶ Open the flow clamp and regulate the flow to the desired rate. To regulate the rate using a volumetric infusion pump, follow the manufacturer's directions for setting up the equipment. Most patients receive small amounts initially, with volumes increasing gradually once tolerance is established.

▶ Flush the tube every 4 hours with water to maintain patency and provide hydration. A needle catheter jejunostomy tube may require flushing every 2 hours to prevent formula buildup inside the tube. A Y connector may be useful for frequent flushing. Attach the continuous feeding to the main port and use the side port for flushes.

▶ Change equipment every 24 hours or according to facility policy.

### Special considerations

▶ If the feeding solution doesn't initially flow through a bulb syringe, attach the bulb and squeeze it gently to start the flow. Then remove the bulb. Never use the bulb to force the formula through the tube.

▶ If the patient becomes nauseated or vomits, stop the feeding immediately. The patient may vomit if the stomach becomes distended from overfeeding or delayed gastric emptying.

▶ To reduce oropharyngeal discomfort from the tube, allow the patient to brush his teeth or care for his dentures regularly and encourage frequent gargling. If the patient is unconscious, administer oral care with wet sponge-tipped swabs every 4 hours. Use petroleum jelly on dry, cracked lips. (*Note:* Dry mucous membranes may indicate dehydration, which requires increased fluid intake.) Clean the patient's nostrils with cotton-tipped applicators, apply lubricant along the mucosa, and assess the skin for signs of breakdown.

▶ During continuous feedings, assess the patient frequently for abdominal distention. Flush the tubing by adding about 50 ml of water to the gavage bag or bulb syringe. This maintains the tube's patency by removing excess formula, which could occlude the tube.

▶ If the patient develops diarrhea, administer small, frequent, less concentrated feedings, or administer bolus feedings over a longer time. Also, make sure that the formula isn't cold and that proper storage and sanitation practices have been followed. The loose stools associated with tube feedings make extra perineal and skin care necessary. Giving paregoric, tincture of opium, or diphenoxylate hydrochloride may improve the condition. Changing to a formula with more fiber may eliminate liquid stools.

▶ If the patient becomes constipated, the doctor may increase the fruit, vegetable, or sugar content of the formula. Assess the patient's hydration status because dehydration may produce constipation. Increase fluid intake as necessary. If the condition persists, administer an appropriate drug or enema, as ordered.

▶ Drugs can be administered through the feeding tube. Except for enteric-coated drugs, time-released, or sustained-release medications, crush tablets or open and dilute capsules in water before administering them. Make sure to flush the tubing afterward to ensure full instillation of medication. Keep in mind that some drugs may change the osmolarity of the feeding formula and cause diarrhea.

▶ Small-bore feeding tubes may kink, making instillation impossible. If you suspect this problem, try changing the patient's position, or withdraw the tube a few inches and restart. Never use a guide wire to reposition the tube.

▶ Constantly monitor the flow rate of a blended or high-residue formula to determine if the formula is clogging the tubing as it settles. To prevent such clogging, squeeze the bag frequently to agitate the solution.

▶ Monitor blood glucose levels to assess glucose tolerance. (A patient with a serum glucose level of less than 200 mg/dl is considered stable.) Also monitor serum levels of electrolytes, blood urea nitrogen, and glucose as well as serum osmolality and other pertinent findings to determine the patient's response to therapy and to assess his hydration status.

▶ Check the flow rate hourly to ensure correct infusion. (With an improvised administration set, use a time tape to record the rate because it's difficult to get precise readings from an irrigation container or enema bag.)

▶ For duodenal or jejunal feeding, most patients tolerate a continuous drip better than bolus feedings. Bolus feedings can cause such complications as hyperglycemia and diarrhea.

### Home care
Patient education for home tube feeding includes instructions on an infusion control device to maintain accuracy, use of the syringe or bag and tubing, care of the tube and insertion site, and formula mixing. Formula may be mixed in an electric blender according to package directions. Formula not used within 24 hours must be discarded. If the formula must hang for more than 8 hours, advise the patient to use a gavage or pump administration set with an ice pouch to decrease the incidence of bacterial growth. Tell him to use a new bag daily.

Teach family members signs and symptoms to report to the doctor or home care nurse as well as measures to take in an emergency.

### Complications
Erosion of esophageal, tracheal, nasal, and oropharyngeal mucosa can result if tubes are left in place for a long time. If possible, use smaller-lumen tubes to prevent such irritation. Check your facility's policy regarding the frequency of changing feeding tubes to prevent complications.

Using the gastric route, frequent or large-volume feedings can cause bloating and retention. Dehydration, diarrhea, and vomiting can cause metabolic disturbances. Cramping and abdominal distention usually indicate intolerance.

Using the duodenal or jejunal route, clogging of the feeding tube is common. The patient may experience metabolic, fluid, and electrolyte abnormalities, including hyperglycemia, hyperosmolar dehydration, coma, edema, hypernatremia, and essential fatty acid deficiency.

The patient also may experience dumping syndrome, in which a large amount of hyperosmotic solution in the duodenum causes excessive diffusion of fluid through the semipermeable membrane and results in diarrhea. In a patient with low serum albumin levels, these symptoms may result from low oncotic pressure in the duodenal mucosa. (See *Managing tube feeding problems,* page 466.)

### Documentation
▶ Record the date, volume of formula, and volume of water on the intake and output sheet.

▶ Document abdominal assessment findings (including tube exit site, if appropriate); amount of residual gastric contents; verification of tube placement; amount, type, and time of feeding; and tube patency.

▶ Document the patient's tolerance of the feeding, including nausea, vomiting, cramping, diarrhea, and distention.

▶ Note the result of blood and urine tests, hydration status, and any drugs given through the tube.

▶ Record the date and time of administration set changes, oral and nasal hygiene, and results of specimen collections.

# Managing tube feeding problems

| Complication | Intervention |
|---|---|
| Aspiration of gastric secretions | ▶ Discontinue feeding immediately.<br>▶ Perform tracheal suction of aspirated contents, if possible.<br>▶ Notify the doctor. Prophylactic antibiotics and chest physiotherapy may be ordered.<br>▶ Check tube placement before feeding to prevent complication. |
| Hyperglycemia | ▶ Monitor blood glucose levels.<br>▶ Notify the doctor of elevated levels.<br>▶ Administer insulin, if ordered.<br>▶ Change the formula to one with a lower sugar content, as ordered. |
| Tube obstruction | ▶ Flush the tube with warm water. If necessary, replace the tube.<br>▶ Flush the tube with 50 ml of water after each feeding to remove excess sticky formula, which could occlude the tube. |
| Vomiting, bloating, diarrhea, or cramps | ▶ Reduce the flow rate.<br>▶ Administer metoclopramide to increase GI motility.<br>▶ Warm the formula to prevent GI distress.<br>▶ For 30 minutes after feeding, position the patient on his right side with his head elevated to facilitate gastric emptying.<br>▶ Notify the doctor. He may want to reduce the amount of formula being given during each feeding. |

## REFERENCES

American Gastroenterological Association. "AGA Medical Position Statement: Guidelines for the Use of Enteral Nutrition," *Gastroenterology* 108(4):1280-81, April 1995. *www.harcourthealth.com/gastro/policy/v108n4p1280.html*

Bowers, S. "All About Tubes: Your Guide to Enteral Feeding Devices," *Nursing2000* 30(12):41-47, December 2000.

Craven, R., and Hirnle, C.J. *Fundamentals of Nursing: Human Health and Function,* 4th ed. Philadelphia: Lippincott Williams & Wilkins, 2002.

Guenter, P., and Silkroski, M. *Tube Feeding: Practical Guidelines and Nursing Protocols.* Gaithersburg, Md.: Aspen Pubs., Inc., 2001.

Metheny, N.A., and Titler, M.G. "Assessing Placement of Feeding Tubes," *American Journal of Nursing* 101(5):36-45, May 2001.

Stone, S.J., et al. "Bedside Placement of Post-pyloric Feeding Tubes," *AACN Clinical Issues* 11(4):517-30, November 2000.

# 9

# Renal and urologic care

**B**ECAUSE THE FUNCTION OF THE URINARY (OR RENAL-UROLOGIC) SYSTEM IS TO PRODUCE, transport, collect, and excrete urine, its dysfunction will disrupt fluid, electrolyte, and acid-base balance and impair waste elimination. To restore or promote effective functioning, treatment of a renal or urologic disorder usually involves temporary or permanent insertion of a urinary, peritoneal, or vascular catheter. Catheterization also allows monitoring of renal and urologic function and aids diagnosis of dysfunction.

When caring for a patient with a renal or urologic disorder, one goal is to help him accept an invasive procedure or adjust to an altered body image. To meet this goal, you must begin by assessing the amount and kind of information he needs and can absorb about the procedure. Then you can present or reinforce this information and tell him what to expect.

# Protocols

## Managing the patient experiencing urinary incontinence

### Purpose
To effectively treat the involuntary loss of urine and to prevent or minimize its recurrence

### Collaborative level
Interdependent

### Expected patient outcomes
▶ The patient's involuntary loss of urine will be reduced or prevented.

### Definition of terms
▶ *Kegel exercises:* Pelvic muscle exercises that systematically contract and relax the pubococcygeal muscles.
▶ *Overflow incontinence:* Urine loss caused by bladder overdistention, which may result from an underactive or contractile detrusor muscle or bladder outlet, urethral obstruction, or detrusor-external sphincter dyssynergia.
▶ *Stress incontinence:* Urine leakage during activities that increase abdominal pressure, such as coughing, sneezing, and laughing.
▶ *Urge incontinence:* The inability to delay urination accompanied by an abrupt, strong desire to void.

▶ *Urinary incontinence:* Demonstrable, involuntary urine loss that causes a social or hygiene problem.

### Indications
Treatment
▶ Stress incontinence
▶ Urge incontinence
▶ Overflow incontinence
▶ Benign prostatic hyperplasia (BPH)

Prevention
▶ Urinary tract infections

### Assessment guidance
Signs and symptoms
*BPH*
▶ Weak urine stream, urinary hesitancy, straining to void, post-void leakage
▶ Pelvic mass
▶ Atrophic vaginitis
▶ Fecal impaction
▶ Perineal skin breakdown related to urine leakage

*Overflow incontinence*
▶ Feelings of bladder fullness
▶ Leakage of small amounts of urine

*Stress incontinence*
▶ Urine loss triggered by laughing, coughing, sneezing, or movement
▶ Urinary frequency

*Urge incontinence*
▶ Urinary frequency and urgency
▶ Voiding of small amounts

## Diagnostic studies
### *Laboratory tests*
▶ Blood urea nitrogen level
▶ Creatinine level
▶ Fasting glucose level
▶ Prostate-specific antigen level
▶ Renal function tests
▶ Calcium level
▶ Urinalysis
▶ Urine culture
▶ Urine cytology

### *Imaging tests*
▶ Prostate ultrasonography
▶ Renal ultrasonography
▶ Voiding cystourethrography

### *Other*
▶ Post-void residual
▶ Prostate biopsy
▶ Urodynamic studies (simple and complex)

## Nursing interventions
▶ Encourage the patient to urinate on a regular schedule to help retrain the bladder.
▶ Increase the patient's fluid intake to six to eight 8-oz glasses of water per day, unless contraindicated. Limit his consumption of caffeinated and acidic beverages.
▶ Increase the patient's dietary fiber intake and take other steps to avoid constipation, which can cause urinary incontinence.
▶ Prepare the patient for surgery, such as for bladder neck suspension, obstruction removal, and periurethral injection.
▶ Administer prescribed medications, such as a bladder relaxant, alpha-receptor agonist, and estrogen.
▶ As needed, apply and maintain an external urine-collection device, which may include an incontinence pad, an indwelling urinary catheter, or a new device, such as the Reliance balloon-tipped urethral plug and the Miniguard patch for the urethral meatus.

## Patient teaching
▶ Teach the patient to perform Kegel exercises. If possible, use biofeedback to help ensure proper performance.

▶ Instruct the patient to drink enough water but to avoid caffeinated and acidic fluids.
▶ Show the patient how to retrain his bladder by recording his fluid intake and output, noting his current urination pattern, and then scheduling specific times to urinate.
▶ Teach the patient how to take his medication properly and safely. Stress the importance of continuing the medication regimen, especially if he must take a diuretic.

## Precautions
▶ Ensure that the patient's fluid intake is safe in relation to other diseases that may coexist.
▶ Observe the patient for signs and symptoms of fluid overload.
▶ Observe the patient for signs and symptoms of electrolyte imbalances.
▶ Assess the patient for signs of laxative abuse.

## Documentation
▶ Record subjective and objective assessment data, including diagnostic test results, in the patient's chart.
▶ Document the patient's fluid intake and output, including the type of fluid intake, frequency of urination, and volume and characteristics of urine.
▶ Record the patient's skin condition.
▶ Record doctor notification and all treatments and interventions performed.
▶ Note the patient's response to treatment.
▶ Document all patient teaching, especially your teaching of Kegel exercises and the patient's ability to perform them correctly.

## Related procedures
▶ Blood glucose tests
▶ Catheter irrigation, urinary
▶ Credé's maneuver
▶ Hand washing
▶ Male incontinence device
▶ Oral drugs
▶ Physical assessment
▶ Postoperative care
▶ Preoperative care
▶ Self-catheterization
▶ Standard precautions
▶ Urine collection
▶ Urine glucose and ketone tests
▶ Urine specific gravity
▶ Vaginal examination

## REFERENCES

Barkley, T., and Myers, T. *Practice Guidelines for Acute Care Nurse Practitioners.* Philadelphia: W.B. Saunders Co., 2001.

Bates, P. "Renal and Urological Problems," in *Medical Surgical Nursing,* 5th ed. Edited by Lewis, S.M., et al. St. Louis: Mosby–Year Book, Inc., 2000.

Bates, P. "Urinary System," in *Medical Surgical Nursing,* 5th ed. Edited by Lewis, S.M., et al. St. Louis: Mosby–Year Book, Inc., 2000.

Brunier, G., and Bartucci, M. "Acute and Chronic Renal Failure," in *Medical Surgical Nursing,* 5th ed. Edited by Lewis, S.M., et al. St. Louis: Mosby–Year Book, Inc., 2000.

Kegel, A.H. "Progressive Resistance Exercises in the Functional Restoration of the Perineal Muscles," *American Journal of Obstetrics and Gynecology* 56:238-49, 1948.

King, B. "Meds and the Dialysis Patient," *RN* 63(7):55-60, July 2001.

Kolcaba, K., et al. "Kegel Exercises. Strengthening the Weak Pelvic Floor Muscles that May Cause Urinary Incontinence." *AJN,* 100(11):59, November 2000.

Smoger, S.H., et al. "Urinary Incontinence Among Male Veterans Receiving Care in Primary Care Clinics," *Annals of Internal Medicine* 132(7):547-41, April 2000.

Thomas, S. "Continence Focus: Good Practice in Continence Services," *Nursing Standards* 14(47):9-15, August 2000.

## ORGANIZATIONS

National Institute of Diabetes and Digestive and Kidney Diseases: *www.niddk.nih.gov*

# Managing the patient requiring dialysis

## Purpose

To remove the end products of protein metabolism from the blood and to maintain fluid and electrolyte balance

## Collaborative level

Interdependent

## Expected patient outcomes

▶ The patient will demonstrate fewer or no signs and symptoms of fluid and electrolyte imbalance.

▶ The patient will show signs and symptoms that reflect removal of the end products of metabolism.

## Definition of terms

▶ *Hemodialysis:* The process of removing metabolic wastes and substances from the bloodstream by removing the blood, circulating it through a purifying dialyzer, and then returning it to the body.

▶ *Peritoneal dialysis:* The process of repeatedly instilling dialysate into the peritoneal cavity; the dialysate attracts end products, fluids, and electrolytes into it and then is withdrawn from the body.

## Indications

Treatment
▶ End-stage renal disease
▶ Drug toxicity
▶ Chemical toxicity

Prevention
▶ Electrolyte imbalance
▶ Acidosis
▶ Renal damage
▶ Platelet dysfunction
▶ Uremic encephalopathy

## Assessment guidance

Signs and symptoms
▶ Anorexia
▶ Cardiomegaly
▶ Crackles
▶ Decreased libido
▶ Easy bruising
▶ Edema
▶ Epistaxis
▶ Forgetfulness
▶ Hypertension
▶ Iso-osmolar urine
▶ Metallic taste in mouth
▶ Myoclonus
▶ Nausea
▶ Peripheral neuropathy (if associated with diabetes)
▶ Pleural effusion
▶ Pruritus
▶ Sallow complexion
▶ Shortness of breath
▶ Weakness

Diagnostic studies
*Laboratory tests*
▶ Antistreptolysin-O titer (to detect glomerulonephritis)
▶ Blood urea nitrogen level
▶ Complete blood count
▶ Creatinine level
▶ Cytology
▶ Fasting blood glucose level

▶ Renal function tests
▶ Calcium level
▶ Phosphate level
▶ Potassium level
▶ Urinalysis
▶ Urine culture
▶ Urine specific gravity

*Imaging tests*
▶ Computed tomography scan (performed with caution because of use of radioiodinated contrast media)
▶ Cystourethrography
▶ Excretory urography
▶ Kidney-ureter-bladder radiography
▶ Renal ultrasonography

## Nursing interventions
▶ Modify the patient's diet based on his disease and type of dialysis. Expect to regulate his fluid and sodium intake to control fluid balance, restrict his protein intake to prevent waste product accumulation, and limit his potassium intake to prevent weakness and cardiac conduction abnormalities.
▶ Assess the patient's fluid intake and output to detect altered urinary elimination.
▶ Use strict sterile technique.
▶ Monitor the patient's vital signs every 10 to 15 minutes for the first hour of exchanges, then every 2 to 4 hours, or more frequently, if necessary.
▶ For the patient receiving hemodialysis, maintain his vascular access device. For the patient receiving peritoneal dialysis, perform in-and-out catheterization as needed.
▶ Provide emotional support for the patient and his family.
▶ Provide preoperative and postoperative care for the patient who requires surgery.
▶ Always monitor outflow fluid (effluent) for color and clarity.
▶ Administer prescribed medications.
▶ Provide pain relief and comfort measures and discuss inadequate pain relief with the doctor.
▶ Perform dressing changes, as needed; assess the site for drainage and the tissue around the site for redness and swelling.

## Patient teaching
▶ Teach the patient about his underlying disease, which may be acute or chronic.
▶ Instruct the patient to follow a diet high in calories but low in protein, sodium,

potassium, and phosphorus to avoid taxing his kidneys further.
▶ Advise the patient about fluid restrictions.
▶ Teach the patient to recognize signs and symptoms of infection, such as redness and swelling.
▶ Tell the patient about his medication regimen and stress the importance of following it exactly as prescribed.
▶ Teach the family about the patient's dialysis and their involvement in it.
▶ Suggest coping strategies, and refer the patient and his family to support groups, as needed.

## Precautions
▶ Assess the patient for sensitivity to medication before administration.
▶ Assess the patient for anticoagulation therapy before he undergoes an invasive procedure.
▶ Avoid the use of contrast media because the patient's kidneys may not be able to filter it.
▶ Closely monitor the patient with heart failure or a respiratory or neurologic disorder.

## Documentation
▶ Record subjective and objective assessment data, including diagnostic test results, in the patient's chart.
▶ Document the patient's fluid intake and output, including the type of fluid intake, frequency of urination, and volume and characteristics of urine.
▶ Note the patient's vital signs frequently; note his body weight daily.
▶ Record all I.M. and I.V. bolus injections.
▶ Record doctor notification and all treatments and interventions performed.
▶ Note the patient's response to treatment.
▶ Document all precautions taken to prevent latex allergy.
▶ Document all teaching about the patient's diagnosis, treatment, and self-care, especially the low-protein, high-calorie diet.
▶ Document maintenance of dietary electrolytes, as indicated by diagnostic indicators.

## Related procedures
▶ Arteriovenous shunt care
▶ Autotransfusion
▶ Blood glucose tests
▶ Cardiac monitoring

▶ Care of the dying patient
▶ Catheter irrigation, urinary
▶ Continuous ambulatory peritoneal dialysis
▶ Hand washing
▶ Male incontinence device
▶ Oral drugs
▶ Peritoneal dialysis
▶ Physical assessment
▶ Postoperative care
▶ Preoperative care
▶ Seizure precautions
▶ Self-catheterization
▶ Standard precautions
▶ Urine collection
▶ Urine glucose and ketone tests
▶ Urine specific gravity
▶ Venipuncture

## REFERENCES

Barkley, T., and Myers, T. *Practice Guidelines for Acute Care Nurse Practitioners.* Philadelphia: W.B. Saunders Co., 2001.
Bates, P. "Renal and Urological Problems," in *Medical Surgical Nursing,* 5th ed. Edited by Lewis, S.M., et al. St. Louis: Mosby–Year Book, Inc., 2000.
Bates, P. "Urinary System," in *Medical Surgical Nursing,* 5th ed. Edited by Lewis, S.M., et al. St. Louis: Mosby–Year Book, Inc., 2000.
Brunier, G., and Bartucci, M. "Acute and Chronic Renal Failure," in *Medical Surgical Nursing,* 5th ed. Edited by Lewis, S.M., et al. St. Louis: Mosby–Year Book, Inc., 2000.
King, B. "Meds and the Dialysis Patient," *RN* 63(7):55-60, July 2001.

## ORGANIZATIONS

National Institute of Diabetes and Digestive and Kidney Diseases: *www.niddk.nih.gov*
Hypertension, Dialysis, and Clinical Nephrology: *www.hdcn.com*

# Managing the patient with altered fluid volume

## Purpose
To promote physiologic homeostasis in a patient with fluid volume alteration

## Collaborative level
Interdependent

## Expected patient outcomes
▶ The patient will maintain balance among the fluid compartments.

## Definition of terms
▶ *Extracellular fluid:* Water found outside the cells, which includes interstitial fluid and intravascular fluid.
▶ *Interstitial space:* The area outside of the vascular fluid and cells.
▶ *Intracellular fluid:* Water found inside the cells.

## Indications
Treatment
▶ Burns
▶ Coma
▶ Renal disease
▶ Gastric feedings
▶ Ascites, especially that caused by cancer or cirrhosis
▶ Hydronephrosis
▶ Hepatic encephalopathy
▶ Hormonal imbalances, especially those caused by antidiuretic hormone, aldosterone, natriuretic peptides, and prostaglandins
▶ Suction
▶ Fistula
▶ Hyperthyroidism
▶ Cushing's disease
▶ Hyperventilation
▶ Blood loss
▶ Diaphoresis

Prevention
▶ Electrolyte imbalance
▶ Acidosis
▶ Renal damage

## Assessment guidance
Signs and symptoms
*Fluid volume deficit*
▶ Confusion
▶ Decreased number of and moisture in stools
▶ Decreased skin turgor
▶ Dry skin
▶ Dry mouth
▶ Flattened neck veins in a supine position
▶ Headache
▶ Heart pounding
▶ Muscle weakness
▶ Oliguria
▶ Orthostatic hypotension
▶ Tachycardia

*Fluid volume excess*
- Cough
- Dyspnea
- Edema
- Elevated hematocrit
- Hyperglycemia
- Hypertension
- Increased blood urea nitrogen level
- Increased osmolality
- Increased sodium level
- Increased specific gravity (greater than 1.030)
- Pitting edema
- Rapid heart rate
- Weight gain

## Diagnostic studies
*Laboratory tests*
- Blood urea nitrogen level
- Complete blood count
- Blood glucose level
- Sodium level
- Plasma electrolyte levels
- Urinalysis
- Urine specific gravity

## Nursing interventions
- Check the patient's vital signs frequently (every 2 hours) and report your findings to the doctor. When measuring blood pressure, note orthostatic changes.
- Perform a neurologic assessment every 2 hours and report your findings to the doctor.
- Closely monitor all oral and I.V. intake and output to assess for fluid balance.
- Assess the patient's cardiac and respiratory systems regularly.
- Evaluate for edema periodically.
- Weigh the patient daily, particularly noting changes in body weight.
- Provide medications and I.V. therapy, as indicated.

## Patient teaching
- Teach the patient about his underlying disease and how it has caused his fluid imbalance.
- Educate the patient about his medication regimen and stress the importance of following it exactly as prescribed.
- Instruct the patient to follow the prescribed diet.
- Advise the patient about fluid restrictions.
- Teach the family about the patient's disorder and their involvement in his care.

## Precautions
- Assess the patient for diuretic use.
- Assess for digoxin toxicity in an older patient.
- Be alert to variances in fluid balance related to a disease such as diabetes insipidus.

## Documentation
- Record subjective and objective assessment data, including diagnostic test results, in the patient's chart.
- Document the patient's fluid intake and output, including the type of fluid intake (hypotonic, hypertonic, and isotonic), frequency of urination, and volume and characteristics of urine.
- Note the patient's vital signs frequently; note his body weight daily.
- Document the patient's neurologic, cardiac, and respiratory status periodically.
- Note the condition of the patient's skin regularly.
- Record doctor notification and all treatments and interventions performed.
- Note the patient's response to treatment.
- Document all teaching about the patient's diagnosis and treatment.
- Document maintenance of dietary electrolytes, as indicated by diagnostic indicators.

## Related procedures
- Autotransfusion
- Blood glucose tests
- Burn care
- Cardiac monitoring
- Care of the dying patient
- Continuous ambulatory peritoneal dialysis
- Hand washing
- I.M. injection
- I.V. bolus injection
- Latex allergy precautions
- Mechanical ventilation
- Nasogastric tube care
- Oral drugs
- Peritoneal dialysis
- Physical assessment
- Postoperative care
- Preoperative care
- Pressure ulcer care
- Seizure precautions

- Standard precautions
- Thoracentesis
- Traumatic wound care
- Tube feedings
- Urine collection
- Urine glucose and ketone tests
- Urine specific gravity

## REFERENCES

Barkley, T., and Myers, T. *Practice Guidelines for Acute Care Nurse Practitioners.* Philadelphia: W.B. Saunders Co., 2001.

Bates, P. "Renal and Urological Problems," in *Medical Surgical Nursing,* 5th ed. Edited by Lewis, S.M., et al. St. Louis: Mosby–Year Book, Inc., 2000.

Bates, P. "Urinary System," in *Medical Surgical Nursing,* 5th ed. Edited by Lewis, S.M., et al. St. Louis: Mosby–Year Book, Inc., 2000.

Brunier, G., and Bartucci, M. "Acute and Chronic Renal Failure," in *Medical Surgical Nursing,* 5th ed. Edited by Lewis, S.M., et al. St. Louis: Mosby–Year Book, Inc., 2000.

Edwards, S. "Regulation of Water, Sodium and Potassium: Implications for Practice," *Nursing Standard* 15(22):36-42, February 2001.

Iggulden, I. "Dehydration and Electrolyte Disturbance," *Nursing Standard* 13(19):48-56, February 1999.

King, B. "Meds and the Dialysis Patient," *RN* 63(7):55-60, July 2001.

Smoger, S.H., et al. "Urinary Incontinence Among Male Veterans Receiving Care in Primary Care Clinics," *Annals of Internal Medicine* 132(7):547-41, April 2000.

## ORGANIZATIONS

Nephrology Channel:
*www.nephrologychannel.com*

# Managing the patient with impaired urinary elimination

## Purpose

To provide effective interventions and treatment for impaired urinary elimination

## Collaborative level

Interdependent

## Expected patient outcomes

- The patient will display normal or improved urinary elimination.

## Definition of terms

- *Bladder neoplasm:* A papillomatous growth in the bladder urothelium.
- *Urinary calculi:* Calcifications or stones in the urinary system.
- *Urinary reflux:* Backward flow of urine in the urinary tract.
- *Urine retention:* The holding of urine in the bladder even as urine production continues.

## Indications

### Treatment

- Bladder neoplasm
- Urinary reflux
- Urinary calculi
- Urine retention
- Benign prostatic hyperplasia (BPH)

### Prevention

- Urinary tract infections
- Renal damage
- Urine stasis

## Assessment guidance

### Signs and symptoms

#### Bladder neoplasms

- Gross painless hematuria
- Bladder irritability
- Dysuria
- Urinary frequency

#### Urinary reflux

- Painful urination
- Urinary frequency
- Bladder distention

#### Urinary calculi

- Severe flank pain, right lower quadrant pain
- Bladder distention
- Nausea, vomiting, diarrhea, or constipation

#### Urine retention or BPH

- Inability to void, straining to void
- Dysuria
- Weak urine stream
- Post-void leakage
- Bladder displacement from midline
- Restlessness, diaphoresis

### Diagnostic studies

#### Laboratory tests

- Blood urea nitrogen level
- Creatinine level
- Fasting blood glucose level

▶ Prostate-specific antigen level
▶ Renal function tests
▶ Calcium level
▶ Urinalysis
▶ Urine culture
▶ Urine cytology

*Imaging tests*
▶ Computed tomography scan
▶ Excretory urography
▶ Kidney-ureter-bladder radiography
▶ Prostate ultrasonography
▶ Renal ultrasonography
▶ Voiding cystourethrography

*Other*
▶ Post-void residual
▶ Prostate biopsy
▶ Urodynamic studies (simple and complex)

## Nursing interventions

▶ Assess the patient's fluid intake and output carefully to evaluate urinary elimination.
▶ Monitor the patient's fluid intake and output.
▶ Modify the patient's diet based on his disorder. For example, provide a diet that will reduce the urine pH and decrease calculi formation in the patient with urinary calculi.
▶ Assess the patient for signs of dehydration.
▶ Maintain the patient's indwelling urinary catheter or provide in-and-out catheterization as needed.
▶ Help the patient avoid constipation by administering a laxative, increasing his fiber and fluid intake, and encouraging regular exercise.
▶ Provide preoperative and postoperative care related to surgery such as for neoplasm removal or urinary calculi lithotripsy.
▶ Administer prescribed medications, such as diuretics and potassium supplements.
▶ As needed, apply and maintain an external urine-collection device, which may include an incontinence pad, indwelling urinary catheter, or a new device, such as the Reliance balloon-tipped urethral plug and the Miniguard patch for the urethral meatus.

## Patient teaching

▶ Show the patient how to perform self-catheterization, if indicated.
▶ Teach the patient to increase fluid intake to 1 to 3 qt (2 to 3 L) per day.
▶ Instruct the patient to record his fluid intake and output and to notice changes in his urinary elimination pattern.
▶ Demonstrate how to care for the surgical wound, if indicated.
▶ Teach the patient how to take his medication properly and safely. Stress the importance of continuing the regimen, especially if he must take a diuretic.
▶ Explain to the patient how to recognize the signs and symptoms of his underlying disorder so that it can be detected early if it recurs.

## Precautions

▶ Ensure that the patient's fluid intake is safe in relation to other diseases that may coexist.
▶ Observe the patient for signs and symptoms of fluid overload.
▶ Observe the patient for signs and symptoms of electrolyte imbalances.
▶ Assess the patient for signs of laxative abuse.
▶ Modify treatments based on the patient's diagnosis and age.

## Documentation

▶ Record subjective and objective assessment data, including diagnostic test results, in the patient's chart.
▶ Document the patient's fluid intake and output, including the type of fluid intake, frequency of urination, and volume and characteristics of urine.
▶ Note the condition of the patient's skin regularly.
▶ Record doctor notification and all treatments and interventions performed.
▶ Note the patient's response to treatment.
▶ Document all teaching about the patient's diagnosis and treatment.

## Related procedures

▶ Blood glucose tests
▶ Catheter irrigation, urinary
▶ Credé's maneuver
▶ Hand washing
▶ Male incontinence device
▶ Oral drugs
▶ Physical assessment
▶ Postoperative care

▶ Preoperative care
▶ Self-catheterization
▶ Standard precautions
▶ Urine collection
▶ Urine glucose and ketone tests
▶ Urine specific gravity

## REFERENCES

Barkley, T., and Myers, T. *Practice Guidelines for Acute Care Nurse Practitioners.* Philadelphia: W.B. Saunders Co., 2001.

Bates, P. "Renal and Urological Problems," in *Medical Surgical Nursing,* 5th ed. Edited by Lewis, S.M., et al. St. Louis: Mosby–Year Book, Inc., 2000.

Bates, P. "Urinary System," in *Medical Surgical Nursing,* 5th ed. Edited by Lewis, S.M., et al. St. Louis: Mosby–Year Book, Inc., 2000.

Brunier, G., and Bartucci, M. "Acute and Chronic Renal Failure," in *Medical Surgical Nursing,* 5th ed. Edited by Lewis, S.M., et al. St. Louis: Mosby–Year Book, Inc., 2000.

Gray, M. "Urinary Retention: Management in the Acute Care Setting: Part 1," *American Journal of Nursing* 100(7):40-48, July 2000.

Gray, M. "Urinary Retention: Management in the Acute Care Setting: Part 2," *American Journal of Nursing* 100(8):36-44, August 2000.

King, B. "Meds and the Dialysis Patient," *RN* 63(7):55-60, July 2001.

## ORGANIZATIONS

National Institute of Diabetes and Digestive and Kidney Diseases: *www.niddk.nih.gov*

Nephrology Channel: *www.nephrologychannel.com*

# Procedures

## Arteriovenous shunt care

An arteriovenous (AV) shunt consists of two segments of tubing joined (in a U-shape) to divert blood from an artery to a vein. Inserted surgically, usually in a forearm or (rarely) an ankle, the AV shunt provides access to the circulatory system for hemodialysis. After insertion, the shunt requires regular assessment for patency and examination of the surrounding skin for signs of infection.

AV shunt care also includes aseptically cleaning the arterial and venous exit sites, applying antiseptic ointment, and dressing the sites with sterile bandages. When done just before hemodialysis, this procedure prolongs the life of the shunt, helps prevent infection, and allows early detection of clotting. Shunt site care is done more often if the dressing becomes wet or nonocclusive.

### Equipment

Drape ● stethoscope ● sterile gloves ● sterile 4″ × 4″ gauze pads ● sterile cotton-tipped applicators ● antiseptic (usually povidone-iodine solution) ● bulldog clamps ● plasticized or hypoallergenic tape ● optional: swab specimen kit, prescribed antimicrobial ointment (usually povidone-iodine), sterile elastic gauze bandage, 2″ × 2″ gauze pads, hydrogen peroxide

Kits containing all the necessary equipment can be prepackaged and stored for use.

### Implementation

▶ Explain the procedure to the patient. Provide privacy and wash your hands.
▶ Place the drape on a stable surface, such as a bedside table, to reduce the risk of traumatic injury to the shunt site. Then place the shunted extremity on the draped surface.
▶ Remove the two bulldog clamps from the elastic gauze bandage and unwrap the bandage from the shunt area.
▶ Carefully remove the gauze dressing covering the shunt and the 4″ × 4″ gauze pad under the shunt.
▶ Assess the arterial and venous exit sites for signs of infection, such as erythema, swelling, excessive tenderness, or drainage.

Obtain a swab specimen of any purulent drainage and notify the doctor immediately of any signs of infection.

▶ Check blood flow through the shunt by inspecting the color of the blood and comparing the warmth of the shunt with that of the surrounding skin. The blood should be bright red; the shunt should feel as warm as the skin.

◆◆ **ALERT!** If the blood is dark purple or black and the temperature of the shunt is lower than the surrounding skin, clotting has occurred. Notify the doctor immediately.

▶ Use the stethoscope to auscultate the shunt between the arterial and venous exit sites. A bruit confirms normal blood flow. Palpate the shunt for a thrill (by lightly placing your fingertips over the access site and feeling for vibration), which also indicates normal blood flow. Don't use a Doppler device to auscultate because it will detect peripheral blood flow as well as shunt-related sounds.

▶ Open a few packages of 4″ × 4″ gauze pads and cotton-tipped applicators, and soak them with the antiseptic. Put on the sterile gloves.

▶ Using a soaked 4″ × 4″ gauze pad, start cleaning the skin at one of the exit sites. Wipe away from the site to remove bacteria and reduce the chance of contaminating the shunt.

▶ Use the soaked cotton-tipped applicators to remove any crusted material from the exit site because the encrustations provide a medium for bacterial growth.

▶ Clean the other exit site, using fresh, soaked 4″ × 4″ gauze pads and cotton-tipped applicators.

▶ Clean the rest of the skin that was covered by the gauze dressing with fresh, soaked 4″ × 4″ gauze pads.

▶ If ordered, apply antimicrobial ointment to the exit sites to help prevent infection.

▶ Place a dry, sterile 4″ × 4″ gauze pad under the shunt. This prevents the shunt from contacting the skin, which could cause skin irritation and breakdown.

▶ Cover the exit sites with a dry, sterile 4″ × 4″ gauze pad, and tape the pad securely to keep the exit sites clean and protected.

▶ For routine daily care, wrap the shunt with an elastic gauze bandage. Leave a small portion of the shunt cannula exposed so the patient can check for patency without removing the dressing.

▶ Place the bulldog clamps on the edge of the elastic gauze bandage so that the patient can use them quickly to stop hemorrhage in case the shunt separates.

▶ For care before hemodialysis, don't redress the shunt, but keep the bulldog clamps readily accessible.

## Special considerations

◆◆ **ALERT!** Make sure the AV junction of the shunt is secured with plasticized or hypoallergenic tape. This prevents separation of the two halves of the shunt, minimizing the risk of hemorrhage.

▶ Avoid blood pressure measurement and venipuncture in the affected arm to prevent shunt occlusion.

▶ Always handle the shunt and dressings carefully. Don't use scissors or other sharp instruments to remove the dressing because you may accidentally cut the shunt. Never remove the tape securing the AV junction during dressing changes.

▶ When cleaning the shunt exit sites, use each 4″ × 4″ gauze pad only once and avoid wiping any area more than once to minimize the risk of contamination. When redressing the site, make sure that the tape doesn't kink or occlude the shunt. If the exit sites are heavily encrusted, place a 2″ × 2″ hydrogen peroxide-soaked gauze pad on the area for about 1 hour to loosen the crust. Make sure the patient isn't allergic to iodine before using povidone-iodine solution or ointment.

## Home care

Ask the patient how he cares for the shunt at home. Then teach proper home care, if necessary.

## Documentation

▶ Record that shunt care was administered, the condition of the shunt and surrounding skin, any ointment used, and any instructions given to the patient.

### REFERENCES

Hayes, D. "Caring for Your Patient with a Permanent Hemodialysis Access," *Nursing2000* 30(3):41-46, March 2000.

*Instructor's Resource Manual for the AACN Core Curriculum for Critical Care Nursing,* 5th ed. Edited by Alspach, J.G. Philadelphia: W.B. Saunders Co., 2001.

# Catheter irrigation, urinary

To avoid introducing microorganisms into the bladder, the nurse irrigates an indwelling catheter only to remove an obstruction such as a blood clot that develops after bladder, kidney, or prostate surgery.

## Equipment

Ordered irrigating solution (such as normal saline solution) • sterile graduated receptacle or emesis basin • sterile bulb syringe or 50-ml catheter tip syringe • two alcohol pads • sterile gloves • linen-saver pad • intake-output sheet • optional: basin of warm water

Commercially packaged kits containing sterile irrigating solution, a graduated receptacle, and a bulb or 50-ml catheter tip syringe are available. If the volume of irrigating solution instilled must be measured, use a graduated syringe instead of a noncalibrated bulb syringe.

### Preparation of equipment

Check the expiration date on the irrigating solution. To prevent vesical spasms during instillation of solution, warm it to room temperature. If necessary, place the container in a basin of warm water. Never heat the solution on a burner or in a microwave oven. Hot irrigating solution can injure the patient's bladder.

## Implementation

▶ Wash your hands and assemble the equipment at the bedside. Explain the procedure to the patient and provide privacy.
▶ Place the patient in the dorsal recumbent position. Then place a linen-saver pad under the patient's buttocks to protect the bed linens.
▶ Create a sterile field at the patient's bedside by opening the sterile equipment tray or commercial kit. Using aseptic technique, clean the lip of the solution bottle by pouring a small amount into a sink or waste receptacle. Then pour the prescribed amount of solution into the graduated receptacle or emesis basin.
▶ Place the tip of the syringe into the solution. Squeeze the bulb or pull back the plunger (depending on the type of syringe) and fill the syringe with the appropriate amount of solution (usually 30 ml).

▶ Open the package of alcohol pads; then put on sterile gloves. Clean the juncture of the catheter and drainage tube with an alcohol pad to remove as many bacterial contaminants as possible.
▶ Disconnect the catheter and drainage tube by twisting them in opposite directions and carefully pulling them apart without creating tension on the catheter. Don't let go of the catheter—hold it in your nondominant hand. Then place the end of the drainage tube on the sterile field, making sure not to contaminate the tube. Keep the end of the drainage tube sterile by placing sterile gauze over it and securing the gauze with a piece of tape.
▶ Twist the bulb syringe or catheter-tip syringe onto the catheter's distal end.
▶ Squeeze the bulb or slowly push the plunger of the syringe to instill the irrigating solution through the catheter. If necessary, refill the syringe and repeat this step until you've instilled the prescribed amount of irrigating solution.
▶ Remove the syringe and direct the return flow from the catheter into a graduated receptacle or emesis basin. Don't let the catheter end touch the drainage in the receptacle or become contaminated in any other way.
▶ Wipe the end of the drainage tube and catheter with the remaining alcohol pad.
▶ Wait a few seconds until the alcohol evaporates; then reattach the drainage tubing to the catheter.
▶ Dispose of all used supplies properly.

## Special considerations

▶ Catheter irrigation requires strict aseptic technique to prevent bacteria from entering the bladder. The ends of the catheter and drainage tube and the tip of the syringe must be kept sterile throughout the procedure.
▶ If you encounter any resistance during instillation of the irrigating solution, don't try to force the solution into the bladder. Instead, stop the procedure and notify the doctor. If an indwelling catheter becomes totally obstructed, obtain an order to remove it and replace it with a new one to prevent bladder distention, acute renal failure, urinary stasis, and subsequent infection.
▶ The doctor may order a continuous irrigation system. This decreases the risk of in-

fection by eliminating the need to disconnect the catheter and drainage tube repeatedly.
▶ Encourage catheterized patients not on restricted fluid intake to increase intake to 3,000 ml per day to help flush the urinary system and reduce sediment formation. To keep the patient's urine acidic and help prevent calculus formation, tell the patient to eat foods containing ascorbic acid, including citrus fruits and juices, cranberry juice, and dark green and deep yellow vegetables.

## Documentation
▶ Note the amount, color, and consistency of return urine flow and document the patient's tolerance for the procedure.
▶ Note any resistance during instillation of the solution. If the return flow volume is less than the amount of solution instilled, note this on the intake and output balance sheets and in your notes.

### REFERENCES
Joanna Briggs Institute. "Management of Short-Term Indwelling Urethral Catheters to Prevent Urinary Tract Infections," *Best Practice* 4(1), 2000. *www.joannabriggs.edu.au/bpmenu.html*
Potter, P.A., and Perry, A.G. *Fundamentals of Nursing,* 5th ed. St. Louis: Mosby–Year Book, Inc., 2001.

# Continuous ambulatory peritoneal dialysis

Continuous ambulatory peritoneal dialysis (CAPD) requires insertion of a permanent peritoneal catheter (such as a Tenckhoff catheter) to circulate dialysate in the peritoneal cavity constantly. Inserted under local anesthetic, the catheter is sutured in place and its distal portion is tunneled subcutaneously to the skin surface. There it serves as a port for the dialysate, which flows in and out of the peritoneal cavity by gravity. (See *Three major steps of continuous ambulatory peritoneal dialysis,* page 480.)

CAPD is used most commonly for patients with end-stage renal disease. CAPD can be a welcome alternative to hemodialysis, because it gives the patient more independence and requires less travel for treatments. It also provides more stable fluid and electrolyte levels than conventional hemodialysis.
▶ Renal function has been shown to decline over months or years on dialysis. Therefore, the number or volume of exchanges will likely increase for the patient on CAPD to maintain control over waste products.

Patients or family members can usually learn to perform CAPD after only 2 weeks of training. In addition, because the patient can resume normal daily activities between solution changes, CAPD helps promote independence and a return to a near-normal lifestyle. It also costs less than hemodialysis.

Conditions that may prohibit CAPD include recent abdominal surgery, abdominal adhesions, an infected abdominal wall, diaphragmatic tears, ileus, and respiratory insufficiency.

## Equipment
*To infuse dialysate*
Prescribed amount of dialysate (usually in 2-L [2-qt] bags) ● heating pad or commercial warmer ● three face masks ● 42" connective tubing with drain clamp ● six to eight packages of sterile 4" × 4" gauze pads ● medication, if ordered ● povidone-iodine pads ● hypoallergenic tape ● plastic snap-top container ● povidone-iodine solution ● sterile basin ● container of alcohol ● sterile gloves ● belt or fabric pouch ● two sterile waterproof paper drapes (one fenestrated) ● optional: syringes, labeled specimen container

*To discontinue dialysis temporarily*
Three sterile waterproof paper barriers (two fenestrated) ● 4" × 4" gauze pads (for cleaning and dressing the catheter) ● two face masks ● sterile basin ● hypoallergenic tape ● povidone-iodine solution ● sterile gloves ● sterile rubber catheter cap

All equipment for infusing the dialysate and discontinuing the procedure must be sterile. Commercially prepared sterile CAPD kits are available.

### Preparation of equipment
Check the concentration of the dialysate against the doctor's order. Also check the expiration date and appearance of the solution — it should be clear, not cloudy. Warm

# Three major steps of continuous ambulatory peritoneal dialysis

A bag of dialysate is attached to the tube entering the patient's abdominal area so the fluid flows into the peritoneal cavity.

While the dialysate remains in the peritoneal cavity, the patient can roll up the bag, place it under his shirt, and go about his normal activities.

Unrolling the bag and suspending it below the pelvis allows the dialysate to drain from the peritoneal cavity back into the bag.

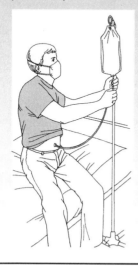
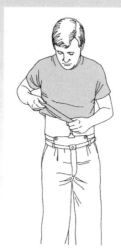
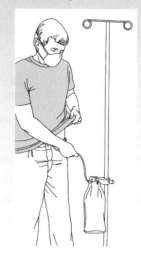

the solution to body temperature with a heating pad or a commercial warmer if one is available. Don't warm the solution in a microwave oven because the temperature is unpredictable.

To minimize the risk of contaminating the bag's port, leave the dialysate container's wrapper in place. This also keeps the bag dry, which makes examining it for leakage easier after you remove the wrapper.

Wash your hands and put on a surgical mask. Remove the dialysate container from the warming setup, and remove its protective wrapper. Squeeze the bag firmly to check for leaks.

If ordered, use a syringe to add any prescribed medication to the dialysate, using sterile technique to avoid contamination. (The ideal approach is to add medication under a laminar flow hood.) Disinfect multiple-dose vials in a 5-minute povidone-iodine soak. Insert the connective tubing into the dialysate container. Open the drain clamp to prime the tube. Then close the clamp.

Place a povidone-iodine pad on the dialysate container's port. Cover the port with a dry gauze pad, and secure the pad with tape. Remove and discard the surgical mask. Tear the tape so it will be ready to secure the new dressing. Commercial devices with povidone-iodine pads are available for covering the dialysate container and tubing connection.

## Implementation

▶ Weigh the patient to establish a baseline level. Weigh him at the same time every day to help monitor fluid balance.

### Infusing dialysate

▶ Assemble all equipment at the patient's bedside, and explain the procedure to him. Prepare the sterile field by placing a waterproof, sterile paper drape on a dry surface near the patient. Take care to maintain the drape's sterility.
▶ Fill the snap-top container with povidone-iodine solution and place it on the sterile field. Place the basin on the sterile field. Then place four pairs of sterile

gauze pads in the sterile basin and saturate them with the povidone-iodine solution. Drop the remaining gauze pads on the sterile field. Loosen the cap on the alcohol container and place it next to the sterile field.

▶ Put on a clean surgical mask and provide one for the patient.

▶ Carefully remove the dressing covering the peritoneal catheter and discard it. Be careful not to touch the catheter or skin. Check skin integrity at the catheter site and look for signs of infection, such as purulent drainage. If drainage is present, obtain a swab specimen, put it in a labeled specimen container, and notify the doctor.

▶ Put on the sterile gloves and palpate the insertion site and subcutaneous tunnel route for tenderness or pain. If these symptoms occur, notify the doctor.

**ALERT!** If the patient experiences drainage, tenderness, or pain, don't proceed with the infusion without specific orders.

▶ Wrap one gauze pad saturated with povidone-iodine solution around the distal end of the catheter and leave it in place for 5 minutes. Clean the catheter and insertion site with the rest of the gauze pads, moving in concentric circles away from the insertion site. Use straight strokes to clean the catheter, beginning at the insertion site and moving outward. Use a clean area of the pad for each stroke. Loosen the catheter cap one notch and clean the exposed area. Place each used pad at the base of the catheter to help support it. After using the third pair of pads, place the fenestrated paper drape around the base of the catheter. Continue cleaning the catheter for another minute with one of the remaining pads soaked with povidone-iodine.

▶ Remove the povidone-iodine pad on the catheter cap, remove the cap, and use the remaining povidone-iodine pad to clean the end of the catheter hub. Attach the connective tubing from the dialysate container to the catheter. Be sure to secure the luer-lock connector tightly.

▶ Open the drain clamp on the dialysate container to allow solution to enter the peritoneal cavity by gravity over a period of 5 to 10 minutes. Leave a small amount of fluid in the bag to make folding it easier. Close the drain clamp.

▶ Fold the bag and secure it with a belt, or tuck it in the patient's clothing or a small fabric pouch.

▶ After the prescribed dwell time (usually 4 to 6 hours), unfold the bag, open the clamp, and allow peritoneal fluid to drain back into the bag by gravity.

▶ When drainage is complete, attach a new bag of dialysate and repeat the infusion.

▶ Discard used supplies appropriately.

## Discontinuing dialysis temporarily

▶ Wash your hands, put on a surgical mask, and provide one for the patient. Explain the procedure to him.

▶ Using sterile gloves, remove and discard the dressing over the peritoneal catheter.

▶ Set up a sterile field next to the patient by covering a clean, dry surface with a waterproof drape. Be sure to maintain the drape's sterility. Place all equipment on the sterile field and place the 4″ × 4″ gauze pads in the basin. Saturate them with the povidone-iodine solution. Open the 4″ × 4″ gauze pads to be used as the dressing and drop them onto the sterile field. Tear pieces of tape as needed.

▶ Tape the dialysate tubing to the side rail of the bed to keep the catheter and tubing off the patient's abdomen.

▶ Change to another pair of sterile gloves. Then place one of the fenestrated drapes around the base of the catheter.

▶ Use a pair of povidone-iodine pads to clean about 6″ (15 cm) of the dialysis tubing. Clean for 1 minute, moving in one direction only, away from the catheter. Then clean the catheter, moving from the insertion site to the junction of the catheter and dialysis tubing. Place used pads at the base of the catheter to prop it up. Use two more pairs of pads to clean the junction for a total of 3 minutes.

▶ Place the second fenestrated paper drape over the first at the base of the catheter. With the fourth pair of pads, clean the junction of the catheter and 6″ of the dialysate tubing for another minute.

▶ Disconnect the dialysate tubing from the catheter. Pick up the catheter cap and fasten it to the catheter, making sure it fits securely over both notches of the hard plastic catheter tip.

▶ Clean the insertion site and a 2″ (5-cm) radius around it with povidone-iodine pads, working from the insertion site out-

# Continuous-cycle peritoneal dialysis

Continuous ambulatory peritoneal dialysis is easier for the patient who uses an automated continuous cycler system. When set up, this system runs the dialysis treatment automatically until all the dialysate is infused. The system remains closed throughout the treatment, which cuts the risk of contamination. Continuous-cycle peritoneal dialysis (CCPD) can be performed while the patient is awake or asleep. The system's alarms warn about general system, dialysate, and patient problems.

The cycler can be set to an intermittent or continuous dialysate schedule at home or in a health care facility. The patient typically initiates CCPD at bedtime and undergoes three to seven exchanges depending on individual prescriptions. Upon awakening, the patient infuses the prescribed dialysis volume, disconnects himself from the unit, and carries the dialysate in his peritoneal cavity during the day.

The continuous cycler follows the same aseptic care and maintenance procedures as the manual method.

---

ward. Let the skin air-dry before applying the dressing.
▶ Discard used supplies appropriately.

## Special considerations
▶ If inflow and outflow are slow or absent, check the tubing for kinks. You can also try raising the solution or repositioning the patient to increase the inflow rate. Repositioning the patient or applying manual pressure to the lateral aspects of the patient's abdomen may also help increase drainage.

## Home care
Teach the patient and family how to use sterile technique throughout the procedure, especially for cleaning and dressing changes, to prevent complications, such as peritonitis. Also teach them the signs and symptoms of peritonitis—cloudy fluid, fever, abdominal pain, and tenderness—and stress the importance of notifying the doctor immediately if such signs or symptoms arise. Also encourage them to call the doctor immediately if redness and drainage occur; these are also signs of infection.

Inform the patient about the advantages of an automated continuous cycler system for home use. (See *Continuous-cycle peritoneal dialysis.*)

Instruct the patient to record his weight and blood pressure daily and to check regularly for swelling of the extremities. Teach him to keep an accurate record of intake and output.

## Complications
Peritonitis is the most frequent complication of CAPD. Although treatable, it can permanently scar the peritoneal membrane, decreasing its permeability and reducing the efficiency of dialysis. Untreated peritonitis can cause septicemia and death.

Excessive fluid loss may result from a concentrated (4.25%) dialysate solution, improper or inaccurate monitoring of inflow and outflow, or inadequate oral fluid intake. Excessive fluid retention may result from improper or inaccurate monitoring of inflow and outflow, or excessive salt or oral fluid intake.

## Documentation
▶ Record the type and amount of fluid instilled and returned for each exchange, the time and duration of the exchange, and any medications added to the dialysate.
▶ Note the color and clarity of the returned exchange fluid and check it for mucus, pus, and blood.
▶ Note any discrepancy in the balance of fluid intake and output, as well as any signs of fluid imbalance, such as weight changes, decreased breath sounds, peripheral edema, ascites, and changes in skin turgor.
▶ Record the patient's weight, blood pressure, and pulse rate after his last fluid exchange for the day.

**REFERENCES**
Halstead, J.C., et al. "Acute Hydrothorax in CAPD: Early Thoracoscopic (VATS) Intervention Allows Return to Peritoneal Dialysis," *Nephron* 92(3):725-27, November 2002.

Pearson, S., et al. "Sclerosing Peritonitis Complicating Continuous Ambulatory Peritoneal Dialysis Managed by Hemodialysis and Home Parenteral Nutrition," *Clinical Nephrology* 58(3):244-46, September 2002.

# Continuous bladder irrigation

Continuous bladder irrigation can help prevent urinary tract obstruction by flushing out small blood clots that form after prostate or bladder surgery. It may also be used to treat an irritated, inflamed, or infected bladder lining.

This procedure requires placement of a triple-lumen catheter. One lumen controls balloon inflation, one allows irrigant inflow, and one allows irrigant outflow. The continuous flow of irrigating solution through the bladder also creates a mild tamponade that may help prevent venous hemorrhage. Although the patient typically receives the catheter while he's in the operating room after prostate or bladder surgery, he may have it inserted at bedside if he isn't a surgical patient.

## Equipment
One 4,000-ml container or two 2,000-ml containers of irrigating solution (usually normal saline solution) or the prescribed amount of medicated solution ● Y-type tubing made specifically for bladder irrigation ● alcohol or povidone-iodine pad ● infusion pump

Normal saline solution is usually prescribed for bladder irrigation after prostate or bladder surgery. Large volumes of irrigating solution are usually required during the first 24 to 48 hours after surgery. This explains the use of Y-type tubing, which allows immediate irrigation with reserve solution.

### Preparation of equipment
Before starting continuous bladder irrigation, double-check the irrigating solution against the doctor's order. If the solution contains an antibiotic, check the patient's chart to make sure he isn't allergic to the drug. Unless specified otherwise, the patient should remain on bed rest throughout continuous bladder irrigation.

## Implementation
▶ Wash your hands. Assemble all equipment at the patient's bedside. Explain the procedure and provide privacy.
▶ Insert the spike of the Y-type tubing into the container of irrigating solution. (If you have a two-container system, insert one spike into each container.)
▶ Squeeze the drip chamber on the spike of the tubing.
▶ Open the flow clamp and flush the tubing to remove air, which could cause bladder distention. Then close the clamp.
▶ To begin, hang the bag of irrigating solution on the I.V. pole.
▶ Clean the opening to the inflow lumen of the catheter with the alcohol or povidone-iodine pad.
▶ Insert the distal end of the Y-type tubing securely into the inflow lumen (third port) of the catheter.
▶ Make sure the catheter's outflow lumen is securely attached to the drainage bag tubing.
▶ Open the flow clamp under the container of irrigating solution and set the drip rate, as ordered, or connect to an infusion pump.
▶ To prevent air from entering the system, don't let the primary container empty completely before replacing it.
▶ If you have a two-container system, simultaneously close the flow clamp under the nearly empty container and open the flow clamp under the reserve container. This prevents reflux of irrigating solution from the reserve container into the nearly empty one. Hang a new reserve container on the I.V. pole and insert the tubing, maintaining asepsis.
▶ Empty the drainage bag about every 4 hours, or as often as needed. Use sterile technique to avoid the risk of contamination.
▶ Monitor vital signs at least every 4 hours during irrigation; increase the frequency if the patient becomes unstable.

## Special considerations
▶ Check the inflow and outflow lines periodically for kinks to make sure the solution is running freely. If the solution flows rapidly, check the lines frequently.
▶ Measure the outflow volume accurately. It should, allowing for urine production, exceed inflow volume. If inflow volume exceeds outflow volume postoperatively, suspect bladder rupture at the suture lines or renal damage, and notify the doctor immediately.
▶ Also assess outflow for changes in appearance and for blood clots, especially if irrigation is being performed postoperative-

ly to control bleeding. If drainage is bright red, irrigating solution should usually be infused rapidly with the clamp wide open until drainage clears. Notify the doctor at once if you suspect hemorrhage. If drainage is clear, the solution is usually given at a rate of 40 to 60 drops/minute. The doctor typically specifies the rate for antibiotic solutions.

▶ Encourage oral fluid intake of 2 to 3 L/day unless contraindicated by another medical condition.

## Complications

Interruptions in a continuous irrigation system can predispose the patient to infection. Obstruction in the catheter's outflow lumen can cause bladder distention.

## Documentation

▶ Each time you finish a container of solution, record the date, time, and amount of fluid given on the intake and output record.
▶ Record the time and amount of fluid each time you empty the drainage bag.
▶ Note the appearance of the drainage and any complaints the patient has.

### REFERENCES

Coveney, V.A., et al. "Optimization of Debris Removal During Bladder Irrigation," *Physiological Measurement* 22(3):523-34, August 2001.

Ng, C. "Assessment and Intervention Knowledge of Nurses in Managing Catheter Patency in Continuous Bladder Irrigation Following TURP," *Urology Nursing* 21(2): 97-98, 101-107, 110-11, April 2001.

# Continuous renal replacement therapy

Formerly called continuous arteriovenous hemofiltration, continuous renal replacement therapy (CRRT) is used to treat patients who suffer from acute renal failure. Unlike the more traditional intermittent hemodialysis (IHD), CRRT is administered around the clock, providing patients with continuous therapy and sparing them the destabilizing hemodynamic and electrolytic changes characteristic of IHD. CRRT is used for patients, such as those who have hypotension, who are unable to tolerate traditional hemodialysis. For such patients,

CRRT is often the only choice of treatment; however, it can also be used on many patients who can tolerate IHD. CRRT methods vary in complexity. The techniques include the following:

▶ Slow continuous ultrafiltration (SCUF) uses arteriovenous access and the patient's blood pressure to circulate blood through a hemofilter. Since the goal with this therapy is the removal of fluids, the patient doesn't receive any replacement fluids.
▶ Continuous arteriovenous hemofiltration (CAVH) uses the patient's blood pressure and arteriovenous access to circulate blood through a flow resistance hemofilter. However, to maintain the patency of the filter and the systemic blood pressure, the patient receives replacement fluids.
▶ Continuous venovenous hemofiltration (CVVH) fuses SCUF and CAVH. A double-lumen catheter is used to provide access to a vein and a pump moves blood through the hemofilter.
▶ Continuous arteriovenous hemodialysis (CAVH-D) combines hemodialysis with hemofiltration. In this technique, the infusion pump moves dialysate solution concurrent to blood flow, adding the ability to continuously remove solute while removing fluid. Like CAVH, it can also be performed in patients with hypotension and fluid overload.
▶ Continuous venovenous hemodialysis (CVVH-D) is similar to CAVH-D, except that a vein provides the access while a pump is used to move dialysate solution concurrent with blood flow.
▶ CVVH or CVVH-D is being used instead of CAVH or CAVH-D in many facilities to treat critically ill patients. CVVH has several advantages over CAVH: it doesn't require arterial access, can be performed in patients with low mean arterial pressures, and has a better solute clearance than CAVH.

## Equipment

CRRT equipment ● heparin flush solution ● occlusive dressings for catheter insertion sites ● sterile gloves ● sterile mask ● povidone-iodine solution ● sterile 4″ × 4″ gauze pads ● tape ● filtration replacement fluid (FRF), as ordered ● infusion pump.

### Preparation of equipment

Prime the hemofilter and tubing according to the manufacturer's instructions.

## CAVH setup

During continuous arteriovenous hemofiltration (CAVH), the patient's arterial blood pressure serves as a natural pump, driving blood through the arterial line. A hemofilter removes water and toxic solutes (ultrafiltrate) from the blood. Replacement fluid is infused into a port on the arterial side; this same port can be used to infuse heparin. The venous line carries the replacement fluid, along with purified blood, to the patient.

This illustration shows one of several CAVH setups.

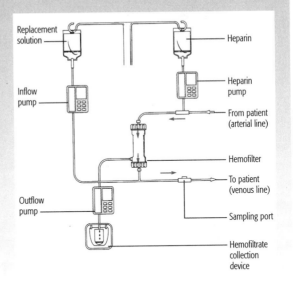

## Implementation

▶ Wash your hands. Assemble your equipment at the patient's bedside, and explain the procedure. (See *CAVH setup.*)

▶ If necessary, assist with inserting the catheters into the femoral artery and vein, using strict sterile technique. (In some cases, an internal arteriovenous fistula or external arteriovenous shunt may be used instead of the femoral route.) If ordered, flush both catheters with the heparin flush solution to prevent clotting.

▶ Apply occlusive dressings to the insertion sites, and mark the dressings with the date and time. Secure the tubing and connections with tape.

▶ Assess all pulses in the affected leg every hour for the first 4 hours, then every 2 hours afterward.

▶ Weigh the patient, take baseline vital signs, and make sure that all necessary laboratory studies have been done (usually, electrolyte levels, coagulation factors, complete blood count, blood urea nitrogen, and creatinine studies). Monitor the patient's weight and vital signs hourly.

▶ Put on the sterile gloves and mask. Prepare the connection sites by cleaning them with gauze pads soaked in povidone-iodine solution, then connect them to the exit port of each catheter.

▶ Using sterile technique, connect the arterial and venous lines to the hemofilter.

▶ Turn on the hemofilter and monitor the blood flow rate through the circuit. The flow rate is usually kept between 500 and 900 ml/hour.

▶ Inspect the ultrafiltrate during the procedure. It should remain clear yellow, with no gross blood. Pink-tinged or bloody ultrafiltrate may signal a membrane leak in the hemofilter, which permits bacterial contamination. If a leak occurs, notify the doctor so he can have the hemofilter replaced.

▶ Assess the affected leg for signs of obstructed blood flow, such as coolness, pallor, and weak pulse. Check the groin area on the affected side for signs of hematoma. Ask the patient if he has pain at the insertion sites.

▶ Calculate the amount of FRF every hour, or as ordered, according to policy. Infuse the prescribed amount and type of FRF through the infusion pump into the arterial side of the circuit.

# Preventing complications of CRRT

Measures to avoid complications are listed below.

| Complication | Interventions |
|---|---|
| Hypotension | ▶ Monitor blood pressure.<br>▶ Temporarily decrease the blood pump's speed for transient hypotension.<br>▶ Increase the vasopressor support. |
| Hypothermia | ▶ Use an inline fluid warmer placed on the blood return line to the patient or an external warming blanket. |
| Fluid and electrolyte imbalances | ▶ Monitor the patient's fluid levels every 4 to 6 hours.<br>▶ Monitor the patient's sodium, lactate, potassium, and calcium levels and replace as necessary. |
| Acid-base imbalances | ▶ Monitor the patient's bicarbonate and arterial blood gas levels. |
| Air embolism | ▶ Observe for air in the system.<br>▶ Use luer-lock devices on catheter openings. |
| Hemorrhage | ▶ Check all connections and keep the dialysis lines visible. |
| Infection | ▶ Perform sterile dressing changes. |

## Special considerations

▶ Because blood flows through an extracorporeal circuit during CAVH and CVVH, the blood in the hemofilter may need to be anticoagulated. To do this, infuse heparin in low doses (usually starting at 500 units/hour) into an infusion port on the arterial side of the setup. Measure thrombin clotting time or the activated clotting time (ACT). This ensures that the circuit, not the patient, is anticoagulated. A normal ACT is 100 seconds; during CRRT, keep it between 100 and 300 seconds, depending on the patient's clotting times. If the ACT is too high or too low, the doctor will adjust the heparin dose accordingly.

▶ Another way to prevent clotting in the hemofilter is to infuse medications or blood through another line rather than the venous line, if possible.

▶ A third way to help prevent clots in the hemofilter, and also to prevent kinks in the catheter, is to make sure the patient doesn't bend the affected leg more than 30 degrees at the hip.

▶ To prevent infection, perform skin care at the catheter insertion sites every 48 hours, using sterile technique. Cover the sites with an occlusive dressing.

▶ If the ultrafiltrate flow rate decreases, raise the bed to increase the distance between the collection device and the hemofilter. Lower the bed to decrease the flow rate.

◆ **ALERT!** Clamping the ultrafiltrate line is contraindicated with some types of hemofilters because pressure may build up in the filter, clotting it and collapsing the blood compartment.

## Complications

Possible complications include bleeding, hemorrhage, hemofilter occlusion, infection, and thrombosis. (See *Preventing complications of CRRT.*)

## Documentation

▶ Record the time the treatment began and ended, fluid balance information, times of dressing changes, complications, medications given, and the patient's tolerance.

## REFERENCES

Dirkes, S.M. "Continuous Renal Replacement Therapy: Dialytic Therapy for Acute Renal Failure in Intensive Care," *Nephrology Nursing Journal* 27(6);581-89, 2000.

Ronco, C., et al. "Continuous Renal Replacement Therapy: Opinions and Evidence," *Advances in Renal Replacement Therapy* 9(4):229-44, October 2002.

Schetz, M., et al. "The Acute Dialysis Quality Initiative-Part VII: Fluid Composition and Management in CRRT," *Advances in Renal Replacement Therapy* 9(4):282-89, October 2002.

*Instructor's Resource Manual for the AACN Core Curriculum for Critical Care Nursing,* 5th ed. Edited by Alspach, J.G. Philadelphia: W.B. Saunders Co., 2001.

## Credé's maneuver

When lower motor neuron damage impairs the voiding reflex, the bladder may become flaccid or areflexic. Because the bladder fails to contract properly, urine collects inside it, causing distention. Credé's maneuver—application of manual pressure over the lower abdomen—promotes complete emptying of the bladder. After appropriate instruction, the patient can perform the maneuver himself, unless he can't reach his lower abdomen or lacks sufficient strength and dexterity. Even when performed properly, however, Credé's maneuver isn't always successful and doesn't always eliminate the need for catheterization.

Credé's maneuver can't be used after abdominal surgery if the incision isn't completely healed. When a patient uses Credé's maneuver, close monitoring of urine output is necessary to help detect possible infection from accumulation of residual urine.

### Equipment
Bedpan, urinal, or bedside commode

### Implementation
▶ Explain the procedure to the patient and wash your hands.
▶ If allowed, place the patient in Fowler's position and position the bedpan or urinal.

## Performing Credé's maneuver

Credé's maneuver is performed by applying manual pressure over the lower abdomen as shown below. This procedure promotes complete emptying of the bladder in the patient with lower motor neuron damage that impairs the voiding reflex.

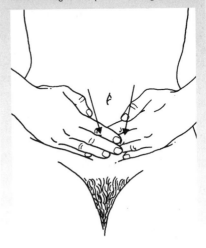

Alternatively, if the patient's condition permits, assist him onto the bedside commode.
▶ Place your hands flat on the patient's abdomen just below the umbilicus. Ask the female patient to bend forward from the hips. Then firmly stroke downward toward the bladder about six times to stimulate the voiding reflex.
▶ Place one hand on top of the other above the pubic arch. Press firmly inward and downward to compress the bladder and expel residual urine. (See *Performing Credé's maneuver.*)
▶ If a portable bladder scanner is available, use this to document if residual urine volume is present after procedure.

### Patient teaching
▶ Explain to the patient that Credé's maneuver is a simple exercise that can be done at home. Tell the patient that he can start a stream of urine from his bladder by performing this easy-to-do maneuver. Tell

the male patient to void directly into the toilet from a standing position if possible. The female patient should sit on the toilet as she normally would.

▶ Show the female patient how to lean forward, bending at the hips, to increase pressure on the bladder.

▶ Have the patient place one hand on top of the other in a return demonstration. Explain that the stroking movement compresses the bladder and expels urine.

### Special considerations

▶ Some facilities require a doctor's order for performing Credé's maneuver. This procedure shouldn't be performed on patients with normal bladder tone or bladder spasms.

▶ After the patient has learned the procedure and can use it successfully, measuring the expelled urine may not be necessary. The patient may then use the maneuver to void directly into the toilet.

### Documentation

▶ Record the date and time of the procedure, the amount of urine expelled, and the patient's tolerance of the procedure.

### REFERENCES

Churchill, B.M., et al. "Dysfunction of the Lower Urinary and Distal Gastrointestinal Tracts in Pediatric Patients with Known Spinal Cord Problems," *Pediatric Clinics of North America* 48(6):1587-630, December 2001.

Nomura, S., et al. "Long-term Analysis of Suprapubic Cystostomy Drainage in Patients with Neurogenic Bladder," *Urologia Internationalis* 65(4):185-89, 2000.

## Hemodialysis

Hemodialysis is performed to remove toxic wastes from the blood of patients in renal failure. This potentially life-saving procedure removes blood from the body, circulates it through a purifying dialyzer and then returns the blood to the body. Various access sites can be used for this procedure. (See *Hemodialysis access sites.*) The most common access device for long-term treatment is an arteriovenous (AV) fistula.

The underlying mechanism in hemodialysis is differential diffusion across a semipermeable membrane, which extracts by-products of protein metabolism, such as urea and uric acid, as well as creatinine and excess body water. This process restores or maintains the balance of the body's buffer system and electrolyte level. Hemodialysis thus promotes a rapid return to normal serum values and helps prevent complications associated with uremia. (See *How hemodialysis works,* page 490.)

Hemodialysis provides temporary support for patients with acute reversible renal failure. It's also used for regular long-term treatment of patients with chronic end-stage renal disease. A less common indication for hemodialysis is acute poisoning, such as a barbiturate or analgesic overdose. The patient's condition (such as rate of creatinine accumulation and weight gain) determines the number and duration of hemodialysis treatments.

Specially prepared personnel usually perform this procedure in a hemodialysis unit. However, if the patient is acutely ill and unstable, hemodialysis can be done at the bedside in the intensive care unit. Special hemodialysis units are available for use at home.

### Equipment

*For preparing the hemodialysis machine*
Hemodialysis machine with appropriate dialyzer ● I.V. solution, administration sets, lines, and related equipment ● dialysate ● optional: heparin, 3-ml syringe with needle, medication label, and hemostat

*For hemodialysis with a double-lumen catheter*
Povidone-iodine pads ● two sterile 4″ × 4″ gauze pads ● two 3-ml and two 5-ml syringes ● tape ● heparin bolus syringe ● gloves

*For hemodialysis with an AV fistula*
Two winged fistula needles (each attached to a 10-ml syringe filled with heparin flush solution) ● linen-saver pad ● povidone-iodine pads ● sterile 4″ × 4″ gauze pads ● tourniquet ● gloves ● adhesive tape

*For hemodialysis with an AV shunt*
Povidone-iodine pads ● alcohol pads ● sterile gloves ● two sterile shunt adapters ● sterile Teflon connector ● two bulldog clamps ● two 10-ml syringes ● normal

# Hemodialysis access sites

Hemodialysis requires vascular access. The site and type of access may vary, depending on the expected duration of dialysis, the surgeon's preference, and the patient's condition.

## Subclavian vein catheterization

Using the Seldinger technique, the doctor or surgeon inserts an introducer needle into the subclavian vein. He then inserts a guide wire through the introducer needle and removes the needle. Using the guide wire, he then threads a 5" to 12" (12.5 to 30.5 cm) plastic or Teflon catheter (with a Y hub) into the patient's vein.

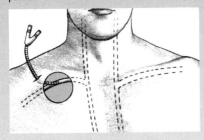

## Femoral vein catheterization

Using the Seldinger technique, the doctor or surgeon inserts an introducer needle into the left or right femoral vein. He then inserts a guide wire through the introducer needle and removes the needle. Using the guide wire, he then threads a 5" to 12" plastic or Teflon catheter with a Y hub or two catheters, one for inflow and another placed about ½" (1.3 cm) distal to the first for outflow.

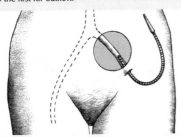

## Arteriovenous fistula

To create a fistula, the surgeon makes an incision into the patient's wrist or lower forearm, then a small incision in the side of an artery and another in the side of a vein. He sutures the edges of the incisions together to make a common opening 3 to 7 mm long.

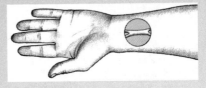

## Arteriovenous shunt

To create a shunt, the surgeon makes an incision in the patient's wrist, lower forearm, or (rarely) an ankle. He then inserts a 6" to 10" transparent Silastic cannula into an artery and another into a vein. Finally, he tunnels the cannulas out through stab wounds and joins them with a piece of Teflon tubing.

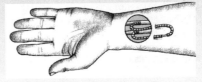

## Arteriovenous graft

To create a graft, the surgeon makes an incision in the patient's forearm, upper arm, or thigh. He then tunnels a natural or synthetic graft under the skin and sutures the distal end to an artery and the proximal end to a vein.

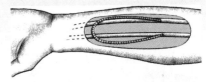

---

saline solution ● four short strips of adhesive tape ● optional: sterile shunt spreader

*For discontinuing hemodialysis with a double-lumen catheter*
Sterile 4" × 4" gauze pads ● povidone-iodine pad ● precut gauze dressing ● clean

# How hemodialysis works

In hemodialysis, blood flows from the patient to an external dialyzer (or artificial kidney) through an arterial access site. Inside the dialyzer, blood and dialysate flow countercurrently divided by a semipermeable membrane. The composition of the dialysate resembles normal extracellular fluid. The blood contains an excess of specific solutes (such as metabolic waste products and some electrolytes), and the dialysate contains electrolytes that may be at abnormal levels in the patient's bloodstream. The dialysate's electrolyte composition can be modified to raise or lower electrolyte levels, depending on need.

Excretory function and electrolyte homeostasis are achieved by *diffusion,* the movement of a molecule across the dialyzer's semipermeable membrane from an area of higher solute concentration to an area of lower concentration. Water (solvent) crosses the membrane from the blood into the dialysate by *ultrafiltration.* This process removes excess water, waste products, and other metabolites through *osmotic pressure* and *hydrostatic pressure.* Osmotic pressure is the movement of water across the semipermeable membrane from an area of lesser solute concentration to one of greater solute concentration. Hydrostatic pressure forces water from the blood compartment into the dialysate compartment. Cleaned of impurities and excess water, the blood returns to the body through a venous site.

## Types of dialyzers

There are three types of dialyzers: the hollow-fiber, the flat-plate or parallel flow-plate, and the coil.

The *hollow-fiber dialyzer,* the most common type, contains fine capillaries, with a semipermeable membrane enclosed in a plastic cylinder. Blood flows through these capillaries as the system pumps dialysate in the opposite direction on the outside of the capillaries.

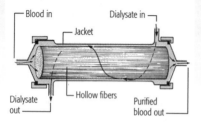

The *flat-plate* or *parallel flow-plate dialyzer* has two or more layers of semipermeable membrane, bound by a semirigid or rigid structure. Blood ports are located at both ends, between the membranes. Blood flows between the membranes, and dialysate flows in the opposite direction along the outside of the membranes.

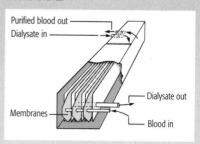

The *coil dialyzer* (no longer widely used) consists of one or more semipermeable membrane tubes supported by mesh and wrapped concentrically around a central core. Blood passes through the coils as dialysate circulates at high speed around the coils and meshwork.

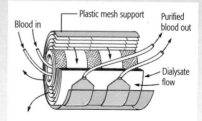

The flat-plate and hollow-fiber dialyzers may be used several times on each patient. Heparin is used to prevent clot formation during hemodialysis.

Three system types can be used to deliver dialysate. The *batch system* uses a reservoir for recirculating dialysate. The *regenerative system* uses sorbents to purify and regenerate recirculating dialysate. The *proportioning system* (the most common) mixes concentrate with water to form dialysate, which then circulates through the dialyzer and goes down a drain after a single pass, followed by fresh dialysate.

and sterile gloves ● normal saline solution ● alcohol pads ● heparin flush solution ● luer-lock injection caps ● optional: transparent occlusive dressing, skin barrier preparation, tape, and materials for culturing drainage

*For discontinuing hemodialysis with an AV fistula*
Gloves ● sterile 4″ × 4″ gauze pads ● two adhesive bandages ● two hemostats ● optional: sterile absorbable gelatin sponges (Gelfoam)

*For discontinuing hemodialysis with an AV shunt*
Sterile gloves ● two bulldog clamps ● two hemostats ● povidone-iodine solution ● sterile 4″ × 4″ gauze pads ● alcohol pads ● elastic gauze bandages ● plasticized or hypoallergenic tape

### Preparation of equipment
Prepare the hemodialysis equipment following the manufacturer's instructions and your facility's protocol. Maintain strict sterile technique to prevent introducing pathogens into the patient's bloodstream during dialysis. Make sure you test the dialyzer and dialysis machine for residual disinfectant after rinsing, and test all the alarms.

### Implementation
▶ Weigh the patient. To determine ultrafiltration requirements, compare his present weight to his weight after the last dialysis and his target weight. Record his baseline vital signs, taking his blood pressure while he's sitting and standing. Auscultate his heart for rate, rhythm, and abnormalities. Observe respiratory rate, rhythm, and quality. Auscultate the lungs for crackles, which is a sign of fluid overload. Assess for edema. Check his mental status and the condition and patency of the access site. Also check for problems since the last dialysis and evaluate previous laboratory data.
▶ Help the patient into a comfortable position (such as supine or sitting in recliner chair with feet elevated). Make sure the access site is well supported and resting on a clean drape.
▶ If the patient is undergoing hemodialysis for the first time, explain the procedure in detail.

▶ Use standard precautions in all cases to prevent transmission of infection. Wash your hands before beginning.

### Beginning hemodialysis with a double-lumen catheter
▶ Prepare venous access. If extension tubing isn't already clamped, clamp it to prevent air from entering the catheter. Then clean each catheter extension tube, clamp, and luer-lock injection cap with povidone-iodine pads to remove contaminants. Next, place a sterile 4″ × 4″ gauze pad under the extension tubing and place two 5-ml syringes and two sterile gauze pads on the drape.
▶ Prepare the anticoagulant regimen as ordered.
▶ Identify arterial and venous blood lines and place them near the drape.
▶ To remove clots and ensure catheter patency, remove catheter caps, attach syringes to each catheter port, open one clamp, and aspirate 1.5 to 3 ml of blood. Close the clamp and repeat the procedure with the other port. Flush each port with 5 ml of heparin flush solution.
▶ Attach blood lines to patient access. First, remove the syringe from the arterial port, and attach the line to the arterial port. Then administer the heparin according to protocol. This prevents clotting in the extracorporeal circuit.
▶ Grasp the venous blood line and attach it to the venous port. Open the clamps on the extension tubing, and secure the tubing to the patient's extremity with tape to reduce tension on the tube and minimize trauma to the insertion site.
▶ Begin hemodialysis according to your unit's protocol.

### Beginning hemodialysis with an AV fistula
▶ Flush the fistula needles, using attached syringes containing heparin flush solution, and set them aside.
▶ Place a linen-saver pad under the patient's arm.
▶ Using aseptic technique, clean a 3″ × 10″ (7.6 × 25 cm) area of skin over the fistula with povidone-iodine pads. Discard each pad after one wipe. (If the patient is sensitive to iodine, use chlorhexidine gluconate [Hibiclens] or alcohol instead.)
▶ Apply a tourniquet above the fistula to distend the veins and facilitate venipuncture. Make sure you avoid occluding the

fistula.

▶ Put on gloves. Perform the venipuncture with a fistula needle. Remove the needle guard and squeeze the wing tips firmly together. Insert the arterial needle at least 1″ (2.5 cm) above the anastomosis, being careful not to puncture the fistula.

▶ Release the tourniquet and flush the needle with heparin flush solution to prevent clotting. Clamp the arterial needle tubing with a hemostat and secure the wing tips of the needle to the skin with adhesive tape to prevent it from dislodging within the vein.

▶ Perform another venipuncture with the venous needle a few inches above the arterial needle. Flush the needle with heparin flush solution. Clamp the venous needle tubing, and secure the wing tips of the venous needle as you did the arterial needle.

▶ Remove the syringe from the end of the arterial tubing, uncap the arterial line from the hemodialysis machine, and connect the two lines. Tape the connection securely to prevent it from separating during the procedure. Repeat these two steps for the venous line.

▶ Release the hemostat and start hemodialysis.

### Beginning hemodialysis with an AV shunt

▶ Remove the bulldog clamps and place them within easy reach of the sterile field. Remove the shunt dressing and clean the shunt, using sterile technique, as you would for daily care. Clean the bulldog clamps with an alcohol pad.

▶ Assemble the shunt adapters according to the manufacturer's directions.

▶ Clean the arterial and venous shunt connection with povidone-iodine pads to remove contaminants. Use a separate pad for each tube and wipe in one direction only, from the insertion site to the connection sites. Allow the tubing to air-dry.

▶ Put on sterile gloves.

▶ Clamp the arterial side of the shunt with a bulldog clamp to prevent blood from flowing through it. Clamp the venous side to prevent leakage when the shunt is opened.

▶ Open the shunt by separating its sides with your fingers or with a sterile shunt spreader, if available. Both sides of the shunt should be exposed. Always inspect the Teflon connector on one side of the shunt to see if it's damaged or bent. If necessary, replace it before proceeding. Note

which side contains the connector so you can use the new one to close the shunt after treatment.

▶ To adapt the shunt to the lines of the machine, attach a shunt adapter and 10-ml syringe filled with about 8 ml of normal saline solution to the side of the shunt containing the Teflon connector. Attach the new Teflon connector to the other side of the shunt with the second adapter. Attach the second 10-ml syringe filled with about 8 ml of normal saline solution to the same side.

▶ Flush the shunt's arterial tubing by releasing its clamp and gently aspirating it with the normal saline solution-filled syringe. Then flush the tubing slowly, observing it for signs of fibrin buildup. Repeat the procedure on the venous side of the shunt.

▶ Secure the shunt to the adapter connection with adhesive tape to prevent separation during treatment.

▶ Connect the arterial and venous lines to the adapters and secure the connections with tape. Tape each line to the patient's arm to prevent unnecessary strain on the shunt during treatment.

▶ Begin hemodialysis according to your unit's protocol.

### Discontinuing hemodialysis with a double-lumen catheter

▶ Wash your hands.

▶ Clamp the extension tubing to prevent air from entering the catheter. Clean all connection points on the catheter and blood lines as well as the clamps to reduce the risk of systemic or local infections.

▶ Place a clean drape under the catheter and place two sterile 4″ × 4″ gauze pads on the drape beneath the catheter lines. Soak the pads with povidone-iodine solution. Then prepare the catheter flush solution with normal saline or heparin flush solution, as ordered.

▶ Put on clean gloves. Grasp each blood line with a gauze pad and disconnect each line from the catheter.

▶ Flush each port with normal saline solution to clean the extension tubing and catheter of blood. Administer additional heparin flush solution, as ordered, to ensure catheter patency. Then attach luer-lock injection caps to prevent entry of air or loss of blood.

▶ Clamp the extension tubing.

▶ When hemodialysis is complete, redress the catheter insertion site; also redress it if it's occluded, soiled, or wet. Place the patient in a supine position with his face turned away from the insertion site so that he doesn't contaminate the site by breathing on it.

▶ Wash your hands and remove the outer occlusive dressing. Then put on sterile gloves, remove the old inner dressing, and discard the gloves and the inner dressing.

▶ Set up a sterile field and observe the site for drainage. Obtain a drainage sample for culture if necessary. Notify the doctor if the suture appears to be missing.

▶ Put on sterile gloves and clean the insertion site with an alcohol pad to remove skin oils. Then clean the site with a povidone-iodine pad and allow it to air-dry.

▶ Put a precut gauze dressing over the insertion site and under the catheter, and place another gauze dressing over the catheter.

▶ Apply a skin barrier preparation to the skin surrounding the gauze dressing. Then cover the gauze and catheter with a transparent occlusive dressing.

▶ Apply a 4″ to 5″ piece of 2″ tape over the cut edge of the dressing to reinforce the lower edge.

### Discontinuing hemodialysis with an AV fistula

▶ Wash your hands. Turn the blood pump on the hemodialysis machine to 50 to 100 ml/minute.

▶ Put on gloves and remove the tape from the connection site of the arterial lines. Clamp the needle tubing with the hemostat and disconnect the lines. The blood in the machine's arterial line will continue to flow toward the dialyzer, followed by a column of air. Just before the blood reaches the point where the normal saline solution enters the line, clamp the blood line with another hemostat.

▶ Unclamp the normal saline solution to allow a small amount to flow through the line. Unclamp the hemostat on the machine line. This allows all blood to flow into the dialyzer where it passes through the filter and back to the patient through the venous line.

▶ After blood is retransfused, clamp the venous needle tubing and the machine's venous line with hemostats. Turn off the blood pump.

▶ Remove the tape from the connection site of the venous lines and disconnect the lines.

▶ Remove the venipuncture needle, and apply pressure to the site with a folded 4″ × 4″ gauze pad until all bleeding stops, usually within 10 minutes. Apply an adhesive bandage. Repeat the procedure on the arterial line.

▶ When hemodialysis is complete, assess the patient's weight, vital signs (including standing blood pressure), and mental status. Then compare your findings with your predialysis assessment data. Document your findings.

▶ Disinfect and rinse the delivery system according to the manufacturer's instructions.

### Discontinuing hemodialysis with an AV shunt

▶ Wash your hands. Turn the blood pump on the hemodialysis machine to 50 to 100 ml/minute.

▶ Put on the sterile gloves and remove the tape from the connection site of the arterial lines. Clamp the arterial cannula with a bulldog clamp, and then disconnect the lines. The blood in the machine's arterial line will continue to flow toward the dialyzer, followed by a column of air. Just before the blood reaches the point where the normal saline solution enters the line, clamp the blood line with a hemostat.

▶ Unclamp the normal saline solution to allow a small amount to flow through the line. Reclamp the normal saline solution line and unclamp the hemostat on the machine line. This allows all blood to flow into the dialyzer where it's circulated through the filter and back to the patient through the venous line.

▶ Just before the last volume of blood enters the patient, clamp the venous cannula with a bulldog clamp and the machine's venous line with a hemostat.

▶ Remove the tape from the connection site of the venous lines. Turn off the blood pump and disconnect the lines.

▶ Reconnect the shunt cannula. Remove the older of the two Teflon connectors and discard it. Connect the shunt, taking care to position the Teflon connector equally between the two cannulas. Remove the bulldog clamps.

▶ Secure the shunt connection with plasticized or hypoallergenic tape to prevent accidental disconnection.

▶ Clean the shunt and its site with the povidone-iodine pads. When the cleaning procedure is finished, remove the povidone-iodine with alcohol pads.

▶ Make sure blood flows through the shunt adequately.

▶ Apply a dressing to the shunt site and wrap it securely (but not too tightly) with elastic gauze bandages. Attach the bulldog clamps to the outside dressing.

▶ When hemodialysis is complete, assess the patient's weight, vital signs, and mental status. Then compare your findings with your predialysis assessment data. Document your findings.

▶ Disinfect and rinse the delivery system according to the manufacturer's instructions.

## Special considerations

▶ Obtain blood samples from the patient as ordered. Samples are usually drawn before beginning hemodialysis.

▶ To avoid pyrogenic reactions and bacteremia with septicemia resulting from contamination, use strict sterile technique during preparation of the machine. Discard equipment that has fallen on the floor or that has been disconnected and exposed to the air.

▶ Immediately report any machine malfunction or equipment defect.

▶ Avoid unnecessary handling of shunt tubing. However, make sure you inspect the shunt carefully for patency by observing its color. Also look for clots and serum and cell separation, and check the temperature of the Silastic tubing. Assess the shunt insertion site for signs of infection, such as purulent drainage, inflammation, and tenderness, which may indicate the body's rejection of the shunt. Also check to see if the shunt insertion tips are exposed.

▶ Make sure you complete each step in this procedure correctly. Overlooking a single step or performing it incorrectly can cause unnecessary blood loss or inefficient treatment from poor clearances or inadequate fluid removal. For example, never allow a saline solution bag to run dry while priming and soaking the dialyzer. This can cause air to enter the patient portion of the dialysate system. Ultimately, failure to perform hemodialysis accurately can lead to patient injury and even death.

▶ If bleeding continues after you remove an AV fistula needle, apply pressure with a sterile, absorbable gelatin sponge. If bleeding persists, apply a similar sponge soaked in topical thrombin solution.

▶ Throughout hemodialysis, carefully monitor the patient's vital signs. Read blood pressure at least hourly or as often as every 15 minutes, if necessary. Monitor the patient's weight before and after the procedure to ensure adequate ultrafiltration during treatment. (Many dialysis units are now equipped with bed scales.)

▶ Perform periodic tests for clotting time on the patient's blood samples and samples from the dialyzer. If the patient receives meals during treatment, make sure they're light.

▶ Continue necessary drug administration during dialysis unless the drug would be removed in the dialysate; if so, administer the drug after dialysis.

## Home care

Before the patient leaves the facility, teach him how to care for his vascular access site. Instruct him to keep the incision clean and dry to prevent infection, and to clean it daily until it heals completely and the sutures are removed (usually 10 to 14 days after surgery). He should notify the doctor of pain, swelling, redness, or drainage in the accessed arm. Teach him how to use a stethoscope to auscultate for bruits and how to palpate a thrill.

Explain that after the access site heals, he may use the arm freely. In fact, exercise is beneficial because it helps stimulate vein enlargement. Remind him not to allow any treatments or procedures on the accessed arm, including blood pressure monitoring or needle punctures. Also tell him to avoid putting excessive pressure on the arm. He shouldn't sleep on it, wear constricting clothing over it, or lift heavy objects or strain with it. He also should avoid getting wet for several hours after dialysis.

Teach the patient exercises for the affected arm to promote vascular dilation and enhance blood flow. He may start by squeezing a small rubber ball or other soft object for 15 minutes, when advised by the doctor.

If the patient will be performing hemodialysis at home, thoroughly review all aspects of the procedure with the patient and his family. Give them the phone number of the dialysis center. Emphasize that training for home hemodialysis is a complex process requiring 2 to 3 months to ensure that the patient or family member performs it safely and competently. Keep in mind that this procedure is stressful.

## Complications

Bacterial endotoxins in the dialysate may cause fever. Rapid fluid removal and electrolyte changes during hemodialysis can cause early dialysis disequilibrium syndrome. Signs and symptoms include headache, nausea, vomiting, restlessness, hypertension, muscle cramps, backache, and seizures.

Excessive removal of fluid during ultrafiltration can cause hypovolemia and hypotension. Diffusion of the sugar and sodium content of the dialysate solution into the blood can cause hyperglycemia and hypernatremia. These conditions, in turn, can cause hyperosmolarity.

Cardiac arrhythmias can occur during hemodialysis as a result of electrolyte and pH changes in the blood. They can also develop in patients taking antiarrhythmic drugs because the dialysate removes these drugs during treatment. Angina may develop in patients with anemia or preexisting arteriosclerotic cardiovascular disease because of the physiologic stress on the blood during purification and ultrafiltration. Reduced oxygen levels due to extracorporeal blood flow or membrane sensitivity may require increasing oxygen administration during hemodialysis.

Some complications of hemodialysis can be fatal. For example, an air embolism can result if the dialyzer retains air, if tubing connections become loose, or if the saline solution container empties. Symptoms include chest pain, dyspnea, coughing, and cyanosis.

Hemolysis can result from obstructed flow of the dialysate concentrate or from incorrect setting of the conductivity alarm limits. Symptoms include chest pain, dyspnea, cherry red blood, arrhythmias, acute decrease in hematocrit, and hyperkalemia.

Hyperthermia, another potentially fatal complication, can result if the dialysate becomes overheated. Exsanguination can result from separations of the blood lines or

from rupture of the blood lines or dialyzer membrane.

## Documentation

▶ Record the time treatment began and any problems with it. Note the patient's vital signs and weight before and during treatment.
▶ Note the time blood samples were taken for testing, the test results, and treatment for complications.
▶ Record the time the treatment was completed and the patient's response to it.

## REFERENCES

American Nephrology Nurses Association (2001). "Position Statement: Daily Hemodialysis/Nocturnal Hemodialysis" [Online]. Available: *www.anna.inurse.com* [2001, October 8].

Herrine, S.K., et al. "Development of an HCV Infection Risk Stratification Algorithm for Patients on Chronic Hemodialysis," *American Journal of Gastroenterology* 97(10): 2619-22, October 2002.

*Instructor's Resource Manual for the AACN Core Curriculum for Critical Care Nursing,* 5th ed. Edited by Alspach, J.G. Philadelphia: W.B. Saunders Co., 2001.

Morgan, L. "A Decade Review: Methods to Improve Adherence to the Treatment Regimen Among Hemodialysis Patients," *Nephrology Nursing Journal* 27(3):299-304, June 2000.

O'Keefe, A., and Daigle, N.W. "A New Approach to Classifying Malnutrition in the Hemodialysis Patient," *Journal of Renal Nutrition* 12(4):248-55, October 2002.

Pfettscher, S.A. "Chronic Renal Failure and Renal Transplant," in *Critical Care Nursing.* Edited by Bucher, L., and Melander, S. Philadelphia: W.B. Saunders Co., 1999.

# Indwelling catheter care and removal

Intended to prevent infection and other complications by keeping the catheter insertion site clean, routine catheter care typically is performed daily after the patient's morning bath and immediately after perineal care. (Bedtime catheter care may have to be performed before perineal care.)

Because some studies suggest that catheter care increases rather than lowers the risk of infection and other complications, many health care facilities don't recommend daily catheter care. Thus, individual facility policy dictates whether a patient will receive such care. Regardless of the catheter care policy, the equipment and the patient's genitalia require inspection twice daily.

An indwelling urinary catheter should be removed when bladder decompression is no longer necessary, when the patient can resume voiding, or when the catheter is obstructed. Depending on the length of the catheterization, the doctor may order bladder retraining before catheter removal.

## Equipment

*For catheter care*
Soap and water ● sterile gloves ● eight sterile 4″ × 4″ gauze pads ● basin ● washcloth ● leg bag ● collection bag ● adhesive tape or leg band ● waste receptacle ● optional: safety pin, rubber band, gooseneck lamp or flashlight, adhesive remover, and specimen container

*For perineal cleaning*
Washcloth ● additional basin ● soap and water

*For catheter removal*
Gloves ● alcohol pad ● 10-ml syringe with a luer-lock ● bedpan ● linen-saver pad ● optional: clamp for bladder retraining

### Preparation of equipment
Wash your hands and bring all equipment to the patient's bedside. Open the gauze pads, place several in the first basin, and pour some povidone-iodine or other cleaning agent over them.

Some facilities specify that, after wiping the urinary meatus with cleaning solution, you should wipe it off with wet, sterile gauze pads to prevent possible irritation from the cleaning solution. If this is your facility's policy, pour water into the second basin, and moisten three more gauze pads.

## Implementation
▶ Explain the procedure and its purpose to the patient.
▶ Provide privacy.

### Catheter care
▶ Make sure that the lighting is adequate so that you can see the perineum and catheter tubing clearly. Place a gooseneck lamp or flashlight at the bedside, if needed.
▶ Inspect the catheter for any problems and check the urine drainage for mucus, blood clots, sediment, and turbidity. Then pinch the catheter between two fingers to determine if the lumen contains any material. If you notice any of these conditions (or if your facility's policy requires it), obtain a urine specimen (collect at least 3 ml of urine, but don't fill the specimen cup more than halfway) and notify the doctor.
▶ Inspect the outside of the catheter where it enters the urinary meatus for encrusted material and suppurative drainage. Also inspect the tissue around the meatus for irritation or swelling.
▶ Remove the leg band, or if adhesive tape was used to secure the catheter, remove the adhesive tape. Inspect the area for signs and symptoms of adhesive burns — redness, tenderness, or blisters.
▶ Put on the gloves. Clean the outside of the catheter and the tissue around the meatus using soap and water. To avoid contaminating the urinary tract, always clean by wiping away from — never toward — the urinary meatus. Use a dry gauze pad to remove encrusted material.

◆ **ALERT!** Don't pull on the catheter while you're cleaning it. This can injure the urethra and the bladder wall. It can also expose a section of the catheter that was inside the urethra, so that when you release the catheter, the newly contaminated section will reenter the urethra, introducing potentially infectious organisms.

▶ Remove your gloves, reapply the leg band, and reattach the catheter to the leg band. If a leg band isn't available, tear a piece of adhesive tape from the roll.
▶ To prevent skin hypersensitivity or irritation, retape the catheter on the opposite side.

◆ **ALERT!** Provide enough slack before securing the catheter to prevent tension on the tubing, which could injure the urethral lumen or bladder wall.

▶ Most drainage bags have a plastic clamp on the tubing to attach them to the sheet. If this isn't available, wrap a rubber band around the drainage tubing, insert the safety pin through a loop of the rubber band, and pin the tubing to the sheet below blad

der level. Then attach the collection bag, below bladder level, to the bed frame.
▶ If necessary, clean residue from the previous tape site with adhesive remover. Dispose of all used supplies in a waste receptacle.

## Catheter removal

▶ Wash your hands. Assemble the equipment at the patient's bedside. Explain the procedure and tell him that he may feel slight discomfort. Tell him that you'll check him periodically during the first 6 to 24 hours after catheter removal to make sure he resumes voiding.
▶ Put on gloves. Place a linen-saver pad under the patient's buttocks. Attach the syringe to the luer-lock mechanism on the catheter.
▶ Pull back on the plunger of the syringe. This deflates the balloon by aspirating the injected fluid. The amount of fluid injected is usually indicated on the tip of the catheter's balloon lumen and on the plan of care and the patient's chart.
▶ Because urine may leak as the catheter is removed, offer the patient a bedpan. Grasp the catheter and pinch it firmly with your thumb and index finger to prevent urine from flowing back into the urethra. Gently pull the catheter from the urethra. If you meet resistance, don't apply force, instead notify the doctor. Remove the bedpan.
▶ Measure and record the amount of urine in the collection bag before discarding it. Remove and discard gloves, and wash your hands. For the first 24 hours after catheter removal, note the time and amount of each voiding.

## Special considerations

▶ Your facility may require the use of specific cleaning agents for catheter care, so check the policy manual before beginning this procedure.
▶ Avoid raising the drainage bag above bladder level. This prevents reflux of urine, which may contain bacteria. To avoid damaging the urethral lumen or bladder wall, always disconnect the drainage bag and tubing from the bed linen and bed frame before helping the patient out of bed.
▶ When possible, attach a leg bag to allow the patient greater mobility. If the patient will be discharged with an indwelling catheter, teach him how to use a leg bag.

(See *Teaching patients about leg bags,* page 498.)
▶ Encourage patients with unrestricted fluid intake to increase intake to at least 3 qt (3 L)/day. This helps flush the urinary system and reduces sediment formation. To prevent urinary sediment and calculi from obstructing the drainage tube, some patients are placed on an acid-ash diet to acidify the urine. Cranberry juice, for example, may help to promote urinary acidity.
▶ After catheter removal, assess the patient for incontinence (or dribbling), urgency, persistent dysuria or bladder spasms, fever, chills, or palpable bladder distention. Report these to the doctor.
▶ When changing catheters after long-term use (usually 30 days), you may need a larger size catheter because the meatus enlarges, causing urine to leak around the catheter.

## Home care

Instruct patients discharged with indwelling catheters to wash the urinary meatus and perineal area with soap and water twice daily and the anal area after each bowel movement.

## Complications

Sediment buildup can occur anywhere in a catheterization system, especially in bedridden and dehydrated patients. To prevent this, keep the patient well hydrated if he isn't on fluid restriction. Change the indwelling catheter as ordered or when malfunction, obstruction, or contamination occurs.

Acute renal failure may result from a catheter obstructed by sediment. Be alert for sharply reduced urine flow from the catheter. Assess for bladder discomfort or distention.

Urinary tract infection can result from catheter insertion or from intraluminal or extraluminal migration of bacteria up the catheter. Signs and symptoms may include cloudy urine, foul-smelling urine, hematuria, fever, malaise, tenderness over the bladder, and flank pain.

Major complications in removing an indwelling catheter are failure of the balloon to deflate and rupture of the balloon. If the balloon ruptures, cystoscopy is usually performed to ensure removal of any balloon fragments.

# Teaching patients about leg bags

A urine drainage bag attached to the leg provides the catheterized patient with greater mobility. Because the bag is hidden under clothing, it may also help him feel more comfortable about catheterization. Leg bags are usually worn during the day and are replaced with a standard collection device at night.

If the patient is discharged with an indwelling catheter, teach him how to attach and remove a leg bag. To demonstrate, you'll need a bag with a short drainage tube, two straps, an alcohol pad, adhesive tape, and a screw clamp or hemostat.

### Attaching the leg bag

▶ Provide privacy and explain the procedure. Describe the advantages of a leg bag, but caution the patient that a leg bag is smaller than a standard collection device and may have to be emptied more frequently.

▶ Remove the protective covering from the tip of the drainage tube. Then show the patient how to clean the tip with an alcohol pad, wiping away from the opening to avoid contaminating the tube. Show him how to attach the tube to the catheter.

▶ Place the drainage bag on the patient's calf or thigh. Have him fasten the straps securely (as shown), and show him how to tape the catheter to his leg. Emphasize that he must leave slack in the catheter to minimize pressure on the bladder, urethra, and related structures. Excessive pressure or tension can lead to tissue breakdown.

▶ Also tell the patient not to fasten the straps too tightly to avoid interfering with his circulation.

### Avoiding complications

▶ Although most leg bags have a valve in the drainage tube that prevents urine reflux into the bladder, urge the patient to keep the drainage bag lower than his bladder at all times because urine in the bag is a perfect growth medium for bacteria. Also, caution him not to go to bed or take long naps while wearing the drainage bag.

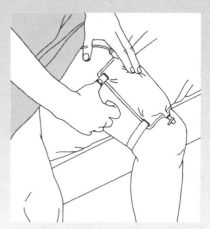

▶ To prevent a full leg bag from damaging the bladder wall and urethra, encourage the patient to empty the bag when it's only half full. He should also inspect the catheter and drainage tube periodically for compression or kinking, which could obstruct urine flow and result in bladder distention.

▶ Tell the patient to wash the leg bag with soap and water or a bacteriostatic solution before each use to prevent infection.

## Documentation

▶ Record the care you performed, any modifications, patient complaints, and the condition of the perineum and urinary meatus.

▶ Note the character of the urine in the drainage bag, any sediment buildup, and whether a specimen was sent for laboratory analysis.

▶ Record fluid intake and output. An hourly record is usually necessary for critically ill patients and those with renal insufficiency who are hemodynamically unstable.

▶ For bladder retraining, record the date and time the catheter was clamped, the time it was released, and the volume and appearance of the urine.

▶ For catheter removal, record the date and time and the patient's tolerance of the procedure.

▶ Record when and how much he voided after catheter removal and any associated problems.

▶ For bladder retraining, record the date and time the catheter was clamped, the time it was released, and the volume and appearance of the urine.

## REFERENCES

Joanna Briggs Institute. "Management of Short-Term Indwelling Urethral Catheters to Prevent Urinary Tract Infections," *Best Practice* 4(1), 2000. *www.joannabriggs.edu.au/bpmenu.html*

Lai, K.K., and Fontecchio, S.A. "Use of Silver-Hydrogel Urinary Catheters on the Incidence of Catheter-Associated Urinary Tract Infections in Hospitalized Patients. *American Journal of Infection Control.* 30(4):221-25, June 2002.

Munasinghe, R.L., et al. "Appropriateness of Use of Indwelling Urinary Catheters in Patients Admitted to the Medical Service. *Infection Control Hospital Epidemiology* 22(10):647-49, October 2001.

Potter, P.A., and Perry, A.G. *Fundamentals of Nursing,* 5th ed. St. Louis: Mosby–Year Book, Inc., 2001.

# Indwelling catheter insertion

Also known as a Foley or retention catheter, an indwelling urinary catheter remains in the bladder to provide continuous urine drainage. A balloon inflated at the catheter's distal end prevents it from slipping out of the bladder after insertion.

Indwelling catheters are used most commonly to relieve bladder distention caused by urine retention and to allow continuous urine drainage when the urinary meatus is swollen from childbirth, surgery, or local trauma. Other indications for an indwelling catheter include urinary tract obstruction (caused by a tumor or enlarged prostate), urine retention or infection from neurogenic bladder paralysis caused by spinal cord injury or disease, and any illness in which the patient's urine output must be monitored closely.

An indwelling catheter is inserted using sterile technique and only when absolutely necessary. Insertion should be performed with extreme care to prevent injury and infection.

**EVIDENCE BASE** Research has indicated that silicone catheters cause fewer infections and obstruction for patients requiring catheterization at home.

## Equipment

Sterile indwelling catheter (latex or silicone #10 to #22 French [average adult sizes are #16 to #18 French]) ● syringe filled with 5 to 8 ml of sterile water (normal saline solution is sometimes used) ● washcloth ● towel ● soap and water ● two linen-saver pads ● sterile gloves ● sterile drape ● sterile fenestrated drape ● sterile cotton-tipped applicators (or cotton balls and plastic forceps) ● povidone-iodine or other antiseptic cleaning agent ● urine receptacle ● sterile water-soluble lubricant ● sterile drainage collection bag ● intake and output sheet ● adhesive tape ● optional: urine specimen container and laboratory request form, leg band with Velcro closure, gooseneck lamp or flashlight, pillows or rolled blankets or towels.

Prepackaged sterile disposable kits that usually contain all the necessary equipment are available. The syringes in these kits are prefilled with 10 ml of normal saline solution.

### Preparation of equipment

Check the order on the patient's chart to determine if a catheter size or type has been specified. Then wash your hands, select the appropriate equipment and assemble it at the patient's bedside.

## Implementation

▶ Explain the procedure to the patient and provide privacy. Check his chart and ask when he voided last. Percuss and palpate the bladder to establish baseline data. Ask if he feels the urge to void.

▶ Have a coworker hold a flashlight or place a gooseneck lamp next to the patient's bed so that you can see the urinary meatus clearly in poor lighting.

▶ Place the female patient in the supine position, with her knees flexed and separated and her feet flat on the bed, about 2 feet (0.6 m) apart. If she finds this position uncomfortable, have her flex one knee and keep the other leg flat on the bed.

**ALERT!** The elderly patient may need pillows or rolled blankets or towels to provide support with positioning.

▶ You may need an assistant to help the patient stay in position or to direct the light. Place the male patient in the supine position with his legs extended and flat on the bed. Ask the patient to hold the position to give you a clear view of the urinary meatus and to prevent contamination of the sterile field.

▶ Use the washcloth to clean the patient's genital area and perineum thoroughly with soap and water. Dry the area with the towel. Then wash your hands.

▶ Place the linen-saver pads on the bed between the patient's legs and under the hips. To create the sterile field, open the prepackaged kit or equipment tray and place it between the female patient's legs or next to the male patient's hip. If the sterile gloves are the first item on the top of the tray, put them on. Place the sterile drape under the patient's hips. Drape the patient's lower abdomen with the sterile fenestrated drape so only the genital area remains exposed. Take care not to contaminate your gloves.

▶ Open the rest of the kit or tray. Put on the sterile gloves if you haven't already done so.

▶ Make sure the patient isn't allergic to iodine solution; if he is allergic, another antiseptic cleaning agent must be used.

▶ Tear open the packet of povidone-iodine or other antiseptic cleaning agent and use it to saturate the sterile cotton balls or applicators. Be careful not to spill the solution on the equipment.

▶ Open the packet of water-soluble lubricant and apply it to the catheter tip; attach the drainage collection bag to the other end of the catheter. (If you're using a commercial kit, the drainage bag may be attached.) Make sure all tubing ends remain sterile and make sure the clamp at the emptying port of the drainage bag is closed to prevent urine leakage from the bag. Some drainage systems have an air-lock chamber to prevent bacteria from traveling to the bladder from urine in the drainage bag.

*Note:* Some urologists and nurses use a syringe prefilled with water-soluble lubricant and instill the lubricant directly into the male urethra, instead of on the catheter tip. This method helps prevent trauma to the urethral lining as well as possible urinary tract infection. Check your facility's policy.

▶ Before inserting the catheter, inflate the balloon with sterile water or normal saline solution to inspect it for leaks. To do this,

attach the prefilled syringe to the luer-lock, then push the plunger and check for seepage as the balloon expands. Aspirate the solution to deflate the balloon. Also inspect the catheter for resiliency. Rough, cracked catheters can injure the urethral mucosa during insertion, which can predispose the patient to infection.

▶ For the female patient, separate the labia majora and labia minora as widely as possible with the thumb, middle, and index fingers of your nondominant hand so you have a full view of the urinary meatus. Keep the labia well separated throughout the procedure (as shown below), so they don't obscure the urinary meatus or contaminate the area after it's cleaned.

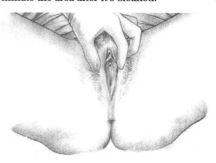

▶ With your dominant hand, use a sterile, cotton-tipped applicator (or pick up a sterile cotton ball with the plastic forceps) and wipe one side of the urinary meatus with a single downward motion (as shown below).

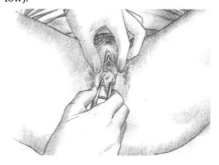

▶ Wipe the other side with another sterile applicator or cotton ball in the same way. Then wipe directly over the meatus with still another sterile applicator or cotton ball. Take care not to contaminate your sterile glove.

▶ For the male patient, hold the penis with your nondominant hand. If he's uncircumcised, retract the foreskin. Then gently lift and stretch the penis to a 60- to 90-degree angle. Hold the penis this way throughout the procedure to straighten the urethra and maintain a sterile field (as shown below).

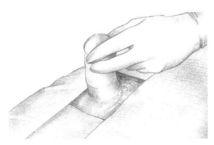

▶ Use your dominant hand to clean the glans with a sterile cotton-tipped applicator or a sterile cotton ball held in the forceps. Clean in a circular motion, starting at the urinary meatus and working outward.
▶ Repeat the procedure, using another sterile applicator or cotton ball and taking care not to contaminate your sterile glove.
▶ Pick up the catheter with your dominant hand and prepare to insert the lubricated tip into the urinary meatus. To facilitate insertion by relaxing the sphincter, ask the patient to cough as you insert the catheter. Tell him to breathe deeply and slowly to further relax the sphincter and prevent spasms. Hold the catheter close to its tip to ease insertion and control its direction.

■ **ALERT!** Never force a catheter during insertion. Maneuver the catheter gently, angling it slightly toward the symphysis pubis as the patient bears down or coughs. If you still meet resistance, stop and notify the doctor. Sphincter spasms, strictures, misplacement in the vagina (in females), or an enlarged prostate (in males) may cause resistance.
▶ For the female patient, advance the catheter 2″ to 3″ (5 to 7.5 cm)—while continuing to hold the labia apart—until urine begins to flow (as shown below).

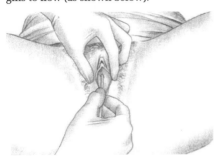

If the catheter is inadvertently inserted into the vagina, leave it there as a landmark. Then begin the procedure over again using new supplies.
▶ For the male patient, advance the catheter to the bifurcation 5″ to 7½″ (13 to 19 cm) and check for urine flow (as shown below). If the foreskin was retracted, replace it to prevent compromised circulation and painful swelling.

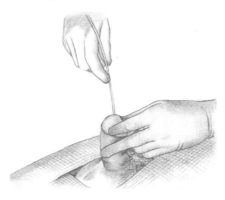

▶ When urine stops flowing, attach the saline-filled syringe to the luer-lock.
▶ Push the plunger and inflate the balloon (as shown below) to keep the catheter in place in the bladder.

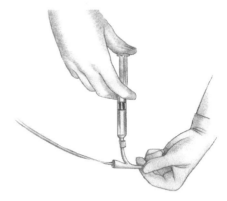

■ **ALERT!** Never inflate a balloon without first establishing urine flow, which assures you that the catheter is in the bladder.
▶ Hang the collection bag below bladder level to prevent urine reflux into the bladder, which can cause infection, and to facilitate gravity drainage of the bladder. Make sure the tubing doesn't get tangled in the bed's side rails.

▶ Tape the catheter to the female patient's thigh to prevent possible tension on the urogenital trigone (as shown below).

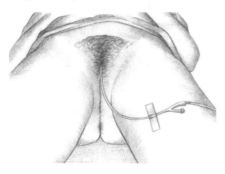

▶ Tape the catheter to the male patient's anterior thigh to prevent pressure on the urethra at the penoscrotal junction, which can lead to formation of urethrocutaneous fistulas. Taping this way also prevents traction on the bladder and alteration in the normal direction of urine flow in males.
▶ As an alternative, secure the catheter to the patient's thigh using a leg band with a Velcro closure (as shown below). This decreases skin irritation, especially in patients with long-term indwelling catheters.

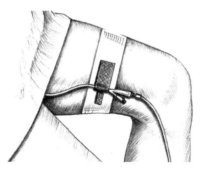

▶ Dispose of all used supplies properly.

### Special considerations
▶ Several types of catheters are available with balloons of various sizes. Each type has its own method of inflation and closure. For example, in one type of catheter, sterile solution or air is injected through the inflation lumen, then the end of the injection port is folded over itself and fastened with a clamp or rubber band.
   *Note:* Injecting a catheter with air makes identifying leaks difficult and doesn't guarantee deflation of the balloon for removal.

▶ A similar catheter is inflated when a seal in the end of the inflation lumen is penetrated with a needle or the tip of the solution-filled syringe. Another type of balloon catheter self-inflates when a prepositioned clamp is loosened. The balloon size determines the amount of solution needed for inflation, and the exact amount is usually printed on the distal extension of the catheter used for inflating the balloon.
▶ If necessary, ask the female patient to lie on her side with her knees drawn up to her chest during the catheterization procedure (as shown below).

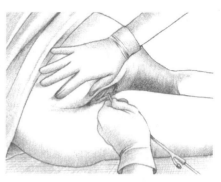

   This position may be especially helpful for elderly or disabled patients such as those with severe contractures.
▶ If the doctor orders a urine specimen for laboratory analysis, obtain it from the urine receptacle with a specimen collection container at the time of catheterization and send it to the laboratory with the appropriate laboratory request form. Connect the drainage bag when urine stops flowing.
▶ Inspect the catheter and tubing periodically while they're in place to detect compression or kinking that could obstruct urine flow. Explain the basic principles of gravity drainage so that the patient realizes the importance of keeping the drainage tubing and collection bag lower than his bladder at all times. If necessary, provide the patient with detailed instructions for performing clean intermittent self-catheterization.
▶ For monitoring purposes, empty the collection bag at least every 8 hours. Excessive fluid volume may require more frequent emptying to prevent traction on the catheter, which would cause the patient discomfort, and to prevent injury to the urethra and bladder wall. Some facilities encour-

age changing catheters at regular intervals, such as every 30 days, if the patient will have long-term continuous drainage.

**◆ ALERT!** Observe the patient carefully for adverse reactions caused by removing excessive volumes of residual urine, such as hypovolemic shock. Check your facility's policy beforehand to determine the maximum amount of urine that may be drained at one time. (Some facilities limit the amount to 700 to 1,000 ml). Whether to limit the amount of urine drained is currently controversial. Clamp the catheter at the first sign of an adverse reaction and notify the doctor.

## Home care
If the patient will be discharged with a long-term indwelling catheter, teach him and his family all aspects of daily catheter maintenance, including care of the skin and urinary meatus, signs and symptoms of urinary tract infection or obstruction, how to irrigate the catheter (if appropriate), and the importance of adequate fluid intake to maintain patency. Explain that a home care nurse should visit every 4 to 6 weeks, or more often if needed, to change the catheter.

## Complications
Urinary tract infection can result from the introduction of bacteria into the bladder. Improper insertion can cause traumatic injury to the urethral and bladder mucosa. Bladder atony or spasms can result from rapid decompression of a severely distended bladder.

## Documentation
▶ Record the date, time, and size and type of indwelling catheter used.
▶ Describe the amount, color, and other characteristics of urine emptied from the bladder. Your hospital may require only the intake and output sheet for fluid-balance data.
▶ If large volumes of urine have been emptied, describe the patient's tolerance for the procedure.
▶ Note whether a urine specimen was sent for laboratory analysis.

## REFERENCES
Joanna Briggs Institute. "Management of Short-Term Indwelling Urethral Catheters to Prevent Urinary Tract Infections," *Best Practice* 4(1), 2000. *www.joannabriggs.edu.au/bpmenu.html*
Potter, P.A., and Perry, A.G. *Fundamentals of Nursing,* 5th ed. St. Louis: Mosby–Year Book, Inc., 2001.

# Male incontinence device

Many patients don't require an indwelling urinary catheter to manage their incontinence. For male patients, a male incontinence device reduces the risk of urinary tract infection from catheterization, promotes bladder retraining when possible, helps prevent skin breakdown, and improves the patient's self-image. The device consists of a condom catheter secured to the shaft of the penis and connected to a leg bag or drainage bag. It has no contraindications but can cause skin irritation and edema.

## Equipment
Condom catheter ● drainage bag ● extension tubing ● hypoallergenic tape or incontinence sheath holder ● commercial adhesive strip or skin-bond cement ● elastic adhesive or Velcro, if needed ● gloves ● razor, if needed ● basin ● soap ● washcloth ● towel

### Preparation of equipment
Fill the basin with lukewarm water. Then bring the basin and the remaining equipment to the patient's bedside.

## Implementation
▶ Explain the procedure to the patient, wash your hands thoroughly, put on gloves, and provide privacy.

### Applying the device
▶ If the patient is circumcised, wash the penis with soap, water, and a washcloth, rinse well, and pat dry with a towel. If the patient is uncircumcised, gently retract the foreskin and clean beneath it. Rinse well but don't dry because moisture provides lubrication and prevents friction during foreskin replacement. Replace the foreskin to avoid penile constriction. Then, if necessary, shave the base and shaft of the penis

# How to apply a condom catheter

Apply an adhesive strip to the shaft of the penis about 1″ (2.5 cm) from the scrotal area.

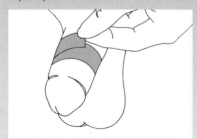

Roll the condom catheter onto the penis past the adhesive strip, leaving about ½″ (1 cm) clearance at the end. Press the sheath gently against the strip until it adheres.

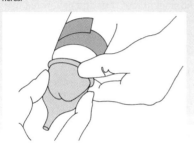

to prevent the adhesive strip or skin-bond cement from pulling pubic hair.

▶ If you're using a precut commercial adhesive strip, insert the glans penis through its opening, and position the strip 1″ (2.5 cm) from the scrotal area. If you're using uncut adhesive, cut a strip to fit around the shaft of the penis. Remove the protective covering from one side of the adhesive strip and press this side firmly to the penis to enhance adhesion. Then remove the covering from the other side of the strip. If a commercial adhesive strip isn't available, apply skin-bond cement and let it dry for a few minutes.

▶ Position the rolled condom catheter at the tip of the penis, leaving 1″ between the condom and the tip of the penis, with the drainage opening at the urinary meatus.

▶ Unroll the catheter upward, past the adhesive strip on the shaft of the penis. Gently press the sheath against the strip until it adheres. (See *How to apply a condom catheter.*)

▶ After the condom catheter is in place, secure it with hypoallergenic tape or an incontinence sheath holder.

▶ Using extension tubing, connect the condom catheter to the leg bag or drainage bag. Remove and discard your gloves.

### Removing the device

▶ Put on gloves and simultaneously roll the condom catheter and adhesive strip off the penis and discard them. If you've used skin-bond cement rather than an adhesive strip, remove it with solvent. Also remove and discard the hypoallergenic tape or incontinence sheath holder.

▶ Clean the penis with lukewarm water, rinse thoroughly, and dry. Check for swelling or signs of skin breakdown.

▶ Remove the leg bag by closing the drain clamp, unlatching the leg straps, and disconnecting the extension tubing at the top of the bag. Discard your gloves.

## Special considerations

▶ If hypoallergenic tape or an incontinence sheath holder isn't available, secure the condom with a strip of elastic adhesive or Velcro. Apply the strip snugly—but not too tightly—to prevent circulatory constriction.

▶ Inspect the condom catheter for twists and the extension tubing for kinks to prevent obstruction of urine flow, which could cause the condom to balloon, eventually dislodging it.

## Documentation

Record the date and time of application and removal of the incontinence device. Also note skin condition and the patient's response to the device, including voiding pattern, to assist with bladder retraining.

### REFERENCES

Edward, D. *Bedside Critical Care Manual.* Philadelphia: Lippincott Williams & Wilkins, 2001.

Hughes, S. "Do Continence Aids Help To Maintain Skin Integrity?" *Journal of Wound Care* 11(6):235-39, June 2002. (Review.)

# Urinary diversion techniques

A cystostomy or a nephrostomy can be used to create a permanent diversion, to relieve obstruction from an inoperable tumor, or to provide an outlet for urine after cystectomy. A temporary diversion can relieve obstruction from a calculus or ureteral edema.

In a cystostomy, a catheter is inserted percutaneously through the suprapubic area into the bladder. In a nephrostomy, a catheter is inserted percutaneously through the flank into the renal pelvis.

**CYSTOSTOMY**

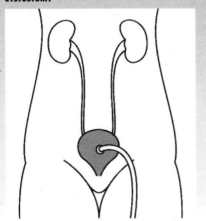

**NEPHROSTOMY**

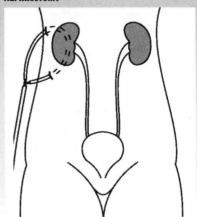

# Nephrostomy and cystostomy tube care

Two urinary diversion techniques—nephrostomy and cystostomy—ensure adequate drainage from the kidneys or bladder and help prevent urinary tract infection or kidney failure. (See *Urinary diversion techniques.*)

A nephrostomy tube drains urine directly from a kidney when a disorder inhibits the normal flow of urine. The tube is usually placed percutaneously, though sometimes it's surgically inserted through the renal cortex and medulla into the renal pelvis from a lateral incision in the flank. The usual indication is obstructive disease, such as calculi in the ureter or ureteropelvic junction, or an obstructing tumor. Draining urine with a nephrostomy tube also allows kidney tissue damaged by obstructive disease to heal.

A cystostomy tube drains urine from the bladder, diverting it from the urethra. This type of tube is used after certain gynecolog-

ic procedures, bladder surgery, prostatectomy, and for severe urethral strictures or traumatic injury. Inserted about 2″ (5 cm) above the symphysis pubis, a cystostomy tube may be used alone or with an indwelling urethral catheter.

## Equipment

Commercially prepared sterile dressing kits may be available.

*For dressing changes*
Povidone-iodine solution or povidone-iodine pads ● 4″ × 4″ gauze pads ● sterile cup or emesis basin ● paper bag ● linen-saver pad ● clean gloves (for dressing removal) ● sterile gloves (for new dressing) ● precut 4″ × 4″ drain dressings or transparent semipermeable dressings ● adhesive tape (preferably hypoallergenic)

*For nephrostomy-tube irrigation*
3-ml syringe ● alcohol pad or povidone-iodine pad ● normal saline solution ● optional: hemostat

# Taping a nephrostomy tube

To tape a nephrostomy tube directly to the skin, cut a wide piece of hypoallergenic adhesive tape twice lengthwise to its midpoint.

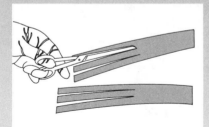

Apply the uncut end of the tape to the skin so that the midpoint meets the tube. Wrap the middle strip around the tube in a spiral fashion. Tape the other two strips to the patient's skin on both sides of the tube.

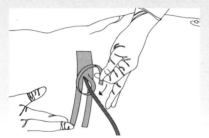

For greater security, repeat this step with a second piece of tape, applying it in the reverse direction. You may also apply two more strips of tape perpendicular to and over the first two pieces.

Always apply another strip of tape lower down on the tube in the direction of the drainage tube to further anchor the tube. Don't put tension on sutures that prevent tube distention.

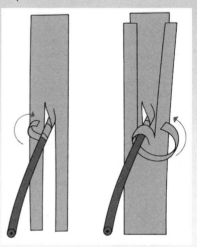

## Preparation of equipment

Wash your hands and assemble all equipment at the patient's bedside. Open several packages of gauze pads, place them in the sterile cup or emesis basin, and pour the povidone-iodine solution over them. Or, if available, open several packages of povidone-iodine pads. If you're using a commercially packaged dressing kit, open it using aseptic technique. Fill the cup with antiseptic solution.

Open the paper bag and place it away from the other equipment to avoid contaminating the sterile field.

## Implementation

▶ Wash your hands, provide privacy, and explain the procedure to the patient.

## Changing a dressing

▶ Help the patient to lie on his back (for a cystostomy tube) or on the side opposite the tube (for a nephrostomy tube) so that you can see the tube clearly and change the dressing more easily.

▶ Place the linen-saver pad under the patient to absorb excess drainage and keep him dry.

▶ Put on the clean gloves. Carefully remove the tape around the tube and then remove the wet or soiled dressing. Discard the tape and dressing in the paper bag. Remove the gloves and discard them in the bag.

▶ Put on the sterile gloves. Pick up a saturated pad or dip a dry one into the cup of antiseptic solution.

▶ To clean the wound, wipe only once with each pad, moving from the insertion site outward. Discard the used pad in the paper bag. Don't touch the bag to avoid contaminating your gloves.

▶ Pick up a sterile 4″ × 4″ drain dressing and place it around the tube. If necessary, overlap two drain dressings to provide maximum absorption. Or, depending on your facility's policy, apply a transparent semipermeable dressing over the site and tubing to allow observation of the site without removing the dressing.

▶ Secure the dressing with hypoallergenic tape. Then tape the tube to the patient's lateral abdomen to prevent tension on the tube. (See *Taping a nephrostomy tube.*)

▶ Dispose of all equipment appropriately. Clean the patient as necessary.

### Irrigating a nephrostomy tube

▶ Fill the 3-ml syringe with the normal saline solution.

▶ Clean the junction of the nephrostomy tube and drainage tube with the alcohol pad or povidone-iodine pad and disconnect the tubes.

▶ Insert the syringe into the nephrostomy tube opening and instill 2 to 3 ml of saline solution into the tube.

▶ Slowly aspirate the solution back into the syringe. To avoid damaging the renal pelvis tissue, never pull back forcefully on the plunger.

▶ If the solution doesn't return, remove the syringe from the tube and reattach it to the drainage tubing to allow the solution to drain by gravity.

▶ Dispose of all equipment appropriately.

## Special considerations

▶ Change dressings once a day or more often, if needed.

◆ **ALERT!** Never irrigate a nephrostomy tube with more than 5 ml of solution because the capacity of the renal pelvis is usually between 4 and 8 ml. (Remember: The purpose of irrigation is to keep the tube patent, not to lavage the renal pelvis.)

▶ When necessary, irrigate a cystostomy tube as you would an indwelling urinary catheter. Perform the irrigation gently to avoid damaging any suture lines.

▶ Check a nephrostomy tube frequently for kinks or obstructions. Kinks are likely to occur if the patient lies on the insertion site. Suspect an obstruction when the amount of urine in the drainage bag decreases or the amount of urine around the

insertion site increases. Pressure created by urine backing up in the tube can damage nephrons. Gently curve a cystostomy tube to prevent kinks.

▶ If a blood clot or mucus plug obstructs a nephrostomy or cystostomy tube, try milking the tube to restore its patency. With your nondominant hand, hold the tube securely above the obstruction to avoid pulling the tube out of the incision. Then place the flat side of a closed hemostat under the tube, just above the obstruction, pinch the tube against the hemostat, and slide both your finger and the hemostat toward you, away from the patient.

▶ Typically, cystostomy tubes for postoperative urologic patients should be checked hourly for 24 hours to ensure adequate drainage and tube patency. To check tube patency, note the amount of urine in the drainage bag and check the patient's bladder for distention.

▶ Keep the drainage bag below the level of the kidney at all times to prevent reflux of urine.

▶ If the tube becomes dislodged, cover the site with a sterile dressing and notify the doctor immediately.

▶ The doctor may order the nephrostomy tube clamped before removal to determine readiness for removal. While the tube is clamped, assess the patient for flank pain and fever and monitor urine output.

## Home care

Tell the home care patient to clean the insertion site with soap and water, check for skin breakdown, and change the dressing daily; then show him how to take these steps. Also, teach him how to change the leg bag or drainage bag. He can use a leg bag during the day and a larger drainage bag at night. Whether he uses a drainage bag or larger container, tell him to wash it daily with a 1:3 vinegar and water solution, rinse it with plain water, and dry it on a clothes hanger or over the towel rack. This prevents crystalline buildup.

Stress the importance of reporting to the doctor signs of infection (red skin or white, yellow, or green drainage at the insertion site) or tube displacement (drainage that smells like urine).

## Complications

The patient has an increased risk of infection because nephrostomy and cystostomy tubes provide a direct opening to the kidneys and bladder.

## Documentation

▶ Describe the color and amount of drainage from the nephrostomy or cystostomy tube and record any color changes as they occur.

▶ Similarly, if the patient has more than one tube, describe the drainage (color, amount, and character) from each tube separately.

▶ If irrigation is necessary, record the amount and type of irrigant used and whether or not you obtained a complete return.

### REFERENCES

Park, D.S., et al. "Percutaneous Nephrostomy Versus Indwelling Ureteral Stents in Patients with Bilateral Nongenitourinary Malignant Extrinsic Obstruction," *Journal of Endourology* 16(3):153-54, April 2002.

Singh, I., et al. "Efficacy and Outcome of Surgical Intervention in Patients with Nephrolithiasis and Chronic Renal Failure," *International Urology and Nephrology* 33(2):293-98, 2001.

# Pediatric urine collection

Collection of a urine specimen for laboratory analysis allows screening for urinary tract infection and renal disorders, evaluation of treatment, and detection of systemic and metabolic disorders.

Although a child without bladder control can't provide a clean-catch midstream urine specimen, the pediatric urine collection bag provides a simple, effective alternative. It offers minimal risk of specimen contamination without resorting to catheterization or suprapubic aspiration. Because the collection bag is secured with adhesive flaps, its use is contraindicated in a patient with extremely sensitive or excoriated perineal skin. Alternative methods of collecting urine from small children include the use of an inside-out disposable diaper.

## Equipment

*For a random specimen*
Pediatric urine collection bag (individually packaged) ● urine specimen container ● label ● laboratory request form ● two disposable diapers of appropriate size ● scissors ● gloves ● washcloth ● soap ● water ● towel ● bowl ● linen-saver pad

*For a culture and sensitivity specimen*
Sterile pediatric urine collection bag ● sterile urine specimen container ● label ● laboratory request form ● two disposable diapers of appropriate size ● scissors ● gloves ● sterile bowl ● sterile or distilled water ● sterile 4″ × 4″ gauze pads ● antiseptic skin cleaner ● alcohol pad ● 3-ml syringe with needle ● linen-saver pad

*For a timed specimen*
24-hour pediatric urine collection bag (individually packaged) with evacuation tubing ● 24-hour urine specimen container ● label ● laboratory request form ● scissors ● two disposable diapers of appropriate size ● gloves ● washcloth ● soap ● water ● bowl ● towel ● sterile 4″ × 4″ gauze pads ● compound benzoin tincture ● small medicine cup ● 35-ml luer-lock syringe or urometer ● tubing stopper ● specimen preservative (such as formaldehyde solution) ● linen-saver pad

Kits containing sterile supplies for clean-catch collections are commercially available and may be used to obtain a culture and sensitivity specimen.

## Preparation of equipment

Check the doctor's order for the type of specimen needed and assemble the appropriate equipment. Check the patient's chart for allergies (for example, to iodine or latex). Complete the laboratory request form to avoid delay in sending the specimen to the laboratory. Wash your hands.

With scissors, make a 2″ (5.1-cm) slit in one diaper, cutting from the center point toward one of the shorter edges. Later, you'll pull the urine collection bag through this slit when you position the bag and diaper on the patient. Pour water into the bowl; use sterile water and a sterile bowl if you need to collect a specimen for culture and sensitivity.

If you need a culture and sensitivity specimen, check the expiration date on each sterile package and inspect for tears. Put on new gloves and open several packages of sterile 4″ × 4″ gauze pads.

If you need a timed specimen and will use benzoin in liquid form, pour it into the medicine cup. Cut the tubing on the urine collection bag so that only 6″ (15.2 cm) remain attached. Discard the excess. Place the stopper in the severed end of the tubing. If you're going to use a urinometer for the patient who voids large amounts, don't cut the tubing; simply attach the device.

## Implementation
▶ Explain the procedure to the patient, if he's old enough, and his parents. Provide privacy, especially if the patient is beyond infancy.

### Collecting a random specimen
▶ Wash your hands.
▶ Place the patient on a linen-saver pad.
▶ Clean the perineal area with soap, water, and a washcloth, working from the urinary meatus outward to prevent contamination of the urine specimen. Wipe gently to prevent tissue trauma and stimulation of urination. Separate the labia of the female patient or retract the foreskin of the uncircumcised male patient to expose the urinary meatus. Thoroughly rinse the area with clear water and dry with a towel. Don't use powders, lotions, or cream because these counteract the adhesive.
▶ Place the patient in the frog position, with his legs separated and knees flexed. If necessary, have the patient's parent hold him while you apply the collection bag.
▶ Remove the protective coverings from the collection bag's adhesive flaps. For the female patient, first separate the labia and gently press the bag's lower rim to the perineum. Then, working upward toward the pubis, attach the rest of the adhesive rim inside the labia majora. For the male patient, place the bag over the penis and scrotum and press the adhesive rim to the skin.
▶ Once the bag is attached, gently pull it through the slit in the diaper to prevent compression of the bag by the diaper and to allow observation of the specimen immediately after the patient voids. Fasten the diaper on the patient.
▶ When urine appears in the bag, put on gloves and gently remove the diaper and the bag. Hold the bag's bottom port over the collection container, remove the tab from the port, and let the urine flow into the container.
▶ Measure the output if necessary.
▶ Label the specimen and attach the laboratory request form to the container. Send it directly to the laboratory. Remove and discard gloves.
▶ Put the second diaper on the patient and make sure he's comfortable.

### Collecting a culture and sensitivity specimen
Follow the procedure for collecting a random specimen, with these modifications:
▶ Use sterile or distilled water, an antiseptic skin cleaner, and sterile 4″ × 4″ gauze pads to clean the perineal area.
▶ After putting on gloves, clean the urinary meatus; then work outward. Wipe only once with each gauze pad; then discard it.
▶ After the patient urinates, remove the bag and use an alcohol pad to clean a small area of the bag's surface. Puncture the clean area with the needle, and aspirate urine into the syringe.
▶ Inject the urine into the sterile specimen container. Be careful to keep the needle from touching the container's sides to maintain sterility. Remember, a large volume of urine is unnecessary because only about 1 ml of urine is needed to perform this test. Remove and discard your gloves.

### Collecting a timed specimen
▶ Check the doctor's order for the duration of the collection and the indication for the procedure. Prepare the patient, put on gloves, and clean the perineum as for random specimen collection.
▶ If getting the bag to adhere is difficult, apply compound benzoin tincture to the perineal area, if ordered, so that the collection bag will adhere better and you won't have to reapply it during the collection period. If using liquid benzoin, dip a gauze pad into the medicine cup containing it. If using benzoin spray, cover the genitalia with a gauze pad before spraying to prevent tissue trauma.
▶ Allow the benzoin to dry. Then apply the collection bag, pull the bottom of the bag and the tubing through the slit in the diaper and fasten the diaper. Remove and discard your gloves.
▶ Check the collection bag and tubing every 30 minutes to ensure a proper seal because any leakage prevents collection of a complete specimen.
▶ When urine appears in the bag, put on gloves and remove the stopper in the bag's tubing. Then attach the syringe to the end of the tubing and aspirate the urine. Re-

move the syringe and insert the stopper into the tubing.

▶ Discard the specimen and begin timing the collection.

▶ When the next urine specimen is obtained, add the preservative to the 24-hour specimen container along with the specimen and refrigerate it, if ordered, to keep the sample stable.

▶ Periodically empty the collection bag to prevent dislodgment of the collection bag. Each time you remove urine, add it to the specimen container; then use the syringe to inject a small amount of air into the collection bag to prevent a vacuum, which can block urine drainage.

▶ When the prescribed collection period has elapsed (or as nearly as possible), stop the collection and send the total accumulated specimen to the laboratory.

▶ Put on gloves and wash the perineal area thoroughly with soap and water to remove the benzoin; then put the second diaper on the patient.

### Special considerations
▶ Whatever the collection method used, avoid forcing fluids to prevent dilution of the specimen, which can alter test results. For a random collection or a culture and sensitivity collection, obtain a first-voided morning specimen, if possible.

▶ If the collection bag becomes dislodged during timed collection, immediately reapply benzoin and attach another collection bag to prevent loss of the specimen and the need to restart the collection.

### Complications
Adhesive from the rim of the collection bag can cause skin excoriation.

### Documentation
▶ Record the date, time, and method of collection.

▶ Record the name of the test, the amount of urine collected (if necessary), and the time of specimen transport to the laboratory.

▶ Document any use of restraints, any complications, and the patient's tolerance of the procedure.

▶ Note the patient's and family's responses to any teaching.

**REFERENCES**
Assadi, F.K. "Quantitation of Microalbuminuria Using Random Urine Samples,"*Pediatric Nephrology* 17(2):107-10, February 2002.
Liao, J.C., and Churchill, B.M. "Pediatric Urine Testing," *Pediatric Clinics of North America* 48(6):1425-40; vii-viii, December 2001.

# Peritoneal dialysis

Peritoneal dialysis is indicated for patients with chronic renal failure who have cardiovascular instability, vascular access problems that prevent hemodialysis, fluid overload, or electrolyte imbalances. In this procedure, dialysate—the solution instilled into the peritoneal cavity by a catheter—draws waste products, excess fluid, and electrolytes from the blood across the semipermeable peritoneal membrane. (See *Principles of peritoneal dialysis.*)

After a prescribed period, the dialysate is drained from the peritoneal cavity, removing impurities with it. The dialysis procedure is then repeated, using a new dialysate each time, until waste removal is complete and fluid, electrolyte, and acid-base balance has been restored.

The catheter is inserted in the operating room or at the patient's bedside with a nurse assisting. With special preparation, the nurse may perform dialysis, either manually or using an automatic or semiautomatic cycle machine.

### Equipment
All equipment must be sterile. Commercially packaged dialysis kits or trays are available.

*For catheter placement and dialysis*
Prescribed dialysate (in 1- or 2-L bottles or bags, as ordered) ● warmer, heating pad, or water bath ● at least three face masks ● medication, such as heparin, if ordered ● dialysis administration set with drainage bag ● two pairs of sterile gloves ● I.V. pole ● fenestrated sterile drape ● vial of 1% or 2% lidocaine ● povidone-iodine pads ● 3-ml syringe with 25G 1″ needle ● ordered type of multi-eyed, nylon, peritoneal catheter (see *Comparing peritoneal dialysis catheters,* pages 512 and 513) ● scalpel

# Principles of peritoneal dialysis

Peritoneal dialysis works through a combination of diffusion and osmosis.

### Diffusion

In diffusion, particles move through a semipermeable membrane from an area of high-solute concentration to an area of low-solute concentration.

In peritoneal dialysis, the water-based dialysate being infused contains glucose, sodium chloride, calcium, magnesium, acetate or lactate, and no waste products. Therefore, the waste products and excess electrolytes in the blood cross through the semipermeable peritoneal membrane into the dialysate. Removing the waste-filled dialysate and replacing it with fresh solution keeps the waste concentration low and encourages further diffusion.

### Osmosis

In osmosis, fluids move through a semipermeable membrane from an area of low-solute concentration to an area of high-solute concentration. In peritoneal dialysis, dextrose is added to the dialysate to give it a higher solute concentration than the blood, creating a high osmotic gradient. Water migrates from the blood through the membrane at the beginning of each infusion, when the osmotic gradient is highest.

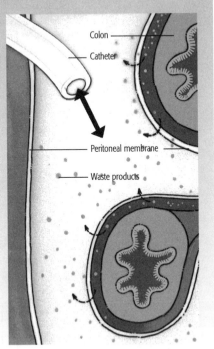

(with #11 blade) • peritoneal stylet • sutures or hypoallergenic tape • povidone-iodine solution (to prepare abdomen) • precut drain dressings • protective cap for catheter • 4″ × 4″ gauze pads • small, sterile plastic clamp • optional: 10-ml syringe with 22G 1½″ needle, protein or potassium supplement, specimen container, label, and laboratory request form

*For dressing changes*
One pair of sterile gloves • 10 sterile cotton-tipped applicators or sterile 2″ × 2″ gauze pads • povidone-iodine ointment • two precut drain dressings • adhesive tape • povidone-iodine solution or normal saline solution • two sterile 4″ × 4″ gauze pads

### Preparation of equipment

Bring all equipment to the patient's bedside. Make sure the dialysate is at body temperature. This decreases patient discomfort during the procedure and reduces vasoconstriction of the peritoneal capillaries. Dilated capillaries enhance blood flow to the peritoneal membrane surface, increasing waste clearance into the peritoneal cavity. Place the container in a warmer or a water bath, or wrap it in a heating pad set at 98.6° F (37° C) for 30 to 60 minutes to warm the solution.

### Implementation

▶ Explain the procedure to the patient. Assess and record vital signs, weight, and abdominal girth to establish baseline levels.
▶ Review recent laboratory values (blood urea nitrogen, serum creatinine, sodium, potassium, and complete blood count).
▶ Identify the patient's hepatitis B virus and human immunodeficiency virus status, if known.

# Comparing peritoneal dialysis catheters

The first step in any type of peritoneal dialysis is insertion of a catheter to allow instillation of dialyzing solution. The surgeon may insert one of the three different catheters described here.

### Tenckhoff catheter

To implant a Tenckhoff catheter, the surgeon inserts the first 6" (17 cm) of the catheter into the patient's abdomen. The next 2¾" (7 cm) segment, which may have a Dacron cuff at one or both ends, is imbedded subcutaneously. Within a few days after insertion, the patient's tissues grow around the cuffs, forming a tight barrier against bacterial infiltration. The remaining 3⅞" (10 cm) of the catheter extends outside of the abdomen and is equipped with a metal adapter at the tip that connects to dialyzer tubing.

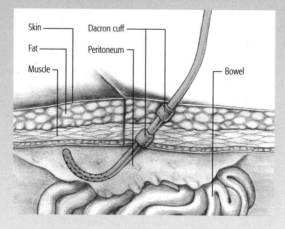

### Flanged-collar catheter

To insert this kind of catheter, the surgeon positions its flanged collar just below the dermis so that the device extends through the abdominal wall. He keeps the distal end of the cuff from extending into the peritoneum, where it could cause adhesions.

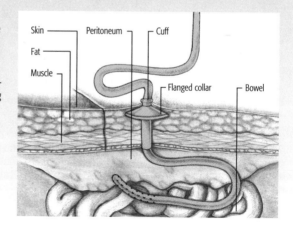

## Catheter placement and dialysis

▶ Have the patient try to urinate. This reduces the risk of bladder perforation during insertion of the peritoneal catheter. If he can't urinate and you suspect that his bladder isn't empty, obtain an order for straight catheterization to empty his bladder.

▶ Place the patient in the supine position, and have him put on one of the sterile face masks.

▶ Wash your hands.

▶ Inspect the warmed dialysate, which should appear clear and colorless.

▶ Put on a sterile face mask. Prepare to add any prescribed medication to the dialysate, using strict sterile technique to avoid contaminating the solution. Medications should be added immediately before the solution will be hung and used. Disinfect multiple-dose vials by soaking them in povidone-iodine solution for 5 minutes. Heparin is typically added to the dialysate

# Comparing peritoneal dialysis catheters *(continued)*

### Column-disk peritoneal catheter

To insert a column-disk peritoneal catheter (CDPC), the surgeon rolls up the flexible disk section of the implant, inserts it into the peritoneal cavity, and retracts it against the abdominal wall. The implant's first cuff rests just outside the peritoneal membrane, while its second cuff rests just underneath the skin. Because the CDPC doesn't float freely in the peritoneal cavity, it keeps inflowing dialyzing solution from being directed at the sensitive organs, which increases patient comfort during dialysis.

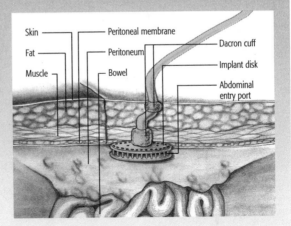

to prevent accumulation of fibrin in the catheter.

▶ Prepare the dialysis administration set. (See *Setup for peritoneal dialysis,* page 514.)

▶ Close the clamps on all lines. Place the drainage bag below the patient to facilitate gravity drainage, and connect the drainage line to it. Connect the dialysate infusion lines to the bottles or bags of dialysate. Hang the bottles or bags on the I.V. pole at the patient's bedside. To prime the tubing, open the infusion lines and allow the solution to flow until all lines are primed. Then close all clamps.

▶ At this point, the doctor puts on a mask and a pair of sterile gloves. He cleans the patient's abdomen with povidone-iodine solution and drapes it with a sterile drape.

▶ Wipe the stopper of the lidocaine vial with povidone-iodine and allow it to dry. Invert the vial and hand it to the doctor so he can withdraw the lidocaine, using the 3-ml syringe with the 25G 1″ needle.

▶ The doctor anesthetizes a small area of the patient's abdomen below the umbilicus. He then makes a small incision with the scalpel, inserts the catheter into the peritoneal cavity, using the stylet to guide

the catheter, and sutures or tapes the catheter in place.

▶ If the catheter is already in place, clean the site with povidone-iodine solution in a circular outward motion, according to your facility's policy, before each dialysis treatment.

▶ Connect the catheter to the administration set, using strict aseptic technique to prevent contamination of the catheter and the solution, which could cause peritonitis.

▶ Open the drain dressing and the 4″ × 4″ gauze pad packages. Put on the other pair of sterile gloves. Apply the precut drain dressings around the catheter. Cover them with the gauze pads and tape them securely.

▶ Unclamp the lines to the patient. Rapidly instill 500 ml of dialysate into the peritoneal cavity to test the catheter's patency.

▶ Clamp the lines to the patient. Immediately unclamp the lines to the drainage bag to allow fluid to drain into the bag. Outflow should be brisk.

▶ Having established the catheter's patency, clamp the lines to the drainage bag and unclamp the lines to the patient to infuse the prescribed volume of solution over a period of 5 to 10 minutes. As soon as the dialysate container empties, clamp the

# Setup for peritoneal dialysis

The illustration below shows the proper setup for peritoneal dialysis.

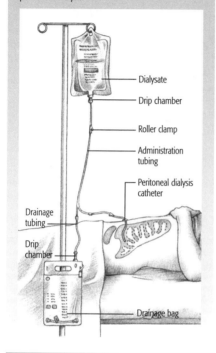

- Dialysate
- Drip chamber
- Roller clamp
- Administration tubing
- Peritoneal dialysis catheter
- Drainage tubing
- Drip chamber
- Drainage bag

---

lines to the patient immediately to prevent air from entering the tubing.

▶ Allow the solution to dwell in the peritoneal cavity for the prescribed time (10 minutes to 4 hours). This lets excess fluid, electrolytes, and accumulated wastes move from the blood through the peritoneal membrane and into the dialysate.

▶ Warm the solution for the next infusion.

▶ At the end of the prescribed dwell time, unclamp the line to the drainage bag and allow the solution to drain from the peritoneal cavity into the drainage bag (normally 20 to 30 minutes).

▶ Repeat the infusion-dwell-drain cycle immediately after outflow until the prescribed number of fluid exchanges have been completed.

▶ If the doctor or your facility's policy requires a dialysate specimen, you'll usually collect one after every 10 infusion-dwell-

drain cycles (*always* during the drain phase), after every 24-hour period, or as ordered. To do this, attach the 10-ml syringe to the 22G 1½" needle. Clean the injection port with iodine or Betadine solution. Then, insert the needle into the injection port on the drainage line, using strict sterile technique, and aspirate the drainage sample. Transfer the sample to the specimen container, label it appropriately, and send it to the laboratory with a laboratory request form.

▶ After completing the prescribed number of exchanges, clamp the catheter and put on sterile gloves. Disconnect the administration set from the peritoneal catheter. Place the sterile protective cap over the catheter's distal end.

▶ Dispose of all used equipment appropriately.

## Dressing changes

▶ Explain the procedure to the patient and wash your hands.

▶ If necessary, carefully remove the old dressings to avoid putting tension on the catheter and accidentally dislodging it and to avoid introducing bacteria into the tract through movement of the catheter.

▶ Put on the sterile gloves.

▶ Saturate the sterile applicators or the 2" × 2" gauze pads with povidone-iodine or normal saline solution, and clean the skin around the catheter, moving in concentric circles from the catheter site outward. Remove any crusted material carefully.

▶ Inspect the catheter site for drainage and the tissue around the site for redness and swelling.

▶ Apply povidone-iodine ointment to the catheter site with a sterile gauze pad.

▶ Place two precut drain dressings around the catheter site. Tape the 4" × 4" gauze pads over them to secure the dressings.

## Special considerations

▶ During and after dialysis, monitor the patient and his response to treatment. Peritoneal dialysis is usually contraindicated in patients who have had extensive abdominal or bowel surgery or extensive abdominal trauma or who have severe vascular disease, obesity, or respiratory distress.

▶ Monitor the patient's vital signs every 10 to 15 minutes for the first 1 to 2 hours of exchanges, then every 2 to 4 hours, or more frequently if necessary. Notify the doctor of any abrupt changes in the patient's condition.

▶ To reduce the risk of peritonitis, use strict sterile technique during catheter insertion, dialysis, and dressing changes. Masks should be worn by all personnel in the room whenever the dialysis system is opened or entered. Change the dressing at least every 24 hours or whenever it becomes wet or soiled. Frequent dressing changes will also help prevent skin excoriation from any leakage.

▶ To prevent respiratory distress, position the patient for maximal lung expansion. Promote lung expansion through turning and deep-breathing exercises.

◆ **ALERT!** If the patient suffers severe respiratory distress during the dwell phase of dialysis, drain the peritoneal cavity and notify the doctor. Monitor any patient on peritoneal dialysis who is being weaned from a ventilator.

▶ To prevent protein depletion, the doctor may order a high-protein diet or a protein supplement. He will also monitor serum albumin levels.

▶ Dialysate is available in three concentrations: 4.25% dextrose, 2.5% dextrose, and 1.5% dextrose. The 4.25% solution usually removes the largest amount of fluid from the blood because its glucose concentration is highest. If your patient receives this concentrated solution, monitor him carefully to prevent excess fluid loss. Also, some of the glucose in the 4.25% solution may enter the patient's bloodstream, causing hyperglycemia severe enough to require an insulin injection or an insulin addition to the dialysate.

▶ Patients with low serum potassium levels may require the addition of potassium to the dialysate solution to prevent further losses.

▶ Monitor fluid volume balance, blood pressure, and pulse to help prevent fluid imbalance. Assess fluid balance at the end of each infusion-dwell-drain cycle. Fluid balance is positive if less than the amount infused was recovered; it's negative if more than the amount infused was recovered. Notify the doctor if the patient retains 500 ml or more of fluid for three consecutive cycles or if he loses at least 1 L of fluid for three consecutive cycles.

▶ Weigh the patient daily to help determine how much fluid is being removed

during dialysis treatment. Note the time and any variations in the weighing technique next to his weight on his chart.

▶ If inflow and outflow are slow or absent, check the tubing for kinks. You can also try raising the I.V. pole or repositioning the patient to increase the inflow rate. Repositioning the patient or applying manual pressure to the lateral aspects of the patient's abdomen may also help increase drainage. If these maneuvers fail, notify the doctor. Improper positioning of the catheter or an accumulation of fibrin may obstruct the catheter.

▶ Always examine outflow fluid (effluent) for color and clarity. Normally it's clear or pale yellow, but pink-tinged effluent may appear during the first three or four cycles. If the effluent remains pink-tinged, or if it's grossly bloody, suspect bleeding into the peritoneal cavity and notify the doctor. Also notify the doctor if the outflow contains feces, which suggests bowel perforation, or if it's cloudy, which suggests peritonitis. Obtain a sample for culture and Gram stain. Send the sample in a labeled specimen container to the laboratory with a laboratory request form.

▶ Patient discomfort at the start of the procedure is normal. If the patient experiences pain during the procedure, determine when it occurs, its quality and duration, and whether it radiates to other body parts. Then notify the doctor. Pain during infusion usually results from a dialysate that is too cool or acidic. Pain may also result from rapid inflow; slowing the inflow rate may reduce the pain. Severe, diffuse pain with rebound tenderness and cloudy effluent may indicate peritoneal infection. Pain that radiates to the shoulder often results from air accumulation under the diaphragm. Severe, persistent perineal or rectal pain can result from improper catheter placement.

▶ The patient undergoing peritoneal dialysis will require a great deal of assistance in his daily care. To minimize his discomfort, perform daily care during a drain phase in the cycle, when the patient's abdomen is less distended.

## Complications

Peritonitis, the most common complication, usually follows contamination of the dialysate, but it may develop if solution leaks from the catheter exit site and flows back into the catheter tract. Respiratory distress may result when dialysate in the peritoneal cavity increases pressure on the diaphragm, which decreases lung expansion.

Protein depletion may result from the diffusion of protein in the blood into the dialysate solution through the peritoneal membrane. As much as ½ oz (14 g) of protein may be lost daily—more in patients with peritonitis.

Constipation is a major cause of inflow-outflow problems; therefore, to ensure regular bowel movements, give a laxative or stool softener as needed.

Excessive fluid loss from the use of 4.25% solution may cause hypovolemia, hypotension, and shock. Excessive fluid retention may lead to blood volume expansion, hypertension, peripheral edema, and even pulmonary edema and heart failure.

Other possible complications include electrolyte imbalance and hyperglycemia, which can be identified by frequent blood tests.

## Documentation

▶ Record the amount of dialysate infused and drained, any medications added to the solution, and the color and character of effluent.
▶ Record the patient's daily weight and fluid balance. Use a peritoneal dialysis flowchart to compute total fluid balance after each exchange.
▶ Note the patient's vital signs and tolerance of the treatment as well as other pertinent observations.

### REFERENCES

National Institute of Diabetes and Digestive and Kidney Diseases. Peritoneal Dialysis Dose and Adequacy. (NIH Publication No. 01-4578). National Kidney and Urologic Diseases Information Clearinghouse, April 2001. *www.niddk.nih.gov/health/kidney/pubs/kidney-failure/peritoneal-dose/peritoneal-dose.htm*
National Kidney Foundation "K-DOQI Clinical Practice Guidelines for Peritoneal Dialysis Adequacy 2000," *American Journal of Kidney Disease* 37(Suppl. 1):S65-S136, 2001.
Pfettscher, S.A. "Chronic Renal Failure and Renal Transplant," in *Critical Care Nursing.* Edited by Bucher, L., and Melander, S. Philadelphia: W.B. Saunders Co., 1999.

# Self-catheterization

A patient with impaired or absent bladder function may catheterize himself for routine bladder drainage. Self-catheterization requires thorough and careful teaching by the nurse. The patient will probably use clean technique for self-catheterization at home, but he must use sterile technique in the facility because of the increased risk of infection.

■ **EVIDENCE BASE** Clean intermittent catheterization is safer than use of an indwelling catheter in terms of preventing urinary tract infections, and is a recommended alternative by the Centers for Disease Control and Prevention for the patient requiring urinary catheterization.

## Equipment

Rubber catheter ● washcloth ● soap and water ● small packet of water-soluble lubricant ● plastic storage bag ● optional: drainage container, paper towels, cornstarch, rubber or plastic sheets, gooseneck lamp, catheterization record, and mirror

### Preparation of equipment

Instruct the patient to keep a supply of catheters at home and to use each catheter only once before cleaning it. Advise him to wash the used catheter in warm, soapy water, rinse it inside and out, and then dry it with a clean towel and store it in a plastic bag until the next time it's needed. Because catheters become brittle with repeated use, tell the patient to check them often and to order a new supply well in advance.

## Implementation

▶ Tell the patient to begin by trying to urinate into the toilet or, if a toilet isn't available or he needs to measure urine quantity, into a drainage container. Then he should wash his hands thoroughly with soap and water and dry them.
▶ Demonstrate how the patient should perform the catheterization, explaining each step clearly and carefully. Position a gooseneck lamp nearby if room lighting is inadequate to make the urinary meatus clearly visible. Arrange the patient's clothing so that it's out of the way.

### Teaching a woman

▶ Demonstrate and explain to the female patient that she should separate the vaginal folds as widely as possible with the fingers of her nondominant hand to obtain a full view of the urinary meatus. She may need to use a mirror to visualize the meatus. Ask if she's right- or left-handed and then tell her which is her nondominant hand. While holding her labia open with the nondominant hand, she should use the dominant hand to wash the perineal area thoroughly with a soapy washcloth, using downward strokes. Tell her to rinse the area with the washcloth, using downward strokes as well.

▶ Show her how to squeeze some lubricant onto the first 3″ (7.6 cm) of the catheter and then how to insert the catheter. (See *Teaching self-catheterization.*)

▶ When the urine stops draining, tell her to remove the catheter slowly, get dressed, and wash the catheter with warm, soapy water. Then she should rinse it inside and out and dry it with a paper towel.

### Teaching a man

▶ Tell a male patient to wash and rinse the end of his penis thoroughly with soap and water, pulling back the foreskin, if appropriate. He should keep the foreskin pulled back during the procedure.

▶ Show him how to squeeze lubricant onto a paper towel and have him roll the first 7″ to 10″ (18 to 25.5 cm) of the catheter in the lubricant. Tell him that copious lubricant will make the procedure more comfortable for him. Then show him how to insert the catheter.

▶ When the urine stops draining, tell him to remove the catheter slowly and, if necessary, pull the foreskin forward again. Have him get dressed and have him wash and dry the catheter as described above.

### Special considerations

▶ Impress upon the patient that the timing of catheterization is critical to prevent overdistention of the bladder, which can lead to infection. Self-catheterization is usually performed every 4 to 6 hours around the clock (or more often at first).

▶ Female patients should be able to identify the body parts involved in self-catheterization, such as the labia majora, labia minora, vagina, and urinary meatus.

## Teaching self-catheterization

Teach a woman to hold the catheter in her dominant hand as if it were a pencil or a dart, about ½″ (1.5 cm) from its tip. Keeping the vaginal folds separated, she should slowly insert the lubricated catheter about 3″ (7.5 cm) into the urethra. Tell her to press down with her abdominal muscles to empty the bladder, allowing all urine to drain through the catheter and into the toilet or drainage container.

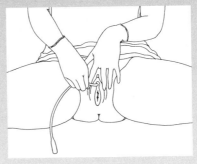

Teach a man to hold his penis in his nondominant hand, at a right angle to his body. He should hold the catheter in his dominant hand as if it were a pencil or a dart and slowly insert it 7″ to 10″ (18 to 25.5 cm) into the urethra until urine begins flowing. Then he should gently advance the catheter about 1″ (2.5 cm) farther, allowing all urine to drain into the toilet or drainage container.

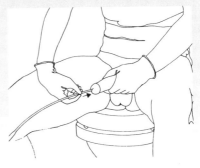

▶ Keep in mind the difference between boiling and sterilization. Boiling kills bacteria, viruses, and fungi but doesn't kill spores, whereas sterilization does. However, for catheter cleaning done in the patient's home, boiling is a sufficient safeguard against spreading infections.

▶ Advise the patient to hold off storing the cleaned catheters in a plastic bag until after they're completely dry to prevent growth of gram-negative organisms.

▶ Stress the importance of regulating fluid intake as ordered to prevent incontinence while maintaining adequate hydration. However, explain that incontinent episodes may occur occasionally. For managing incontinence, the doctor or a home health care nurse can help develop a plan such as more frequent catheterizations. After an incontinent episode, tell the patient to wash with soap and water, pat himself dry with a towel, and expose the skin to the air for as long as possible. He can reduce urine odor by putting methylbenzethonium (Diaparene) or cornstarch on his skin. Bedding and furniture can be protected by covering them with rubber or plastic sheets and then covering the rubber or plastic with fabric.

▶ Also, stress the importance of taking medications, as ordered, to increase urine retention and help prevent incontinence. Advise the patient to avoid calcium-rich and phosphorus-rich foods, as ordered, to reduce the chance of renal calculus formation.

### Complications

Overdistention of the bladder can lead to urinary tract infection and urine leakage. Improper hand washing or equipment cleaning can also cause urinary tract infection. Incorrect catheter insertion can injure the urethral or bladder mucosa.

### Documentation

▶ Record the date and times of catheterization, character of the urine (such as color, odor, clarity, and presence of particles or blood), the amount of urine (such as increase, decrease, or no change), and any problems encountered during the procedure.

▶ Note whether the patient has difficulty performing a return demonstration.

### REFERENCES

Joanna Briggs Institute. "Management of Short-Term Indwelling Urethral Catheters to Prevent Urinary Tract Infections," *Best Practice* 4(1), 2000.
*www.joannabriggs.edu.au/bpmenu.html*

Potter, P.A., and Perry, A.G. *Fundamentals of Nursing,* 5th ed. St. Louis: Mosby–Year Book, Inc., 2001.

# Timed urine collection

Because hormones, proteins, and electrolytes are excreted in small, variable amounts in urine, specimens for measuring these substances must typically be collected over an extended period to yield quantities of diagnostic value.

A 24-hour specimen is used most commonly because it provides an average excretion rate for substances eliminated during this period. Timed specimens may also be collected for shorter periods, such as 2 or 12 hours, depending on the specific information needed.

A timed urine specimen may also be collected after administering a challenge dose of a chemical—insulin, for example—to detect various renal disorders.

### Equipment

Large collection container with a cap or stopper or a commercial plastic container ● preservative, if necessary ● gloves ● bedpan or urinal if patient doesn't have an indwelling catheter ● graduated container if patient is on intake and output measurement ● ice-filled container if a refrigerator isn't available ● label ● laboratory request form ● four patient-care reminders

Check with the laboratory to find out which preservatives may need to be added to the specimen or whether a dark collection container is required.

### Implementation

▶ Explain the procedure to the patient and his family, as necessary, to enlist their cooperation and prevent accidental disposal of urine during the collection period. Emphasize that failure to collect even one specimen during the collection period invalidates the test and requires that it begin again.

▶ Place patient-care reminders over the patient's bed, in his bathroom, on the bedpan hopper in the utility room, and on the urinal or indwelling catheter collection bag. Include the patient's name and room number, the date, and the collection interval.

▶ Instruct the patient to save all urine during the collection period, to notify you after each voiding, and to avoid contaminating the urine with stool or toilet tissue. Explain any dietary or drug restrictions and make sure he understands and is willing to comply with them.

### For 2-hour collection

▶ If possible, instruct the patient to drink two to four 8-oz (470- to 950- ml) glasses of water about 30 minutes before collection begins. After 30 minutes, tell him to void. Put on gloves and discard this specimen so the patient starts the collection period with an empty bladder.

▶ If ordered, administer a challenge dose of medication (such as glucose solution or corticotropin) and record the time.

▶ After each voiding, put on gloves and add the specimen to the collection container.

▶ Instruct the patient to void about 15 minutes before the end of the collection period, if possible, and add this specimen to the collection container.

▶ At the end of the collection period, remove and discard your gloves and send the appropriately labeled collection container to the laboratory immediately, along with a properly completed laboratory request form.

### For 12- or 24-hour collection

▶ Put on gloves and ask the patient to void. Discard this urine so the patient starts the collection period with an empty bladder. Record the time.

▶ After putting on gloves and pouring the first urine specimen into the collection container, add the required preservative. Refrigerate the bottle or keep it on ice until the next voiding, as appropriate.

▶ Collect all urine voided during the prescribed period. Just before the collection period ends, ask the patient to void again, if possible. Add this last specimen to the collection container, pack it in ice to inhibit deterioration of the specimen and remove and discard your gloves. Label the collection container and send it to the laboratory with a properly completed laboratory request form.

### Special considerations

▶ Keep the patient well hydrated before and during the test to ensure adequate urine flow.

▶ Before collection of a timed specimen, make sure the laboratory will be open when the collection period ends to help ensure prompt, accurate results. Never store a specimen in a refrigerator that contains food or medication to avoid contamination. If the patient has an indwelling catheter in place, put the collection bag in an ice-filled container at his bedside.

▶ Instruct the patient to avoid exercise and ingestion of coffee, tea, or any drugs (unless directed otherwise by the doctor) before the test to avoid altering test results.

### Home care

If the patient must continue collecting urine at home, provide written instructions for the appropriate method. Tell the patient that he can keep the collection container in a brown bag in his refrigerator at home, separate from other refrigerator contents.

### Documentation

▶ Record the date and intervals of specimen collection and when the collection container was sent to the laboratory.

### REFERENCES

Kouri, T., et al. "Reference Intervals for the Markers of Proteinuria with a Standardised Bed-rest Collection of Urine," *Clinical Chemistry and Laboratory Medicine* 39(5):418-25, May 2001.

Jelliffe, R. "Estimation of Creatinine Clearance in Patients with Unstable Renal Function, Without a Urine Specimen," *American Journal of Nephrology* 22(4):320-24, July-August 2002.

# Urinary diversion stoma care

Urinary diversions provide an alternative route for urine flow when a disorder, such as an invasive bladder tumor, impedes normal drainage. A permanent urinary diversion is indicated in any condition that requires a total cystectomy. In conditions requiring temporary urinary drainage or diversion, a suprapubic or urethral catheter is usually inserted to divert the flow of urine temporarily. The catheter remains in place until the incision heals.

Urinary diversions may also be indicated for patients with neurogenic bladder, congenital anomaly, traumatic injury to the

# Types of permanent urinary diversion

The steps involved in creating an ileal conduit or a continent urinary diversion are described here.

### Ileal conduit
A segment of the ileum is excised, and the two ends of the ileum that result from excision of the segment are sutured closed. Then the ureters are dissected from the bladder and anastomosed to the ileal segment. One end of the ileal segment is closed with sutures; the opposite end is brought through the abdominal wall, thereby forming a stoma.

### Continent urinary diversion
A tube is formed from part of the ascending colon and ileum. One end of the tube is brought to the skin to form the stoma. At the internal end of this tube, a nipple valve is constructed so urine won't drain out unless a catheter is inserted through the stoma into the newly formed bladder pouch. The urethral neck is sutured closed.

Another recently developed type of continent urinary diversion (not pictured here) is "hooked" back to the urethra, obviating the need for a stoma.

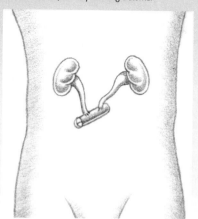
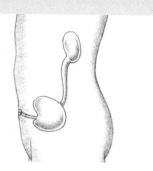

---

lower urinary tract, or severe chronic urinary tract infection.

Ileal conduit and continent urinary diversion are the two types of permanent urinary diversions with stomas. (See *Types of permanent urinary diversion*.)

These procedures usually require the patient to wear a urine-collection appliance and to care for the stoma created during surgery.

## Equipment
Soap and warm water • waste receptacle (such as an impervious or wax-coated bag) • linen-saver pad • hypoallergenic paper tape • povidone-iodine solution • urine collection container • rubber catheter (usually #14 or #16 French) • ruler • scissors • urine-collection appliance (with or without antireflux valve) • graduated cylinder • cottonless gauze pads (some rolled, some flat) • washcloth • skin barrier in liquid, paste, wafer, or sheet form • appliance belt

• stoma covering (nonadherent gauze pad or panty liner) • two pairs of gloves • optional: adhesive solvent, irrigating syringe, tampon, hair dryer, electric razor, regular gauze pads, vinegar, and deodorant tablets

Commercially packaged stoma care kits are available. In place of soap and water, you can use adhesive remover pads, if available, or cotton gauze saturated with adhesive solvent.

## Preparation of equipment
Assemble all the equipment on the patient's overbed table. Tape the waste receptacle to the table for ready access. Provide privacy for the patient and wash your hands. Measure the diameter of the stoma with a ruler. Cut the opening of the appliance with the scissors—it shouldn't be more than ⅛″ to ⅙″ (0.3 to 0.4 cm) larger than the diameter of the stoma. Moisten the faceplate of the appliance with a small amount of solvent or water to prepare it for

adhesion. Performing these preliminary steps at the bedside allows you to demonstrate the procedure and show the patient that it isn't difficult, which will help him relax.

## Implementation

▶ Wash your hands again. Explain the procedure to the patient as you go along and offer constant reinforcement and reassurance to counteract negative reactions that may be elicited by stoma care.

▶ Place the bed in low Fowler's position so the patient's abdomen is flat. This position eliminates skin folds that could cause the appliance to slip or irritate the skin and allows the patient to observe or participate.

▶ Put on the gloves and place the linen-saver pad under the patient's side, near the stoma. Open the drain valve of the appliance being replaced to empty the urine into the graduated cylinder. Then, to remove the appliance, use a washcloth to apply soap and water or adhesive solvent as you gently push the skin back from the pouch. If the appliance is disposable, discard it into the waste receptacle. If it's reusable, clean it with soap and lukewarm water and let it air-dry.

◆ **ALERT!** To avoid irritating the patient's stoma, avoid touching it with adhesive solvent. If adhesive remains on the skin, gently rub it off with a dry gauze pad. Discard used gauze pads in the waste receptacle.

▶ To prevent a constant flow of urine onto the skin while you're changing the appliance, wick the urine with an absorbent, lint-free material. (See *Wicking urine from a stoma.*)

▶ Use water to carefully wash off any crystal deposits that may have formed around the stoma. If urine has stagnated and has a strong odor, use soap to wash it off. Be sure to rinse thoroughly to remove any oily residue that could cause the appliance to slip.

▶ Follow your facility's skin care protocol to treat any minor skin problems.

▶ Dry the peristomal area thoroughly with a gauze pad because moisture will keep the appliance from sticking. Use a hair dryer if you wish. Remove any hair from the area with scissors or an electric razor to prevent hair follicles from becoming irritated when the pouch is removed, which can cause folliculitis.

## Wicking urine from a stoma

Use a piece of rolled, cottonless gauze or a tampon to wick urine from a stoma. Working by capillary action, wicking absorbs urine while you prepare the patient's skin to hold a urine-collection appliance.

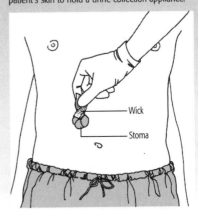

▶ Inspect the stoma to see if it's healing properly and to detect complications. Check the color and the appearance of the suture line and examine any moisture or effluent. Inspect the peristomal skin for redness, irritation, and intactness.

▶ Apply the skin barrier. If you apply a wafer or sheet, cut it to fit over the stoma. Remove any protective backing and set the barrier aside with the adhesive side up. If you apply a liquid barrier (such as Skin-Prep), saturate a gauze pad with it and coat the peristomal skin. Move in concentric circles outward from the stoma until you've covered an area 2″ (5.1 cm) larger than the wafer. Let the skin dry for several minutes; it should feel tacky. Gently press the wafer around the stoma, sticky side down, smoothing from the stoma outward.

▶ If you're using a barrier paste, open the tube, squeeze out a small amount, and then discard it. Then squeeze a ribbon of paste directly onto the peristomal skin about ½″ (1.5 cm) from the stoma, making a complete circle. Make several more concentric circles outward. Dip your fingers into lukewarm water and smooth the paste until the skin is completely covered from the edge of the stoma to 3″ to 4″ (7.5 to 10 cm) out-

ward. The paste should be ¼" to ½" (0.5 to 1.5 cm) thick. Discard the gloves, wash your hands, and put on new gloves.
▶ Remove the material used for wicking urine and place it in the waste receptacle.
▶ Now place the appliance over the stoma, leaving only a small amount (⅜" to ¾" [1 to 2 cm]) of skin exposed.
▶ Secure the faceplate of the appliance to the skin with paper tape, if recommended. To do this, place a piece of tape lengthwise on each edge of the faceplate so that the tape overlaps onto the skin.
▶ Apply the appliance belt, making sure that it's on a level with the stoma. If the belt is applied above or below the stoma, it could break the bag's seal or rub or injure the stoma. The belt should be loose enough for you to insert two fingers between the skin and the belt. If the belt is too tight, it could irritate the skin or cause internal damage. Some devices don't require a belt. Instead, the pouch has a ridge that fits over the rim of barrier adhesive and snaps securely into place.
▶ Dispose of the used materials appropriately.

## Special considerations
▶ The patient's attitude toward his urinary diversion stoma plays a big part in determining how well he'll adjust to it. To encourage a positive attitude, help him get used to the idea of caring for his stoma and the appliance as though they're natural extensions of himself. When teaching him to perform the procedure, give him written instructions and provide positive reinforcement after he completes each step. Suggest that he perform the procedure in the morning when urine flows most slowly.
▶ Help the patient choose between disposable and reusable appliances by telling him the advantages and disadvantages of each. Emphasize the importance of correct placement and of a well-fitted appliance to prevent seepage of urine onto the skin. When positioned correctly, most appliances remain in place for at least 3 days and for as long as 5 days if no leakage occurs. After 5 days, the appliance should be changed. With the improved adhesives and pouches available, belts aren't always necessary.
▶ Because urine flows constantly, it accumulates quickly, becoming even heavier than stools. To prevent the weight of the urine from loosening the seal around the stoma and separating the appliance from the skin, tell the patient to empty the appliance through the drain valve when it is one-third to one-half full.
▶ Instruct the patient to connect his appliance to a urine-collection container before he goes to sleep. The continuous flow of urine into the container during the night prevents the urine from accumulating and stagnating in the appliance.
▶ Teach the patient sanitary and dietary measures that can protect the peristomal skin and control the odor that commonly results from alkaline urine, infection, or poor hygiene. Reusable appliances should be washed with soap and lukewarm water, then air-dried thoroughly to prevent brittleness. Soaking the appliance in vinegar and water or placing deodorant tablets in it can further dissipate stubborn odors. An acid-ash diet that includes ascorbic acid and cranberry juice may raise urine acidity, thereby reducing bacterial action and fermentation (the underlying causes of odor). Generous fluid intake also helps to reduce odors by diluting the urine.
▶ Tell the patient that mucus may be present in the urine.
▶ If the patient has a continent urinary diversion, make sure you know how to meet his special needs. (See *Caring for the patient with a continent urinary diversion*.)
▶ Inform the patient about support services provided by ostomy clubs and the American Cancer Society.

## Home care
The patient or a family member can learn to care for a urinary diversion stoma at home. However, the patient's emotional adjustment to the stoma must be given special consideration before he can be expected to maintain it properly. Arrange for a visiting nurse or an enterostomal therapist to assist the patient at home.

## Complications
Because the intestinal mucosa is delicate, an ill-fitting appliance can cause bleeding. This is especially likely to occur with an ileal conduit, the most common type of urinary diversion stoma, because a segment of the intestine forms the conduit. Peristomal skin may become reddened or excoriated from too-frequent changing or improper placement of the appliance, poor skin care, or allergic reaction to the appli-

# Caring for the patient with a continent urinary diversion

In this procedure, an alternative to the traditional ileal conduit, a pouch created from the ascending colon and terminal ileum serves as a new bladder, which empties through a stoma. To drain urine continuously, several drains are inserted into this reconstructed bladder and left in place for 3 to 6 weeks until the new stoma heals. The patient will be discharged from the hospital with the drains in place. He'll return to have them removed and to learn to catheterize his stoma

### First hospitalization
▶ Immediately after surgery, monitor intake and output from each drain. Be alert for decreased output, which may indicate that urine flow is obstructed.
▶ Watch for common postoperative complications, such as infection or bleeding. Also watch for signs of urinary leakage, which include increased abdominal distention and urine appearing around the drains or midline incision.
▶ Irrigate the drains as ordered.
▶ Clean the area around the drains daily, first with povidone-iodine solution and then with sterile water. Apply a dry, sterile dressing to the area. Use precut 4″ × 4″ drain dressings around the drain to absorb leakage.
▶ To increase the patient's mobility and comfort, connect the drains to a leg bag.

### Second hospitalization or outpatient
▶ After the patient's drains are removed, teach him how to catheterize the stoma. Begin by gathering the following equipment on a clean towel: rubber catheter (usually #14 or #16 French), water-soluble lubricant, washcloth, stoma covering (nonadherent gauze pad or panty liner), hypoallergenic adhesive tape, and an irrigating solution (optional).
▶ Apply water-soluble lubricant to the catheter tip to facilitate insertion.
▶ Remove and discard the stoma cover. Using the washcloth, clean the stoma and the area around it, starting at the stoma and working outward in a circular motion.

▶ Hold the urine-collection container under the catheter; then slowly insert the catheter into the stoma. Urine should then begin to flow into the container. If it doesn't, gently rotate the catheter or redirect its angle. If the catheter drains slowly, it may be plugged with mucus. Irrigate it with sterile saline solution or sterile water to clear it. When the flow stops, pinch the catheter closed and remove it.

### Home care
▶ Teach the patient how to care for the drains and their insertion sites during the 3 to 6 weeks he'll be at home before their removal and teach him how to attach them to a leg bag. Also teach him how to recognize the signs of infection and obstruction.
▶ After the drains are removed, teach the patient how to empty the pouch and establish a schedule. Initially, he should catheterize the stoma and empty the pouch every 2 to 3 hours. Later, he should catheterize every 4 hours while awake and also irrigate the pouch each morning and evening, if ordered. Instruct him to empty the pouch whenever he feels a sensation of fullness.
▶ Tell the patient that the catheters are reusable, but only after they've been cleaned. He should clean the catheter thoroughly with warm, soapy water, rinse it thoroughly, and hang it to dry over a clean towel. He should store cleaned and dried catheters in plastic bags. Tell him he can reuse catheters for up to 1 month before discarding them. However, he should immediately discard any catheter that becomes discolored or cracked.

---

ance or adhesive. Constant leakage around the appliance can result from improper placement of the appliance or from poor skin turgor.

## Documentation
▶ Record the appearance and color of the stoma and whether it's inverted, flush with the skin, or protruding. If it protrudes, note how much it protrudes above the skin. (The normal range is ½″ to ¾″ [1.5 to 2 cm].)
▶ Record the appearance and condition of the peristomal skin, noting any redness or irritation or complaints by the patient of itching or burning.

**REFERENCES**

Black, P. "Practical Stoma Care," *Nursing Standard* 14(41):47-53; quiz 54-55, June-July 2000. (Review.)

Winter, W.E. 3rd, et al. "Modified Technique for Urinary Diversion with Incontinent Conduits," *Gynecologic Oncology* 86(3): 351-53, September 2002.

# Urine collection

A random urine specimen, usually collected as part of the physical examination or at various times during hospitalization, permits laboratory screening for urinary and systemic disorders as well as for drug screening. A clean-catch midstream specimen is replacing random collection because it provides a virtually uncontaminated specimen without the need for catheterization.

An indwelling catheter specimen—obtained either by clamping the drainage tube and emptying the accumulated urine into a container or by aspirating a specimen with a syringe—requires sterile collection technique to prevent catheter contamination and urinary tract infection. This method is contraindicated after genitourinary surgery.

## Equipment

*For a random specimen*
Bedpan or urinal with cover, if necessary ● gloves ● graduated container ● specimen container with lid ● label ● laboratory request form

*For a clean-catch midstream specimen*
Soap and water ● gloves ● graduated container ● three sterile 2″ × 2″ gauze pads ● povidone-iodine solution ● sterile specimen container with lid ● label ● bedpan or urinal, if necessary ● laboratory request form

Commercial clean-catch kits containing antiseptic towelettes, sterile specimen container with lid and label, and instructions for use in several languages are widely used.

*For an indwelling catheter specimen*
Gloves ● Betadine swab ● 10-ml syringe ● 21G or 22G 1½″ needle ● tube clamp ● sterile specimen container with lid ● label ● laboratory request form

## Implementation

▶ Tell the patient you need a urine specimen for laboratory analysis. Explain the procedure to him and his family, if necessary, to promote cooperation and prevent accidental disposal of specimens.

### Collecting a random specimen

▶ Provide privacy. Instruct the patient on bed rest to void into a clean bedpan or urinal or ask the ambulatory patient to void into either one in the bathroom.

▶ Put on gloves. Pour at least 120 ml of urine into the specimen container and cap the container securely. If the patient's urine output must be measured and recorded, pour the remaining urine into the graduated container. Otherwise, discard the remaining urine. If you inadvertently spill urine on the outside of the container, clean and dry it to prevent cross-contamination.

▶ After you label the specimen container with the patient's name and room number and the date and time of collection, attach the request form and send it the laboratory immediately. Delayed transport of the specimen may alter test results.

▶ Clean the graduated container and urinal or bedpan and return them to their proper storage. Discard disposable items.

▶ Wash your hands thoroughly to prevent cross-contamination. Offer the patient a washcloth and soap and water to wash his hands.

### Collecting a clean-catch midstream specimen

▶ Because the goal is a virtually uncontaminated specimen, explain the procedure to the patient carefully. Provide illustrations to emphasize the correct collection technique, if possible.

▶ Tell the patient to remove all clothing from the waist down and to stand in front of the toilet as for urination or, if female, to sit far back on the toilet seat and spread her legs. Then have the patient clean the periurethral area (tip of the penis or labial folds, vulva, and urinary meatus) with soap and water and wipe the area three times, each time with a fresh 2″ × 2″ gauze pad soaked in povidone-iodine solution or with the wipes provided in a commercial kit. Instruct the female patient to separate her labial folds with the thumb and forefinger. Tell her to wipe down one side with the first pad and discard it, to wipe the other side with the second pad and discard it and, finally, to wipe down the center over the urinary meatus with the third pad and discard it. Stress the importance of cleaning from front to back to avoid contaminating the genital area with fecal matter. For the uncircumcised male patient, emphasize the need to retract his foreskin to effectively clean the meatus and to keep it retracted during voiding.

▶ Tell the female patient to straddle the bedpan or toilet to allow labial spreading and to keep her labia separated while voiding.

▶ Instruct the patient to begin voiding into the bedpan, urinal, or toilet. Then, without stopping the urine stream, the patient should move the collection container into the stream, collecting 30 to 50 ml at the midstream portion of the voiding. He can then finish voiding into the bedpan, urinal, or toilet.

▶ Put on gloves before discarding the first and last portions of the voiding and measure the remaining urine in a graduated container for intake and output records, if necessary. Be sure to include the amount in the specimen container when recording the total amount voided.

▶ Take the sterile container from the patient and cap it securely. Avoid touching the inside of the container or the lid. If the outside of the container is soiled, clean it and wipe it dry. Remove gloves and discard them properly.

▶ Wash your hands thoroughly. Tell the patient to wash his hands and urethral area to remove the cleansing solution to avoid skin irritation.

▶ Label the container with the patient's name and room number, name of test, type of specimen, collection time, and suspected diagnosis, if known. If a urine culture has been ordered, note any current antibiotic therapy on the laboratory request form. Send the container to the laboratory immediately or place it on ice to prevent specimen deterioration and altered test results.

### Collecting an indwelling catheter specimen

▶ About 30 minutes before collecting the specimen, clamp the drainage tube to allow urine to accumulate.

▶ Put on gloves. If the drainage tube has a built-in sampling port, wipe the port with an alcohol pad. Uncap the needle on the syringe and insert the needle into the sam-

## Aspirating a urine specimen

If the patient has an indwelling urinary catheter in place, clamp the tube distal to the aspiration port for about 30 minutes. Wipe the port with an alcohol pad and insert a needle and a 20- or 30-ml syringe into the port perpendicular to the tube. Aspirate the required amount of urine and expel it into the specimen container. Remove the clamp on the drainage tube.

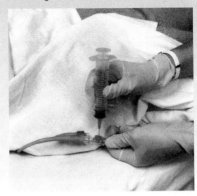

pling port at a 90-degree angle to the tubing. Aspirate the specimen into the syringe. (See *Aspirating a urine specimen*.)

▶ If the drainage tube doesn't have a sampling port and the catheter is made of rubber, obtain the specimen from the catheter. Other types of catheters will leak after you withdraw the needle. To withdraw the specimen from a rubber catheter, wipe it with an alcohol pad just above where it connects to the drainage tube. Insert the needle into the rubber catheter at a 45-degree angle and withdraw the specimen. Never insert the needle into the shaft of the catheter because this may puncture the lumen leading to the catheter balloon.

▶ Transfer the specimen to a sterile container, label it, and send it to the laboratory immediately or place it on ice. If a urine culture is to be performed, be sure to list any current antibiotic therapy on the laboratory request form.

▶ If the catheter isn't made of rubber or has no sampling port, wipe the area where the catheter joins the drainage tube with an alcohol pad. Disconnect the catheter and allow urine to drain into the sterile specimen container. Avoid touching the inside of the sterile container with the catheter and don't touch anything with the catheter drainage tube to avoid contamination. When you've collected the specimen, wipe both connection sites with an alcohol pad and join them. Cap the specimen container, label it, and send it to the laboratory immediately or place it on ice.

■◆■ **ALERT!** Make sure you unclamp the drainage tube after collecting the specimen to prevent urine backflow, which may cause bladder distention and infection.

### Home care

Instruct the patient to collect the specimen in a clean container with a tight-fitting lid and to keep it on ice or in the refrigerator (separate from food items) for up to 24 hours.

### Documentation

▶ Record the times of specimen collection and transport to the laboratory. Specify the test as well as the appearance, odor, and color and any unusual characteristics of the specimen.
▶ If necessary, record the urine volume in the intake and output record.

**REFERENCES**

Cherry, R.A., et al. "Accuracy of Short-duration Creatinine Clearance Determinations in Predicting 24-hour Creatinine Clearance in Critically Ill and Injured Patients," *The Journal of Trauma* 53(2):267-71, August 2002.

Edward, D., et al. *Bedside Critical Care Manual.* Philadelphia: Lippincott Williams & Wilkins, 2001.

# Urine specific gravity

The kidneys maintain homeostasis by varying urine output and urine concentration of dissolved salts. Urine specific gravity measures the concentration of urine solutes, which reflects the kidneys' capacity to concentrate urine. The capacity to concentrate urine is among the first functions lost when renal tubular damage occurs.

Urine specific gravity is determined by comparing the weight of a urine specimen with that of an equivalent volume of distilled water, which is 1.000. Because urine contains dissolved salts and other substances, it's heavier than 1.000. Urine specific gravity ranges from 1.003 (very dilute) to 1.035 (highly concentrated); normal values range from 1.010 to 1.025. Specific gravity is measured with a urinometer (a specially calibrated hydrometer designed to float in a cylinder of urine), a refractometer, which measures the refraction of light as it passes through a urine specimen, or a reagent strip test.

Elevated specific gravity reflects an increased concentration of urine solutes, which occurs in conditions that cause renal hypoperfusion, and may indicate heart failure, dehydration, hepatic disorders, or nephrosis. Low specific gravity reflects failure to reabsorb water and concentrate urine; it may indicate hypercalcemia, hypokalemia, alkalosis, acute renal failure, pyelonephritis, glomerulonephritis, or diabetes insipidus.

### Equipment

Calibrated urinometer and cylinder, refractometer, or reagent strips (Multistix) ● gloves ● specimen container

### Implementation

▶ Explain the procedure to the patient and tell him when you'll need the specimen. Explain why you're withholding fluids and for how long to ensure his cooperation.

Measuring with a refractometer
▶ Put on gloves and collect a random or controlled urine specimen.
▶ Place a single drop of urine on the refractometer slide.
▶ Turn on the light and look through the eyepiece to see the specific gravity indicated on a scale. (Some instruments have a digital display.)

Measuring with a reagent strip
▶ Put on gloves and obtain a random or controlled urine specimen.
▶ Dip the reagent end of the test strip into the specimen for 2 seconds.
▶ Tap the strip on the rim of the specimen container to remove excess urine and compare the resultant color change with the color chart supplied with the kit.

## Special considerations

Test the urinometer in distilled water at room temperature to ensure that its calibration is 1.000. If necessary, correct the urinometer reading for temperature effects; add 0.001 to your observed reading for every 5.4° F (3° C) above the calibration temperature of 71.6° F (22° C); subtract 0.001 for every 5.4° F below 71.6° F.

## Documentation

▶ Record the specific gravity, volume, color, odor, and appearance of the collected urine specimen.
▶ Indicate whether the doctor was made aware of the test results.

### REFERENCES

Edward, D., et al. *Bedside Critical Care Manual*. Philadelphia: Lippincott Williams & Wilkins, 2001.

Parikh, C.R., et al. "Screening for Microalbuminuria Simplified by Urine Specific Gravity," *American Journal of Nephrology* 22(4):315-19, July-August 2002.

# 10

# Musculoskeletal care

TRADITIONALLY, NURSES CARING FOR PATIENTS WITH MUSCULOSKELETAL DISORDERS HAVE needed to operate special mechanical and traction equipment. Today, they need to understand the principals of internal and external fixation, prosthetics, orthotics, immobilization, and implantation.

This chapter will help you manage the patient who's undergoing an amputation, has a fracture, or is experiencing minor trauma. In addition, this chapter will help you understand the step-by-step procedures that will allow you to provide up-to-date care for the patient with musculoskeletal disorders.

# Protocols

## Managing the patient undergoing amputation

### Purpose
To provide preoperative and postoperative care related to an amputation and to prevent or minimize its physical and psychological sequelae

### Collaborative level
Interdependent

### Expected patient outcomes
▶ The patient will report satisfactory pain control.
▶ The patient will display no signs or symptoms of infection.
▶ The patient will adapt to changes in his body image.

### Definition of terms
▶ *Flap (or closed) amputation:* A type of amputation in which the surgeon closes the open end of a stump with a skin flap. The wound is sutured to cover the bone end.
▶ *Guillotine (or open) amputation:* A type of amputation in which the surgeon doesn't leave a skin flap. Instead, the wound is left open to promote drainage. The main indication is wound contamination or infection.

### Indications
Treatment
▶ Gangrene
▶ Trauma, such as severe crush, mangled extremity, and electrical burn injuries; irreversible neurovascular compromise; and frostbite
▶ Peripheral vascular disease with chronic limb ischemia and intractable pain
▶ Malignancy
▶ Congenital deformity

Prevention
▶ Hypovolemia
▶ Hemorrhage
▶ Infection
▶ Skin breakdown
▶ Venous thromboembolism
▶ Myoglobinuria, which can lead to acute renal failure
▶ Maladaptive psychological response to loss of body part

### Assessment guidance
Signs and symptoms
▶ Extremity pain
▶ Burning sensation
▶ Numbness
▶ Destructive trauma to extremity (after injury)
▶ Discoloration, as with pallor, necrotic skin changes, gangrene
▶ Weak or absent distal pulses
▶ Loss of sensory function, motor function, or both

Diagnostic studies
*Laboratory tests*
▶ White blood cell count
▶ Serum hemoglobin level
▶ Hematocrit
▶ Urine myoglobin level
▶ Blood urea nitrogen level
▶ Serum creatinine level

*Imaging tests*
▶ X-rays
▶ Computed tomography scan
▶ Arteriography
▶ Doppler ultrasonography

*Other*
▶ Ankle-brachial index (ABI)

## Nursing interventions
### Preoperative care
▶ Assess the patient's neurovascular status to detect signs and symptoms of limb ischemia. Compare his limbs bilaterally, noting skin color, location and quality of distal pulses, thrills, skin temperature, capillary refill, and sensory and motor function. Investigate patient reports of pain, burning, or numbness.
▶ Report changes in the patient's neurovascular status to the doctor immediately.
▶ Maintain a patent I.V. line.
▶ Assess the patient's ABI by comparing the systolic blood pressure in his dorsalis pedis or posterior tibialis artery with that in his brachial artery. The ratio of these pressures helps detect vascular insufficiency in an injured limb. An ABI below 0.9 suggests vascular insufficiency.
▶ If surgery may be delayed, pack a gangrenous limb in ice to prevent free circulation of toxins and sepsis.
▶ For extremity trauma or a crush injury, prevent movement of the injury site to decrease pain, injury, and blood loss. Use appropriate wound dressings and splinting or immobilization techniques. Monitor the patient for evidence of myoglobinuria and take measures to prevent the subsequent development of acute renal failure.
▶ Give a narcotic analgesic and other medication to control pain.
▶ Assess the patient's skin integrity, noting areas of breakdown or drainage.
▶ Assess the patient for signs and symptoms of infection or worsening infection.
▶ For an infected or contaminated extremity wound, give tetanus prophylaxis and an I.V. antibiotic.
▶ Assess the patient's nutritional status. If you discover deficiencies, consult a dietitian or nutritionist so that the patient's nutrition can be optimized before surgery, if possible.
▶ Identify and address coexisting conditions that could negatively affect the surgical outcome, such as diabetes mellitus, cardiovascular disease, anemia, and dehydration.
▶ Assess the patient's psychological response to the anticipated procedure and his use of coping skills.
▶ Promote open and honest dialogue with the patient about the planned amputation. Provide information, answer questions, address his concerns and fears, and discuss phantom limb sensations and pain, the rehabilitation plan, and the timing of prosthesis fitting, as indicated.
▶ Arrange for physical and occupational therapy for preoperative physical conditioning, if possible.
▶ Prepare the patient for surgery as required.
▶ Make the patient as comfortable as possible; provide reassurance.

### Postoperative care
▶ Monitor the patient's vital signs, as indicated.
▶ Support the patient's airway, breathing, and circulation, as indicated.
▶ Maintain a patent I.V. line. Be prepared to give I.V. fluid boluses and blood products.
▶ Give an I.V. narcotic analgesic to control pain.
▶ Closely monitor the patient's fluid intake and output, hemoglobin level, and hematocrit to assess for signs of myoglobinuria, hypovolemia, hemorrhagic shock, and acute renal failure.
▶ Inspect the surgical dressing; notify the surgeon immediately if you detect bleeding or hemorrhage.
▶ Place the stump in the position ordered by the surgeon. Typically, the joint should be elevated in an extended position to prevent contracture.
▶ Assess the patient's psychological state. Encourage him to express his feelings; provide emotional support, as needed.
▶ Dress the stump, as ordered by the surgeon. Expect to use an elastic compression dressing to decrease edema and to condition the stump for a prosthetic device. Use strict sterile technique to prevent wound infection.
▶ Assess the patient's skin integrity, noting areas of impaired wound healing in or around the stump.
▶ Assess the patient for signs and symptoms of infection in the stump.
▶ Facilitate the rehabilitation plan by working with the multidisciplinary health

care team to achieve the patient's goals, providing or reinforcing information, and offering encouragement.
▶ To prevent venous thromboembolism, give prophylactic anticoagulants, as ordered.

## Patient teaching
▶ Explain the purpose of amputation to the patient and his family.
▶ Discuss all treatments and nursing interventions and tell how they promote optimal recovery or relieve pain.
▶ Teach the patient about all diagnostic studies he must undergo to identify limb viability, neurovascular compromise, and complications.
▶ Review and reinforce all aspects of the patient's rehabilitation plan.
▶ Inform the patient about possible complications, such as hypovolemia, hemorrhage, infection, skin breakdown, and venous thromboembolism. Instruct him to recognize and report their signs and symptoms as soon as they are detected.

## Precautions
▶ In the patient with severe extremity trauma, be alert for hemorrhagic shock in the acute preoperative period.
▶ If an amputation produces significant blood loss, expect the patient to have an increased risk of hemorrhagic shock in the postoperative period.
▶ Wound contamination or infection generally requires guillotine (open) amputation. If this occurs, prepare the patient for stump revisions in the operating room before a prosthesis is fitted.
▶ Be alert for signs and symptoms of infection or ischemia in the stump, which may require additional surgery for a higher level of amputation.
▶ A crush injury predisposes the patient to rhabdomyolysis and myoglobinuria. Therefore, observe for evidence of acute renal failure.

## Documentation
▶ Record subjective and objective assessment data in the patient's medical record.
▶ Document all specimens obtained and the date and time they were sent to the laboratory.
▶ Note the results of all diagnostic studies.
▶ Document the patient's fluid intake and output; be sure to include infused fluids, blood, and blood products.

▶ Record all treatments and nursing interventions, notification of the doctor, and subsequent care.
▶ Document the patient's response to each treatment.
▶ Summarize the results of teaching sessions with the patient and his family.

## Related procedures
▶ Arterial puncture for blood gas analysis
▶ Cardiac monitoring
▶ Central venous pressure monitoring
▶ I.V. bolus injection
▶ Indwelling urinary catheter insertion
▶ Oxygen administration
▶ Physical assessment
▶ Postoperative care
▶ Preoperative care
▶ Pulse and ear oximetry
▶ Sequential compression therapy
▶ Splint application
▶ Stump and prosthesis care
▶ Transfusion of whole blood and packed cells
▶ Venipuncture

## REFERENCES
Bayley, E., and Turke, S. *A Comprehensive Curriculum for Trauma Nursing.* Boston: Jones & Bartlett, 1999.

Emergency Nurses Association. *Trauma Nursing Core Course,* 5th ed. Park Ridge, Ill.: Emergency Nurses Association, 2000.

Hoover, T.J., and Siefert, J.A. "Soft Tissue Complications of Orthopedic Emergencies." *Emergency Medicine Clinics of North America* 18(1):115-39, February 2000.

Laskowski-Jones, L. "Managing Hemorrhage," *Nursing* 27(9):36-41, September 1997.

Moore, E., et al. *Trauma,* 4th ed. New York: McGraw-Hill Book Co., 2000.

Treat-Jacobson, D., et al. "A Patient-Derived Perspective of Health-Related Quality of Life with Peripheral Arterial Disease," *Journal of Nursing Scholarship* 34(1):55-60, 2002.

Walton, J. "Helping High-Risk Surgical Patients Beat the Odds," *Nursing* 31(3):54-59, March 2001.

## ORGANIZATIONS
American College of Surgeons: *www.facs.org*
Emergency Nurses Association: *www.ena.org*
National Amputation Foundation: *www.nationalamputation.org*

# Managing the patient with a fracture

## Purpose
To treat a fracture rapidly and effectively-cand to prevent or minimize its complications

## Collaborative level
Interdependent

## Expected patient outcomes
▶ The patient will maintain hemodynamic stability.
▶ The patient will demonstrate preservation of neurovascular function.
▶ The patient will report satisfactory control of pain.

## Definition of terms
▶ *Closed fracture:* A fracture that isn't associated with disrupted skin integrity and doesn't communicate with external environment.
▶ *Open fracture:* A fracture that disrupts skin integrity and allows the fracture to communicate with the external environment, resulting in a high infection risk.
▶ *Immobilization methods:* Interventions that restrict movement of an injured body part.
▶ *Compartment syndrome:* A condition in which pressure within an osteofascial compartment increases (usually because of muscle compartment edema or hemorrhage) and compromises circulation and tissue function, leading to myoneural necrosis.
▶ *Fat embolism syndrome:* A condition in which fats and free fatty acids are liberated into the systemic circulation and pulmonary vessels, which may impair neurologic, circulatory, and respiratory function. The syndrome is associated with fractures of the long bones, pelvis, and ribs; multiple trauma; and orthopedic surgery.

## Indications
Treatment
▶ Closed fractures
▶ Open fractures

Prevention
▶ Hypovolemic shock
▶ Infection
▶ Fat embolism syndrome

▶ Venous thromboembolism, which may lead to deep vein thrombosis or pulmonary embolus
▶ Compartment syndrome
▶ Avascular necrosis
▶ Skin breakdown

## Assessment guidance
Signs and symptoms
*Closed and open fractures*
▶ Pain, point tenderness, tingling, and numbness in or around the injury site
▶ Deformity
▶ Discoloration
▶ Edema
▶ Crepitus
▶ Loss of function
▶ Tachycardia, hypotension, and oliguria (with significant blood loss)
▶ Nausea, dizziness, dry mouth, and thirst (if hypovolemia results from blood loss)

*Open fracture*
▶ Disruption in skin integrity, such as a puncture wound, laceration, and bleeding, over the injury site
▶ Exposed bone

Diagnostic studies
*Laboratory tests*
▶ Hemoglobin
▶ Hematocrit
▶ White blood cell (WBC) count
▶ Urine myoglobin level
▶ Blood urea nitrogen level
▶ Serum creatinine level
▶ Creatinine kinase level

*Imaging tests*
▶ X-rays
▶ Computed tomography scan
▶ Arteriography
▶ Doppler ultrasonography

*Other*
▶ Ankle-brachial index (ABI)

## Nursing interventions
Care related to fractures
▶ Assess the patient's airway, breathing, and circulation to prioritize interventions. Plan to manage fractures after acute threats to life are addressed.
▶ For a suspected or actual spinal column fracture, apply a cervical collar; maintain the patient in a supine position and perform a coordinated logroll with extra per-

sonnel, as indicated, assuring that the head and spine are aligned at all times. To maintain optimal spinal immobilization, use a backboard with head blocks if the patient must be transported to a trauma center or other facility.

▶ Maintain a patent I.V. line with normal saline solution.

▶ For open fractures, control hemorrhage with gentle direct pressure. Cover exposed bone with a sterile saline-soaked dressing, and then stabilize the patient, as indicated.

▶ Report any change in neurovascular status to the doctor immediately.

▶ Prevent movement of the fracture site to decrease pain, injury, and blood loss. Use an appropriate splinting or immobilization technique as an initial emergency intervention.

▶ Splint the injury to immobilize the joints above and below the fracture site.

▶ Immobilize a long bone fracture in anatomic alignment unless a gross deformity is present.

▶ Immobilize a fractured joint in the position found.

▶ Consider applying a traction splint for a midshaft femur fracture.

▶ If an open fracture appears grossly contaminated, irrigate the wound with sterile normal saline solution.

▶ For a pelvic fracture, minimize patient movement and transfers to decrease blood loss; for an "open book" pelvic fracture, apply a pneumatic antishock garment or other pelvic stabilization device to compress the pelvis and reduce internal pelvic hemorrhage. If such devices aren't available, swaddle the pelvis snugly with a bath blanket.

▶ Assess the patient's ABI by comparing the systolic blood pressure in his dorsalis pedis or posterior tibialis artery with that in his brachial artery. The ratio of these pressures helps detect vascular insufficiency in an injured limb. An ABI below 0.9 suggests vascular insufficiency.

▶ Manage inflammation by applying an ice pack (or chemical cold pack) and elevating the injured limb above heart level, when possible.

▶ Give a narcotic analgesic and nonsteroidal anti-inflammatory drug to control pain.

▶ For an open fracture, give tetanus prophylaxis and an I.V. antibiotic.

▶ Give conscious sedation during interventions to reduce and immobilize a fracture.

▶ As needed, assist with more definitive fracture reduction and immobilization methods, such as skin traction, skeletal traction, casting, and external fixation.

▶ Prepare the patient for surgery when surgical debridement or open reduction-internal fixation is required.

▶ Assess the patient's skin integrity, noting areas of breakdown or drainage on dressings or casts.

▶ Assess the patient for signs and symptoms of infection, such as fever, elevated WBC count, foul odor, purulent drainage, and excessive pain.

▶ Monitor the patient for signs and symptoms of deep vein thrombosis, such as calf pain, edema, and Homan's sign.

▶ To prevent venous thromboembolism, apply a pneumatic compression device and give a low-molecular-weight heparin or other anticoagulant.

▶ Monitor the patient for signs and symptoms of compartment syndrome, such as unusually severe pain, pain with passive muscle stretching, sensory hyperesthesia or paresthesia, loss of function, palpable tenseness of the muscle compartment, paralysis (late sign), and absent pulses (very late sign). If you detect such findings, report them to the doctor immediately. If compartment syndrome is present, anticipate fasciotomy.

▶ Assess the patient for signs and symptoms of fat embolism syndrome, such as agitation, restlessness, dyspnea, tachypnea, tachycardia, fever, petechiae (on the neck, chest, axillae, and conjunctivae), altered mental status (including seizures and coma), hypoxemia, free fat in the urine, and fluffy exudates on chest X-ray. If you detect such findings, report them to the doctor immediately.

▶ Monitor the patient for signs and symptoms of pulmonary embolism, such as dyspnea, tachypnea, chest pain, anxiety or apprehension, cough, hemoptysis, hypoxemia, low-grade fever, and thrombophlebitis. If you detect such findings, report them to the doctor immediately.

▶ Monitor the patient's urine color to detect myoglobinuria, especially after a crush injury. Dark red, orange, or tea-colored urine suggests myoglobinuria.

## Care related to hypovolemia or hemorrhagic shock

▶ Assess and manage the patient's airway, breathing, and circulation. Then prioritize resuscitation interventions as needed.
▶ Give supplemental oxygen, as indicated.
▶ Assist with endotracheal intubation if respiratory insufficiency is present.
▶ Monitor the patient's vital signs every 15 minutes, or as indicated.
▶ Establish large-bore I.V. access (14 or 16 G in peripheral sites; 8.0 F or larger for central venous access).
▶ Begin aggressive fluid resuscitation with a crystalloid solution, such as normal saline or lactated Ringer's solution, to restore circulating blood volume.
▶ Draw blood for laboratory tests, including hemoglobin level, hematocrit, serum lactate level, and type and crossmatch. Also obtain blood for arterial blood gas analysis.
▶ Insert an indwelling urinary catheter to continuously measure urine output.
▶ Closely monitor the patient's fluid intake and output. Promptly report oliguria or anuria because myoglobin deposition in the renal tubules can precipitate acute renal failure.
▶ Make the patient as comfortable as possible; provide reassurance.
▶ Prepare the patient for surgery, as indicated.

## Patient teaching

▶ Explain the purpose of immobilization and splinting to the patient and his family.
▶ Discuss all treatments and nursing interventions and tell how they correct the fracture, decrease inflammation, or relieve pain.
▶ Teach the patient about all diagnostic studies he must undergo to identify fractures and complications.
▶ Review and reinforce all aspects of the patient's rehabilitation plan.
▶ Inform the patient about possible complications, such as venous thromboembolism, compartment syndrome, infection, and skin breakdown. Instruct him to recognize and report signs and symptoms as soon as they are detected.
▶ Suggest strategies to prevent trauma and avoid or minimize future injuries.

## Precautions

▶ Expect fractures to produce significant blood loss. For example, blood loss from a humerus fracture may be 1 to 2 L; forearm fracture, 0.5 to 1 L; pelvic fracture, 1.5 to 4.5 L; femur fracture, 1 to 2 L; tibia fracture, 0.5 to 1.5 L; and spine or rib fracture, 1 to 3 L. Femur, pelvic, and multiple fractures predispose the patient to hemorrhagic shock.
▶ A fracture accompanied by joint dislocation is likely to be associated with neurovascular compromise. Expect the doctor to reduce a dislocation as soon as possible to prevent avascular necrosis.
▶ Don't attempt to straighten a fractured joint.
▶ Assess the patient's neurovascular function *before* and *after* splinting. If neurovascular compromise results after splint application, adjust or remove the splint to help restore adequate neurovascular function. If function remains impaired, notify the doctor immediately.
▶ Give an I.V. narcotic analgesic for optimal pain control in the acute phase of care.

## Documentation

▶ Document the mechanism of injury that caused the patient's fracture.
▶ Record subjective and objective assessment data in the patient's medical record.
▶ Note all specimens obtained and the date and time they were sent to the laboratory.
▶ Document the results of all diagnostic studies.
▶ Record the patient's fluid intake and output; be sure to include infused fluids, blood, and blood products.
▶ Write down all treatments and nursing interventions, notification of the doctor, and subsequent care.
▶ Document the patient's response to each treatment.
▶ Record all teaching sessions with the patient and his family.

## Related procedures

▶ Arterial puncture for blood gas analysis
▶ Bryant's traction
▶ Cardiac monitoring
▶ Cast preparation
▶ Central venous pressure monitoring
▶ Cervical collar application
▶ Clavicle strap application
▶ Cold application
▶ Endotracheal intubation

▶ Endotracheal tube care
▶ End-tidal carbon dioxide monitoring
▶ External fixation
▶ Hip-spica cast care
▶ Indwelling catheter insertion
▶ Internal fixation
▶ I.V. bolus injection
▶ Manual ventilation
▶ Mechanical traction
▶ Mechanical ventilation
▶ Oxygen administration
▶ Physical assessment
▶ Postoperative care
▶ Preoperative care
▶ Pulse and ear oximetry
▶ Sequential compression therapy
▶ Splint application
▶ Transfusion of whole blood and packed cells
▶ Triangular sling application
▶ Urine collection
▶ Venipuncture

## REFERENCES

Hoover, T.J., and Siefert, J.A. "Soft Tissue Complications of Orthopedic Emergencies," *Emergency Medicine Clinics of North America.* 18(1):115-39, February 2000.

Laskowski-Jones, L. "Multisystem Problems: Trauma," in *Critical Care Nursing.* Edited by Bucher, L., and Melander, S.D. Philadelphia: W.B. Saunders Co., 1999.

Matthews, B.D., et al. "Fatal Cerebral Fat Embolism After Open Reduction and Internal Fixation of Femur Fracture," *Journal of Trauma* 50(3):585, March 2001.

Moore, E., et al. *Trauma,* 4th ed. New York: McGraw-Hill Book Co., 2000.

Mosley-Koehler, K. "Postoperative Pain Management in the Patient with a Tibial Fracture," *Journal of Orthopaedic Nursing* 3(4): 197-202, 1999.

Perron, A.D., et al. "Orthopedic Pitfalls in the ED: Acute Compartment Syndrome," *American Journal of Emergency Medicine* 19(5):413-16, September 2001.

## ORGANIZATIONS

American College of Surgeons: *www.facs.org*
Emergency Nurses Association: *www.ena.org*

# Managing the patient with minor trauma

## Purpose

To treat minor trauma rapidly and effectively and to prevent or minimize its complications

## Collaborative level

Interdependent

## Expected patient outcomes

▶ The patient will preserve neurovascular function.
▶ The patient will report satisfactory control of pain.
▶ The patient will preserve functional independence.

## Definition of terms

▶ *Contusion:* Bleeding into soft tissue from broken blood vessels associated with trauma; skin discoloration and bruising results.
▶ *Sprain:* Ligament injury from twisting or wrenching forces applied to a joint; the joint moves beyond its normal range of motion.
▶ *Strain:* A muscular injury caused by overstretching or overuse.
▶ *Compartment syndrome:* A condition in which pressure within an osteofascial compartment increases (usually because of muscle compartment edema or hemorrhage) and compromises circulation and tissue function, leading to myoneural necrosis.

## Indications

Treatment
▶ Contusions
▶ Sprains
▶ Strains

Prevention
▶ Infection
▶ Neurovascular compromise
▶ Compartment syndrome

## Assessment guidance

Signs and symptoms
▶ Pain or point tenderness at or around the injury site
▶ Muscle spasm
▶ Discoloration
▶ Edema

▶ Impaired or limited function of the injured area

## Diagnostic studies
### Laboratory tests
▶ Hemoglobin
▶ Hematocrit
▶ White blood cell count
▶ Urine myoglobin level
▶ Creatinine kinase level

### Imaging
▶ X-rays
▶ Computed tomography scan
▶ Magnetic resonance imaging
▶ Arteriography
▶ Doppler ultrasonography

### Other
▶ Ankle-brachial index (ABI)

## Nursing interventions
▶ Assess the patient's airway, breathing, and circulation. Treat minor musculoskeletal injuries only after physiologic compromise and major injuries are addressed.
▶ Perform a thorough patient assessment to identify the mechanism of injury and injury sites.
▶ While assessing and treating minor musculoskeletal trauma, assume that a fracture exists until diagnostic studies prove otherwise. As needed, apply a splint or use another stabilization technique.
▶ Assess the patient's neurovascular status and report changes to the doctor immediately.
▶ Assess the patient's ABI by comparing the systolic blood pressure in his dorsalis pedis or posterior tibialis artery with that in his brachial artery. The ratio of these pressures helps detect vascular insufficiency in an injured limb. An ABI below 0.9 suggests vascular insufficiency.
▶ Manage inflammation by applying an ice pack (or chemical cold pack) to the injury site for 20 minutes every 2 to 3 hours for the first 24 to 72 hours after the injury.
▶ Elevate the injured limb above the heart level while swelling is present.
▶ For a sprain or strain, apply a compression bandage and limit the patient's weight-bearing or non-weight-bearing activity, as appropriate.
▶ Provide crutches or other assistive devices, as needed.

▶ Give a narcotic analgesic and nonsteroidal anti-inflammatory drug to control pain.
▶ For an injury that disrupts skin integrity, give tetanus prophylaxis and an antibiotic.
▶ Assess the patient for signs and symptoms of infection.
▶ Monitor the patient for signs and symptoms of compartment syndrome, such as unusually severe pain, pain with passive muscle stretching, sensory hyperesthesia or paresthesia, loss of function, palpable tenseness of the muscle compartment, paralysis (late sign), and absent pulses (very late sign). If you detect such findings, report them to the doctor immediately. If compartment syndrome is present, anticipate fasciotomy.
▶ Make the patient as comfortable as possible; provide reassurance.

## Patient teaching
▶ Explain the purpose of immobilization and splinting to the patient and his family.
▶ Discuss all treatments and nursing interventions and tell how they decrease inflammation or relieve pain.
▶ Teach the patient about all diagnostic studies he must undergo to identify musculoskeletal injuries and complications.
▶ Advise the patient to limit or restrict activity, as ordered.
▶ Teach the patient how to use crutches or other assistive devices, as indicated.
▶ Inform the patient about possible complications, such as compartment syndrome and infection. Instruct him to recognize and report signs and symptoms as soon as they are detected.
▶ Suggest strategies to prevent trauma and avoid or minimize future injuries.

## Precautions
▶ Anticipate that contusions may produce significant blood loss if they're large or involve multiple body areas.
▶ A hematoma may become infected over time (usually several days). Assess areas of contusion for evidence of abscess formation, such as a palpable mass, increased pain, warmth over the site, and fever.
▶ Even minor trauma can produce compartment syndrome. Therefore, assess the patient's neurovascular status carefully.

## Documentation
▶ Document the mechanism of injury that was responsible for the patient's injury.
▶ Record subjective and objective assessment data in the patient's medical record.
▶ Note all specimens obtained and the date and time they were sent to the laboratory.
▶ Document the results of all diagnostic studies.
▶ Write down all treatments and nursing interventions, notification of the doctor, and subsequent care.
▶ Document the patient's response to each treatment.
▶ Record all teaching sessions with the patient and his family.

## Related procedures
▶ Cast preparation
▶ Cervical collar application
▶ Clavicle strap application
▶ Cold application
▶ Physical assessment
▶ Splint application
▶ Triangular sling application

### REFERENCES
Bayley, E., and Turke, S. *A Comprehensive Curriculum for Trauma Nursing.* Boston: Jones & Bartlett, 1999.
Emergency Nurses Association. *Trauma Nursing Core Course,* 5th ed. Park Ridge, Ill.: Emergency Nurses Association, 2000.
Hoover, T.J., and Siefert, J.A. "Soft Tissue Complications of Orthopedic Emergencies," *Emergency Medicine Clinics of North America* 18(1):115-39, 2000.
Moore, E., et al. *Trauma,* 4th ed. New York: McGraw-Hill, 2000
Perron, A.D., et al. "Orthopedic Pitfalls in the ED: Acute Compartment Syndrome," *American Journal of Emergency Medicine* 19(5):413-16, September 2001.

### ORGANIZATIONS
American College of Surgeons: *www.facs.org*
Emergency Nurses Association: *www.ena.org*

# Procedures

# Bryant's traction

Also called vertical suspension, Bryant's traction is used primarily to reduce developmental hip dislocations in children. With the patient lying supine in a bed or crib, the traction extends the legs vertically at a 90-degree angle to the body. Even if the disorder affects only one leg, the patient will have traction applied to both legs to prevent hip rotation and to ensure equal stress on the legs and even, bilateral bone growth.

Bryant's traction continues for 2 to 4 weeks. Afterward, the patient may be immobilized in a hip-spica cast. (See *Maintaining body alignment and traction,* page 538.)

Usually chosen for children under age 2 who weigh 25 to 30 lb (11.5 to 14 kg), Bryant's traction is contraindicated for heavier children because the risk of positional hypertension rises with increased weight.

## Equipment
Traction setup (supplied by the orthopedic department) ● moleskin traction straps ● elastic bandages ● foam rubber padding ● cotton balls ● compound benzoin tincture ● adhesive tape ● jacket restraint ● optional: safety razor, cotton batting, convoluted foam mattress, and sheepskin pad

### Preparation of equipment
Assist the doctor and orthopedic technician with measuring and cutting the moleskin straps and with assembling the traction equipment.

## Implementation
▶ Thoroughly explain the purpose and function of the traction to enhance learning and alleviate patient and family anxiety. If

## Maintaining body alignment and traction

Keeping the patient's body in the correct position with Bryant's traction requires precision and continual supervision and adjustment.

At the same time that the traction apparatus holds the patient's legs perpendicular to the mattress, you'll need to ensure that the patient's buttocks stay slightly elevated to provide countertraction and that his shoulders stay flat and in the same position on the mattress to maintain body alignment.

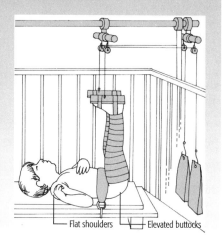

Flat shoulders — — Elevated buttocks

possible, use visual aids to illustrate your teaching. Keep a diagram handy for parents and a doll in traction for the patient.

▶ Ask the parents whether their child is sensitive or allergic to rubber or to adhesive tape.

▶ If the patient has hairy legs, shave or clip the hair with a safety razor to ensure good contact between the moleskin traction straps and the skin. Use soap, warm water, and long, downward strokes to minimize nicking.

▶ Use cotton balls to apply the compound benzoin tincture, if ordered, to the patient's legs to protect the skin.

▶ Assist the doctor or orthopedic technician with placing foam rubber padding and moleskin traction straps against the patient's legs and securing the straps with elastic bandages from foot to thigh. Secure the elastic bandages with adhesive tape. If the patient is allergic to rubber or to adhesive tape, wrap the legs in cotton batting before applying the straps.

▶ If necessary to keep the patient positioned properly, apply a jacket restraint to keep the weights from pulling the patient forward and altering the tractional force.

▶ Carefully monitor the circulatory status of the patient's legs 15 minutes and 30 minutes after applying initial traction. Then check circulatory status every 4 hours to detect any impairment caused by

traction. Assess capillary refill, skin color, sensation, movement, temperature, peripheral pulses, and bandage tightness. If you detect circulatory compromise, loosen the elastic bandages and notify the patient's doctor.

▶ Take care to position the elastic bandages precisely. Unless contraindicated, periodically remove the bandages from the unaffected leg to assess circulation and provide skin care. When doing so, have another person hold the traction straps in place to prevent slipping. Don't unwrap the affected leg unless ordered to do so by the patient's doctor.

▶ Check the patient's position regularly to ensure optimum traction. Make sure to raise the patient's buttocks high enough off the mattress to allow one hand to slide between the skin and the mattress. Avoid raising the buttocks too high, though, because this may reduce the effectiveness of traction.

▶ Try marking the bed sheet with an "X" at the correct shoulder position as a guide to correct body alignment. Near the patient's bed, post an illustration of the correct alignment to guide other nurses and caregivers.

▶ Provide skin care every 4 hours, focusing especially on the back, buttocks, and elbows, the areas most prone to breakdown. Place a convoluted foam mattress, a sheepskin pad, or both beneath the patient to help prevent or alleviate skin problems.

▶ Inspect the traction apparatus at least every 2 hours to ensure the correct weight. Make sure that the weights hang freely, the pulleys glide easily, the ropes aren't frayed, and the knots remain snugly tied and taped.

▶ Encourage the patient to take deep breaths at least every 2 hours to minimize his risk of developing hypostatic pneumonia.

▶ Review the patient's diet to ensure that he consumes enough fiber and fluid to prevent constipation and urinary stasis. (Infants should consume about 130 ml of fluid for each kilogram of body weight every 24 hours; toddlers should consume about 115 ml/kg.)

▶ Promote safety by keeping the side rails raised on the patient's bed whenever you aren't at the bedside.

### Special considerations

▶ To promote regular deep breathing and guard against pneumonia, allow the patient to blow a horn, whistle, pinwheel, or bubbles heartily or encourage him to sing. This promotes lung expansion and enjoyment at the same time.

▶ Because a child can't always tell you that he's in pain, carefully observe his behavior, facial expression, and cry to judge his discomfort level. In addition to needing an analgesic or sedative, the patient may need an antispasmodic medication to relieve irritable muscles and prevent muscle spasms.

▶ To foster development, diversion, and mobility, provide age-appropriate games and activities as permitted within the confines of traction. For infants, this can include mobiles, music boxes, and rattles. Toddlers may enjoy puppets, large-pieced puzzles, and dolls. Involve the family in their child's care and recreational activities to increase the patient's sense of security and to minimize the family's sense of anxiety. If facility policy permits, consider moving the infant's crib to the playroom so that he can be around other children.

▶ Eating and drinking are difficult and inconvenient for the patient in Bryant's traction because of the head-down position. To facilitate digestion and encourage eating, especially if the patient refuses food, place a small pillow under his head at mealtime.

If possible, allow him to choose his own foods and encourage his family to bring food from home.

▶ To minimize patient movement, change bed linens every other day unless the linens get wet or soiled. Keep sheets taut and wrinkle-free to help prevent skin breakdown.

### Complications

Although generally safe, Bryant's traction may lead to pneumonia from restricted lung expansion resulting from the head-down position. Skin necrosis may result from bandages wrapped too tightly. Other complications include urinary stasis and constipation.

### Documentation

▶ Record the date and time that traction was applied, the amount of weight applied, and the patient's circulatory status, skin condition, and position.

▶ Note whether weights hang freely.

▶ Document changes in the patient's status and describe the patient's and family's responses to the traction.

▶ Note the patient's and family's responses to any patient teaching.

### REFERENCES

Edward, D., et al. *Bedside Critical Care Manual.* Philadelphia: Lippincott Williams & Wilkins, 2001.

Pape, H.C., et al. "Changes in the Management of Femoral Shaft Fractures in Polytrauma Patients: From Early Total Care to Damage Control Orthopedic Surgery," *The Journal of Trauma* 53(3):452-61, September 2002.

# Cast preparation

A cast is a hard mold that encases a body part, usually an extremity, to provide immobilization of bones and surrounding tissue. It can be used to treat injuries (including fractures), correct orthopedic conditions (such as deformities), or promote healing after general or plastic surgery, amputation, or nerve and vascular repair.

Casts may be constructed of plaster, fiberglass, or other synthetic materials. Plaster, a commonly used material, is inexpensive, nontoxic, nonflammable, easy to

## Types of cylindrical casts

Made of plaster, fiberglass, or synthetic material, casts may be applied almost anywhere on the body to support a single finger or the entire body. Common casts are shown here.

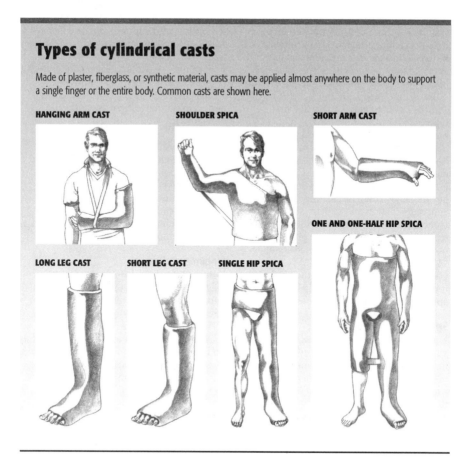

**HANGING ARM CAST**

**SHOULDER SPICA**

**SHORT ARM CAST**

**ONE AND ONE-HALF HIP SPICA**

**LONG LEG CAST**   **SHORT LEG CAST**   **SINGLE HIP SPICA**

mold, and rarely causes allergic reactions or skin irritation. However, fiberglass is lighter, stronger, and more resilient than plaster. Because fiberglass dries rapidly, it is more difficult to mold, but it can bear body weight immediately if needed. (See *Types of cylindrical casts.*)

Typically, a doctor applies a cast and a nurse prepares the patient and the equipment and assists during the procedure. With special preparation, a nurse may apply or change a standard cast, but an orthopedist must reduce the fracture and set the fracture.

Contraindications for casting may include skin diseases, peripheral vascular disease, diabetes mellitus, open or draining wounds, overwhelming edema, and susceptibility to skin irritations. However, these aren't strict contraindications; the doctor must weigh the potential risks and benefits for each patient.

### Equipment

Tubular stockinette ● casting material ● plaster rolls ● plaster splints (if necessary) ● bucket of water ● sink equipped with plaster trap ● linen-saver pad ● sheet wadding ● sponge or felt padding (if necessary) ● pillows or bath blankets ● cast scissors, cast saw, and cast spreader (for removing a cast) ● optional: rubber gloves, cast stand, moleskin or adhesive tape

Gather the tubular stockinette, cast material, and plaster splints in the appropriate sizes. Tubular stockinettes range from 2″ to 12″ (5 to 30.5 cm) wide; plaster rolls, from 2″ to 6″ (5 to 15 cm) wide; and plaster splints, from 3″ to 6″ (8 to 15 cm) wide. Wear rubber gloves, especially if applying a fiberglass cast.

### Preparation of equipment

Gently squeeze the packaged casting material to make sure the envelopes don't have any air leaks. Humid air penetrating such leaks can cause plaster to become stale, which can make it set too quickly, form lumps, fail to bond with lower layers, or set as a soft, friable mass. (Baking a stale plaster roll at a medium temperature for 1 hour can make it usable again.)

Follow the manufacturer's directions for water temperature when preparing plaster. Usually, room temperature or slightly warmer water is best because it allows the cast to set in about 7 minutes without excessive exothermia. (Cold water retards the rate of setting and may be used to facilitate difficult molding; warm water speeds the rate of setting and raises skin temperature under the cast.) Place all equipment within the doctor's reach.

## Implementation

▶ To ease the patient's fears, explain the procedure. If plaster is being used, make sure he understands that heat will build under the cast because of a chemical reaction between the water and plaster. Also begin explaining some aspects of proper cast care to prepare him for patient teaching and to assess his knowledge level.
▶ Cover the appropriate parts of the patient's bedding and gown with a linen-saver pad.
▶ If the cast is applied to the wrist or arm, remove rings that may interfere with circulation in the fingers.
▶ Assess the condition of the skin in the affected area, noting any redness, contusions, or open wounds. This will make it easier to evaluate any complaints the patient may have after the cast is applied.
▶ If the patient has an open wound, prepare him for a local anesthetic if the doctor will administer one. Clean the wound. Assist the doctor as he closes the wound and applies a dressing.
▶ To establish baseline measurements, assess neurovascular status. Palpate the distal pulses; assess the color, temperature, and capillary refill of the appropriate fingers or toes; and check neurologic function, including sensation and motion in the affected and unaffected extremities.
▶ Help the doctor position the limb as ordered. (Commonly, the limb is immobilized in the neutral position.)
▶ Support the limb in the prescribed position while the doctor applies the tubular stockinette and sheet wadding. The stock-

inette should extend beyond the ends of the cast to pad the edges. (If the patient has an open wound or a severe contusion, the doctor may not use the stockinette.) He then wraps the limb in sheet wadding, starting at the distal end, and applies extra wadding to the distal and proximal ends of the cast area, as well as any points of prominence. As he applies the sheet wadding, check for wrinkles.
▶ Prepare the various cast materials, as ordered.

### Preparing a plaster cast

▶ Place a roll of plaster casting on its end in the bucket of water. Make sure to immerse it completely. When air bubbles stop rising from the roll, remove it, gently squeeze out the excess water and hand the casting material to the doctor, who will begin applying it to the extremity. As he applies the first roll, prepare a second roll in the same manner. (Stay at least one roll ahead of the doctor during the procedure.)
▶ After the doctor applies each roll, he'll smooth it to remove wrinkles, spread the plaster into the cloth webbing, and empty air pockets. If he's using plaster splints, he'll apply them in the middle layers of the cast. Before wrapping the last roll, he'll pull the ends of the tubular stockinette over the cast edges to create padded ends, prevent cast crumbling, and reduce skin irritation. He'll then use the final roll to keep the ends of the stockinette in place.

### Preparing a fiberglass cast

▶ If you're using water-activated fiberglass, immerse the tape rolls in tepid water for 10 to 15 minutes to initiate the chemical reaction that causes the cast to harden. Open one roll at a time. Avoid squeezing out excess water before application.
▶ If you're using light-cured fiberglass, you can unroll the material more slowly. This casting remains soft and malleable until it's exposed to ultraviolet light, which sets it.

### Completing the cast

▶ As necessary, "petal" the cast's edges to reduce roughness and to cushion pressure points. (See *How to petal a cast,* page 542.)
▶ Use a cast stand or your palm to support the cast in the therapeutic position until it becomes firm (usually 6 to 8 minutes) to prevent indentations in the cast. Place the cast on a firm smooth surface to continue

## How to petal a cast

Rough cast edges can be cushioned by petaling them with adhesive tape or moleskin. To do this, first cut several 4" × 2" (10 × 5 cm) strips. Round off one end of each strip to keep it from curling. Then, making sure the rounded end of the strip is on the outside of the cast, tuck the straight end just inside the cast edge.

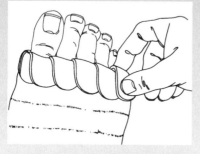

Smooth the moleskin with your finger until you're sure it's secured inside and out. Repeat the procedure, overlapping the moleskin pieces until you've gone all the way around the cast edge.

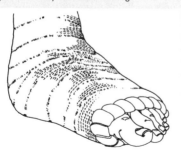

drying. Place pillows under joints to maintain flexion, if necessary.

▶ To check circulation in the casted limb, palpate the distal pulse and assess the color, temperature, and capillary refill of the fingers or toes. Determine neurologic status by asking the patient if he's experiencing paresthesia in the extremity or decreased motion of the extremity's uncovered joints. Assess the unaffected extremity in the same manner and compare findings.

▶ Elevate the limb above heart level with pillows or bath blankets as ordered to facilitate venous return and reduce edema.

▶ The doctor will then send the patient for X-rays to ensure proper positioning.

▶ Instruct the patient to notify the doctor of any pain, foul odor, drainage, or burning sensation under the cast. (After the cast hardens, the doctor may cut a window in it to inspect the painful or burning area.)

▶ Pour water from the plaster bucket into a sink containing a plaster trap. Don't use a regular sink because plaster will block the plumbing.

### Special considerations

▶ A fiberglass cast dries immediately after application. A plaster extremity cast dries in approximately 24 to 48 hours; a plaster spica or body cast, in 48 to 72 hours. During this drying period, the cast must be properly positioned to prevent a surface depression that could cause pressure areas or dependent edema. Neurovascular status must be assessed, drainage monitored, and the condition of the cast checked periodically.

▶ After the cast dries completely, it looks white and shiny and no longer feels damp or soft. Care consists of monitoring for changes in the drainage pattern, preventing skin breakdown near the cast, and averting the complications of immobility.

▶ Patient teaching must begin immediately after the cast is applied and should continue until the patient or a family member can care for the cast.

▶ Never use the bed or a table to support the cast as it sets because molding can result, causing pressure necrosis of underlying tissue. Also, don't use rubber- or plastic-covered pillows before the cast hardens because they can trap heat under the cast.

▶ If a cast is applied after surgery or traumatic injury, remember that the most accurate way to assess for bleeding is to monitor vital signs. A visible blood spot on the cast can be misleading: One drop of blood can produce a circle 3" (7.6 cm) in diameter.

▶ The doctor usually removes the cast at the appropriate time, with a nurse assisting. (See *Removing a cast.*)

Tell the patient that when the cast is removed, his casted limb will appear thinner and flabbier than the uncasted limb. In addition, his skin will appear yellowish or gray from the accumulated dead skin and oils from the glands near the skin surface.

# Removing a cast

Typically, a cast is removed when a fracture heals or requires further manipulation. Less common indications include cast damage, a pressure ulcer under the cast, excessive drainage or bleeding, and a constrictive cast.

Explain the procedure to the patient. Tell him he'll feel some heat and vibration as the cast is split with the cast saw. If the patient is a child, tell him that the saw is very noisy but won't cut the skin beneath. Warn the patient that when the padding is cut, he'll see discolored skin and signs of poor muscle tone. Reassure him that you'll stay with him. The illustrations here show how a plaster cast is removed.

| | | |
|---|---|---|
| The doctor cuts one side of the cast, then the other. As he does so, closely monitor the patient's anxiety level. | Next, the doctor opens the cast pieces with a spreader. | Finally, using cast scissors, the doctor cuts through the cast padding. |

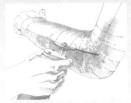 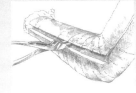 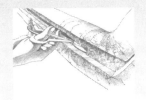

When the cast is removed, provide skin care to remove accumulated dead skin and to begin restoring the extremity's normal appearance.

---

Reassure him that with exercise and good skin care, his limb will return to normal.

▶ A procedure called "windowing" may be initiated on a cast to allow the nurse or physician to visualize wounds under the cast or to remove drains. Additionally, windowing can allow pulse assessment.

▶ Bivalving is cutting the cast lengthwise along both sides and then applying a device such as an Ace wrap or splint. Bivalving is generally done to decrease pressure on underlying tissue.

## Home care

Before the patient goes home, teach him how to care for his cast. Tell him to keep the casted limb elevated above heart level to minimize swelling. Raise a casted leg by having the patient lie in a supine position with his leg on top of pillows. Prop a casted arm so that the hand and elbow are higher than the shoulder.

Instruct the patient to call the doctor if he can't move his fingers or toes, if he has numbness or tingling in the affected limb, or if he has signs or symptoms of infection, such as fever, unusual pain, or a foul odor from the cast. Advise him to maintain muscle strength by continuing any recommended exercises.

If the cast needs repair (if it loosens, cracks, or breaks) or if the patient has any questions about cast care, advise him to notify his doctor. Warn him not to get the cast wet. Moisture will weaken or destroy it. If the doctor approves, have the patient cover the cast with a plastic bag or cast cover for showering or bathing.

Urge the patient not to insert anything (such as a back scratcher or powder) into the cast to relieve itching. Foreign matter can damage the skin and cause an infection. Tell him, though, that he can apply alcohol on the skin at the cast edges. Warn the patient not to chip, crush, cut, or otherwise break any area of the cast and not to bear weight on the cast unless instructed to do so by the doctor.

If the patient must use crutches, instruct him to remove throw rugs from the floor and to rearrange furniture to reduce the risk of tripping and falling. If the patient has a cast on his dominant arm, he may need help with bathing, toileting, eating, and dressing.

## Complications

Complications of improper cast application include compartment syndrome, palsy, paresthesia, ischemia, ischemic myositis, pressure necrosis and, eventually, misalignment or nonunion of fractured bones.

## Documentation

Record the date and time of cast application and skin condition of the extremity before the cast was applied. Note contusions, redness, or open wounds; results of neurovascular checks, before and after application, for the affected and unaffected extremities; location of any special devices, such as felt pads or plaster splints; and any patient teaching.

### REFERENCES

Armstrong, D.G., et al. "Technique for Fabrication of an 'Instant Total-contact Cast' for Treatment of Neuropathic Diabetic Foot Ulcers," *Journal of the American Podiatric Medical Association* 92(7):405-408, July-August 2002.

Kowalski, K.L., et al. "Evaluation of Fiberglass Versus Plaster of Paris for Immobilization of Fractures of the Arm and Leg," *Military Medicine* 167(8):657-61, August 2002.

## Cervical collar application

A cervical collar may be used for an acute injury (such as strained cervical muscles) or a chronic condition (such as arthritis or cervical metastasis). Or it may augment such splinting devices as a spine board to prevent potential cervical spine fracture or spinal cord damage.

Designed to hold the neck straight with the chin slightly elevated and tucked in, the collar immobilizes the cervical spine, decreases muscle spasms, and reduces pain; it also prevents further injury and promotes healing. As symptoms of an acute injury subside, the patient may gradually discontinue wearing the collar, alternating periods of wear with increasing periods of removal, until he no longer needs the collar.

## Equipment

Cervical collar in the appropriate size • optional: cotton (for padding) (See *Types of cervical collars*.)

## Types of cervical collars

Cervical collars are used to support an injured or weakened cervical spine and to maintain alignment during healing.

Made of rigid plastic, the molded cervical collar holds the patient's neck firmly, keeping it straight, with the chin slightly elevated and tucked in.

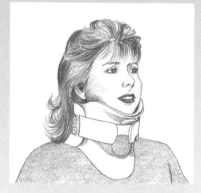

The soft cervical collar, made of spongy foam, provides gentler support and reminds the patient to avoid cervical spine motion.

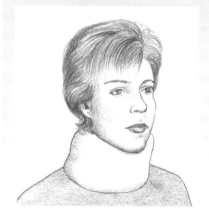

## Implementation

▶ Check the patient's neurovascular status before application.
▶ Instruct the patient to position his head slowly to face directly forward.
▶ Place the cervical collar in front of the patient's neck to ensure that the size is correct.

▶ Fit the collar snugly around the neck and attach the Velcro fasteners or buckles at the back of the neck.
▶ Check the patient's airway and his neurovascular status to ensure that the collar isn't too tight.

## Special considerations
▶ For a sprain or a potential cervical spine fracture, make sure the collar isn't too high in front because this may hyperextend the neck. In a neck sprain, such hyperextension may cause ligaments to heal in a shortened position. In a potential cervical spine fracture, hyperextension may cause serious neurologic damage.
▶ If the patient complains of pressure, the collar may be too tight. Remove and reapply it. If the patient complains of skin irritation or friction, the collar itself may be irritating him. Apply protective cotton padding between the irritated skin and the collar.

## Home care
Teach the patient how to apply the collar and how to do a neurovascular check. Have the patient demonstrate how to apply the collar after you have instructed him. Some collars are complex and the patient (or caregiver) may need to practice if he will be responsible for application. If indicated, advise sleeping without a pillow.

## Documentation
▶ Note the type and size of the cervical collar and the time and date of application in your notes. Record the results of neurovascular checks.
▶ Document patient comfort, the collar's snugness, and all patient instructions.

### REFERENCES
March, J.A., et al. "Changes in Physical Examination Caused by Use of Spinal Immobilization," *Prehospital Emergency Care* 6(4):421-24, October-December 2002.
Webber-Jones, J.E., et al. "The Management and Prevention of Rigid Cervical Collar Complications," *Orthopedic Nursing* 21(4): 19-25; quiz 25-27, July-August 2002. (Review.)

# Clavicle strap application

Also called a figure-eight strap, a clavicle strap reduces and immobilizes fractures of the clavicle. It does this by elevating, extending, and supporting the shoulders in position for healing, known as the position of attention. A commercially available figure-eight strap or a 4″ elastic bandage may serve as a clavicle strap. This strap is contraindicated for an uncooperative patient.

## Equipment
Powder or cornstarch ● figure-eight clavicle strap or 4″ elastic bandage ● safety pins, if necessary ● tape ● cotton batting or padding ● marking pen ● analgesics as ordered ● optional: scissors

## Implementation
▶ Explain the procedure to the patient and provide privacy.
▶ Help the patient take off his shirt or cut off the shirt if movement is too painful.
▶ Assess neurovascular integrity by palpating skin temperature; noting the color of the hand and fingers; palpating the radial, ulnar, and brachial pulses bilaterally; and then comparing the affected side with the unaffected side. Ask the patient about any numbness or tingling distal to the injury and assess his motor function.
▶ Determine the patient's degree of comfort and administer analgesics, as ordered.
▶ Demonstrate how to assume the position of attention. Instruct the patient to sit upright and assume this position gradually to minimize pain.
▶ Gently apply powder as appropriate to the axillae and shoulder area to reduce friction from the clavicle strap. You can use cornstarch if the patient is allergic to powder.

### Applying a figure-eight strap
▶ Place the apex of the triangle between the scapulae and drape the straps over the shoulders. Bring the strap with the Velcro or buckle end under one axilla and through the loop; then pull the other strap under the other axilla and through the loop. (See *Types of clavicle straps*, page 546.)
▶ Gently adjust the straps so they support the shoulders in the position of attention.
▶ Bring the straps back under the axillae toward the anterior chest, making sure that they maintain the position of attention.

# Types of clavicle straps

Clavicle straps provide support to the shoulder to help heal a fractured clavicle. These straps are available ready-made. They can also be made from a bandage.

Commercially made clavicle straps have a short back panel and long straps that extend around the patient's shoulders and axillae. They have Velcro pads or buckles on the ends for easy fastening.

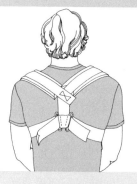

When making a clavicle strap with a wide elastic bandage, start in the middle of the patient's back. After wrapping the bandage around the shoulders, fasten the ends with safety pins.

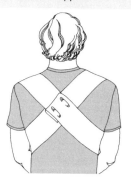

### Applying a 4″ elastic bandage

▶ Roll both ends of the elastic bandage toward the middle, leaving between 12″ and 18″ (30.5 to 46 cm) unrolled.

▶ Place the unrolled portion diagonally across the patient's back, from right shoulder to left axilla.

▶ Bring the lower end of the bandage under the left axilla and back over the left shoulder; loop the upper end over the right shoulder and under the axilla.

▶ Pull the two ends together at the center of the back so that the bandage supports the position of attention.

### Completing a figure-eight strap or elastic bandage

▶ Secure the ends using safety pins, Velcro pads, or a buckle, depending on the equipment. Make sure a buckle or any sharp edges face away from the skin. Tape the secured ends to the underlying strap or bandage.

▶ Place cotton batting or padding under the straps, as well as under the buckle or pins, to avoid skin irritation.

▶ Use a pen to mark the strap at the site of the loop of the figure-eight strap or the site where the elastic bandage crosses on the patient's back. If the strap loosens, this mark helps you tighten it to the original position.

▶ Assess neurovascular integrity, which may be impaired by a strap that is too tight. If neurovascular integrity is compromised when the strap is correctly applied, notify the doctor. He may want to change the treatment.

### Special considerations

▶ If possible, perform the procedure with the patient standing. However, this may not be feasible because the pain from the fracture can cause syncope. If the patient can't stand, have him sit upright.

▶ An adult with a clavicle strap made from an elastic bandage may require a triangular sling to help support the weight of the arm, enhance immobilization, and reduce pain. For a small child or a confused adult, a well-molded plaster jacket is needed to ensure immobilization. Inadequate immobilization can cause improper healing.

▶ Instruct the patient not to remove the clavicle strap. Explain that, with help, he can maintain proper hygiene by lifting segments of the strap to remove the cotton and by washing and powdering the skin daily. Explain that fresh cotton should be applied after cleaning.

▶ For a hospitalized patient, monitor the position of the strap by checking the pen markings every 8 hours. Also assess neurovascular integrity. Teach the outpatient how to assess his own neurovascular in-

tegrity and to recognize symptoms to report promptly to the doctor.
> Clavicle straps are typically worn for 4 to 8 weeks.

## Documentation
> In the appropriate section of the emergency department sheet or in your notes, record the date and time of strap application, type of clavicle strap, use of powder and padding, bilateral neurovascular integrity before and after the procedure, and instructions to the patient.

### REFERENCES
Edward, D., et al. *Bedside Critical Care Manual.* Philadelphia: Lippincott Williams & Wilkins, 2001.
Wentz, S., et al. "Reconstruction Plate Fixation with Bone Graft for Mid-shaft Clavicular Non-union in Semi-professional Athletes," *Journal of Orthopaedic Science* 4(4): 269-72, 1999.

## Electrical bone growth stimulation

By imitating the body's natural electrical forces, electrical bone growth stimulation initiates or accelerates the healing process in a fractured bone that fails to heal. About 1 in 20 fractures may fail to heal properly, possibly as a result of infection, insufficient reduction or fixation, pseudarthrosis, or severe tissue trauma around the fracture.

Recent discoveries about the stimulating effects of electrical currents on osteogenesis have led to using electrical bone stimulation to promote healing. The technique is also being investigated for treating spinal fusions.

Three basic electrical bone stimulation techniques are available: fully implantable direct current stimulation, semi-invasive percutaneous stimulation, and noninvasive electromagnetic coil stimulation. (See *Methods of electrical bone growth stimulation.*)

Choice of technique depends on the fracture type and location, the doctor's preference, and the patient's ability and willingness to comply. The invasive device requires little or no patient involvement. With the other two methods, however, the patient must manage his own treatment

## Methods of electrical bone growth stimulation

Electrical bone growth stimulation may be invasive or noninvasive.

### Invasive system
An invasive system involves placing a spiral cathode inside the bone at the fracture site. A wire leads from the cathode to a battery-powered generator, also implanted in local tissues. The patient's body completes the circuit.

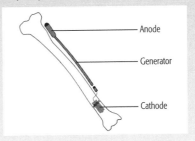

- Anode
- Generator
- Cathode

### Noninvasive system
A noninvasive system may include a cufflike transducer or fitted ring that wraps around the patient's limb at the level of the injury. Electric current penetrates the limb.

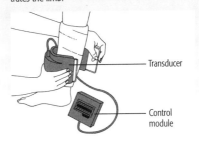

- Transducer
- Control module

schedule and maintain the equipment. Treatment time averages 3 to 6 months.

## Equipment
*For direct current stimulation*
Equipment set (a small generator with leadwires that connect to a titanium cathode wire that is surgically implanted into the nonunited bone site)

*For percutaneous stimulation*
Equipment set (an external anode skin pad with a leadwire, lithium battery pack, and

one to four Teflon-coated stainless steel cathode wires that are surgically implanted)

*For electromagnetic stimulation*
Equipment set (a generator that plugs into a standard 110-V outlet and two strong electromagnetic coils, which can be incorporated into a cast, cuff, or orthotic device, that are placed on either side of the injured area)

### Preparation of equipment

All equipment comes in sets with instructions provided by the manufacturer. Follow the instructions carefully. Make sure that all parts are included and are sterilized according to facility policy and procedure.

## Implementation

▶ Tell the patient whether he'll have an anesthetic and, if possible, which kind.

### Direct current stimulation

▶ Implantation is performed under general anesthesia. Afterward, the doctor may apply a cast or external fixator to immobilize the limb. The patient is usually hospitalized for 2 to 3 days after implantation. Weight bearing may be ordered, as tolerated.

▶ After the bone fragments join, the generator and leadwire can be removed under local anesthesia. The titanium cathode remains implanted.

### Percutaneous stimulation

▶ Remove excessive body hair from the injured site before applying the anode pad. Avoid stressing or pulling on the anode wire. Instruct the patient to change the anode pad every 48 hours. Tell him to report any local pain to his doctor and not to bear weight for the duration of treatment.

### Electromagnetic stimulation

▶ Show the patient where to place the coils and tell him to apply them for 3 to 10 hours each day as ordered by his doctor. Many patients find it most convenient to perform the procedure at night.

▶ Urge the patient not to interrupt the treatments for more than 10 minutes at a time.

▶ Teach the patient how to use and care for the generator.

▶ Relay the doctor's instructions for weight bearing. Usually, the doctor will advise against bearing weight until evidence of healing appears on X-rays.

## Special considerations

▶ A patient who receives direct current electrical bone stimulation shouldn't undergo electrocauterization, diathermy, or magnetic resonance imaging. Electrocautery may short the system; diathermy may potentiate the electrical current, possibly causing tissue damage; and magnetic resonance imaging will interfere with or stop the current.

▶ Percutaneous electrical bone stimulation is contraindicated in patients with any kind of inflammatory process. Ask the patient if he's sensitive to nickel or chromium; both are present in the electrical bone stimulation system.

▶ Electromagnetic coils are contraindicated for a pregnant patient, a patient with a tumor, or a patient with an arm fracture and a pacemaker.

## Home care

Teach the patient how to care for his cast or external fixation devices and for the electrical generator. Urge him to follow treatment instructions faithfully.

## Complications

Complications associated with any surgical procedure, including increased risk of infection, may occur with direct current electrical bone stimulation equipment. Local irritation or skin ulceration may occur around cathode pin sites with percutaneous devices. No complications are associated with the use of electromagnetic coils.

## Documentation

▶ Record the type of electrical bone stimulation equipment provided, including date, time, and location, as appropriate.

▶ Note the patient's skin condition and tolerance of the procedure.

▶ Record instructions given to the patient and family members as well as their ability to understand and act on those instructions.

### REFERENCES

Evans, R.D., et al. "Electrical Stimulation with Bone and Wound Healing," *Clinics in Podiatric Medicine and Surgery* 18(1):79-95, January 2001.

Patterson, M. "What's the Buzz on External Bone Growth Stimulators?" *Nursing* 30(6): 44-45, June 2000.

## External fixation

In external fixation, a doctor inserts metal pins through skin and muscle layers into the broken bones and affixes them to an adjustable external frame that maintains their proper alignment. (See *Types of external fixation devices*.)

This procedure is used most commonly to treat open, unstable fractures with extensive soft tissue damage, comminuted closed fractures, and septic, nonunion fractures and to facilitate surgical immobilization of a joint. Specialized types of external fixators may be used to lengthen leg bones or immobilize the cervical spine.

An advantage of external fixation over other immobilization techniques is that it stabilizes the fracture while allowing full visualization and access to open wounds. It also facilitates early ambulation, thus reducing the risk of complications from immobilization.

The Ilizarov fixator is a special type of external fixation device. This device is a combination of rings and tensioned transosseous wires used primarily in limb lengthening, bone transport, and limb salvage. Highly complex, it provides gradual distraction resulting in good-quality bone formation with a minimum of complications.

### Equipment

Sterile cotton-tipped applicators • prescribed antiseptic cleaning solution • ice bag • sterile gauze pads • povidone-iodine solution • analgesic or narcotic • optional: antimicrobial ointment

Equipment varies with the type of fixator and the type and location of the fracture. Typically, sets of pins, stabilizing rods, and clips are available from manufacturers. Don't reuse pins.

### Preparation of equipment

Make sure that the external fixation set includes all the equipment it's supposed to include and that the equipment has been sterilized according to your facility's procedure.

## Types of external fixation devices

The doctor's selection of an external fixation device depends on the severity of the patient's fracture and the type of bone alignment needed.

### Universal day frame

This device is used to manage tibial fractures. The frame allows the doctor to readjust the position of bony fragments by angulation and rotation. The compression-distraction device allows compression and distraction of bony fragments.

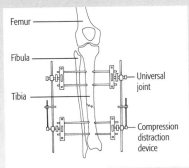

### Portsmouth external fixation bar

This device is used to manage complicated tibial fractures. The locking nut adjustment on the mobile carriage only allows bone compression, so the doctor must accurately reduce bony fragments before applying the device.

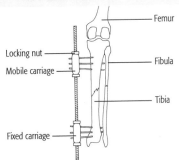

### Implementation

❯ Explain the procedure to the patient to reduce his anxiety. Assure him that he'll feel little pain after the fixation device is in place and that he'll be able to adjust to the apparatus.

▶ Tell the patient that he'll be able to move about with the apparatus in place, which may help him resume normal activities more quickly.

▶ After the fixation device is in place, perform neurovascular checks every 2 to 4 hours for 24 hours, then every 4 to 8 hours, as appropriate, to assess for possible neurologic damage. Assess color, motion, sensation, digital movement, edema, capillary refill, and pulses of the affected extremity. Compare with the unaffected side.

▶ Apply an ice bag to the surgical site, as ordered, to reduce swelling, relieve pain, and lessen bleeding.

▶ Administer analgesics or narcotics as ordered before exercising or mobilizing the affected extremity to promote comfort.

▶ Monitor the patient for pain not relieved by analgesics or narcotics and for burning, tingling, or numbness, which may indicate nerve damage or circulatory impairment.

▶ Elevate the affected extremity, if appropriate, to minimize edema.

▶ Perform pin-site care as ordered, to prevent infection. Pin-site care varies but you'll usually follow guidelines such as these: use sterile technique; avoid digging at pin sites with the cotton-tipped applicator; if ordered, clean the pin site and surrounding skin with a cotton-tipped applicator dipped in ordered antiseptic solution; if ordered, apply an antimicrobial ointment to the pin site; apply a loose sterile dressing, or dress with sterile gauze pads soaked in povidone-iodine solution. Perform pin-site care as often as necessary, depending on the amount of drainage.

▶ Also check for redness, tenting of the skin, prolonged or purulent drainage from the pin site, swelling, elevated body or pin-site temperature, and any bowing or bending of pins, which may stress the skin.

### For the patient with an Ilizarov fixator

▶ When the device has been placed and preliminary calluses have begun to form at the insertion sites (in 5 to 7 days), gentle distraction is initiated by turning the appropriate screws one-quarter turn (1 mm) every 4 to 6 hours, as ordered.

▶ Teach the patient that he must be consistent in turning the screws every 4 to 6 hours around the clock. Make sure he understands that he must be strongly committed to compliance with the protocol for the procedure to be successful. Because the treatment period may be prolonged (4 to 10 months), discuss with the patient and family members the psychological effects of long-term care.

▶ Don't administer nonsteroidal anti-inflammatory drugs (NSAIDs) to patients who are being treated with the Ilizarov fixator. NSAIDs may decrease the necessary inflammation caused by the distraction, resulting in delayed bone formation.

## Special considerations

▶ Before discharge, teach the patient and family members how to provide pin-site care. This is a sterile procedure in the facility, but clean technique can be used at home. Teach them how to recognize signs of pin-site infection.

▶ Tell the patient to keep the affected limb elevated when sitting or lying down.

## Complications

Complications of external fixation include loosening of pins and loss of fracture stabilization, infection of the pin tract or wound, skin breakdown, nerve damage, and muscle impingement.

Ilizarov fixator pin sites are more prone to infection because of the extended treatment period and because of the pins' movement to accomplish distraction. The pins are also more likely to break because of their small diameter. Also, the large number of pins used increases the patient's risk of neurovascular compromise.

## Documentation

▶ Assess and document the condition of the pin sites and skin.

▶ Document the patient's reaction to the apparatus and to ambulation as well as his understanding of teaching instructions.

### REFERENCES

Maher, A., et al. *Orthopaedic Nursing,* 3rd ed. Philadelphia: W.B. Saunders Co., 2002.

McKenzie, L.L. "In Search of a Standard for Pin Site Care," *Orthopaedic Nursing* 18(2):73-78, March-April 1999.

Schoen, D.C. *Core Curriculum for Orthopaedic Nursing,* 4th ed. Pitman, N.J.: National Association of Orthopaedic Nurses, 2001.

Sims, M., and Whiting, J. "Pin Site Care," *Nursing Times* 96(48):46, November-December 2000.

Smith, S., ed. *Orthopaedic Nursing Care Competencies: Adult Acute Care.* Pitman, N.J.: National Association of Orthopaedic Nurses, 1999.

## Hip-spica cast care

After orthopedic surgery to correct a fracture or deformity, a patient may need a hip-spica cast to immobilize both legs. Occasionally, the doctor may apply a hip-spica cast to treat an orthopedic deformity that doesn't require surgery.

Caring for a patient in a hip-spica cast poses several challenges, including protecting the cast from urine and feces, keeping the cast dry, ensuring proper blood supply to the legs, and teaching the patient and his parents how to care for the cast at home.

Infants usually adapt more easily to the cast than older children but both need encouragement, support, and diversionary activity during their prolonged immobilization.

### Equipment

Waterproof adhesive tape ● moleskin or plastic petals ● cast cutter or saw ● scissors ● nonabrasive cleaner ● hair dryer ● damp sponge or cloth ● optional: disposable diaper or perineal pad

### Implementation

❯ Before the doctor applies the cast, describe the procedure to the patient and his parents. For patients ages 3 to 12, illustrate your explanation. Draw a picture, present a diagram, or use a doll with a cast or an elastic gauze dressing wrapped around its trunk and limbs. (See *Understanding the hip-spica cast.*)

❯ After the doctor constructs the cast, keep all but the perineal area uncovered. Provide privacy by draping a small cover over this opening. Turn the patient every 1 to 2 hours to speed drying time. Make sure you turn the patient to his unaffected side to prevent adding pressure to the affected side. If the patient is an infant, you can turn him by yourself. If the patient is an older child or an adolescent, seek assistance before attempting to turn him. When turning the patient, don't use the stabilizer

### Understanding the hip-spica cast

As you talk with parents about their child's hip-spica cast, describe how it will extend from the child's lower rib margin (or sometimes from the nipple line) down to the tips of the toes on the affected side and to the knee on the opposite unaffected side. Also mention that it expands at the waist to allow the child to eat comfortably. A stabilizer bar positioned between the legs keeps the hips in slight abduction and separates the legs.

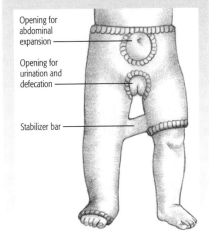

Opening for abdominal expansion

Opening for urination and defecation

Stabilizer bar

bar between his legs for leverage. Excessive pressure on this bar may disrupt the cast. Handle a damp cast only with your palms to avoid misshaping the cast material.

❯ After the cast dries, inspect the inside edges of the cast for stray pieces of casting material that can irritate the skin. (A traditional hip-spica cast requires 24 to 48 hours to dry. However, a hip-spica cast made from newer, quick-drying substances takes only 8 to 10 hours to dry. If made of fiberglass, it will dry in less than 1 hour.)

❯ Cut several petal-shaped pieces of moleskin using the scissors and place them, overlapping, around the open edges of the cast to protect the patient's skin. Use waterproof adhesive tape around the perineal area.

❯ Bathe the patient to remove any cast fragments from his skin.

▶ Assess the patient's legs for coldness, swelling, cyanosis, or mottling. Also assess pulse strength, toe movement, sensation (such as numbness, tingling, and burning), and capillary refill. Perform these circulatory assessments every 1 to 2 hours while the cast is wet and every 2 to 4 hours after the cast dries.

▶ If the cast is applied after surgery, remember that the most accurate way to assess for bleeding is to monitor vital signs. A visible blood spot on the cast can be misleading: One drop of blood can produce a circle 3″ (7.6 cm) in diameter.

▶ Check the patient's exposed skin for redness or irritation, and observe the patient for pain or discomfort caused by hot spots (pressure-sensitive areas under the cast). Also be alert for a foul odor. These signs and symptoms suggest a pressure ulcer or infection.

▶ To relieve itching, set a handheld hair dryer on "cool" and blow air under the cast. Warn the patient and his parents not to insert any object (such as a ruler, coat hanger, or knitting needle) into the cast to relieve itching by scratching because these objects could disrupt the suture line, break adjacent skin, and introduce infection. Also, be vigilant in ensuring that small objects or food particles don't become lodged under the cast and cause skin breakdown and infection.

▶ Encourage the patient's family to visit and participate in his care and recreation. This increases the patient's sense of security and enhances the parents' sense of participation and control.

### Special considerations

▶ If the patient is incontinent (or not toilet-trained), protect the cast from soiling. Tuck a folded disposable diaper or perineal pad around the perineal edges of the cast. Then apply a second diaper to the patient, over the top of the cast, to hold the first diaper in place. Also, tuck plastic petals into the cast to channel urine and feces into a bedpan. If the cast still becomes soiled, wipe it with a nonabrasive cleaner and a damp sponge or cloth. Then air-dry it with a hair dryer set on "cool."

▶ Keep a cast cutter or saw available at all times to remove the cast quickly in case of an emergency.

▶ During mealtimes, position older children on their abdomens to promote safer eating and swallowing.

▶ Before removing the cast, reassure the parents and the patient that the noisy sawing process is painless. If necessary, explain how the saw works.

### Home care

Before discharge, teach the parents how to care for the cast and give them an opportunity to demonstrate their understanding. Include instructions for checking circulatory status, recognizing signs of circulatory impairment, and notifying the doctor. Also demonstrate how to turn the child, apply moleskin, clean the cast, and ensure adequate nourishment.

Teach the parents to treat dry, scaly skin around the cast by washing the child's skin frequently. After the cast is removed, they may apply baby oil or other lotion to soothe the skin. Urge them to schedule and keep all follow-up medical appointments.

Teach the parents how to use a car restraint device, such as the E-Z-ON Vest, because the child won't be able to use a conventional car seat.

### Complications

Complications associated with a hip-spica cast come from immobility. They include constipation, urinary stasis, renal calculi, skin breakdown, respiratory compromise, and contractures. Frequent turnings, range-of-motion exercises, and adequate hydration and nutrition can minimize complications. Using an incentive spirometer can avoid respiratory complications.

### Documentation

▶ Record the date and time of cast care.
▶ Describe the circulatory status in the patient's legs and record measurements of any bleeding or drainage.
▶ Note the condition of the cast and the patient's skin. Describe all skin care given.
▶ Record findings of bowel and bladder assessments.
▶ Note patient and family tolerance of the cast.
▶ Document patient- and family-teaching topics discussed as well.

**REFERENCES**

Norman-Taylor, F.H., et al. "Risk of Refracture Through Unicameral Bone," *Journal of Pediatric Orthopedics* 22(2):249-54, March-April 2002.

Pasque, C.B., and Harbach, G.P. "Hip Spica Application Using an Operating Table Armboard," *Journal of Pediatric Orthopedics* 20(6):757-58, November-December 2000.

# Internal fixation

In internal fixation, also known as surgical reduction or open reduction-internal fixation, the doctor implants fixation devices to stabilize the fracture. Internal fixation devices include nails, screws, pins, wires, and rods, all of which may be used in combination with metal plates. These devices remain in the body indefinitely unless the patient experiences adverse reactions after the healing process is complete. (See *Reviewing internal fixation devices*, page 554.)

Internal fixation is typically used to treat fractures of the face and jaw, spine, arm or leg bones, and fractures involving a joint (most commonly, the hip). Internal fixation permits earlier mobilization and can shorten hospitalization, particularly in elderly patients with hip fractures.

## Equipment

Ice bag ● pain medication (analgesic or narcotic) ● incentive spirometer ● elastic stockings

Patients with leg fractures may also need: overhead frame with trapeze ● pressure-relief mattress ● crutches or walker ● pillow (hip fractures may require abductor pillows).

### Preparation of equipment

Equipment is collected and prepared in the operating room.

## Implementation

▶ Explain the procedure to the patient to allay his fears. Tell him what to expect during postoperative assessment and monitoring, teach him how to use an incentive spirometer, and prepare him for proposed exercise and progressive ambulation regimens if necessary. Instruct him to tell the doctor if he feels pain.

▶ After the procedure, monitor the patient's vital signs every 2 to 4 hours for 24 hours, then every 4 to 8 hours, according to your facility's protocol. Changes in vital signs may indicate hemorrhage or infection.

▶ Monitor fluid intake and output every 4 to 8 hours.

▶ Perform neurovascular checks every 2 to 4 hours for 24 hours, then every 4 to 8 hours as appropriate. Assess color, motion, sensation, digital movement, edema, capillary refill, and pulses of the affected area. Compare findings with the unaffected side.

▶ Apply an ice bag to the operative site, as ordered, to reduce swelling, relieve pain, and lessen bleeding.

▶ To promote comfort, administer analgesics or narcotics, as ordered, before exercising or mobilizing the affected area. If the patient is using patient-controlled analgesia, instruct him to administer a dose before exercising or mobilizing.

▶ Monitor the patient for pain unrelieved by analgesics or narcotics and for burning, tingling, or numbness, which may indicate infection or impaired circulation.

▶ Elevate the affected limb on a pillow, if appropriate, to minimize edema.

▶ Check surgical dressings for excessive drainage or bleeding. Also check the incision site for signs of infection, such as erythema, drainage, edema, and unusual pain.

▶ Assist and encourage the patient to perform range-of-motion and other muscle strengthening exercises, as ordered, to promote circulation, improve muscle tone, and maintain joint function.

▶ Teach the patient to perform progressive ambulation and mobilization using an overhead frame with trapeze, or crutches or a walker, as appropriate.

## Special considerations

▶ To avoid the complications of immobility after surgery, have the patient use an incentive spirometer.

▶ Apply elastic stockings and a sequential compression device, as appropriate. The patient may also require a pressure-relief mattress.

## Home care

Before discharge, teach the patient and family members how to care for the incision site and recognize signs and symptoms of wound infection. Also teach them

# Reviewing internal fixation devices

Choice of a specific internal fixation device depends on the location, type, and configuration of the fracture.

In trochanteric or subtrochanteric fractures, the surgeon may use a hip pin or nail, with or without a screw plate. A pin or plate with extra nails stabilizes the fracture by impacting the bone ends at the fracture site.

In an uncomplicated fracture of the femoral shaft, the surgeon may use an intramedullary rod. This device permits early ambulation with partial weight bearing.

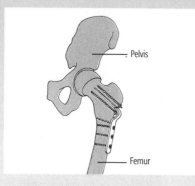

Pelvis

Femur

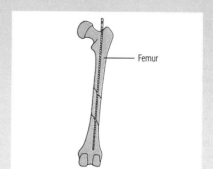

Femur

Another choice for fixation of a long-bone fracture is a screw plate, shown here on the tibia.

In an arm fracture, the surgeon may fix the involved bones with a plate, rod, or nail. Most radial and ulnar fractures may be fixed with plates, whereas humeral fractures are commonly fixed with rods.

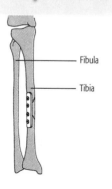

Fibula

Tibia

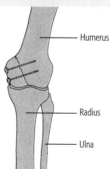

Humerus

Radius

Ulna

---

about administering pain medication, practicing an exercise regimen (if any), and using assistive ambulation devices (such as crutches or a walker), if appropriate.

## Complications

Wound infection and, more critically, infection involving metal fixation devices may require reopening the incision, draining the suture line, and possibly removing the fixation device. Any such infection

would require wound dressings and antibiotic therapy. Other complications may include malunion, nonunion, fat or pulmonary embolism, and neurovascular impairment.

## Documentation

▶ In the patient record, document perioperative findings on cardiovascular, respiratory, and neurovascular status.

❱ Note which pain management techniques were used.

❱ Describe wound appearance and alignment of the affected bone.

❱ Note the patient's response to teaching about appropriate exercise, care of the infection site, use of assistive devices (if appropriate), and symptoms that should be reported to the doctor.

## REFERENCES

Maher, A., et al. *Orthopaedic Nursing,* 3rd ed. Philadelphia: W.B. Saunders Co., 2002.

McKenzie, L.L. "In Search of a Standard for Pin Site Care," *Orthopaedic Nursing* 18(2):73-78, March-April 1999.

Schoen, D.C. *Core Curriculum for Orthopaedic Nursing,* 4th ed. Pitman, N.J.: National Association of Orthopaedic Nurses, 2001.

Sims, M., and Whiting, J. "Pin Site Care," *Nursing Times* 96(48):46, November-December 2000.

Smith, S., ed. *Orthopaedic Nursing Care Competencies: Adult Acute Care.* Pitman, N.J.: National Association of Orthopaedic Nurses, 1999.

# Mechanical traction

Mechanical traction exerts a pulling force on a part of the body, usually the spine, pelvis, or long bones of the arms and legs. It can be used to reduce fractures, treat dislocations, correct or prevent deformities, improve or correct contractures, or decrease muscle spasms. Depending on the injury or condition, an orthopedist may order either skin or skeletal traction.

Applied directly to the skin and thus indirectly to the bone, skin traction is ordered when a light, temporary, or noncontinuous pulling force is required. Contraindications for skin traction include a severe injury with open wounds, an allergy to tape or other skin traction equipment, circulatory disturbances, dermatitis, and varicose veins. In skeletal traction, an orthopedist inserts a pin or wire through the bone and attaches the traction equipment to the pin or wire to exert a direct, constant, longitudinal pulling force. Indications for skeletal traction include fractures of the tibia, femur, and humerus. Infections such as osteomyelitis contraindicate skeletal traction. Although physical therapy or

an orthopedic technician will probably set up the traction frames, you will need to be familiar with basic traction frames. (See *Traction frames,* page 556.)

The design of the patient's bed usually dictates whether to use a claw clamp or I.V.-post-type frame. (However, the claw-type Balkan frame is rarely used.) Setup of the specific traction can be done by a nurse with special skills, an orthopedic technician, or the doctor. Instructions for setting up these traction units usually accompany the equipment.

After the patient is placed in the specific type of traction ordered by the orthopedist, the nurse is responsible for preventing complications from immobility; for routinely inspecting the equipment; for adding traction weights, as ordered; and, in patients with skeletal traction, for monitoring the pin insertion sites for signs of infection. (See *Comparing types of traction,* page 557.)

## Equipment

*For a claw-type basic frame*
102″ (259 cm) plain bar ● two 66″ (168-cm) swivel-clamp bars ● two upper-panel clamps ● two lower-panel clamps

*For an I.V.-type basic frame*
102″ plain bar ● 27″ (69-cm) double-clamp bar ● 48″ (122-cm) swivel-clamp bar ● two 36″ (91.4-cm) plain bars ● four 4″ (10-cm) I.V. posts with clamps ● cross clamp

*For an I.V.-type Balkan frame*
Two 102″ plain bars ● two 27″ double-clamp bars ● two 48″ swivel-clamp bars ● five 36″ plain bars ● four 4″ I.V. posts with clamps ● eight cross clamps

*For all frame types*
Trapeze with clamp ● wall bumper or roller

*For skeletal traction care*
Sterile cotton-tipped applicators ● prescribed antiseptic solution ● sterile gauze pads ● povidone-iodine solution ● optional: antimicrobial ointment

## Preparation of equipment
Arrange with central supply or the appropriate department to have the traction equipment transported to the patient's room on a traction cart. If appropriate,

# Traction frames

You may encounter three types of traction frames, as described below.

### Claw-type basic frame
With this frame, claw attachments secure the uprights to the footboard and headboard.

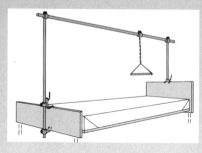

### I.V.-type basic frame
With this frame, I.V. posts, placed in I.V. holders, support the horizontal bars across the foot and head of the bed. These horizontal bars then support the two uprights.

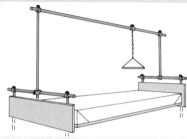

### I.V.-type Balkan frame
This frame features I.V. posts and horizontal bars (secured in the same manner as those for the I.V.-type basic frame) that support four uprights.

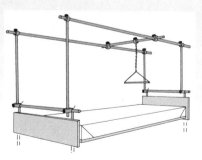

gather the equipment for pin-site care at the patient's bedside. Pin-site care protocols may vary with each facility or doctor.

## Implementation
Explain the purpose of traction to the patient. Emphasize the importance of maintaining proper body alignment after the traction equipment is set up.

■ **EVIDENCE BASE** Regardless of the type of traction used, several principles should be followed:
▶ Countertraction must always be provided by the patient's body weight, pull of weights in the opposite direction, or elevation of the bed.
▶ The line of the pull should be maintained at all times.
▶ The weights should hang freely at all times.
▶ Friction should be prevented on the traction apparatus.

### Setting up a claw-type basic frame
▶ Attach one lower-panel and one upper-panel clamp to each 66″ swivel-clamp bar.
▶ Fasten one bar to the footboard and one to the headboard by turning the clamp

knobs clockwise until they're tight and then pulling back on the upper clamp's rubberized bar until it's tight.
▶ Secure the 102″ horizontal plain bar atop the two vertical bars, making sure that the clamp knobs point up.
▶ Using the appropriate clamp, attach the trapeze to the horizontal bar about 2′ (60 cm) from the head of the bed.

### Setting up an I.V.-type basic frame
▶ Attach one 4″ I.V. post with clamp to each end of both 36″ horizontal plain bars.
▶ Secure an I.V. post in each I.V. holder at the bed corners. Using a cross clamp, fasten the 48″ vertical swivel-clamp bar to the middle of the horizontal plain bar at the foot of the bed.
▶ Fasten the 27″ vertical double-clamp bar to the middle of the horizontal plain bar at the head of the bed.
▶ Attach the 102″ horizontal plain bar to the tops of the two vertical bars, making sure the clamp knobs point up.
▶ Using the appropriate clamp, attach the trapeze to the horizontal bar about 2′ from the head of the bed.

### Setting up an I.V.-type Balkan frame
▶ Attach one 4″ I.V. post with clamp to each end of two 36″ horizontal plain bars.
▶ Secure an I.V. post in each I.V. holder at the bed corners.
▶ Attach a 48″ vertical swivel-clamp bar, using a cross clamp, to each I.V. post clamp on the horizontal plain bar at the foot of the bed.
▶ Fasten one 36″ horizontal plain bar across the midpoints of the two 48″ swivel-clamp bars, using two cross clamps.
▶ Attach a 27″ vertical double-clamp bar to each I.V. post clamp on the horizontal bar at the head of the bed.
▶ Using two cross clamps, fasten a 36″ horizontal plain bar across the midpoints of two 27″ double-clamp bars.
▶ Clamp a 102″ horizontal plain bar onto the vertical bars on each side of the bed, making sure the clamp knobs point up.
▶ Use two cross clamps to attach a 36″ horizontal plain bar across the two overhead bars, about 2′ from the head of the bed.
▶ Attach the trapeze to this 36″ horizontal bar.

## Comparing types of traction

Traction therapy applies a pulling force to an injured or diseased limb. For traction to be effective, it must be combined with an equal mix of countertraction. Weights provide the pulling force. Countertraction is produced by positioning the patient's body weight against the traction pull.

### Skin traction
This procedure immobilizes a body part intermittently over an extended period through direct application of a pulling force on the patient's skin. The force may be applied using adhesive or nonadhesive traction tape or other skin traction devices, such as a boot, belt, or halter.
    This traction exerts a light pull and uses up to 8 lb per extremity for an adult.

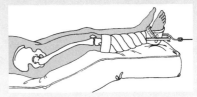

### Skeletal traction
This procedure immobilizes a body part for prolonged periods by attaching weighted equipment directly to the patient's bones. This may be accomplished with pins, screws, wires, or tongs. The amount of weight applied is determined by the patient's body size and extent of injury.

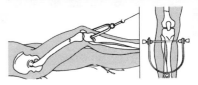

### After setting up any frame
▶ Attach a wall bumper or roller to the vertical bar or bars at the head of the bed. This protects the walls from damage caused by the bed or equipment.

### Caring for the traction patient
▶ Show the patient how much movement he's allowed and instruct him not to readjust the equipment. Also tell him to report

any pain or pressure from the traction equipment.

▶ At least once per shift, make sure that the traction equipment connections are tight. Check for impingements, such as ropes rubbing on the footboard or getting caught between pulleys. Friction and impingement reduce the effectiveness of traction.

▶ Inspect the traction equipment to ensure the correct alignment.

▶ Inspect the ropes for fraying, which can eventually cause a rope to break.

▶ Make sure the ropes are positioned properly in the pulley track. An improperly positioned rope changes the degree of traction.

▶ To prevent tampering and aid stability and security, make sure that all rope ends are taped above the knot.

▶ Inspect the equipment regularly to make sure that the traction weights hang freely. Weights that touch the floor, bed, or each other reduce the amount of traction.

▶ About every 2 hours, check the patient for proper body alignment and reposition the patient as necessary. Misalignment causes ineffective traction and may keep the fracture from healing properly.

▶ To prevent complications from immobility, assess neurovascular integrity routinely. The patient's condition, the hospital routine, and the doctor's orders determine the frequency of neurovascular assessments.

▶ Provide skin care, encourage coughing and deep breathing exercises, and assist with ordered range-of-motion exercises for unaffected extremities. Apply and maintain elastic support stockings, if they are used. Check elimination patterns and provide laxatives, as ordered.

▶ For the patient with skeletal traction, make sure that the protruding pin or wire ends are covered with cork to prevent them from tearing the bedding or injuring the patient and staff.

▶ Check the pin site and surrounding skin regularly for signs of infection.

▶ If ordered, clean the pin site and surrounding skin. Pin-site care varies, but you'll usually follow guidelines like these: use sterile technique; avoid digging at pin sites with the cotton-tipped applicator; if ordered, clean the pin site and surrounding skin with a cotton-tipped applicator dipped in ordered antiseptic; if ordered, apply antimicrobial ointment to the pin sites; apply a loose sterile dressing, or dress with sterile gauze pads soaked in povidone-iodine solution. Perform pin-site care as often as necessary, depending on the amount of drainage.

## Special considerations

▶ When using skin traction, apply ordered weights slowly and carefully to avoid jerking the affected extremity. To avoid injury in case the ropes break, arrange the weights so they don't hang over the patient.

▶ When applying Buck's traction, make sure the line of pull is always parallel to the bed and not angled downward to prevent pressure on the heel. Placing a flat pillow under the extremity may be helpful as long as it doesn't alter the line of pull.

## Complications

Immobility during traction may result in pressure ulcers; muscle atrophy, weakness, or contractures; and osteoporosis. Immobility can also cause GI disturbances, such as constipation; urinary problems, including stasis and calculi; respiratory problems, such as stasis of secretions and hypostatic pneumonia; and circulatory disturbances, including stasis and thrombophlebitis. Prolonged immobility, especially after traumatic injury, may promote depression or other emotional disturbances. Skeletal traction may cause osteomyelitis originating at the pin or wire sites.

## Documentation

▶ In the patient record, document the amount of traction weight used daily, noting the application of additional weights and the patient's tolerance.

▶ Document equipment inspections and patient care, including routine checks of neurovascular integrity, skin condition, respiratory status, and elimination patterns.

▶ If applicable, note the condition of the pin site and any care given.

**REFERENCES**

Maher, A.B., et al. *Orthopaedic Nursing,* 3rd ed. Philadelphia: W.B. Saunders Co., 2002.

McKenzie, L.L. "In Search of a Standard for Pin Site Care," *Orthopaedic Nursing* 18(2): 73-78, March-April 1999.

Sims, M., and Whiting, J. "Pin Site Care," *Nursing Times* 96(48):46, November-December 2000.

# Types of splints

Three kinds of splints are commonly used to help provide support for injured or weakened limbs or to help correct deformities.

A rigid splint can be used to immobilize a fracture or dislocation in an extremity. Ideally, two people should apply a rigid splint to an extremity.

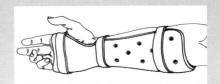

A traction splint immobilizes a fracture and exerts a longitudinal pull that reduces muscle spasms, pain, and arterial and neyral damage. Used primarily for femoral fractures, a traction splint may also be applied for a fractured hip or tibia. Two trained people should apply a traction splint.

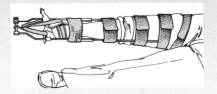

A spine board, applied for a suspected spinal fracture, is a rigid splint that supports the injured person's entire body. Three people should apply a spine board.

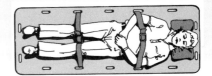

# Splint application

By immobilizing the site of an injury, a splint alleviates pain and allows the injury to heal in proper alignment. It also minimizes possible complications, such as excessive bleeding into tissues, restricted blood flow caused by bone pressing against vessels, and possible paralysis from an unstable spinal cord injury. In cases of multiple serious injuries, a splint or spine board allows caretakers to move the patient without risking further damage to bones, muscles, nerves, blood vessels, and skin.

A splint can be applied to immobilize a simple or compound fracture, a dislocation, or a subluxation. (See *Types of splints*.)

During an emergency, any injury suspected of being a fracture, dislocation, or subluxation should be splinted. No contraindications exist for rigid splints; don't use traction splints for upper extremity injuries and open fractures.

## Equipment

Rigid splint, spine board, traction splint, or Velcro support splint • bindings • padding • sandbags or rolled towels or clothing • optional: roller gauze • cloth strips • sterile compress • ice bag

Several commercial splints are widely available. Consult the manufacturer's instructions before applying the device. In an emergency, any long, sturdy object, such as a tree limb, mop handle, or broom—even a magazine—can be used to make a rigid splint for an extremity; a door can be used as a spine board.

An inflatable semirigid splint, called an air splint, sometimes can be used to secure an injured extremity. (See *Using an air splint*, page 560.)

Velcro straps, 2″ roller gauze, or 2″ cloth strips can be used as bindings. When improvising, avoid using twine or rope, if possible, because they can restrict circulation.

## Using an air splint

In an emergency, an air splint can be applied to immobilize a fracture or control bleeding, especially from a forearm or lower leg. This compact, comfortable splint is made of double-walled plastic and provides gentle, diffuse pressure over an injured area. The appropriate splint is chosen, wrapped around the affected extremity, secured with Velcro or other strips, and then inflated. The fit should be snug enough to immobilize the extremity without impairing circulation.

An air splint (shown below) may actually control bleeding better than a local pressure bandage. Its clear plastic construction simplifies inspection of the affected site for bleeding, pallor, or cyanosis. An air splint also allows the patient to be moved without further damage to the injured limb.

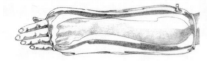

### Implementation

▶ Obtain a complete history of the injury, if possible, and begin a thorough head-to-toe assessment, inspecting for obvious deformities, swelling, or bleeding.
▶ Ask the patient if he can move the injured area (typically an extremity). Compare it bilaterally with the uninjured extremity, where applicable. Gently palpate the injured area; inspect for swelling, obvious deformities, bleeding, discoloration, and evidence of fracture or dislocation.
▶ Remove or cut away clothing from the injury site, if necessary. Check neurovascular integrity distal to the site. Explain the procedure to the patient to allay his fears.
▶ If an obvious bone misalignment causes the patient acute distress or severe neurovascular problems, align the extremity in its normal anatomic position, if possible. Stop, however, if this causes further neurovascular deterioration. Don't try to straighten a dislocation to avoid damaging displaced vessels and nerves. Also, don't attempt reduction of a contaminated bone end because this may cause additional laceration of soft tissues, vessels, and nerves

as well as gross contamination of deep tissues.
▶ Apply a sterile compress to any open wound.
▶ Choose a splint that will immobilize the joints above and below the fracture; pad the splint as necessary to protect bony prominences.

### Applying a rigid splint

▶ Support the injured extremity above and below the fracture site while applying firm, gentle traction.
▶ Have an assistant place the splint under, beside, or on top of the extremity, as ordered.
▶ Tell the assistant to apply the bindings to secure the splint.
▶ Assess the neurovascular status of the extremity; if it's impaired by the bindings, reapply them.

### Applying a spine board

▶ Pad the spine board (or door) carefully, especially the areas that will support the lumbar region and knees, to prevent uneven pressure and discomfort.
▶ If the patient is lying on his back, place one hand on each side of his head and apply gentle traction to the head and neck, keeping the head aligned with the body. Have one assistant logroll the patient onto his side while another slides the spine board under the patient. Then instruct the assistants to roll the patient onto the board while you maintain traction and alignment.
▶ If the patient is prone, logroll him onto the board so he ends up in a supine position.
▶ To maintain body alignment, use strips of cloth to secure the patient on the spine board; to keep head and neck aligned, place sandbags or rolled towels or clothing on both sides of his head.

### Applying a traction splint

▶ Specialized training is required before applying a traction splint.
▶ Place the splint beside the injured leg. (Never use a traction splint on an arm because the major axillary plexus of nerves and blood vessels can't tolerate countertraction.) Adjust the splint to the correct length and then open and adjust the Velcro straps.

▶ Have an assistant keep the leg motionless while you pad the ankle and foot and fasten the ankle hitch around them. (You may leave the shoe on.)

▶ Tell the assistant to lift and support the leg at the injury site as you apply firm, gentle traction.

▶ While you maintain traction, tell the assistant to slide the splint under the leg, pad the groin to avoid excessive pressure on external genitalia, and gently apply the ischial strap.

▶ Have the assistant connect the loops of the ankle hitch to the end of the splint.

▶ Adjust the splint to apply enough traction to secure the leg comfortably in the corrected position.

▶ After applying traction, fasten the Velcro support splints to secure the leg closely to the splint.

**ALERT!** Don't use a traction splint for a severely angulated femur or knee fracture.

### Special considerations

▶ At the scene of an accident, always examine the patient completely for other injuries. Avoid unnecessary movement or manipulation, which might cause additional pain or injury.

▶ Always consider the possibility of cervical injury in an unconscious patient. If possible, apply the splint before repositioning the patient.

▶ If the patient requires a rigid splint but one isn't available, use another body part as a splint. To splint a leg in this manner, pad its inner aspect and secure it to the other leg with roller gauze or cloth strips.

▶ After applying any type of splint, monitor vital signs frequently because bleeding in fractured bones and surrounding tissues may cause shock. Also, monitor the neurovascular status of the fractured limb by assessing skin color, taking the patient's temperature, and checking for pain and numbness in the fingers or toes. Numbness or paralysis distal to the injury indicates pressure on nerves.

▶ Transport the patient as soon as possible to a health care facility. Apply ice to the injury. Regardless of the apparent extent of the injury, don't allow the patient to eat or drink anything until the doctor evaluates him.

▶ Indications for removing a splint include evidence of improper application or vascular impairment. Apply gentle traction and remove the splint carefully under a doctor's direct supervision.

### Complications

Multiple transfers and repeated manipulation of a fracture may result in fat embolism, indicated by shortness of breath, agitation, and irrational behavior. This complication usually occurs 24 to 72 hours after injury or manipulation.

### Documentation

▶ Record the circumstances and cause of the injury.

▶ Document the patient's complaints, noting whether symptoms are localized.

▶ Record neurovascular status before and after applying the splint.

▶ Note the type of wound and the amount and type of drainage, if any.

▶ Document the time of splint application.

▶ If the bone end should slip into surrounding tissue or if transportation causes any change in the degree of dislocation, make sure to note it.

### REFERENCES

Edward, D., et al. *Bedside Critical Care Manual.* Philadelphia: Lippincott Williams & Wilkins, 2001.

Young, C.C., et al. "Treatment of Plantar Fasciitis," *American Family Physician* 63(3): 467-74, 477-78, February 2001. (Review.)

## Stump and prosthesis care

Patient care directly after limb amputation includes monitoring drainage from the stump, positioning the affected limb, assisting with exercises prescribed by a physical therapist, and wrapping and conditioning the stump. Postoperative care of the stump will vary slightly, depending on the amputation site (arm or leg) and the type of dressing applied to the stump (elastic bandage or plaster cast).

After the stump heals, it requires only routine daily care, such as proper hygiene and continued muscle-strengthening exercises. The prosthesis, when in use, also requires daily care. Typically, a plastic prosthesis, the most common type, must be cleaned and lubricated and checked for proper fit. As the patient recovers from the physical and psychological trauma of amputation, he'll need to learn correct procedures for routine daily care of the stump and the prosthesis.

## Equipment

*For postoperative stump care*
Pressure dressing • abdominal (ABD) pad • suction equipment, if ordered • overhead trapeze • 1" adhesive tape, bandage clips or safety pins • sandbags or trochanter roll (for a leg) • elastic stump shrinker or 4" elastic bandage • optional: tourniquet (as a last resort to control bleeding)

*For stump and prosthesis care*
Mild soap or alcohol pads • stump socks or athletic tube socks • two washcloths • two towels • appropriate lubricating oil

## Implementation

▶ Perform routine postoperative care. Frequently assess respiratory status and level of consciousness, monitor vital signs and I.V. infusions, check tube patency, and provide for the patient's comfort and safety.

### Monitoring stump drainage

▶ Because gravity causes fluid to accumulate at the stump, frequently check the amount of blood and drainage on the dressing. Notify the doctor if accumulations of drainage or blood increase rapidly. If excessive bleeding occurs, notify the doctor immediately and apply a pressure dressing or compress the appropriate pressure points. If this doesn't control bleeding, use a tourniquet only as a last resort. Keep a tourniquet available, if needed.
▶ Tape the ABD pad over the moist part of the dressing, as needed. Providing a dry area helps prevent bacterial infection.
▶ Monitor the suction drainage equipment and note the amount and type of drainage.

### Positioning the extremity

▶ Elevate the extremity for the first 24 hours to reduce swelling and promote venous return.
▶ To prevent contractures, position an arm with the elbow extended and the shoulder abducted.
▶ To correctly position a leg, elevate the foot of the bed slightly and place sandbags or a trochanter roll against the hip to prevent external rotation.

**◆ ALERT!** Don't place a pillow under the thigh to flex the hip; this can cause hip flexion contracture. For the same reason, tell the patient to avoid prolonged sitting.
▶ After a below-the-knee amputation, maintain knee extension to prevent hamstring muscle contractures.
▶ After any leg amputation, place the patient on a firm surface in the prone position for at least 2 hours per day with his legs close together and without pillows under his stomach, hips, knees, or stump, unless this position is contraindicated. This position helps prevent hip flexion, contractures, and abduction; it also stretches the flexor muscles.

### Assisting with prescribed exercises

▶ After arm amputation, encourage the patient to exercise the remaining arm to prevent muscle contractures. Help the patient perform isometric and range-of-motion (ROM) exercises for both shoulders as prescribed by the physical therapist because use of the prosthesis requires both shoulders.
▶ After leg amputation, stand behind the patient and, if necessary, support him with your hands at his waist during balancing exercises.
▶ Instruct the patient to exercise the affected and unaffected limbs to maintain muscle tone and increase muscle strength. A patient with a leg amputation may perform push-ups, as ordered, (in the sitting position, arms at his sides) or pull-ups on the overhead trapeze to strengthen his arms, shoulders, and back in preparation for using crutches.

### Wrapping and conditioning the stump

▶ If the patient doesn't have a rigid cast, apply an elastic stump shrinker to prevent edema and shape the limb in preparation for the prosthesis. Wrap the stump so that it narrows toward the distal end. This helps to ensure comfort when the patient wears the prosthesis.
▶ If an elastic stump shrinker isn't available, you can wrap the stump in a 4" elastic bandage. To do this, stretch the bandage to about two-thirds its maximum length as you wrap it diagonally around the stump, with the greatest pressure distally. (Depending on the size of the leg, you may

# Wrapping a stump

Proper stump care helps protect the limb, reduces swelling, and prepares the limb for a prosthesis. As you perform the procedure, teach it to the patient.

Start by obtaining two 4″ elastic bandages. Center the end of the first 4″ bandage at the top of the patient's thigh. Unroll the bandage downward over the stump and to the back of the leg.

Make three figure-eight turns to adequately cover the ends of the stump. As you wrap, include the roll of flesh in the groin area. Use enough pressure to ensure that the stump narrows toward the end so that it fits comfortably into the prosthesis.

Use the second 4″ bandage to anchor the first bandage around the waist. For a below-the-knee amputation, use the knee to anchor the bandage in place. Secure the bandage with clips, safety pins, or adhesive tape. Check the stump bandage regularly and rewrap it if it bunches at the end.

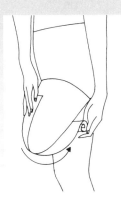 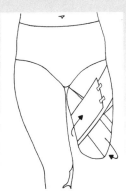 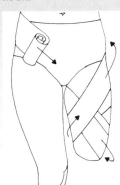

need to use two 4″ bandages.) Secure the bandage with clips, safety pins, or adhesive tape. Make sure the bandage covers all portions of the stump smoothly because wrinkles or exposed areas encourage skin breakdown. (See *Wrapping a stump*.)

▶ If the patient experiences throbbing after the stump is wrapped, the bandage may be too tight; remove the bandage immediately and reapply it less tightly. Throbbing indicates impaired circulation.

▶ Check the bandage regularly. Rewrap it when it begins to bunch up at the end (usually about every 12 hours for a moderately active patient), or as necessary.

▶ After removing the bandage to rewrap it, massage the stump gently, always pushing toward the suture line rather than away from it. This stimulates circulation and prevents scar tissue from adhering to the bone.

▶ When healing begins, instruct the patient to push the stump against a pillow. Then have him progress gradually to pushing against harder surfaces, such as a padded chair, then a hard chair. These conditioning exercises will help the patient adjust to experiencing pressure and sensation in the stump.

■ **EVIDENCE BASE** Avoid applying lotion to the residual stump because it may clog follicles, increasing the risk of infection. In addition, it's a desired goal of the healing process to toughen the area in order to tolerate the prosthesis.

## Caring for the healed stump

▶ Bathe the stump but never shave it to prevent infection. If possible, bathe the stump at the end of the day because the warm water may cause swelling, making reapplication of the prosthesis difficult. Don't soak the stump for long periods.

▶ Inspect the stump for redness, swelling, irritation, and calluses. Report any of these to the doctor. Tell the patient to avoid putting weight on the stump. (The skin should be firm but not taut over the bony end of the limb.)

▶ Continue muscle-strengthening exercises so the patient can build the strength he'll need to control the prosthesis.

▶ Change and wash the patient's elastic bandages every day to avoid exposing the skin to excessive perspiration, which can be irritating. Wash the elastic bandages in warm water and gentle, nondetergent soap; lay them flat on a towel to dry. Machine washing or drying may shrink the elastic bandages. To shape the stump, an elastic bandage should be worn 24 hours per day except while bathing.

### Caring for the plastic prosthesis

▶ Wipe the plastic socket of the prosthesis with a damp washcloth and mild soap or alcohol to prevent bacterial accumulation.

▶ Wipe the insert (if the prosthesis has one) with a dry washcloth.

▶ Dry the prosthesis thoroughly; if possible, allow it to dry overnight.

▶ Maintain and lubricate the prosthesis as instructed by the manufacturer.

▶ Check for malfunctions and adjust or repair the prosthesis as necessary to prevent further damage.

▶ Check the condition of the shoe on a foot prosthesis frequently and change it as necessary.

### Applying the prosthesis

▶ Apply a stump sock. Keep the seams away from bony prominences.

▶ If the prosthesis has an insert, remove it from the socket, place it over the stump, and insert the stump into the prosthesis.

▶ If it has no insert, merely slide the prosthesis over the stump. Secure the prosthesis onto the stump according to the manufacturer's directions.

### Special considerations

▶ If a patient arrives at the facility with a traumatic amputation, the amputated part may be saved for possible reimplantation. (See *Caring for an amputated body part.*)

▶ Teach the patient how to care for his stump and prosthesis properly. Make sure he knows the signs and symptoms of problems in the stump. Explain that a 10-lb (4.5-kg) change in body weight will alter his stump size and require a new prosthesis socket to ensure a correct fit.

▶ Exercise of the remaining muscles in an amputated limb must begin the day after surgery. A physical therapist will direct these exercises. For example, arm exercises progress from isometrics to assisted ROM to active ROM. Leg exercises include rising from a chair, balancing on one leg, and ROM exercises of the knees and hips.

▶ For a below-the-knee amputation, you may substitute an athletic tube sock for a stump sock by cutting off the elastic band. If the patient has a rigid plaster of paris dressing, perform normal cast care. Check the cast frequently to make sure it doesn't slip off. If it does, apply an elastic bandage immediately and notify the doctor because edema will develop rapidly.

### Home care

Emphasize to the patient that proper care of his stump can speed healing. Tell him to inspect his stump carefully every day using a mirror and to continue proper daily stump care. Instruct him to call the doctor if the incision appears to be opening, looks red or swollen, feels warm, is painful to touch, or is seeping drainage.

Tell the patient to massage the stump toward the suture line to mobilize the scar and prevent its adherence to bone. Advise him to avoid exposing the skin around the stump to excessive perspiration, which can be irritating. Tell him to change his elastic bandages or stump socks daily to avoid this.

Tell the patient that he may experience twitching, spasms, or phantom limb pain as his stump muscles adjust to amputation. Advise him that he can decrease these symptoms with heat, massage, or gentle pressure. If his stump is sensitive to touch, tell him to rub it with a dry washcloth for 4 minutes three times per day.

Stress the importance of performing prescribed exercises to help minimize complications, maintain muscle strength and tone, prevent contractures, and promote independence. Also, stress the importance of

# Caring for an amputated body part

After traumatic amputation, the surgeon may be able to reimplant the severed body part through microsurgery. The chance of successful reimplantation is much greater if the amputated part has received proper care.

If the patient arrives at the hospital with a severed body part, first make sure that bleeding at the amputation site has been controlled. Then use the following guidelines for preserving the body part.

▶ Put on sterile gloves. Place several sterile gauze pads and an appropriate amount of sterile roller gauze in a sterile basin, and pour sterile normal saline or sterile lactated Ringer's solution over them. *Note:* never use another solution and don't try to scrub or debride the part.

▶ Holding the body part in one gloved hand, carefully pat it dry with sterile gauze. Place saline-soaked gauze pads over the stump; then wrap the whole body part with saline-soaked roller gauze. Wrap the gauze with a sterile towel, if available. Then put this package in a watertight container or bag and seal it.

▶ Fill another plastic bag with ice and place the part, still in its watertight container, inside. Seal the outer bag. (Always protect the part from direct contact with ice—and never use dry ice—to prevent irreversible tissue damage, which would make the part unsuitable for reimplantation.) Keep this bag ice-cold until the doctor is ready to do the reimplantation surgery.

▶ Label the bag with the patient's name, identification number, identification of the amputated part, the facility's identification number, and the date and time when cooling began.

*Note:* The body part must be wrapped and cooled quickly. Irreversible tissue damage occurs after only 6 hours at ambient temperature. However, hypothermic management seldom preserves tissues for more than 24 hours.

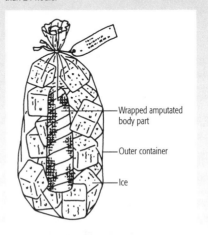

Wrapped amputated body part

Outer container

Ice

---

positioning to prevent contractures and edema.

Note any complaints of phantom limb sensations. These are feelings that the amputated part is still present. Not all these complaints are painful. The patient may describe sensations of warmth, cold, itching, or pain in the missing limb. These sensations are caused from intact peripheral nerves proximal to the amputation site that carried messages between the brain and the amputated part. Interventions for phantom limb sensations include visual imaging and ROM exercises.

## Complications

The most common postoperative complications include hemorrhage, stump infection, contractures, and a swollen or flabby stump. Complications that may develop at

any time after an amputation include skin breakdown or irritation from lack of ventilation; friction from an irritant in the prosthesis; a sebaceous cyst or boil from tight socks; psychological problems, such as denial, depression, or withdrawal; and phantom limb pain caused by stimulation of nerves that once carried sensations from the distal part of the extremity.

## Documentation

▶ Record the date, time, and specific procedures of all postoperative care, including amount and type of drainage, condition of the dressing, need for dressing reinforcement, and appearance of the suture line and surrounding tissue.

▶ Note any signs of skin irritation or infection, any complications and the nursing action taken, the patient's tolerance of exercises, and his psychological reaction to the amputation.

▶ During routine daily care, document the date, time, type of care given, and condition of the skin and suture line, noting any signs or symptoms of irritation, such as redness or tenderness.

▶ Note the patient's progress in caring for the stump or prosthesis.

### REFERENCES

Bryant, G. "Stump Care," *AJN* 101(2):67-71, February 2001.

Goldberg, T., et al. "Postoperative Management of Lower Extremity Amputation," *Physical Medicine and Rehabilitation Clinics of North America* 11(3):559-68, August 2000.

Maher, A.B., et al. *Orthopaedic Nursing*, 3rd ed. Philadelphia: W.B. Saunders Co., 2002.

## Triangular sling application

Made from a triangular piece of muslin, canvas, or cotton, a sling supports and immobilizes an injured arm, wrist, or hand, and thereby facilitates healing. It may be applied to restrict movement of a fracture or dislocation or to support a muscle sprain. A sling can also support the weight of a splint or help secure dressings.

### Equipment

Triangular bandage or commercial sling ● gauze (for padding) ● safety pins (tape for children younger than age 7)

### Implementation

▶ Explain the procedure to the patient and wash your hands.

▶ If you anticipate prolonged use of a sling, pad the area under the knot with gauze to prevent skin irritation. Place the sling outside the shirt collar to reduce direct pressure on the neck and shoulder.

▶ If the arm requires complete immobilization, apply a swathe after placing the arm in a sling. (See *Applying a swathe.*)

**◆ ALERT!** If the patient is a child, fold the bandage in half to make a smaller triangle. Then follow the steps shown in *Making a sling.*

At regular intervals, check to be sure that the sling is in proper position. Also assess patient comfort and circulation to the fingers.

## Applying a swathe

To further immobilize an arm after applying a sling, wrap a folded triangular bandage or wide elastic bandage around the patient's upper torso and the upper arm on the injured side. Don't cover the patient's uninjured arm. Make the swathe just tight enough to secure the injured arm to the body. Pin the ends of the bandage just in front of the axilla on the uninjured side.

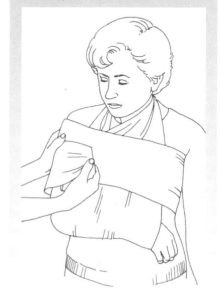

### Special considerations

▶ Before the patient leaves the hospital, provide an extra triangular bandage.

▶ Teach him and a family member or friend how to change the sling. If appropriate, instruct him to change the sling regularly because a soiled sling can cause irritation and infection. Also teach him how to check periodically for axillary and cervical skin breakdown.

### Documentation

▶ In the patient's chart, record the date, time, and location of sling application and describe the patient's tolerance of the procedure.

▶ Document neurovascular status, noting color and temperature.

# Making a sling

Place the apex of a triangular bandage behind the patient's elbow on the injured side. Hold one end of the bandage so it extends up toward the patient's neck on the uninjured side and let the other end hang straight down. The bandage's long side should parallel the midline of the patient's body.

Adjust the bandage so that the forearm and upper arm form an angle of slightly less than 90 degrees to increase venous return from the hand and forearm and to facilitate drainage from swelling. Then tie the two bandage ends at the side of the patient's neck, rather than at the back, to prevent neck flexion and avoid irritation and pressure over a cervical vertebra.

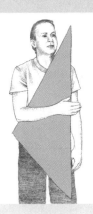

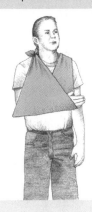

Loop the top corner of the bandage over the shoulder on the uninjured side and around the back of the patient's neck. Then bring the lower end of the bandage over the flexed forearm and up to the shoulder on the injured side.

Carefully secure the sling with a safety pin above and behind the elbow. For a child younger than age 7, use tape instead of a pin to avoid injury.

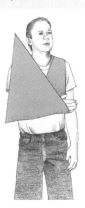

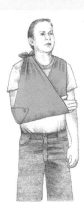

## REFERENCES

Edward, D., et al. *Bedside Critical Care Manual.* Philadelphia: Lippincott Williams & Wilkins, 2001.

Harris, R.I., et al. "Structural Properties of the Intact and the Reconstructed Coracoclavicular Ligament Complex," *The American Journal of Sports Medicine* 28(1):103-108, January-February 2000.

# 11

# Skin care

B ESIDES HELPING TO SHAPE A PATIENT'S SELF-IMAGE, THE SKIN PERFORMS MANY PHYSIO-logic functions. For instance, it protects internal body structures from the environment and pathogens. It also helps regulate body temperature and homeostasis and serves as an organ of sensation and excretion. As a result, meticulous skin care is essential to overall health. When skin integrity is compromised by pressure ulcers, burns, or other lesions, you'll need to take steps to prevent or control infection, promote new skin growth, control pain, and provide emotional support.

To enhance natural healing, skin wounds need regular dressing changes (with extra changes for soiled dressings), thorough cleaning and, if necessary, debridement to remove debris, reduce bacterial growth, and encourage tissue repair.

If you're working with a patient who has impaired skin integrity—such as a patient with burns or pressure ulcers—your primary goal is to prevent or control infection because damage to skin integrity increases the risk of infection, which could delay healing, worsen pain, and possibly threaten the patient's life.

This chapter provides protocols for managing the patient with impaired thermoregulation, burns, pressure ulcers, or a high risk of pressure injury. In addition, this chapter describes step-by-step procedures that will help you maintain the patient's skin integrity and prevent or control infection.

# Protocols

## Managing the patient with altered skin integrity

### Purpose
To identify types of wounds and their appropriate treatment options; to promote healing and minimize complications in the patient with altered skin integrity

### Collaborative level
Interdependent

### Expected patient outcomes
▶ The patient will remain infection-free.
▶ The patient will maintain all limbs intact.
▶ The patient will maintain limb function.
▶ The patient will report adequate pain management.
▶ The patient will display wound healing (or stabilization if healing isn't possible).

### Definition of terms
▶ *Altered skin integrity:* A change in the epidermis, dermis, or subcutaneous tissue unrelated to aging. This includes open wounds or changes in intact skin.

▶ *Arterial ulcer:* A nonhealing or poorly healing wound, usually on the legs and commonly initiated by minor trauma. Poor arterial circulation significantly delays or impairs wound healing.
▶ *Diabetic foot ulcer:* A wound on the plantar surface of the foot over a bony prominence that has been under pressure from walking or footwear. The wound is related to peripheral neuropathy and vascular disease and appears as a deep ulceration with a thick ring of callous (hyperkeratosis) at the wound edges.
▶ *Pressure ulcer:* A partial- or full-thickness wound caused by pressure, friction, or shearing force; it typically occurs over bony prominences.
▶ *Systemic cutaneous manifestation:* A skin manifestation of underlying disease or of a common systemic disease, such as acromegaly, or an extension of an underlying neoplasm that metastasizes to the skin.
▶ *Traumatic wound:* A partial-thickness wound involving the epidermis and partial dermis, such as a skin tear, or a full-thickness wound involving the epidermis, dermis, and subcutaneous tissue.

▶ *Thermal injury:* A cold injury, such as frostbite, or heat injury such as a burn from scalding.
▶ *Venous ulcer:* A partial- or full-thickness wound on the leg caused by venous stasis disease and edema.

## Indications
### Treatment
▶ Diabetic foot ulcer
▶ Arterial ulcer
▶ Venous ulcer
▶ Pressure ulcer
▶ Systemic cutaneous manifestation
▶ Traumatic wound
▶ Thermal injury

### Prevention
▶ Infection
▶ Further tissue injury or breakdown
▶ Loss of limb
▶ Loss of function
▶ Deformity

## Assessment guidance
### Signs and symptoms
▶ Pain
▶ Tenderness
▶ Fever
▶ Chills
▶ Open wound or altered skin integrity
▶ Warmth, erythema, edema, or induration at or around the affected area
▶ Drainage
▶ Odor
▶ Visible tunneling, undermining, or sinus tracts in wound bed
▶ Limited range of motion (ROM) and function in an arm or leg

### Diagnostic studies
#### Laboratory tests
▶ Complete blood count
▶ Hemoglobin level
▶ Hematocrit
▶ Wound culture and sensitivity test
▶ Tissue biopsy culture and sensitivity test
▶ Erythrocyte sedimentation rate
▶ Antinuclear antibody count
▶ Rheumatoid factor test

#### Imaging tests
▶ Arterial Doppler ultrasonography
▶ Venous Doppler ultrasonography
▶ Arteriography
▶ Venography

#### Other
▶ Transcutaneous oxygen measurements
▶ Ankle-brachial index (ABI)
▶ Segmental pressures

## Nursing interventions
▶ Identify and treat the cause of the wound.
▶ Reduce or relieve pressure, friction, and shearing force by repositioning the patient and providing pressure-reducing surfaces, such as seat cushions, mattress overlays, mattress replacement systems, or specialty beds.
▶ Keep the head of the bed at the lowest level that's safe for the patient.
▶ Minimize or eliminate skin irritants, such as drainage, urine, or feces, from the wound and periwound areas by frequent cleaning and the use of moisture-barrier products, as appropriate.
▶ Treat the systemic disorder.
▶ Remove foreign bodies.
▶ Apply compression therapy, such as multilayer wraps or Unna's boot, to treat venous insufficiency.
▶ Monitor the patient's vital signs.
▶ Assess the patient's ABI by comparing the systolic blood pressure in his dorsalis pedis or posterior tibialis artery with that in his brachial artery. The ratio of these pressures helps detect vascular insufficiency in an injured limb. An ABI below 0.9 suggests vascular insufficiency.
▶ Monitor the wound for signs of infection.
▶ Explain all treatments and procedures to the patient before performing them.

### Local wound care
▶ Clean the wound.
▶ Consult the doctor about removing necrotic tissue.
▶ Provide absorptive dressings for draining wounds.
▶ Provide a moist wound environment for dry wounds.
▶ Gently pack cavity wounds to fill dead space.
▶ Provide dressings that don't further injure the wound or periwound tissue.
▶ Collect a specimen for wound culture and sensitivity testing.
▶ Administer pain-relieving medication.
▶ Position the patient to promote comfort and preserve the function of the arm or leg.
▶ Consult a wound, ostomy, or continence nurse to evaluate and recommend inter-

ventions for complex or nonhealing wounds.

▶ Consult a dietitian to obtain a nutritional evaluation.

▶ Consult a physical or occupational therapist, if needed, to help maintain the limb's ROM and function.

▶ Give the patient antibiotics to treat infected wounds.

▶ Institute contact isolation procedures if a wound is infected.

## Patient teaching

▶ Inform the patient and his family, if appropriate, of the wound's severity.

▶ Teach the patient and his family how to relieve pressure and avoid friction and shearing force by positioning the patient properly and using pads and other pressure-reducing devices.

▶ Emphasize the importance of good nutrition in aiding wound healing.

▶ Teach the patient to recognize the signs and symptoms of wound deterioration or infection.

▶ Encourage patient communication to ensure adequate pain relief.

▶ Discuss possible outcomes, including healing and scarring, changes in body image, and functional limitations.

## Precautions

▶ Ensure that written consent is obtained before debridement begins.

▶ Identify all allergies before applying a topical dressing or administering a systemic medication.

▶ Read the product information on all topical dressings to identify ingredients that may cause allergic reactions.

▶ Follow the manufacturer's guidelines for product use.

▶ Assess the patient's vascular status, and confirm adequate arterial circulation before applying compression therapy.

## Contraindications

Contraindications include sensitivity to one or more ingredients in topical treatments; severe arterial insufficiency, unless revascularization is performed before leg debridement; severe arterial insufficiency in the patient who would otherwise undergo compression therapy.

## Documentation

▶ Document the wound status in detail, noting its location, length, width, and depth.

▶ Record the status of the wound bed, including the presence of slough, eschar, tunneling, undermining, sinus tracts, and exposed muscle, fascia, tendon, or bone.

▶ Record the color and type of drainage.

▶ Note the condition of the periwound tissue, including friability, induration, edema, and erythema.

▶ Document all aspects of wound care, including the date and time it was performed as well as the type of treatment or dressing applied.

▶ Document subjective symptoms reported by the patient and objective signs obtained by nursing assessment.

▶ Record the date, time, and type of specimens sent to the laboratory. Also record the results of all diagnostic studies.

▶ Document your notification of the doctor and subsequent interventions ordered.

▶ Note all nursing interventions, particularly administration of pain relief measures and the patient's response to them.

▶ Document each patient-teaching session and the patient's response.

▶ Record the patient's response to each treatment.

## Related procedures

▶ Biological burn dressing
▶ Burn care
▶ Clinitron therapy bed
▶ Mechanical debridement
▶ Oral drugs
▶ Physical assessment
▶ Pressure ulcer care
▶ Skin biopsy
▶ Skin graft care
▶ Skin medications
▶ Skin staple and clip removal
▶ Surgical wound management
▶ Swab specimens
▶ Transcutaneous $PO_2$ monitoring
▶ Transdermal drugs
▶ Traumatic wound care
▶ Unna's boot
▶ Use of isolation equipment
▶ Wound dehiscence and evisceration care
▶ Wound irrigation

**REFERENCES**
Bryant, R.A., ed. *Acute and Chronic Wounds: Nursing Management,* 2nd ed. St. Louis: Mosby–Year Book, Inc., 2000.
Krasner, D., et al., eds. *Chronic Wound Care: A Clinical Source Book for Healthcare Professionals,* 3rd ed. Wayne, Pa.: Health Management Publications, 2001.

**ORGANIZATIONS**
Agency for Healthcare Research and Quality: *www.guidelines.gov/index.asp*
National Pressure Ulcer Advisory Panel: *www.npuap.org*
Wound Healing Society: *www.woundheal.org*
Wound, Ostomy, and Continence Nurses Society: *www.wocn.org*

# Managing the patient with altered thermoregulation

## Purpose
To guide care for the patient with severe hypothermia or hyperthermia

## Collaborative level
Independent

## Expected patient outcomes
▶ The patient will maintain effective airway clearance.
▶ The patient will display hemodynamic stability.
▶ The patient will maintain renal function.
▶ The patient will report adequate pain management.
▶ The patient will maintain a core body temperature within normal limits.

## Definition of terms
▶ *Hyperthermia:* A body temperature significantly above 98.6° F (37° C).
▶ *Hypothermia:* A body temperature significantly below 98.6° F.

## Indications
Treatment
▶ Heat stroke
▶ Heat exhaustion
▶ Sepsis
▶ Cerebral edema
▶ Head injury
▶ Brain tumor
▶ Cerebral hemorrhage
▶ Environmental exposure to extreme or prolonged cold or heat

▶ Central nervous system disorders affecting the hypothalamus

Prevention
▶ Infection
▶ Tissue injury or breakdown
▶ Loss of limb
▶ Loss of function
▶ Deformity
▶ Death

## Assessment guidance
Signs and symptoms
▶ Pain, numbness, paresthesia
▶ Fever
▶ Chills
▶ Shivering
▶ Altered mental status
▶ Headache
▶ Fatigue
▶ Muscle cramps
▶ Thirst
▶ Body temperature significantly above or below 98.6° F
▶ Pallor or cyanosis of the arms and legs
▶ Flushing or erythema of the body
▶ Tachycardia or bradycardia
▶ Hypertension or hypotension
▶ Electrolyte imbalances indicating hyponatremia, acidosis, or dehydration
▶ Oliguria or anuria
▶ Cardiac arrhythmias

Diagnostic studies
*Laboratory tests*
▶ Electrolyte levels
▶ Hemoglobin level
▶ Hematocrit
▶ Arterial blood gas analysis

*Imaging tests*
▶ Electrocardiography

*Other*
▶ Intracranial pressure monitoring

## Nursing interventions
▶ Perform a complete physical assessment and obtain an accurate medical history.
▶ Identify the type and extent of exposure if the cause is environmental.
▶ Support the patient's respiratory and cardiovascular function.
▶ Secure adequate I.V. access.
▶ Administer fluid replacement.
▶ Initiate rewarming or cooling, as indicated.

▶ Prevent pressure, friction, and shearing force to the body and affected arms and legs by providing pressure-reducing surfaces, such as mattress replacement systems or specialty beds.

▶ Monitor the patient's electrolyte levels, intake and output, and vital signs.

▶ Monitor the patient for signs and symptoms of infection or complications.

▶ Explain all treatments and procedures to the patient before performing them.

▶ Provide local wound care as indicated.

▶ Clean the wound.

▶ Consult the doctor about removing necrotic tissue.

▶ Apply a sterile dressing.

▶ Provide absorptive dressings for draining wounds.

▶ Provide a moist wound environment for dry wounds.

▶ Gently pack cavity wounds to fill dead space.

▶ Provide dressings that don't further injure the wound or periwound tissue.

▶ Collect a specimen for wound culture and sensitivity testing.

▶ Administer pain-relieving medication.

▶ Position the patient to promote comfort and preserve the function of his arm or leg.

▶ Consult a dietitian to obtain a nutritional evaluation.

▶ Consult a physical or occupational therapist, if needed, to help maintain the limb's range of motion and function.

▶ Administer antibiotics if wounds are infected.

▶ Institute neutropenic isolation precautions.

## Patient teaching

▶ Inform the patient and his family, if appropriate, of the wound's severity.

▶ Teach the patient and his family how to relieve pressure and avoid friction and shearing force by positioning the patient properly and using pads and other pressure-reducing devices.

▶ Emphasize the importance of good nutrition in aiding wound healing.

▶ Teach the patient to recognize the signs and symptoms of wound deterioration or infection.

▶ Encourage the patient to communicate to ensure adequate pain relief.

▶ Discuss possible outcomes, including healing and scarring, changes in body image, and functional limitations.

## Precautions

▶ Ensure that written consent is obtained before debridement begins.

▶ Identify all allergies before applying a topical dressing or administering a systemic medication.

▶ Read the product information on all topical dressings to identify ingredients that may cause allergic reactions.

▶ Follow the manufacturer's guidelines for product use.

## Contraindications

Contraindications include sensitivity to one or more ingredients in topical treatments.

## Documentation

▶ Record the time, date, type, and amount of fluids or blood products infused.

▶ Document the time, date, type, and amount of analgesics administered.

▶ Document the wound status in detail, noting its location, length, width, and depth.

▶ Record the status of the wound bed, including the presence of slough, eschar, tunneling, undermining, sinus tracts, and exposed muscle, fascia, tendon, or bone.

▶ Record the color and type of drainage.

▶ Note the condition of the periwound tissue, including friability, induration, edema, and erythema.

▶ Document all aspects of wound care, including the date and time it was performed as well as the type of treatment or dressing applied.

▶ Document subjective symptoms reported by the patient and objective signs obtained by nursing assessment.

▶ Record the date, time, and type of specimens sent to the laboratory. Also record the results of all diagnostic studies.

▶ Document your notification of the doctor and subsequent interventions ordered.

▶ Note all nursing interventions, particularly administration of pain relief measures and the patient's response to them.

▶ Document each patient-teaching session and the patient's response.

▶ Record the patient's response to each treatment.

## Related procedures

▶ Biological burn dressing

▶ Burn care

▶ Clinitron therapy bed

◗ Cold application
◗ Direct heat application
◗ Hydrotherapy
◗ Hyperthermia-hypothermia therapy
◗ Mechanical debridement
◗ Oral drugs
◗ Physical assessment
◗ Skin biopsy
◗ Skin graft care
◗ Skin medications
◗ Swab specimens
◗ Transcutaneous $Po_2$ monitoring
◗ Transdermal drugs
◗ Traumatic wound care
◗ Use of isolation equipment
◗ Wound irrigation

### REFERENCES

Bryant, R.A., ed. *Acute and Chronic Wounds: Nursing Management,* 2nd ed. St. Louis: Mosby–Year Book, Inc., 2000.
Krasner, D., et al., eds. *Chronic Wound Care: A Clinical Source Book for Healthcare Professionals,* 3rd ed. Wayne, Pa.: Health Management Publications, 2001.

### ORGANIZATIONS
Wound Healing Society: *www.woundheal.org*

# Managing the patient with drains

## Purpose
To manage various types of tubes and drains and prevent complications

## Collaborative level
Interdependent

## Expected patient outcomes
◗ The patient will maintain intact skin around the tube or drain site.
◗ The patient will display no signs or symptoms of infection.
◗ The patient will have a tube or drain that remains patent.
◗ The patient will have a tube or drain that remains correctly positioned.

## Definition of terms
◗ *Drain:* A device placed during surgery to drain internal fluid.
◗ *Effluent:* Output or drainage from a tube or drain in the GI system.
◗ *Tube:* A hollow device placed in a body organ or space to drain or instill fluid.

## Indications
Treatment
◗ Disorders that require surgical intervention and placement of a drain

Prevention
◗ Skin deterioration around a tube or drain
◗ Infection at a tube or drain site or within a cavity
◗ Obstruction of a tube or drain
◗ Migration of a tube or drain

## Assessment guidance
Signs and symptoms
◗ Pain at or around the tube or drain site
◗ Abdominal pain or distention
◗ Fever
◗ Chills
◗ Altered skin integrity around the tube or drain site
◗ Pain or tenderness around the tube or drain site
◗ Warmth, erythema, edema, or induration at or around the tube or drain site
◗ Lack of drainage or change in expected output
◗ Inability to instill irrigant

Diagnostic studies
*Laboratory tests*
◗ White blood cell count
◗ pH analysis of effluent

*Imaging tests*
◗ Radiology
◗ Flat plate of abdomen
◗ Gastrografin contrast and lower GI X-ray studies
◗ Computed tomography scan

## Nursing interventions
◗ Identify the type and location of the tube or drain.
◗ Identify the tube's expected function, such as drainage or instillation.
◗ Identify the expected effluent and amount of output.
◗ Maintain a closed drainage system or suction.
◗ Assess the tube site and the color, amount, and odor of any drainage.
◗ Assess the patient's skin integrity around the tube or drain site.
◗ Stabilize the tube at the proximal and distal ends to prevent migration or inadvertent removal.
◗ Monitor the patient's vital signs.

▶ Monitor the tube or drain site for signs and symptoms of infection.
▶ Explain all treatments and procedures to the patient before performing them.

### Local tube or drain care
▶ Maintain a tube stabilization device.
▶ When changing a tube stabilizer, clean the area around the tube, assess skin integrity, and apply a skin protectant, as appropriate.
▶ Notify the doctor if you detect skin breakdown or a change in the color, amount, or odor of the effluent and output.
▶ Administer pain-relieving medication.
▶ Position the patient to promote comfort.
▶ Consult a wound, ostomy, or continence nurse to evaluate and recommend interventions for complex tubes or drains or for skin breakdown at the tube entry site.
▶ Institute contact isolation procedures if drainage is infectious.

## Patient teaching
▶ Inform the patient and his family of the tube's or drain's purpose and function.
▶ Educate the patient to avoid tension or pressure on the tube or drain.
▶ Emphasize the importance of good nutrition in aiding wound healing.
▶ Teach the patient to recognize the signs and symptoms of a change in tube or drain patency or location.
▶ Encourage patient communication to ensure adequate pain relief.
▶ Discuss expected outcomes, including pain relief, duration of tube or drain use (temporary or permanent), healing and scarring, changes in body image, and functional limitations.

## Precautions
▶ Identify all allergies before applying adhesives or dressings.
▶ Effluent with a pH below 6.0 can quickly cause severe skin irritation and breakdown; provide adequate skin protection through topical creams, dressings, or pouching to maintain skin integrity.
▶ High-output tubes or drains (more than 200 ml/24 hr) can cause significant fluid and electrolyte changes; closely monitor the patient's fluid intake and output and electrolyte levels.

## Contraindications
Contraindications include sensitivity to one or more ingredients in adhesives or topical treatments.

## Documentation
▶ Document details about the tube or drain, including its location; amount, color, and odor of drainage; the type of tube stabilizer in place; and the date and time of dressing changes and the surrounding skin's condition.
▶ Document subjective symptoms reported by the patient and objective signs obtained by nursing assessment.
▶ Record the date, time, and type of specimens sent to the laboratory. Also record the results of all diagnostic studies.
▶ Document your notification of the doctor and subsequent interventions ordered.
▶ Note all nursing interventions, particularly administration of pain relief measures and the patient's response to them.
▶ Document each patient-teaching session and the patient's response.
▶ Record the patient's response to each treatment.

## Related procedures
▶ Chest tube insertion
▶ Feeding tube insertion and removal
▶ Nasoenteric-decompression tube care
▶ Nasogastric tube care
▶ Nephrostomy and cystostomy tube care
▶ Oral drugs
▶ Physical assessment
▶ Postoperative care
▶ Skin medications
▶ Surgical wound care
▶ Transabdominal tube feedings
▶ Tube feedings
▶ Use of isolation equipment

### REFERENCES
Bryant, R.A., ed. *Acute and Chronic Wounds: Nursing Management,* 2nd ed. St. Louis: Mosby–Year Book, Inc., 2000.
Krasner, D., et al., eds. *Chronic Wound Care: A Clinical Source Book for Healthcare Professionals,* 3rd ed. Wayne, Pa.: Health Management Publications, 2001.

### ORGANIZATIONS
Wound, Ostomy, and Continence Nurses Society: *www.wocn.org*
Wound Healing Society: *www.woundheal.org*

# Managing the patient with pressure ulcers

## Purpose
To guide treatment of the patient with pressure ulcers

## Collaborative level
Independent

## Expected patient outcomes
▶ The patient will explain how to prevent infection.
▶ The patient will maintain all limbs intact.
▶ The patient will maintain limb function.
▶ The patient will report adequate pain management.
▶ The patient will display wound healing (or stabilization if healing isn't possible).

## Definition of terms
▶ *Eschar:* An unstageable pressure ulcer caused by necrotic tissue that prevents the determination of the wound's depth.
▶ *Stage I pressure ulcer:* An observable pressure-related alteration of intact skin that may include changes in skin temperature (warmth or coolness), tissue consistency (firm or boggy), or sensation (pain or itching). The ulcer appears as a defined area of persistent redness in lightly pigmented skin; in darker skin, it may appear persistently red, blue, or purple.
▶ *Stage II pressure ulcer:* A partial-thickness skin loss involving the epidermis, dermis, or both. The ulcer is superficial and appears as an abrasion, blister, or shallow crater.
▶ *Stage III pressure ulcer:* A full-thickness skin loss involving damage to or necrosis of subcutaneous tissue that may extend to, but not through, the underlying fascia. The ulcer appears as a deep crater with or without undermining of adjacent tissue.
▶ *Stage IV pressure ulcer:* A full-thickness skin loss with extensive destruction, tissue necrosis, or damage to muscle, bone, or supporting structures (such as a tendon or joint capsule). Undermining and sinus tracts also may be associated with a stage IV pressure ulcer.

## Indications
Treatment
▶ Wounds caused by pressure, friction, and shearing force

Prevention
▶ Infection
▶ Further tissue injury or breakdown
▶ Loss of limb
▶ Loss of function
▶ Deformity
▶ Tissue death

## Assessment guidance
Signs and symptoms
▶ Pain or tenderness
▶ Fever
▶ Chills
▶ Open wound or altered skin integrity
▶ Pain or tenderness at or around the affected area
▶ Warmth, erythema, edema, or induration at or around the affected area
▶ Drainage
▶ Odor
▶ Visible tunneling, undermining, or sinus tracts in the wound bed
▶ Limited range of motion (ROM) and function of the arm or leg

Diagnostic studies
*Laboratory tests*
▶ White blood cell count
▶ Hemoglobin level
▶ Hematocrit
▶ Wound culture and sensitivity testing
▶ Tissue biopsy culture and sensitivity testing
▶ Albumin level
▶ Prealbumin level
▶ Total protein level

*Imaging tests*
▶ Arterial Doppler ultrasonography
▶ Arteriography
▶ Vascular Doppler ultrasonography

*Other*
▶ Transcutaneous oxygen measurements
▶ Ankle-brachial index (ABI)

## Nursing interventions
▶ Perform a complete physical assessment and obtain an accurate medical history.
▶ Identify and stage the pressure ulcer if possible.
▶ Assess the patient's ABI by comparing the systolic blood pressure in his dorsalis pedis or posterior tibialis artery with that in his brachial artery. The ratio of these pressures helps detect vascular insufficien-

cy in an injured limb. An ABI below 0.9 suggests vascular insufficiency.

## Managing tissue load
▶ Reduce or relieve pressure, friction, and shearing force by repositioning the patient and providing pressure-reducing surfaces, such as seat cushions, mattress overlays, mattress replacement systems, or specialty beds. Choose appropriate devices based on the wound's severity and the patient's general condition.
▶ Avoid positioning the patient on the pressure ulcer.
▶ Establish a written repositioning schedule.
▶ Keep the head of the bed at the lowest level that's safe for the patient.
▶ Minimize or eliminate skin irritants, such as drainage, urine, or feces, in the wound and periwound areas by frequent cleaning and the use of moisture-barrier products, as appropriate.
▶ Use pillows or other positioning devices to prevent direct contact between bony prominences.

## Nutritional care and assessment
▶ Consult a dietitian to obtain a nutritional evaluation.
▶ Monitor the patient's nutritional intake.
▶ Monitor indicators of nutritional status, such as albumin, prealbumin, and total protein levels.

## Ulcer care
▶ Monitor the patient's vital signs.
▶ Monitor the patient for signs and symptoms of wound infection.
▶ Explain all treatments and procedures to the patient before performing them.

## Local wound care
▶ Clean the wound.
▶ Consult the doctor about removing necrotic tissue.
▶ Provide absorptive dressings for draining wounds.
▶ Provide a moist wound environment for dry wounds.
▶ Gently pack cavity wounds to fill dead space.
▶ Provide dressings that don't further injure the wound or periwound tissue.
▶ Collect a specimen for wound culture and sensitivity testing.

▶ Determine the patient's risk for developing additional pressure ulcers.
▶ Administer pain-relieving medication.
▶ Position the patient to promote comfort and preserve the function of his arm or leg.
▶ Consult a wound, ostomy, or continence nurse to evaluate and recommend interventions for complex or nonhealing wounds.
▶ Consult a physical or occupational therapist or both, if needed, to help maintain the limb's ROM and function.
▶ Administer antibiotics to treat an infected wound.
▶ Institute contact isolation procedures if the wound is infected.

## Patient teaching
▶ Inform the patient and his family, if appropriate, of the wound's severity.
▶ Teach the patient and his family how to relieve pressure and avoid friction and shearing force by positioning the patient properly and using pads and other pressure-reducing devices.
▶ Emphasize the importance of good nutrition in aiding wound healing.
▶ Teach the patient to recognize the signs and symptoms of wound deterioration or infection.
▶ Encourage patient communication to ensure adequate pain relief.
▶ Discuss possible outcomes, including healing and scarring, changes in body image, and functional limitations.

## Precautions
▶ Ensure written consent is obtained before debridement begins.
▶ Identify all allergies before applying any topical dressing or administering a systemic medication.
▶ Read the product information on all topical dressings to identify ingredients that may cause allergic reactions.
▶ Follow the manufacturer's guidelines for product use.

## Contraindications
Contraindications include sensitivity to one or more ingredients in topical treatments and severe arterial insufficiency, unless revascularization is performed before leg debridement.

## Documentation

▶ Document the pressure ulcer in detail, noting its stage (if possible), location, length, width, and depth.
▶ Record the status of the wound bed, including the presence of slough, eschar, tunneling, undermining, sinus tracts, and exposed muscle, fascia, tendon, or bone.
▶ Record the color and type of drainage.
▶ Note the condition of the periwound tissue, including friability, induration, edema, and erythema.
▶ Document all aspects of wound care, including the date and time it was performed as well as the type of treatment or dressing applied.
▶ Document subjective symptoms reported by the patient and objective signs obtained by nursing assessment.
▶ Record the date, time, and type of specimens sent to the laboratory. Also record the results of all diagnostic studies.
▶ Document your notification of the doctor and subsequent interventions ordered.
▶ Note all nursing interventions, particularly administration of pain relief measures and the patient's response to them.
▶ Document each patient-teaching session and the patient's response.
▶ Record the patient's response to each treatment.

## Related procedures

▶ Clinitron therapy bed
▶ Mechanical debridement
▶ Oral drugs
▶ Physical assessment
▶ Pressure ulcer care
▶ Skin biopsy
▶ Skin graft care
▶ Skin medications
▶ Swab specimens
▶ Transdermal drugs
▶ Use of isolation equipment
▶ Wound irrigation

**REFERENCES**

Bryant, R.A., ed. *Acute and Chronic Wounds: Nursing Management,* 2nd ed. St. Louis: Mosby–Year Book, Inc., 2000.
Krasner, D., et al., eds. *Chronic Wound Care: A Clinical Source Book for Healthcare Professionals,* 3rd ed. Wayne, Pa.: Health Management Publications, 2001.

**ORGANIZATIONS**

Agency for Healthcare Research and Quality: *www.guidelines.gov/index.asp*
National Pressure Ulcer Advisory Panel: *www.npuap.org*
Wound Healing Society: *www.woundheal.org*
Wound, Ostomy, and Continence Nurses Society: *www.wocn.org*

# Managing the patient at risk for developing pressure ulcers

## Purpose

To guide the prevention of pressure ulcers

## Collaborative level

Interdependent

## Expected patient outcomes

▶ The patient will maintain intact skin and show no signs of skin breakdown.

## Definition of terms

▶ *Dynamic overlay:* A mattress-size pad of air, gel, foam, or a combination with a motor that circulates air through a system of pockets within the device. This device is applied over an existing mattress to reduce pressure from the supporting surface.
▶ *Friction:* Resistance to movement between two surfaces; it occurs when the patient's body moves against bed linens and the supporting surface.
▶ *Maceration:* Overhydration of the epidermis by prolonged exposure to fluid.
▶ *Mattress replacement system:* A full mattress of air, gel, foam, or a combination. The device can be static or dynamic and is applied over a bed frame to reduce pressure from the supporting surface.
▶ *Pressure reduction:* An intervention used to reduce pressure over a bony prominence or affected area.
▶ *Risk assessment:* The use of specific criteria to determine the patient's potential for developing a pressure ulcer. Commonly used tools include the Braden, Norton, and Grosnell scales.
▶ *Shearing force:* A force that occurs when the patient's skin remains stationary and the underlying tissue shifts; it can cause tissue damage and ischemia.
▶ *Specialty bed:* A full dynamic bed system that can provide low-air-loss and alter-

nating pressure, or air-fluidized pressure relief.

▶ *Static overlay:* A mattress-size pad of air, gel, foam, or gel-foam combination applied over an existing mattress to reduce pressure from the supporting surface.

▶ *Tissue load:* The amount of force exerted on a specific body area; it includes the weight of the body and the resistance of the surface on which the area rests. It typically is described in pounds per square inch.

## Indications
### Treatment
▶ Wounds caused by pressure, friction, or shearing force

### Prevention
▶ Infection
▶ Tissue injury or breakdown
▶ Loss of function
▶ Deformity

## Assessment guidance
### Signs and symptoms
▶ Pain or tenderness
▶ Limited movement of an arm, leg, or other body part
▶ Poor nutritional status
▶ Incontinence
▶ Limited function of an arm, leg, or other body part

### Diagnostic studies
#### Laboratory tests
▶ Albumin level
▶ Prealbumin level
▶ Total protein level

#### Other
▶ Ankle-brachial index

## Nursing interventions
▶ Perform a complete physical assessment and obtain an accurate medical history.
▶ Use a risk assessment tool to identify the severity of the risk.
▶ Reassess the risk with any significant change in the patient's status, such as surgery, fever, infection, falls, altered mental status, declining nutritional intake, new onset of incontinence, and increased pain or stress
▶ Reduce or relieve pressure, friction, and shearing force by repositioning the patient and providing pressure-reducing surfaces,

such as seat cushions, mattress overlays, mattress replacement systems, or specialty beds. Choose appropriate devices based on the severity of the risk, the patient's general condition, and history of previous pressure ulcers.

▶ Avoid positioning the patient over a bony prominence.

▶ Establish a written repositioning schedule.

▶ Keep the head of the bed at the lowest level that's safe for the patient.

▶ Minimize or eliminate skin irritants, such as drainage, urine, or feces, in the wound and periwound areas by frequent cleaning and the use of moisture-barrier products, as appropriate.

▶ Use pillows or other positioning devices to prevent direct contact between bony prominences.

▶ Consult a dietitian to obtain a nutritional evaluation.

▶ Monitor the patient's nutritional intake.

▶ Monitor indicators of nutritional status, such as albumin, prealbumin, and total protein levels.

▶ Monitor the patient's vital signs.

▶ Monitor the patient for signs and symptoms of the effects of pressure, friction, shearing force, and maceration.

▶ Explain all interventions to the patient before performing them.

▶ Determine the patient's risk of developing additional pressure ulcers.

▶ Position the patient to provide comfort and preserve the function of his arm or leg.

▶ Consult a wound, ostomy, or continence nurse to evaluate and recommend interventions and pressure-reducing devices to prevent injuries.

▶ Consult a physical or occupational therapist or both, if needed, to help maintain the limb's range of motion and function.

## Patient teaching
▶ Inform the patient and his family of the severity of the risk of developing pressure ulcers.

▶ Teach the patient and his family how to relieve pressure and avoid friction and shearing force by positioning the patient properly and using pads and other pressure-reducing devices.

▶ Emphasize the importance of good nutrition in preventing skin breakdown.

❯ Instruct the patient and his family to recognize the early signs and symptoms of tissue compromise and pressure ulcers.

❯ Encourage patient communication to ensure adequate pain relief.

## Precautions

❯ Support the patient's joints and limbs in correct alignment to prevent pain, muscle spasms, and contractures.

## Documentation

❯ Document the patient's risk assessment score and any reassessment scores.

❯ Record all interventions used to reduce pressure, relieve friction and shearing force, and avoid maceration and chemical skin injuries from drainage, urine, or feces.

❯ Document subjective symptoms reported by the patient and objective signs obtained by nursing assessment.

❯ Record the results of all diagnostic studies.

❯ Document your notification of the doctor and subsequent interventions ordered.

❯ Note all nursing interventions, particularly administration of pain relief measures and the patient's response to them.

❯ Document each patient-teaching session and the patient's response.

## Related procedures

❯ Oral drugs

❯ Physical assessment

❯ Skin medications

❯ Transdermal drugs

### REFERENCES

Bryant, R A., ed. *Acute and Chronic Wounds: Nursing Management,* 2nd ed. St. Louis: Mosby–Year Book, Inc., 2000.

Krasner, D., et al., eds. *Chronic Wound Care: A Clinical Source Book for Healthcare Professionals,* 3rd ed. Third Edition. Wayne, Pa.: Health Management Publications, 2001.

### ORGANIZATIONS

Agency for Healthcare Research and Quality: *www.guidelines.gov/index.asp*

National Pressure Ulcer Advisory Panel: *www.npuap.org*

Wound Healing Society: *www.woundheal.org*

Wound, Ostomy, and Continence Nurses Society: *www.wocn.org*

# Procedures

# Biological burn dressing

Biological dressings provide a temporary protective covering for burn wounds and clean granulation tissue. They also temporarily secure fresh skin grafts and protect graft donor sites. In common use are three organic materials (pigskin, cadaver skin, and amniotic membrane) and one synthetic material (Biobrane). (See *Comparing biological dressings.*) In addition to stimulating new skin growth, these dressings act like normal skin: they reduce heat loss, block infection, and minimize fluid, electrolyte, and protein losses.

Amniotic membrane or fresh cadaver skin usually is applied to the patient in the operating room, although it may be applied in a treatment room. Pigskin or Biobrane may be applied in either the operating room or a treatment room. Before applying a biological dressing, the caregiver must clean and debride the wound. The frequency of dressing changes depends on the type of wound and the dressing's specific function.

## Equipment

Ordered analgesic ● cap ● mask ● two pairs of sterile gloves ● sterile or clean gown ● shoe covers ● biological dressing ● normal saline solution ● sterile basin ● Xeroflo gauze ● sterile forceps ● sterile scissors ● sterile hemostat ● elastic netting

# Comparing biological dressings

| Type | Description and uses | Nursing considerations |
|------|----------------------|------------------------|
| Cadaver (homograft) | ▶ Obtained at autopsy up to 24 hours after death<br>▶ Applied in the operating room or at the bedside to débrided, untidy wounds<br>▶ Available as fresh cryopreserved homografts in tissue banks nationwide<br>▶ Provides protection, especially to granulation tissue after escharotomy<br>▶ May be used in some patients as a test graft for autografting<br>▶ Covers excised wounds immediately | ▶ Observe for exudate.<br>▶ Watch for signs of rejection.<br>▶ Keep in mind that the gauze dressing may be removed every 8 hours to observe the graft. |
| Pigskin (heterograft or xenograft) | ▶ Applied in the operating room or at the bedside<br>▶ Comes fresh or frozen in rolls or sheets<br>▶ Can cover and protect débrided, untidy wounds, mesh autografts, clean (eschar-free) partial-thickness burns, and exposed tendons | ▶ Reconstitute frozen form with normal saline solution 30 minutes before use.<br>▶ Watch for signs of rejection.<br>▶ Cover with gauze dressing or leave exposed to air as ordered. |
| Amniotic membrane (homograft) | ▶ Available from the obstetric department<br>▶ Must be sterile and come from an uncomplicated birth; must have had serologic tests done<br>▶ Antimicrobials not required if in bacteriostatic condition<br>▶ May be used to protect partial-thickness burns or (temporarily) granulation tissue before autografting<br>▶ Applied by the doctor to clean wounds only | ▶ Change the membrane every 48 hours.<br>▶ Cover the membrane with a gauze dressing or leave it exposed as ordered.<br>▶ If you apply a gauze dressing, change it every 48 hours. |
| Biobrane (biosynthetic membrane) | ▶ Comes in sterile, prepackaged sheets in various sizes and in glove form for hand burns<br>▶ Used to cover donor graft sites, superficial partial-thickness burns, débrided wounds awaiting autograft, and meshed autografts<br>▶ Provides significant pain relief<br>▶ Applied by the nurse | ▶ Leave the membrane in place for 3 to 14 days, possibly longer.<br>▶ Don't use this dressing for preparing a granulation bed for subsequent autografting. |

## Preparation of equipment

Place the biological dressing in the sterile basin containing sterile normal saline solution (or open the Biobrane package). Using aseptic technique, open the sterile dressing packages. Arrange the equipment on the dressing cart, and keep the cart readily accessible. Make sure the treatment area has adequate light to allow accurate wound assessment and dressing placement.

## Implementation

▶ If this is the patient's first treatment, explain the procedure to allay his fears and promote cooperation. Provide privacy.

▶ If ordered, give an analgesic to the patient 20 minutes before beginning the procedure or give an analgesic I.V. immediately before the procedure to increase the patient's comfort and tolerance levels.

▶ Wash your hands and put on cap, mask, gown, shoe covers, and sterile gloves.

▶ Clean and debride the wound to reduce bacteria. Remove and dispose of gloves. Wash your hands and put on a fresh pair of sterile gloves.

▶ Place the dressing directly on the wound surface. Apply pigskin dermal (shiny) side down; apply Biobrane nylon-backed (dull) side down. Roll the dressing directly onto the skin, if applicable. Place the dressing strips so that the edges touch but don't overlap. Use sterile forceps, if necessary. Smooth the dressing. Eliminate folds and wrinkles by rolling out the dressing with the hemostat handle, the forceps handle, or your sterile-gloved hand to cover the wound completely and ensure adherence.

▶ Use the scissors to trim the dressing around the wound so that the dressing fits the wound without overlapping adjacent areas.

▶ Place Xeroflo gauze directly over an allograft, pigskin graft, or amniotic membrane. Place a few layers of gauze on top to absorb exudate, and wrap with a roller gauze dressing. Secure the dressing with tape or elastic netting. During daily dressing changes, the dressing will be removed down to the Xeroflo gauze, and the gauze will be replaced after the Xeroflo is inspected for drainage, adherence, and signs of infection.

▶ Place a nonadhesive dressing (such as Exu-dry) over the Biobrane to absorb drainage and provide stability. Wrap the dressing with a roller gauze dressing, and secure it with tape or elastic netting. During daily dressing changes, the dressing will be removed down to the Biobrane and the site inspected for signs of infection. After the Biobrane adheres (usually in 2 to 3 days), it doesn't need to be covered with a dressing.

▶ Position the patient comfortably, elevating the area if possible. This reduces edema, which may prevent the biological dressing from adhering.

## Special considerations

Handle the biological dressing as little as possible.

## Home care

Instruct the patient or caregiver to assess the site daily for signs of infection, swelling, blisters, drainage, and separation. Make sure the patient knows whom to contact if these complications develop.

## Complications

Infection may develop under a biological dressing. Observe the wound carefully during dressing changes for infection signs. If wound drainage appears purulent, remove the dressing, clean the area with normal saline solution or another prescribed cleaning solution, and apply a fresh biological dressing.

## Documentation

▶ Record the time and date of dressing changes.

▶ Note areas of application, quality of adherence, and purulent drainage or other infection signs.

▶ Describe the patient's tolerance of the procedure.

## REFERENCES

Chou, T.D., et al. "Reconstruction of Burn Scar of the Upper Extremities with Artificial Skin," *Plastic and Reconstructive Surgery* 108(2):378-84: discussion 385, August 2001.

Hansen, S.L., et al. "Using Skin Replacement Products To Treat Burns and Wounds," *Advances in Skin & Wound Care* 14(1):37-44; quiz 45-46, January-February 2001. (Review.)

# Burn care

The goals of burn care are to maintain the patient's physiologic stability, repair skin integrity, prevent infection, and promote maximal functioning and psychosocial health. Competent care immediately after a burn occurs can dramatically improve the success of overall treatment. (See *Burn care at the scene.*)

Burn severity is determined by the depth and extent of the burn and the presence of other factors, such as age, complications,

# Burn care at the scene

By acting promptly when a burn injury occurs, you can improve the patient's chance of uncomplicated recovery. Emergency care at the scene should include steps to stop the burn from worsening; assessment of the patient's airway, breathing, and circulation (ABCs); a call for help from an emergency medical service (EMS); and emotional and physiologic support for the patient.

## Stop the burning process

▶ If the victim is on fire, tell him to fall to the ground and roll to put out the flames. (If he panics and runs, air will fuel the flames, worsening the burn and increasing the risk of inhalation injury.) Or, if you can, wrap the victim in a blanket or other large covering to smother the flames and protect the burned area from dirt. Keep his head outside the blanket so that he doesn't breathe toxic fumes. As soon as the flames are out, unwrap the patient so that the heat can dissipate.

▶ Cool the burned area with any nonflammable liquid. This decreases pain and stops the burn from growing deeper or larger.

▶ If possible, remove potential sources of heat, such as jewelry, belt buckles, and some types of clothing. Besides adding to the burning process, these items may cause constriction as edema develops. If the patient's clothing adheres to his skin, don't try to remove it. Rather, cut around it.

▶ Cover the wound with a tablecloth, sheet, or other smooth, nonfuzzy material.

## Assess the damage

▶ Assess the patient's ABCs, and perform cardiopulmonary resuscitation, if necessary. Then check for other serious injuries, such as fractures, spinal cord injury, lacerations, blunt trauma, and head contusions.

▶ Estimate the extent and depth of the burns. If flames caused the burns and the injury occurred in a closed space, assess for signs of inhalation injury: singed nasal hairs, burns on the face or mouth, soot-stained sputum, coughing or hoarseness, wheezing, or respiratory distress.

▶ Call for help as quickly as possible. Send someone to contact the EMS.

▶ If the patient is conscious and alert, try to get a brief medical history as soon as possible.

▶ Reassure the patient that help is on the way. Provide emotional support by staying with him, answering questions, and explaining what's being done for him.

▶ When help arrives, give the EMS a report on the patient's status.

---

and coexisting illnesses. (See *Estimating burn surfaces in adults and children,* pages 584 and 585, and *Evaluating burn severity,* page 586.)

To promote stability, you'll need to carefully monitor your patient's respiratory status, especially if he has suffered smoke inhalation. Be aware that a patient with burns involving more than 20% of his total body surface area usually needs fluid resuscitation, which aims to support the body's compensatory mechanisms without overwhelming them. Patients with burns of 20% to 40% of total body surface area are at increased risk for developing systemic inflammatory syndrome. If the burns are over 40% total body surface area, the patient will suffer a profound inflammatory response syndrome with diffuse capillary leakage in the first 24 hours. Patients will also have increased energy expenditure

and muscle wasting despite adequate caloric intake. Expect to give fluids (such as lactated Ringer's solution) to keep the patient's urine output at 30 to 50 ml/hour, and expect to monitor blood pressure and heart rate. You'll also need to control body temperature because skin loss interferes with temperature regulation. Use warm fluids, heat lamps, and hyperthermia blankets, as appropriate, to keep the patient's temperature above 97° F (36.1° C), if possible. Additionally, you'll frequently review such laboratory values as serum electrolyte levels to detect early changes in the patient's condition.

Infection can increase wound depth, cause rejection of skin grafts, slow healing, worsen pain, prolong hospitalization, and even lead to death. To help prevent infection, use strict aseptic technique during care, dress the burn site, monitor and rotate

# Estimating burn surfaces in adults and children

You need to use different formulas to compute burned body surface area (BSA) in adults and children because the proportion of BSA varies with growth.

### Rule of Nines

You can quickly estimate the extent of an adult patient's burn by using the Rule of Nines. This method quantifies BSA in percentages either in fractions or multiples of nine. To use this method, mentally assess the patient's burns using the body chart shown below. Add the corresponding percentages for each body section burned. Use the total — a rough estimate of burn extent — to calculate initial fluid replacement needs.

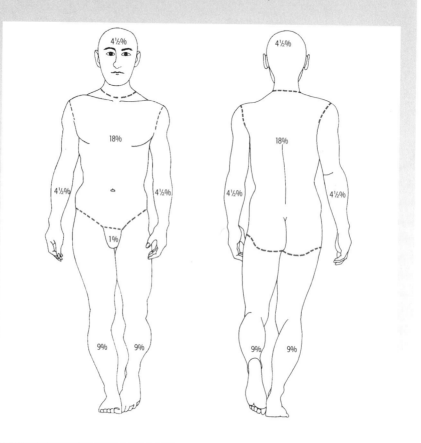

I.V. lines regularly, and carefully assess the burn extent, body system function, and the patient's emotional status.

Other interventions, such as careful positioning and regular exercise for burned extremities, help maintain joint function, prevent contractures, and minimize defor-

mity. (See *Positioning the burn patient to prevent deformity,* page 587.)

Skin integrity is repaired through aggressive wound debridement followed by maintenance of a clean wound bed until the wound heals or is covered with a skin graft. Full-thickness burns and some deep

# Estimating burn surfaces in adults and children *(continued)*

### Lund and Browder chart

The Rule of Nines isn't accurate for infants and children because their body shapes differ from those of adults. An infant's head, for example, accounts for about 17% of his total BSA, compared with 7% for an adult. Instead, use the Lund and Browder chart shown here.

### Percentage of burned body surface by age

| | At birth | 0–1 yr | 1–4 yr | 5–9 yr | 10–15 yr | Adult |
|---|---|---|---|---|---|---|
| **A: Half of head** | $9\frac{1}{2}$% | $8\frac{1}{2}$% | $6\frac{1}{2}$% | $5\frac{1}{2}$% | $4\frac{1}{2}$% | $3\frac{1}{2}$% |
| **B: Half of thigh** | $2\frac{3}{4}$% | $3\frac{1}{4}$% | 4% | $4\frac{1}{4}$% | $4\frac{1}{2}$% | $4\frac{3}{4}$% |
| **C: Half of leg** | $2\frac{1}{2}$% | $2\frac{1}{2}$% | $2\frac{3}{4}$% | 3% | $3\frac{1}{4}$% | $3\frac{1}{2}$% |

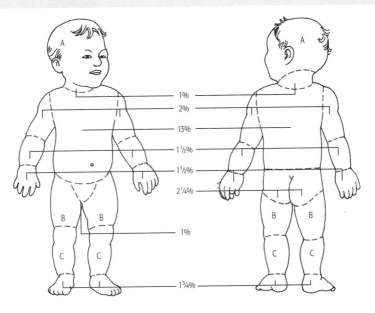

partial-thickness burns must be debrided and grafted in the operating room. The standard of care is to exercise and graft any burn that is judged unlikely to heal within 3 weeks. Surgery takes place as soon as possible after fluid resuscitation. Most wounds are managed with twice-daily dressing changes using topical antibiotics. Burn dressings encourage healing by barring germ entry and by removing exudate, eschar, and other debris that host infection. After thorough wound cleaning, topical antibacterial agents are applied and the wound is covered with absorptive, coarse-

# Evaluating burn severity

To judge a burn's severity, assess its depth and extent as well as the presence of other factors.

### Superficial partial-thickness (first-degree) burn

Does the burned area appear pink or red with minimal edema? Is the area sensitive to touch and temperature changes? If so, the patient most likely has a superficial partial-thickness, or first-degree, burn affecting only the epidermal skin layer.

### Deep partial-thickness (second-degree) burn

Does the burned area appear pink or red, with a mottled appearance? Do red areas blanch when you touch them? Does the skin have large, thick-walled blisters with subcutaneous edema? Does touching the burn cause severe pain? Is the hair still present? If so, the patient most likely has a deep partial-thickness, or second-degree, burn affecting the epidermal and dermal layers.

### Full-thickness (third-degree) burn

Does the burned area appear red, waxy white, brown, or black? Does red skin remain red with no blanching when you touch it? Is the skin leathery with extensive subcutaneous edema? Is the skin insensitive to touch? Does the hair fall out easily? If so, the patient most likely has a full-thickness, or third-degree, burn that affects all skin layers. The patient won't feel pain because the nerve endings are destroyed.

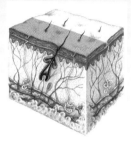 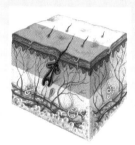 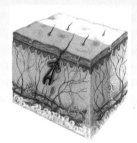

mesh gauze. Roller gauze typically tops the dressing and is secured with elastic netting or tape.

## Equipment

Normal saline solution • sterile bowl • sterile blunt scissors • sterile tissue forceps • ordered topical medication • burn gauze • roller gauze • fine-mesh gauze • elastic gauze • elastic netting or tape • cotton-tipped applicators or sterile tongue depressor • ordered pain medication • three pairs of sterile gloves • sterile gown • mask • surgical cap • heat lamps • impervious plastic trash bag • cotton bath blanket • 4″ × 4″ gauze pads

A sterile field is required, and all equipment and supplies used in the dressing should be sterile.

## Preparation of equipment

Warm normal saline solution by immersing unopened bottles in warm water. Assemble equipment on the dressing table. Make sure the treatment area has adequate light to allow accurate wound assessment. Open equipment packages using aseptic technique. Arrange supplies on a sterile field in order of use.

To prevent cross-contamination, plan to dress the cleanest areas first and the dirtiest or most contaminated last. To help prevent excessive pain or cross-contamination, you may need to perform the dressing in stages to avoid exposing all wounds at the same time.

# Positioning the burn patient to prevent deformity

| Burned area | Potential deformity | Preventive positioning | Nursing interventions |
|---|---|---|---|
| Neck | ▶ Flexion contraction of neck<br>▶ Extensor contraction of neck | ▶ Extension<br>▶ Prone with head slightly elevated | ▶ Remove pillow from bed.<br>▶ Place pillow or rolled towel under upper chest to flex cervical spine, or apply cervical collar. |
| Axilla | ▶ Adduction and internal rotation<br><br>▶ Adduction and external rotation | ▶ Shoulder joint in external rotation and 100- to 103-degree abduction<br>▶ Shoulder in forward flexion and 100- to 130-degree abduction | ▶ Use an I.V. pole, bedside table, or sling to suspend arm.<br>▶ Use an I.V. pole, bedside table, or sling to suspend arm. |
| Pectoral region | ▶ Shoulder protraction | ▶ Shoulders abducted and externally rotated | ▶ Remove pillow from bed. |
| Chest or abdomen | ▶ Kyphosis | ▶ Same as for pectoral region, with hips neutral (not flexed) | ▶ Use no pillow under head or legs. |
| Lateral trunk | ▶ Scoliosis | ▶ Supine; affected arm abducted | ▶ Put pillows or blanket roll at sides. |
| Elbow | ▶ Flexion and pronation | ▶ Arm extended and supinated | ▶ Use an elbow splint, arm board, or bedside table. |
| Wrist | ▶ Flexion<br>▶ Extension | ▶ Splint in 15-degree extension<br>▶ Splint in 15-degree flexion | ▶ Apply a hand splint.<br>▶ Apply a hand splint. |
| Fingers | ▶ Adhesions of the extensor tendons; loss of plantar grip | ▶ Metacarpophalangeal joints in maximum flexion; interphalangeal joints in slight flexion; thumb in maximum abduction | ▶ Apply a hand splint; wrap fingers separately. |
| Hip | ▶ Internal rotation, flexion, and adduction; possibly joint subluxation if contracture is severe | ▶ Neutral rotation and abduction; extension by prone position | ▶ Put a pillow under buttocks (if supine) or use trochanter rolls or knee or long leg splints. |
| Knee | ▶ Flexion | ▶ Extension | ▶ Use a knee splint with no pillows under legs. |
| Ankle | ▶ Plantar flexion if foot muscles are weak or their tendons are divided | ▶ 90-degree dorsiflexion | ▶ Use a footboard or ankle splint. |

## Implementation

▸ Give the ordered pain medication about 20 minutes before beginning wound care to maximize patient comfort and cooperation.
▸ Explain the procedure to the patient and provide privacy.
▸ Turn on overhead heat lamps to keep the patient warm. Make sure that they don't overheat the patient.
▸ Pour warmed normal saline solution into the sterile bowl in the sterile field.
▸ Wash your hands.

### Removing a dressing without hydrotherapy

▸ Put on a gown, a mask, and sterile gloves.
▸ Remove dressing layers down to the innermost layer by cutting the outer dressings with sterile blunt scissors. Lay open these dressings.
▸ If the inner layer appears dry, soak it with warm normal saline solution to ease removal.
▸ Remove the inner dressing with sterile tissue forceps or your sterile gloved hand.
▸ Because soiled dressings harbor infectious microorganisms, dispose of the dressings carefully in the impervious plastic trash bag according to facility policy. Dispose of your gloves and wash your hands.
▸ Put on a new pair of sterile gloves. Using gauze pads moistened with normal saline solution, gently remove any exudate and old topical medication.
▸ Carefully remove all loose eschar with sterile forceps and scissors, if ordered.
▸ Assess wound condition. The wound should appear clean, with no debris, loose tissue, purulence, inflammation, or darkened margins.
▸ Before applying a new dressing, remove your gown, gloves, and mask. Discard them properly, and put on a clean mask, surgical cap, gown, and sterile gloves.

### Applying a wet dressing

▸ Soak fine-mesh gauze and the elastic gauze dressing in a large sterile basin containing the ordered solution (for example, silver nitrate).
▸ Wring out the fine-mesh gauze until it's moist but not dripping and apply it to the wound. Warn the patient that he may feel transient pain when you apply the dressing.

▸ Wring out the elastic gauze dressing, and position it to hold the fine-mesh gauze in place.
▸ Roll an elastic gauze dressing over these two dressings to keep them intact.
▸ Cover the patient with a cotton bath blanket to prevent chills. Change the blanket if it becomes damp. Use an overhead heat lamp, if necessary.
▸ Change the dressings frequently to keep the wound moist, especially if you're using silver nitrate. Silver nitrate becomes ineffective, and the silver ions may damage tissue if the dressings become dry. (To maintain moisture, some protocols call for irrigating the dressing with solution at least every 4 hours through small slits cut into the outer dressing.)

### Applying a dry dressing with a topical medication

▸ Remove old dressings, and clean the wound (as described previously).
▸ Apply the ordered medication to the wound in a thin layer (about 2 to 4 mm thick) with your sterile gloved hand or sterile tongue depressor. Then apply several layers of burn gauze over the wound to contain the medication but allow exudate to escape.
▸ Remember to cut the dry dressing to fit only the wound areas; don't cover unburned areas.
▸ Cover the entire dressing with roller gauze and secure it with elastic netting or tape.
▸ Most dressings should be changed twice daily.

### Providing arm and leg care

▸ Apply the dressings from the distal to the proximal area to stimulate circulation and prevent constriction. Wrap the burn gauze once around the arm or leg so the edges overlap slightly. Continue wrapping in this way until the gauze covers the wound.
▸ Apply a dry roller gauze dressing to hold the bottom layers in place. Secure with elastic netting or tape.

### Providing hand and foot care

▸ Wrap each finger separately with a single layer of a 4″ × 4″ gauze pad to allow the patient to use his hands and to prevent webbing contractures.

▶ Place the hand in a functional position and secure this position using a dressing. Apply splints, if ordered.
▶ Put gauze between each toe as appropriate to prevent webbing contractures.

### Providing chest, abdomen, and back care
▶ Apply the ordered medication to the wound in a thin layer. Then cover the entire burned area with sheets of burn gauze.
▶ Wrap the area with roller gauze or apply a specialty vest dressing to hold the burn gauze in place.
▶ Secure the dressing with elastic netting or tape. Make sure the dressing doesn't restrict respiratory motion, especially in very young or elderly patients or in those with circumferential injuries.

### Providing facial care
▶ If the patient has scalp burns, clip or shave the hair around the burn as ordered. Clip other hair until it's about 2″ (5 cm) long to prevent contamination of burned scalp areas.
▶ Shave facial hair if it comes in contact with burned areas.
▶ Typically, facial burns are managed with milder topical agents (such as triple antibiotic ointment) and are left open to air. If dressings are required, make sure they don't cover the eyes, nostrils, or mouth.

### Providing ear care
▶ Clip or shave the hair around the affected ear.
▶ Remove exudate and crusts with cotton-tipped applicators dipped in normal saline solution.
▶ Place a layer of 4″ × 4″ gauze behind the auricle to prevent webbing.
▶ Apply the ordered medication to 4″ × 4″ gauze pads and place the pads over the burned area. Before securing the dressing with a roller bandage, position the patient's ears normally to avoid damaging the auricular cartilage.
▶ Assess the patient's hearing ability.

### Providing eye care
▶ Clean the area around the eyes and eyelids with a cotton-tipped applicator and normal saline solution every 4 to 6 hours, or as needed, to remove crusts and drainage.
▶ Give ordered eye ointments or eyedrops.

▶ If the eyes can't be closed, apply lubricating ointments or drops.
▶ Be sure to close the patient's eyes before applying eye pads to prevent corneal abrasion. Don't apply any topical ointments near the eyes without a doctor's order.

### Providing nasal care
▶ Check the nostrils for inhalation injury: inflamed mucosa, singed vibrissae, and soot.
▶ Clean the nostrils with cotton-tipped applicators dipped in normal saline solution. Remove crusts.
▶ Apply the ordered ointments.
▶ If the patient has a nasogastric tube, use tracheostomy ties to secure the tube. Be sure to check ties frequently for tightness resulting from swelling of facial tissue. Clean the area around the tube every 4 to 6 hours.

## Special considerations
▶ Thorough assessment and documentation of the wound's appearance are essential to detect infection and other complications. A purulent wound or green-gray exudate indicates infection, an overly dry wound suggests dehydration, and a wound with a swollen, red edge suggests cellulitis. Suspect a fungal infection if the wound is white and powdery. Healthy granulation tissue appears clean, pinkish, faintly shiny, and free of exudate.
▶ Because blisters protect underlying tissue, leave them intact unless they impede joint motion, become infected, or cause patient discomfort.
▶ Keep in mind that the patient with healing burns has increased nutritional needs. He'll require extra protein and carbohydrates to accommodate an almost doubled basal metabolism.
▶ If you must manage a burn with topical medications, exposure to air, and no dressing, watch for such problems as wound adherence to bed linens, poor drainage control, and partial loss of topical medications.

## Home care
Begin discharge planning as soon as the patient enters the facility to help him (and his family) make a smooth transition from facility to home. To encourage therapeutic compliance, prepare him to expect scarring, teach him wound management and

## Successful burn care after discharge

You can help the patient make a successful transition from hospital to home by encouraging him to follow the wound care and self-care guidelines below.

### Wound care

Instruct the patient or his family to follow this procedure when changing dressings:

▶ Clean the bathtub, shower, or washbasin thoroughly; then assemble the required equipment (topical medication, if ordered, and dressing supplies). Open the supplies aseptically on a clean surface.

▶ Wash your hands. Remove the old dressing and discard it.

▶ Using a clean washcloth and mild soap and water, wash the wound to remove all the old medication. Try to remove any loose skin too. Then pat the skin dry with a clean towel.

▶ Check the burned area for signs of infection, such as redness, heat, foul odor, increased pain, and difficulty moving the area. If any of these signs is present, notify the doctor after completing the dressing change.

▶ Wash your hands. If ordered, apply a thin layer of topical medication to the burned area.

▶ Cover the burned area with thin layers of gauze and wrap it with a roller gauze. Finally, secure the dressing with tape or elastic netting.

### Self-care

To enhance healing, instruct the patient to eat well-balanced meals with adequate carbohydrates and proteins, to eat between-meal snacks, and to include at least one protein source in each meal and snack. Tell him to avoid tobacco, alcohol, and caffeine because they constrict peripheral blood flow.

Advise the patient to wash new skin with mild soap and water. To prevent excessive skin dryness, instruct him to use a lubricating lotion and to avoid lotions containing alcohol or perfume. Caution the patient to avoid bumping or scratching regenerated skin tissue.

Recommend nonrestrictive, nonabrasive clothing, which should be laundered in a mild detergent. Advise the patient to wear protective clothing during cold weather to prevent frostbite.

Warn the patient not to expose new skin to strong sunlight and to always wear sunscreen with a sun protection factor of 20 or higher. Also, tell him not to expose new skin to irritants, such as paint, solvents, strong detergents, and antiperspirants. Recommend cool baths or ice packs to relieve itching.

To minimize scar formation, the patient may need to wear a pressure garment, usually for 23 hours per day for 6 months to 1 year. Instruct him to remove it only during daily hygiene. Suspect that the garment is too tight if the patient's fingers or toes are cold, numb, or discolored or if the garment's seams and zippers leave deep, red impressions for more than 10 minutes after the garment is removed.

---

pain control, and urge him to follow the prescribed exercise regimen.

Provide encouragement and emotional support and urge the patient to join a burn survivor support group. Also, teach the family or caregivers how to encourage, support, and provide care for the patient. (See *Successful burn care after discharge*.)

### Complications

Infection is the most common burn complication.

### Documentation

▶ Record the date and time of all care provided.

▶ Describe special dressing-change techniques, wound condition, topical medica-tions given, positioning of the burned area, and the patient's tolerance of the procedure.

### REFERENCES

American Burn Association. "Practice Guidelines for Burn Care," *Journal of Burn Care and Rehabilitation* 22(3 Suppl.), May-June 2001.

Wiebelhaus, P., et al. "Burns: Handle with Care," *RN* 62(11):52-58, November 1999.

# Closed-wound drain management

Typically inserted during surgery in anticipation of substantial postoperative drainage, a closed-wound drain promotes heal-

# Using a closed-wound drainage system

The portable closed-wound drainage system draws drainage from a wound site, such as the chest wall postmastectomy (shown at left), by means of a Y-tube. To empty the drainage, remove the plug and empty it into a graduated cylinder. To reestablish suc- tion, compress the drainage unit against a firm surface to expel air and, while holding it down, replace the plug with your other hand (as shown in the center). The same principle is used for the Jackson-Pratt bulb drain (shown at right).

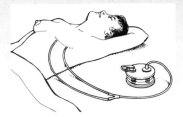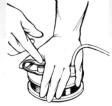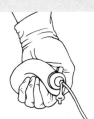

ing and prevents swelling by suctioning the serosanguineous fluid that accumulates at the wound site. By removing this fluid, the closed-wound drain helps reduce the risk of infection and skin breakdown as well as the number of dressing changes. Hemovac and Jackson-Pratt closed drainage systems are used most commonly.

A closed-wound drain consists of perforated tubing connected to a portable vacuum unit. The distal end of the tubing lies within the wound and usually leaves the body from a site other than the primary suture line to preserve the integrity of the surgical wound. The tubing exit site is treated as an additional surgical wound; the drain is usually sutured to the skin.

If the wound produces heavy drainage, the closed-wound drain may be left in place for longer than 1 week. Drainage must be emptied and measured frequently to maintain maximum suction and prevent strain on the suture line.

## Equipment

Graduated biohazard cylinder • sterile laboratory container, if needed • alcohol pads • gloves • gown • face shield • trash bag • sterile gauze pads • antiseptic cleaning agent • prepackaged povidone-iodine swabs • optional: label

## Implementation

▶ Check the doctor's order and assess the patient's condition.

▶ Explain the procedure to the patient, provide privacy, and wash your hands.
▶ Unclip the vacuum unit from the patient's bed or gown.
▶ Using aseptic technique, release the vacuum by removing the spout plug on the collection chamber. The container expands completely as it draws in air.
▶ Empty the unit's contents into a graduated biohazard cylinder, and note the amount and appearance of the drainage. If diagnostic tests will be performed on the fluid specimen, pour the drainage directly into a sterile laboratory container, note the amount and appearance, label the specimen, and send it to the laboratory.
▶ Maintaining aseptic technique, use an alcohol pad to clean the unit's spout and plug.
▶ To reestablish the vacuum that creates the drain's suction power, fully compress the vacuum unit. With one hand holding the unit compressed to maintain the vacuum, replace the spout plug with your other hand. (See *Using a closed-wound drainage system.*)
▶ Check the patency of the equipment. Make sure the tubing is free of twists, kinks, and leaks because the drainage system must be airtight to work properly. The vacuum unit should remain compressed when you release manual pressure; rapid reinflation indicates an air leak. If this occurs, recompress the unit and make sure the spout plug is secure.

▶ Secure the vacuum unit to the patient's gown. Fasten it below wound level to promote drainage. Don't apply tension on drainage tubing when fastening the unit to prevent possible dislodgment. Remove and discard your gloves and wash your hands thoroughly.

▶ Observe the sutures that secure the drain to the patient's skin; look for signs of pulling or tearing and for swelling or infection of surrounding skin. Gently clean the sutures with sterile gauze pads soaked in an antiseptic cleaning agent or with a povidone-iodine swab.

▶ Properly dispose of drainage, solutions, and trash bag and clean or dispose of soiled equipment and supplies according to facility policy.

### Special considerations

▶ Empty the drain and measure its contents once during each shift if drainage has accumulated, more often if drainage is excessive. Removing excess drainage maintains maximum suction and avoids straining the drain's suture line.

▶ Empty the drain and measure its contents before the patient ambulates to prevent the weight of drainage from pulling on the drain as the patient ambulates.

▶ If the patient has more than one closed drain, number the drains so you can record drainage from each site.

**◆◆ ALERT!** Be careful not to mistake chest tubes for closed-wound drains because the vacuum of a chest tube should never be released.

### Complications

Occlusion of the tubing by fibrin, clots, or other particles can reduce or obstruct drainage.

### Documentation

▶ Record the date and time you empty the drain, appearance of the drain site and presence of swelling or signs of infection, equipment malfunction and consequent nursing action, and patient's tolerance of the treatment.

▶ On the intake and output sheet, record drainage color, consistency, type, and amount. If the patient has more than one closed-wound drain, number the drains and record the information above separately for each drainage site.

**REFERENCES**
Edward, D., et al. *Bedside Critical Care Manual.* Philadelphia: Lippincott Williams & Wilkins, 2001.
McConnell, E.A. "Using a Closed-wound Drainage System," *Nursing* 29(6):32, June 1999.

# Cold application

The application of cold constricts blood vessels; inhibits local circulation, suppuration, and tissue metabolism; relieves vascular congestion; slows bacterial activity in infections; reduces body temperature; and may act as a temporary anesthetic during brief, painful procedures. (See *Reducing pain with ice massage.*)

Because treatment with cold also relieves inflammation, reduces edema, and slows bleeding, it may provide effective initial treatment after eye injuries, strains, sprains, bruises, muscle spasms, and burns. Cold doesn't reduce preexisting edema however, because it inhibits reabsorption of excess fluid.

Cold may be applied in dry or moist forms, but ice shouldn't be placed directly on a patient's skin because it may further damage tissue. Moist application is more penetrating than dry because moisture facilitates conduction. Devices for applying cold include an ice bag or collar, K pad (which can produce cold or heat), and chemical cold packs and ice packs. Devices for applying moist cold include cold compresses for small body areas and cold packs for large areas.

Apply cold treatments cautiously on patients with impaired circulation, on children, and on elderly or arthritic patients because of the risk of ischemic tissue damage.

### Equipment

Patient thermometer ● towel ● adhesive tape or roller gauze ● gloves, if necessary

*For an ice bag or collar*
Tap water ● ice chips ● absorbent, protective cloth covering

*For a K pad*
Temperature-adjustment key ● distilled water ● absorbent, protective cloth covering

*For a chemical cold pack*
Single-use packs are available for applying dry cold. These lightweight plastic packs contain a chemical that turns cold when activated. Reusable, sealed cold packs, filled with an alcohol-based solution, are also available. These packs may be stored frozen until use and, after exterior disinfection, may be refrozen and used again. Other chemical packs are activated by striking, squeezing, or kneading them.

*For a cold compress or pack*
Basin of ice chips ● container of tap water ● bath thermometer ● compress material (4″ × 4″ gauze pads or washcloths) or pack material (towels or flannel) ● linen-saver pad ● waterproof covering

## Preparation of equipment
### Ice bag or collar
Select a device of the correct size, fill it with cold tap water, and check for leaks. Then empty the device and fill it about halfway with crushed ice. Using small pieces of ice helps the device mold to the patient's body. Squeeze the device to expel air that might reduce conduction. Fasten the cap and wipe any moisture from the outside of the device. Wrap the bag or collar in a cloth covering, and secure the cover with tape or roller gauze. The protective cover prevents tissue trauma and absorbs condensation.

### K pad
Check the cord for frayed or damaged insulation. Then fill the control unit two-thirds full with distilled water or to the level recommended by the manufacturer. Don't use tap water because it leaves mineral deposits in the unit. Check for leaks and then tilt the unit several times to clear the pad's tubing of air. Tighten the cap. After ensuring that the hoses between the control unit and pad are free of tangles, place the unit on the bedside table, slightly above the patient so that gravity can assist water flow. If the central supply department hasn't preset the temperature, use the temperature-adjustment key to adjust the control unit setting to the lowest temperature. Cover the pad with an absorbent, protective cloth and secure the cover with tape or roller gauze. Plug in the unit and turn it on. Allow the pad to cool for 2 minutes before placing it on the patient.

## Reducing pain with ice massage

In most cases ice shouldn't be applied directly to the patient's skin because it risks damaging the skin surface and underlying tissues. However, when carefully performed, ice massage may help the patient tolerate brief, painful procedures, such as bone marrow aspiration, catheterization, chest tube removal, injection into joints, lumbar puncture, and suture removal.

Prepare for ice massage by gathering the ice, a porous covering to hold it in (if desired), and a cloth for wiping water from the patient as the ice melts. The water may be frozen in a paper cup ahead of time. The paper is then removed from one-half of the cup and the exposed ice is rubbed on the skin.

Just before the procedure begins, rub the ice over the appropriate area to numb it. Assess the site frequently; stop rubbing immediately if you detect signs of tissue intolerance.

As the procedure begins, rub the ice over a point near, but not at the site. This distracts the patient from the procedure itself and gives him another stimulus on which to concentrate.

If the procedure lasts longer than 10 minutes or if you think tissue damage may occur, move the ice to a different site and continue massage.

If you know in advance that the procedure probably will last longer than 10 minutes, massage the site intermittently—2 minutes of massage alternating with a rest period—until the skin regains its normal color. Alternatively, you can divide the area into several sites and apply ice to each for several minutes at a time.

*Chemical cold pack*
Select a pack of the appropriate size, and follow the manufacturer's directions (strike, squeeze, or knead) to activate the cold-producing chemicals. Make certain that the container hasn't been broken during activation. Wrap the pack in a cloth cover and secure the cover with tape or roller gauze.

*Cold compress or pack*
Cool a container of tap water by placing it in a basin of ice or by adding ice to the water. Using a bath thermometer for guidance, adjust the water temperature to 59° F

# Using cold for a muscle sprain

Cold can help relieve pain and reduce edema during the first 24 to 72 hours after a sprain occurs. Tell the patient to apply cold to the area four times daily for 20 to 30 minutes each time.

For each application, instruct the patient to obtain enough crushed ice to cover the painful area, place it in a plastic bag, and place the bag inside a pillowcase or large piece of cloth (as shown below).

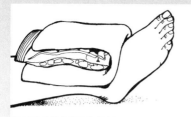

For later applications, the patient may want to fill a paper cup with water, stand a tongue blade in the cup, and place it in the freezer. After the water freezes, he can peel the paper off the ice and hold it with the protruding handle. If he chooses this method, tell him to first cover the area with a cloth. Applying ice directly to the skin can cause frostbite or cold shock.

Instruct the patient to rub the ice over the painful area for the specified treatment time. Warn him that although ice eases pain in a joint that has begun to stiffen, he shouldn't let the analgesic effect encourage overuse of the joint.

After 24 to 72 hours, when heat and swelling have subsided or when cold no longer helps, the patient should switch to heat application.

(15° C) or as ordered. Immerse the compress or pack material in the water.

## Implementation

▶ Check the doctor's order and assess the patient's condition.
▶ Explain the procedure to the patient, provide privacy, and make sure the room is warm and free of drafts. Wash your hands thoroughly.
▶ Record the patient's temperature, pulse, and respirations to serve as a baseline.

▶ Expose only the treatment site to avoid chilling the patient.

### Applying an ice bag or collar, a K pad, or a chemical cold pack
▶ Place the covered cold device on the treatment site and begin timing the application.
▶ Observe the site frequently for signs of tissue intolerance, such as blanching, mottling, cyanosis, maceration, and blisters. Also be alert for shivering and complaints of burning or numbness. If this sign or these symptoms develop, discontinue treatment and notify the doctor.
▶ Refill or replace the cold device as necessary to maintain the correct temperature. Change the protective cover if it becomes wet.
▶ Remove the device after the prescribed treatment period (usually 30 minutes).

### Applying a cold compress or pack
▶ Place a linen-saver pad under the site.
▶ Remove the compress or pack from the water and wring it out to prevent dripping. Apply it to the treatment site and begin timing the application.
▶ Cover the compress or pack with a waterproof covering to provide insulation and to keep the surrounding area dry. Secure the covering with tape or roller gauze to prevent it from slipping.
▶ Check the application site frequently for signs of tissue intolerance and note complaints of burning or numbness. If these symptoms develop, discontinue treatment and notify the doctor.
▶ Change the compress or pack as needed to maintain the correct temperature. Remove it after the prescribed treatment period (usually 20 minutes).

### Concluding all cold applications
▶ Dry the patient's skin and re-dress the treatment site according to the doctor's orders. Then position the patient comfortably and take his temperature, pulse, and respirations for comparison with baseline.
▶ Dispose of liquids and soiled materials properly. If the cold treatment will be repeated, clean and store the equipment in the patient's room, out of his reach; otherwise, return it to storage.

## Special considerations

▶ Apply cold immediately after an injury to minimize edema. (See *Using cold for a muscle sprain.*) Although colder temperatures can be tolerated for a longer time when the treatment site is small, don't continue any application for longer than 1 hour to avoid reflex vasodilation. The application of temperatures below 59° F (15° C) also causes local reflex vasodilation.

▶ Use sterile technique when applying cold to an open wound or to a lesion that may open during treatment. Also maintain sterile technique during eye treatment, with separate sterile equipment for each eye to prevent cross-contamination.

▶ Avoid securing cooling devices with pins because an accidental puncture could allow extremely cold fluids to leak out and burn the patient's skin.

▶ If the patient is unconscious, anesthetized, neurologically impaired, irrational, or otherwise insensitive to cold, stay with him throughout the treatment and check the application site frequently for complications.

▶ Warn the patient against placing ice directly on his skin because the extreme cold can cause burns.

## Complications

Hemoconcentration may cause thrombi. Intense cold may cause pain, burning, or numbness.

## Documentation

▶ Record the time, date, and duration of cold application; type of device used (ice bag or collar, K pad, or chemical cold pack); site of application; temperature or temperature setting; patient's temperature, pulse, and respirations before and after application; skin appearance before, during, and after application; signs or symptoms of complications; and the patient's tolerance of treatment.

### REFERENCES

Edward, D., et al. *Bedside Critical Care Manual.* Philadelphia: Lippincott Williams & Wilkins, 2001.

Kuzu, N., and Ucar, H. "The Effect of Cold on the Occurrence of Bruising, Haematoma and Pain at the Injection Site in Subcutaneous Low Molecular Weight Heparin," *International Journal of Nursing Studies* 38(1):51-59, February 2001.

# Direct heat application

Heat applied directly to the patient's body raises tissue temperature and enhances the inflammatory process by causing vasodilation and increasing local circulation. This promotes leukocytosis, suppuration, drainage, and healing. Heat also increases tissue metabolism, reduces pain caused by muscle spasm, and decreases congestion in deep visceral organs.

Direct heat may be dry or moist. Dry heat can be delivered at a higher temperature and for a longer time. Devices for applying dry heat include the hot-water bottle, electric heating pad, K pad, and chemical hot pack.

Moist heat softens crusts and exudates, penetrates deeper than dry heat, is less drying to the skin, produces less perspiration, and usually is more comfortable for the patient. Devices for applying moist heat include warm compresses for small body areas and warm packs for large areas.

Direct heat treatment can't be used on a patient at risk for hemorrhage. It's also contraindicated if the patient has a sprained limb in the acute stage (because vasodilation would increase pain and swelling) or if he has a condition associated with acute inflammation such as appendicitis. Direct heat should be applied cautiously to pediatric and elderly patients and to patients with impaired renal, cardiac, or respiratory function; arteriosclerosis or atherosclerosis; or impaired sensation. It should be applied with extreme caution to heat-sensitive areas, such as scar tissue and stomas.

## Equipment

Patient thermometer ● towel ● adhesive tape or roller gauze ● absorbent, protective cloth covering ● gloves, if the patient has an open lesion

*For a hot-water bottle*
Hot tap water ● pitcher ● bath thermometer ● absorbent, protective cloth covering

*For an electric heating pad*
Absorbent, protective cloth covering

*For a K pad*
Distilled water ● temperature-adjustment key ● absorbent, protective cloth covering

*For a chemical hot pack (disposable)*
Absorbent, protective cloth covering

*For a warm compress or pack (sterile or nonsterile)*
Basin of hot tap water or container of sterile water, normal saline, or other solution as ordered ● bath thermometer ● hot-water bottle, K pad, or chemical hot pack ● linen-saver pad ● optional: forceps

The following items may be sterile or nonsterile as needed: compress material (such as flannel and 4″ × 4″ gauze pads) or pack material (such as absorbent towels and large absorbent pads) ● cotton-tipped applicators ● forceps ● bowl or basin ● bath thermometer ● waterproof covering ● towel ● dressing

### Preparation of equipment
*Hot-water bottle*
Fill the bottle with hot tap water to detect leaks and warm the bottle; then empty it. Run hot tap water into a pitcher and measure the water temperature with the bath thermometer. Adjust the temperature, usually to 115° to 125° F (46.1° to 51.7° C) for adults.

◆ **ALERT!** Adjust the water temperature to 105° to 115° F (40.6° to 46.1° C) for elderly patients or children younger than age 2.

Next, pour hot water into the bottle, filling it one-half to two-thirds full. Partially filling the bottle keeps it lightweight and flexible to mold to the treatment area. Squeeze the bottle until the water reaches the neck to expel any air that would make the bottle inflexible and reduce heat conduction. Fasten the top and cover the bag with an absorbent cloth. Secure the cover with tape or roller gauze.

*Electric heating pad*
Check the cord for frayed or damaged insulation. Then plug in the pad and adjust the control switch to the desired setting. Wrap the pad in a protective cloth covering and secure the cover with tape or roller gauze.

*K pad*
Check the cord for frayed or damaged insulation and fill the control unit two-thirds full with distilled water, according to the manufacturer's directions. Don't use tap water because it leaves mineral deposits in the unit. Check for leaks and then tilt the unit in several directions to clear the pad's tubing of air. Tighten the cap and then loosen it a quarter turn to allow heat expansion within the unit. After making sure the hoses between the control unit and the pad are free of tangles, place the unit on the bedside table, slightly above the patient so that gravity can assist water flow. If the central supply department hasn't preset the temperature, use the temperature-adjustment key provided to set the temperature on the control unit. The usual temperature is 105° F. Place the pad in a protective cloth covering and secure the cover with tape or roller gauze. Plug in the unit, turn it on, and allow the pad to warm for 2 minutes.

*Chemical hot pack*
Select a pack of the correct size. Follow the manufacturer's directions (strike, squeeze, or knead) to activate the heat-producing chemicals. Place the pack in a protective cloth covering, and secure the cover with tape or roller gauze.

*Sterile warm compress or pack*
Warm the container of sterile water or solution by setting it in a sink or basin of hot water. Measure its temperature with a sterile bath thermometer. If a sterile thermometer is unavailable, pour some heated sterile solution into a clean container, check the temperature with a regular bath thermometer, and then discard the tested solution. Adjust the temperature by adding hot or cold water to the sink or basin until the solution reaches 131° F (55° C) for adults.

Pour the heated solution into a sterile bowl or basin. Then using sterile technique, soak the compress or pack in the heated solution. If necessary, prepare a hot-water bottle, K pad, or chemical hot pack to keep the compress or pack warm.

*Nonsterile warm compress or pack*
Fill a bowl or basin with hot tap water or other solution, and measure the temperature of the fluid with a bath thermometer. Adjust the temperature, usually to 131° F (55° C) for adults.

Soak the compress or pack in the hot liquid. If necessary, prepare a hot-water bottle, K pad, or chemical hot pack to keep the compress or pack warm.

## Implementation
▶ Check the doctor's order and assess the patient's condition.
▶ Explain the procedure to the patient and tell him not to lean or lie directly on the heating device because this reduces air space and increases the risk of burns. Warn him against adjusting the temperature of the heating device or adding hot water to a hot-water bottle. Advise him to report pain immediately and remove the device if necessary.
▶ Provide privacy and make sure the room is warm and free from drafts.
▶ Wash your hands.
▶ Take the patient's temperature, pulse, and respiration to serve as a baseline. If heat treatment is being applied to raise the patient's body temperature, monitor temperature, pulse, and respirations throughout the application.
▶ Expose only the treatment area because vasodilation will make the patient feel chilly.

### Applying a hot-water bottle, an electric heating pad, a K pad, or a chemical hot pack
▶ Before applying the heating device, press it against your inner forearm to test its temperature and heat distribution. If it heats unevenly, obtain a new device.
▶ Apply the device to the treatment area and, if necessary, secure it with tape or roller gauze. Begin timing the application.
▶ Assess the patient's skin condition frequently and remove the device if you observe increased swelling or excessive redness, blistering, maceration, or pallor or if the patient reports discomfort. Refill the hot-water bottle as necessary to maintain the correct temperature.
▶ Remove the device after 20 to 30 minutes, or as ordered.
▶ Dry the patient's skin with a towel and redress the site, if necessary. Take the patient's temperature, pulse, and respiration for comparison with the baseline. Position him comfortably in bed.
▶ If the treatment is to be repeated, store the equipment in the patient's room, out of his reach; otherwise, return it to its proper place.

### Applying a warm compress or pack
▶ Place a linen-saver pad under the site.
▶ Remove the warm compress or pack from the bowl or basin. (Use sterile forceps throughout the procedure if needed.)
▶ Wring excess solution from the compress or pack. Excess moisture increases the risk of burns.
▶ Apply the compress gently to the affected site. After a few seconds, lift the compress and check the skin for excessive redness, maceration, or blistering. When you're sure the compress isn't causing a burn, mold it firmly to the skin to keep air out, which reduces the temperature and effectiveness of the compress. Work quickly so the compress retains its heat.
▶ Apply a waterproof covering (sterile, if necessary) to the compress. Secure it with tape or roller gauze to prevent it from slipping.
▶ Place a hot-water bottle, K pad, or chemical hot pack over the compress and waterproof covering to maintain the correct temperature. Begin timing the application.
▶ Check the patient's skin every 5 minutes for tissue tolerance. Remove the device if the skin shows excessive redness, maceration, or blistering or if the patient experiences pain or discomfort. Change the compress as needed to maintain the correct temperature.
▶ Remove the compress after 15 to 20 minutes, or as ordered. Discard the compress into a waterproof trash bag.
▶ Dry the patient's skin with a towel (sterile, if necessary). Note the condition of the skin and redress the area, if necessary. Take the patient's temperature, pulse, and respiration for comparison with baseline. Make sure the patient is comfortable.

## Special considerations
▶ If the patient is unconscious, anesthetized, irrational, neurologically impaired, or insensitive to heat, stay with him throughout the treatment.
▶ When direct heat is ordered to decrease congestion within internal organs, the application must cover a large enough area to increase blood volume at the skin's surface. For relief of pelvic organ congestion, for example, apply heat over the patient's lower abdomen, hips, and thighs. To achieve local relief, you may concentrate heat only over the specified area. (See *Using moist heat to relieve muscle spasm,* page 598.)

## Using moist heat to relieve muscle spasm

Tell patients to choose moist heat rather than dry heat when attempting to ease muscle tension or spasm. Moist heat is less drying to the skin, less apt to cause burns, less likely to cause excessive fluid and salt loss through sweating, and more likely to penetrate deeper tissues. Instruct the patient to apply heat for 20 to 30 minutes, as follows:

▶ Place a moist towel over the painful area.

▶ Cover the towel with a hot-water bottle properly filled and at the correct temperature.

▶ Remove the hot-water bottle and wet pack after 20 to 30 minutes. Don't continue application for longer than 30 minutes because therapeutic value decreases after that time.

---

▶ As an alternative method of applying sterile moist compresses, use a bedside sterilizer to sterilize the compresses. Saturate the compress with tap water or another solution and wring it dry. Then place it in the bedside sterilizer at 275° F (135° C) for 15 minutes. Remove the compress with sterile forceps or sterile gloves, and wring out the excess solution. Then place the compress in a sterile bowl and measure its temperature with a sterile thermometer.

▶ Currently microwave ovens are being used to heat compresses and packaged hot packs. Be sure to follow the pack directions and don't overheat or underheat the packet. Always check the temperature before placing the device on the affected area.

### Complications

Because tissue damage may result from direct heat application, monitor the temperature of the compress carefully. Frequently assess the condition of the patient's skin under the heat application device.

### Documentation

▶ Record the time and date of heat application including type, temperature or heat setting, duration, and site of application; the patient's temperature, pulse, respirations, and skin condition before, during, and after treatment; signs of complications; and the patient's tolerance of the treatment.

**REFERENCES**
Barillo, D.J., et al. "Burns Caused by Medical Therapy," *The Journal of Burn Care & Rehabilitation* 21(3):269-73; discussion 268, May-June 2000.
Edward, D., et al. *Bedside Critical Care Manual.* Philadelphia: Lippincott Williams & Wilkins, 2001.

# Hydrotherapy

Treating diseases or injuries by immersing part or all of the patient's body in water is known as hydrotherapy. Commonly used to debride serious burns and to hasten healing, hydrotherapy also promotes circulation and comfort in patients with peripheral vascular disease and musculoskeletal disorders such as arthritis. Although hydrotherapy usually involves immersing the patient in a tub of water ("tubbing"), showers or other water-spray techniques may replace tubbing in some health care facilities and burn centers. (See *Positioning the patient for hydrotherapy.*)

The nurse or physical therapist usually assists the patient into the tub or shower area if he's ambulatory. If he isn't ambulatory, he can enter the water using a stretcher or hoist device.

Hydrotherapy is contraindicated in the presence of sudden changes: fever, electrolyte or fluid imbalance, or unstable vital signs. Always follow the standard precautions guidelines.

### Equipment

Water tank or tub or shower table ● plastic tub liner ● chemical additives as ordered ● plinth (padded table for patient to sit or lie on while performing exercises) ● stretcher ● headrest ● hydraulic hoist ● gown ● surgical cap ● mask ● gloves (for removing dressings) ● shoulder-length gloves (for tubbing) ● apron ● debridement instruments ● razor, shaving cream, mild soap, shampoo, and washcloth (for general cleaning) ● fluffed gauze pads ● cotton-tipped applicators ● sterile sheets ● warm, sterile bath blankets ● optional: analgesic

Barriers, sheets, and bath blankets may be sterile or clean, depending on the patient's condition and your facility's infection-control policies.

## Preparation of equipment

Thoroughly clean and disinfect the tub or shower, its equipment, and the tub or shower room before each treatment to prevent cross-contamination. After cleaning, place the tub liner in the tub and fill the tub with warm water (98° to 104° F [36.6° to 40° C]).

Attach the headrest to the sides of the tub. Add prescribed chemicals (such as sodium chloride) to the water to maintain the normal isotonic level (usually 0.9%) and to prevent dialysis and tissue irritation. Also add potassium chloride to prevent potassium loss and calcium hypochlorite detergent as ordered. Warm the bath blankets and ensure that the room is warm enough to avoid chilling the patient.

## Implementation

▶ If this is the patient's first treatment, explain the procedure to him to allay his fears and promote cooperation. As necessary (before debridement, for example), give an analgesic about 20 minutes before the procedure.
▶ Check the patient's vital signs.
▶ If the patient is receiving an I.V. infusion, make sure that he has enough I.V. solution to last through the procedure.
▶ Transfer the patient to a stretcher and transport him to the therapy room. If he's ambulatory, he may walk unassisted, provided that the therapy room is nearby.
▶ Wash your hands and put on your gown, gloves, mask, and surgical cap.
▶ Remove the outer dressings and dispose of them properly before immersing the patient. Leave the inner gauze layer on the wound unless it can be easily removed.
▶ If the patient is ambulatory, position him on the plinth for transfer to the tub, or assist him into the tub and situate him on the already lowered plinth.
▶ If the patient isn't ambulatory, attach the stretcher to the overhead hydraulic hoist. Ensure that the hoist hooks are fastened securely. Use the hoist to transfer the patient to and from the tub.
▶ Lower the patient into the tub. Position him so that the headrest supports his head. Allow him to soak for 3 to 5 minutes.
▶ Remove your gloves, wash your hands, and put on the shoulder-length tubbing gloves and apron.
▶ Remove remaining gauze dressings, if any, from the patient's wounds.

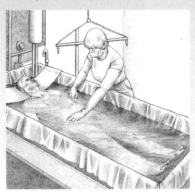
▶ If ordered, place the tub's agitator into the water and turn it on. The motor may burn out if it's turned on out of the water. Some tubs have aerators to agitate the water.
▶ Clean all unburned areas first (encourage the patient to do this if he can). Wash unburned skin, and clip or shave hair near the wound. Shave facial hair, shampoo the scalp, and give mouth care, as appropriate. Provide perineal care, and clean inside the patient's nose and the folds of the ears and eyes with cotton-tipped applicators.
▶ Gently scrub burned areas with fluffed gauze pads to remove topical agents, exudates, necrotic tissue, and other debris. Debride the wound after turning off the agitator.
▶ Exercise the patient's extremities with active or passive range of motion, depending on his condition and exercise tolerance. Alternatively, you may have the physical therapist exercise the patient.
▶ After you've completed the treatment, use the hoist to raise the patient above the water.

▶ With the patient still suspended over the water, spray-rinse his body to remove debris from shaving, cleaning, and debridement.

▶ Transfer the patient to a stretcher covered with a clean sheet and bath blanket, and cover him with a warm sterile sheet (a blanket may be added for warmth). Pat unburned areas dry to prevent chilling.

▶ Remove the wet or damp sheets and cover the patient with dry sheets. Remove your gown, gloves, and mask before transporting the patient to the dressing area for further debridement, if needed, and new sterile dressings.

▶ Have the tub drained, cleaned, and disinfected according to facility policy.

## Special considerations

▶ Remain with the patient at all times to prevent accidents in the tub. Limit hydrotherapy to 20 or 30 minutes. Watch the patient closely for adverse reactions.

▶ Patients with an endotracheal tube may receive hydrotherapy. Spray their wounds while they're suspended over the tub on a plinth. Immerse patients with longstanding tracheostomies only with a doctor's order.

▶ If necessary, weigh the patient during hydrotherapy to assess nutritional status and fluid shift. Use a hoist that has a table scale.

▶ Whirlpool treatments should be discontinued when the wounds are assessed as clean because the whirlpool's agitating water may result in trauma to the regenerating tissue.

## Complications

Incomplete disinfection of tub, drains, and faucets or cross-contamination from members of the tubbing team may cause infection. The patient may chill easily from decreased resistance to temperature changes. A fluid or electrolyte imbalance (or both) may result from a chemical imbalance between the patient and the tub solution.

## Documentation

▶ Record the date, time, and patient's reaction.

▶ Note the patient's condition (including vital signs and wound appearance).

▶ Document any wound infection or bleeding.

▶ Note treatments given, such as debridement and dressing changes.

▶ Record any special treatments in the nursing plan of care.

## REFERENCES

Ahlqvist, J. "Hydrotherapy Has Had and Has a Rationale," *Rheumatology* (Oxford). 41(9):1070-71, September 2002.

Moore, J.E., et al. "Incidence of *Pseudomonas aeruginosa* in Recreational and Hydrotherapy Pool," *Communicable Disease and Public Health* 5(1):23-26, March 2002.

# Hyperthermia-hypothermia therapy

A blanket-sized aquathermia K pad, the hyperthermia-hypothermia blanket raises, lowers, or maintains body temperature through conductive heat or cold transfer between the blanket and the patient. It can be operated manually or automatically.

In manual operation, the nurse or doctor sets the temperature on the unit. The blanket reaches and maintains this temperature regardless of the patient's temperature. The temperature control must be adjusted manually to reach a different setting. The nurse monitors the patient's body temperature with a conventional thermometer.

In automatic operation, the unit directly and continually monitors the patient's temperature by means of a thermistor probe (rectal, skin, or esophageal) and alternates heating and cooling cycles as necessary to achieve and maintain the desired body temperature. The thermistor probe also may be used in conjunction with manual operation but isn't essential. The unit is equipped with an alarm to warn of abnormal temperature fluctuations and a circuit breaker that protects against current overload.

The blanket is most commonly used to reduce high fever when more conservative measures, such as baths, ice packs, and antipyretics, are unsuccessful. Other uses include maintaining normal temperature during surgery or shock; inducing hypothermia during surgery to decrease metabolic activity and thereby reduce oxygen requirements; reducing intracranial pressure; controlling bleeding and intractable pain in patients with amputations, burns, or cancer; and providing warmth in cases of severe hypothermia.

## Equipment

Hyperthermia-hypothermia control unit • operation manual • fluid for the control unit (distilled water or distilled water and 20% ethyl alcohol) • thermistor probe (such as rectal, skin, or esophageal) • patient thermometer • one or two hyperthermia-hypothermia blankets • one or two disposable blanket covers (or one or two sheets or bath blankets) • lanolin or a mixture of lanolin and cold cream • adhesive tape • towel • sphygmomanometer • gloves and gown, if necessary • optional: protective wraps for the patient's hands and feet

Disposable hyperthermia-hypothermia blankets are available for single-patient use.

### Preparation of equipment

First, read the operation manual. Inspect the control unit and each blanket for leaks and the plugs and connecting wires for broken prongs, kinks, and fraying. If you detect or suspect malfunction, don't use the equipment.

Review the doctor's order, and prepare one or two blankets by covering them with disposable covers (or use a sheet or bath blanket when positioning the blanket on the patient). The cover absorbs perspiration and condensation, which could cause tissue breakdown if left on the skin. Connect the blanket to the control unit, and set the controls for manual or automatic operation and for the desired blanket or body temperature. Make sure the machine is properly grounded before plugging it in.

Turn on the machine and add liquid to the unit reservoir, if necessary, as fluid fills the blanket. Allow the blanket to preheat or precool so that the patient receives immediate thermal benefit.

## Implementation

▶ Assess the patient's condition and explain the procedure to him. Provide privacy and make sure the room is warm and free from drafts. Check facility policy and, if necessary, make sure the patient or a responsible family member has signed a consent form.

▶ Wash your hands thoroughly. If the patient isn't already wearing a patient gown, ask him to put one on. Use a gown with cloth ties rather than metal snaps or pins to prevent heat or cold injury.

▶ Take the patient's temperature, pulse, respirations, and blood pressure to serve as a baseline and assess his level of consciousness, pupil reaction, limb strength, and skin condition.

▶ Keeping the bottom sheet in place and the patient recumbent, roll the patient to one side and slide the blanket halfway underneath him so that its top edge aligns with his neck. Then roll the patient back, and pull and flatten the blanket across the bed. Place a pillow under the patient's head. Make sure that his head doesn't lie directly on the blanket because the blanket's rigid surface may be uncomfortable and the heat or cold may lead to tissue breakdown. If necessary, use a sheet or bath blanket as insulation between the patient and the blanket.

▶ Apply lanolin or a mixture of lanolin and cold cream to the patient's skin where it touches the blanket to help protect the skin from heat or cold sensation.

▶ In automatic operation, insert the thermistor probe in the patient's rectum and tape it in place to prevent accidental dislodgment. If rectal insertion is contraindicated, tuck a skin probe deep into the axilla and secure it with tape. If the patient is comatose or anesthetized, insert an esophageal probe. Plug the other end of the probe into the correct jack on the unit's control panel.

▶ Place a sheet or, if ordered, the second hyperthermia-hypothermia blanket over the patient. This increases the thermal benefit by trapping cooled or heated air.

▶ Wrap the patient's hands and feet if he wishes to minimize chilling and promote comfort. Monitor vital signs and perform a neurologic assessment every 5 minutes until the desired body temperature is reached and then every 15 minutes until temperature is stable or as ordered.

▶ Check fluid intake and output hourly or as ordered. Observe the patient regularly for color changes in skin, lips, and nail beds and for edema, induration, inflammation, pain, and sensory impairment. If they occur, discontinue the procedure and notify the doctor.

▶ Reposition the patient every 30 minutes to 1 hour, unless contraindicated, to prevent skin breakdown. Keep the patient's skin, bedclothes, and blanket cover free from perspiration and condensation and

# Using a warming system

Shivering, which is the compensatory response to falling body temperature, may use more oxygen than the body can supply, especially in a surgical patient. In the past, you would cover the patient with blankets to warm his body. Now, health care facilities may supply a warming system such as the Bair Hugger patient-warming system (shown below).

This new system helps to gradually increase body temperature. Like a large hair dryer, the warming unit draws air through a filter, warms the air to the desired temperature, and circulates it through a hose connected to a warming blanket that's placed over the patient.

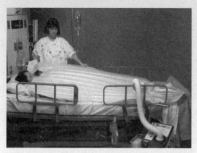

When using the warming system, follow these guidelines:
▶ Use a bath blanket in a single layer over the warming blanket to minimize heat loss.
▶ Place the warming blanket directly over the patient with the paper side facing down and the clear tubular side facing up.
▶ Make sure the connection hose is at the foot of the bed.
▶ Take the patient's temperature during the first 15 to 30 minutes and at least every 30 minutes while the warming blanket is in use.
▶ Obtain guidelines from the patient's doctor for discontinuing use of the warming blanket.

reapply cream to exposed body parts as needed.
▶ After turning off the machine, follow the manufacturer's directions. Some units must remain plugged in for at least 30 minutes to allow the condenser fan to remove water vapor from the mechanism. Continue to monitor the patient's temperature until it stabilizes because body temperature

can fall as much as 5° F (2.8° C) after this procedure.
▶ Remove all equipment from the bed. Dry the patient and make him comfortable. Supply a fresh patient gown, if necessary. Cover him lightly.
▶ Continue to perform neurologic checks and monitor vital signs, fluid intake and output, and general condition every 30 minutes for 2 hours and then hourly or as ordered.
▶ Return the equipment to the central supply department for cleaning, servicing, and storage.

## Special considerations
▶ If the patient shivers excessively during hypothermia treatment, discontinue the procedure and notify the doctor immediately. By increasing metabolism, shivering elevates body temperature.
▶ Avoid lowering the temperature more than 1 degree every 15 minutes to prevent premature ventricular contractions.
▶ Don't use pins to secure catheters, tubes, or blanket covers because an accidental puncture can result in fluid leakage and burns.
▶ With hyperthermia or hypothermia therapy, the patient may experience a secondary defense reaction (such as vasoconstriction or vasodilation, respectively) that causes body temperature to rebound and thus defeat the treatment's purpose.
▶ If the patient requires isolation, place the blanket, blanket cover, and probe in a plastic bag clearly marked with the type of isolation so that the central supply department can give it special handling. If the blanket is disposable, discard it, using appropriate precautions.
▶ To avoid bacterial growth in the reservoir or blankets, always use sterile distilled water and change it monthly. Check to see if facility policy calls for adding a bacteriostatic agent to the water. Avoid using deionized water because it may corrode the system.
▶ To gradually increase body temperature, especially in postoperative patients, the doctor may order a disposable warming system. (See *Using a warming system.*)

## Complications
Use of a hyperthermia-hypothermia blanket can cause shivering, marked changes in vital signs, increased intracranial pressure,

respiratory distress or arrest, cardiac arrest, oliguria, and anuria.

## Documentation

▶ Record the patient's pulse, respirations, blood pressure, neurologic signs, fluid intake and output, skin condition, and position change.

▶ Record the patient's temperature and that of the blanket every 30 minutes while the blanket is in use.

▶ Document the type of hyperthermia-hypothermia unit used; control settings (manual or automatic and temperature settings); date, time, duration, and patient's tolerance of treatment; and signs of complications.

### REFERENCES

Edward, D., et al. *Bedside Critical Care Manual.* Philadelphia: Lippincott Williams & Wilkins, 2001.

Shankaran, S., et al. "Whole-body Hypothermia for Neonatal Encephalopathy: Animal Observations as a Basis for a Randomized, Controlled Pilot Study in Term Infants," *Pediatrics* 110(2 Part 1):377-85, August 2002.

# Laser therapy

Using the highly focused and intense energy of a laser beam, the surgeon can treat various skin lesions. Laser surgery has several advantages. As a surgical instrument, the laser offers precise control. It spares normal tissue, speeds healing, and deters infection by sterilizing the operative site. In addition, by sealing tiny blood vessels as it vaporizes tissue, the laser beam leaves a nearly bloodless operative field. In addition, the procedure can be performed on an outpatient basis.

The lasers used most commonly to treat skin lesions are vascular, pigment, and carbon dioxide ($CO_2$) lasers. (See *Understanding types of laser therapy,* page 604.)

In general, laser surgery is safe, although bleeding and scarring can result. One pronounced hazard to the patient and treatment staff alike is eye damage or other injury caused by unintended laser beam reflection. For this reason, everyone in the surgical suite, including the patient, must wear special goggles to filter laser light. Also, the surgeon must use special nonre-flective instruments. Access to the room must be strictly controlled, and all windows must be covered.

## Equipment

Laser ● filtration face masks ● protective eyewear ● laser vacuum ● extra vacuum filters ● prescribed cleaning solution ● surgical drape ● sterile gauze ● nonadherent dressings ● surgical tape ● cotton-tipped applicators ● nonreflective surgical instruments ● gowns ● sterile gloves

### Preparation of equipment

Before the procedure begins, prepare the tray. It should include a local anesthetic and dry and wet gauze. The gauze will be used to control bleeding, protect healthy tissue, and abrade and remove any eschar, which would otherwise inhibit laser absorption. Prepare surgical instruments as needed.

## Implementation

▶ Put on gown, filtration face mask, and protective eyewear.

▶ Tell the patient how the laser works and review its benefits. Point out the equipment and outline the procedure to help allay the patient's concerns.

▶ Just before the surgeon begins, position the patient comfortably, drape him, and place protective gauze, if needed, around the operative site. Confirm that everyone in the room, including the patient, has protective eyewear on to filter the laser light.

▶ Lock the door to the surgical suite to keep unprotected persons from inadvertently entering the room.

▶ After the surgeon gives the anesthetic and it takes effect, activate the laser vacuum. The $CO_2$ laser has a vacuum hose attached to a separate apparatus. Use this apparatus to clear the surgical site. The vacuum has a filter that traps and collects most of the vaporized tissue. Change the filter whenever suction decreases and follow facility guidelines for filter disposal.

▶ When the surgeon finishes the procedure, apply direct pressure with a sterile gauze pad to any bleeding wound for 20 minutes. (Wear sterile gloves.) If the wound continues to bleed, notify the doctor.

▶ Once the bleeding is controlled, use aseptic technique to clean the area with a cotton-tipped applicator dipped in the prescribed cleaning solution. Then size and

# Understanding types of laser therapy

Laser therapy has become an essential tool for treating many types of skin lesions. The number of lasers used in dermatology is growing, and each type is used for specific conditions. The term *laser* is an acronym for Light Amplification by the Stimulated Emission of Radiation. When directed toward the skin, most of this light energy is absorbed by chromophores, which are substances that absorb specific wavelengths of light. This is the basis of selective photothermolysis, which has revolutionized cutaneous laser surgery. Melanin is the target chromophore in pigmented lesions, and oxyhemoglobin in microvessels is the target chromophore in vascular lesions.

The factors that determine the thermal effect from laser light are energy, density, pulse direction, and heat conduction. The thermal effects of laser light can be changed by changing these factors.

To provide the most effective case, you should be familiar with the various types of lasers and the indications for each.

### Lasers for vascular lesions

The laser most commonly used for vascular lesions is the flashlamp-pumped dye laser (FLPDL). Other types include copper vapor, argon, KTP, krypton, neodymium:yttrium-aluminum-garnet (Nd:YAG), and frequency-doubled Q-switched Nd:YAG lasers. The type of laser used depends on the type of vascular lesion. Port-wine stains, hemangiomas, venous lake, rosacea, telangiectasia, and Kaposi's sarcoma are examples of vascular lesions that are appropriate for laser therapy.

### Lasers for pigmented lesions

Lasers that are effective in treating tattoos and dermal and epidermal pigmented lesions include Q-switched ruby, Q-switched Nd:YAG, Q-switched alexandrite, FLPDL, copper vapor, krypton, and KTP. Among the pigmented lesions appropriate for laser treatment are nevi of Ota, melasma, solar lentigo, café-au-lait spots, Becker's nevi, and epidermal nevi.

### Carbon dioxide laser

Although it's one of the oldest lasers, the carbon dioxide laser is used less commonly since the advent of lasers that work on the principle of selective photothermolysis. This laser causes thermal injury, resulting in ablation in the defocused mode and cut tissue in the focused mode. It's used to treat actinic cheilitis, rhinophyma, warts, keloids, and other lesions.

### Lasers for hair removal

Lasers used to eliminate unwanted hair include ruby, diode, alexondrite, and Nd:YAG. Laser treatment is only effective in removing dark-colored hair; it isn't effective for removing blonde, red, white, or gray hair.

---

cut a nonadherent dressing. Secure the dressing with surgical tape.
▶ Vascular and pigment lasers won't result in a wound; only superficial skin changes will occur.

## Special considerations
▶ The surgeon uses the laser beam much as he would a scalpel to excise the lesion. Explain that the laser causes a burnlike wound that can be deep. Inform the patient that the wound will appear charred. Also, tell the patient that some of the eschar will be removed during the initial postoperative cleaning and that more will gradually dislodge at home.
▶ Warn the patient to expect a burning odor and smoke during the procedure. A machine called a smoke evacuator, which sounds like a vacuum cleaner, will clear it away. Advise the patient that he may sense heat from the laser. Urge him to tell the doctor immediately if pain develops.
▶ The nurse must have thorough knowledge of how each laser operates and of laser safety considerations for both the patient and the health care providers.

## Home care
Teach the patient how to dress his wound or care for his skin daily as ordered by the surgeon. Tell him that he can take showers but shouldn't immerse the wound site in water to promote wound healing and prevent infection.

If the wound bleeds at home, demonstrate how to apply direct pressure on the site with clean gauze or a washcloth for 20 minutes. If pressure doesn't control the bleeding, tell the patient to call his doctor.

If the patient's foot or leg was operated on, urge him to keep the extremity elevated and to use it as little as possible because pressure can inhibit healing.

Warn the patient to protect the treated area from exposure to the sun to avoid changes in pigmentation. Tell him to call the doctor if a fever of 100° F (37.8° C) or higher persists longer than 1 day.

## Complications

Bleeding, scarring, and infection are rare complications of laser surgery.

## Documentation

▶ Note the patient's skin condition before and after the procedure.
▶ Document any bleeding, record the type of dressing applied, and list the patient's complaints of pain.
▶ Note whether the patient comprehends home care instructions.

### REFERENCES

Franz, R. "Laser Therapy and Microdermabrasion Treat Acne Scars," *Dermatology Nursing* 13(5):396, October 2001.
Loo, W.J., and Lanigan, S.W. "Recent Advances in Laser Therapy for the Treatment of Cutaneous Vascular Disorders," *Lasers in Medical Science* 17(1):9-12, 2002.
McBurney, E. "Side Effects and Complications of Laser Therapy," *Dermatology Clinics* 20(1):165-76, January 2002.

# Mechanical debridement

Debridement involves removing necrotic tissue by mechanical, chemical, or surgical means to allow underlying healthy tissue to regenerate. Mechanical debridement procedures include irrigation, hydrotherapy, and excision of dead tissue with forceps and scissors. The procedure may be done at the bedside or in a specially prepared room. Keep in mind that state and facility policies vary as to the nurse's role in debridement.

Depending on the type of burn, a combination of debridement techniques may be used. Other debridement techniques include chemical debridement (with wound-cleaning beads or topical agents that absorb exudate and debris) or surgical excision and skin grafting (usually reserved for deep burns or ulcers). Typically, the patient receives a local or general anesthetic.

Burn wound debridement removes eschar (hardened, dead tissue). This prevents or controls infection, promotes healing, and prepares the wound surface to receive a graft. Ideally, the wound should be debrided daily during the dressing change. Frequent, regular debridement guards against possible hemorrhage resulting from more extensive and forceful debridement. It also reduces the need to conduct extensive debridement under anesthesia.

Closed blisters over partial-thickness burns shouldn't be debrided.

## Equipment

Ordered pain medication ● two pairs of sterile gloves ● two gowns or aprons ● mask ● cap ● sterile scissors ● sterile forceps ● 4″ × 4″ sterile gauze pads ● sterile solutions and medications as ordered ● hemostatic agent, as ordered

Be sure to have the following equipment immediately available to control hemorrhage: needle holder, gut suture with needle, and silver nitrate sticks.

## Implementation

▶ Explain the procedure to the patient to allay his fears and promote cooperation. Teach him distraction and relaxation techniques, if possible, to minimize his discomfort.
▶ Provide privacy. Give an analgesic 20 minutes before debridement begins, or give an I.V. analgesic immediately before the procedure.
▶ Keep the patient warm. Expose only the area to be debrided to prevent chilling and fluid and electrolyte loss.
▶ Wash your hands and put on a cap, mask, gown or apron, and sterile gloves.
▶ Remove the burn dressings and clean the wound.
▶ Remove your gown or apron and dirty gloves and change to another gown or apron and sterile gloves.
▶ Lift loosened edges of eschar with forceps. Use the curved, blunt dissecting scissors to probe the eschar. Care should be taken not to disturb any new epithelium. Cut the dead tissue from the wound with the scissors. Leave a ¼″ (0.6-cm) edge on remaining eschar to avoid cutting into viable tissue.

▶ Because debridement removes only dead tissue, bleeding should be minimal. If bleeding occurs, apply gentle pressure on the wound with sterile 4″ × 4″ gauze pads. Then apply the hemostatic agent. If bleeding persists, notify the doctor and maintain pressure on the wound until he arrives. Excessive bleeding or spurting vessels may require ligation.

▶ Perform additional procedures, such as application of topical medications and dressing replacements as ordered.

### Special considerations

▶ Work quickly, with an assistant, if possible, to complete this painful procedure as soon as possible. Limit the procedure time to 20 minutes, if possible.

▶ Acknowledge the patient's discomfort and provide emotional support.

▶ Debride no more than a 4″ (10.2-cm) square area at one time.

### Complications

Because burns damage or destroy the protective skin barrier, infection may develop despite the use of aseptic technique and equipment. In addition, some blood loss may occur if debridement exposes an eroded blood vessel or if you inadvertently cut a vessel. Fluid and electrolyte imbalances may result from exudate lost during the procedure.

### Documentation

▶ Record the date and time of wound debridement, the area debrided, and solutions and medications used.

▶ Describe wound condition, noting signs of infection or skin breakdown.

▶ Record the patient's tolerance of and reaction to the procedure.

▶ Note indications for additional therapy.

**REFERENCES**

Attinger, C., et al. "Surgical Debridement: The Key to Successful Wound Healing and Reconstruction," *Clinics in Podiatric Medicine and Surgery* 17(4):599-630, October 2000.

Wound, Ostomy, and Continence Nurses Society. *Position Statement: Conservative Sharp Wound Debridement for Registered Nurses.* Costa Mesa, Calif.: WOCN, 1996. *www.wocn.org/publications/posstate/debride.htm.*

Wound, Ostomy, and Continence Nurses Society. *Position Statement: Staging of Pressure Ulcers.* Costa Mesa, Calif.: WOCN, 1996. *www.wocn.org/publications/posstate/staging.htm.*

## Pressure ulcer care

As their name implies, pressure ulcers result when pressure, applied with great force for a short period or with less force over a longer period, impairs circulation, depriving tissues of oxygen and other life-sustaining nutrients. This process damages skin and underlying structures. Untreated, the ischemic lesions that result can lead to serious infection.

Most pressure ulcers develop over bony prominences, where friction and shearing force combine with pressure to break down skin and underlying tissues. Common sites include the sacrum, coccyx, ischial tuberosities, and greater trochanters. Other common sites include the skin over the vertebrae, scapulae, elbows, knees, and heels in bedridden and relatively immobile patients.

Successful pressure ulcer treatment involves relieving pressure, restoring circulation and, if possible, resolving or managing related disorders. Typically, the effectiveness and duration of treatment depend on the pressure ulcer's characteristics. (See *Assessing pressure ulcers.*)

Ideally, prevention is the key to avoiding extensive therapy. Preventive measures include ensuring adequate nourishment and mobility to relieve pressure and promote circulation. (See *Braden scale for predicting pressure ulcer risk,* pages 608 and 609.)

When a pressure ulcer develops despite preventive efforts, treatment includes methods to decrease pressure, such as frequent repositioning to shorten pressure duration and the use of special equipment to reduce pressure intensity. Treatment also may involve special pressure-reducing devices, such as beds, mattresses, mattress overlays, and chair cushions. Other therapeutic measures include risk factor reduction and the use of topical treatments, wound cleansing, debridement, and dressings to support moist wound healing. (See *Guide to topical agents for pressure ulcers,* page 610.)

# Assessing pressure ulcers

To select the most effective treatment for a pressure ulcer, you first need to assess its characteristics. The pressure ulcer staging system described below, used by the National Pressure Ulcer Advisory Panel and the Agency for Healthcare Research and Quality, reflects the anatomic depth of exposed tissue. Keep in mind that if the wound contains necrotic tissue, you won't be able to determine the stage until you can see the wound base.

### Stage 1

The heralding lesion of a pressure ulcer is persistent redness in lightly pigmented skin and persistent red, blue, or purple hues on darker skin. Other indicators include changes in temperature, consistency, or sensation.

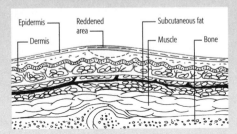

### Stage 2

This stage is marked by partial-thickness skin loss involving the epidermis, the dermis, or both. The ulcer is superficial and appears as an abrasion, a blister, or a shallow crater.

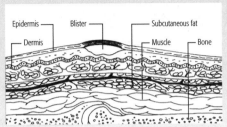

### Stage 3

The ulcer constitutes a full-thickness wound penetrating the subcutaneous tissue, which may extend to – but not through – underlying fascia. The ulcer resembles a deep crater and may undermine adjacent tissue.

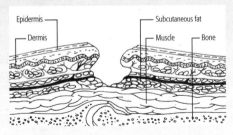

### Stage 4

The ulcer extends through the skin, accompanied by extensive destruction, tissue necrosis, or damage to muscle, bone, or supporting structures (such as tendons and joint capsules).

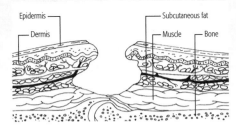

Vacuum-assisted closure (VAC) is a relatively new treatment for wounds that are difficult to heal. Approved by the Food and Drug Administration in 1995, VAC aids wound healing by applying a controlled level of negative pressure to remove blood

(Text continues page 610.)

# Braden scale for predicting pressure ulcer risk

The Braden scale, shown below, is the most reliable of several instruments for assessing the older patient's risk of developing pressure ulcers. The lower the score, the greater the risk.

**Patient's name**_____     **Evaluator's name**_____

| | | |
|---|---|---|
| **Sensory perception** <br> Ability to respond meaningfully to pressure-related discomfort | **1 Completely limited:** Is unresponsive (doesn't moan, flinch, or grasp in response) to painful stimuli because of diminished level of consciousness or sedation <br><br> **OR** <br><br> Has a limited ability to feel pain over most of body surface | **2 Very limited:** Responds only to painful stimuli; can't communicate discomfort except through moaning or restlessness <br><br> **OR** <br><br> Has a sensory impairment that limits ability to feel pain or discomfort over half of body |
| **Moisture** <br> Degree to which skin is exposed to moisture | **1 Constantly moist:** Skin is kept moist almost constantly by perspiration, urine, or other fluid; dampness is detected every time patient is moved or turned | **2 Very moist:** Skin is usually but not always moist; linens must be changed at least once per shift |
| **Activity** <br> Degree of physical activity | **1 Bedridden:** Confined to bed | **2 Confined to chair:** Ability to walk severely limited or nonexistent; can't bear own weight and must be assisted into chair or wheelchair |
| **Mobility** <br> Ability to change and control body position | **1 Completely immobile:** Doesn't make even slight changes in body or extremity position without assistance | **2 Very limited:** Makes occasional slight changes in body or extremity position but can't make frequent or significant changes independently |
| **Nutrition** <br> Usual food intake pattern | **1 Very poor:** Never eats a complete meal; rarely eats more than one-third of any food offered; eats two servings or less of protein (meat or dairy products) per day; takes fluids poorly; doesn't take a liquid dietary supplement <br><br> **OR** <br><br> Is nothing-by-mouth status or maintained on clear liquids or I.V. fluids for more than 5 days | **2 Probably inadequate:** Rarely eats a complete meal and generally eats only about one-half of any food offered; protein intake includes only three servings of meat or dairy products per day; occasionally will take a dietary supplement <br><br> **OR** <br><br> Receives less than optimum amount of liquid diet or tube feeding |
| **Friction and shear** | **1 Problem:** Requires moderate to maximum assistance in moving; complete lifting without sliding against sheets is impossible; frequently slides down in bed or chair, requiring frequent repositioning with maximum assistance; spasticity, contractures, or agitation leads to almost constant friction | **2 Potential problem:** Moves feebly or requires minimum assistance during a move; skin probably slides to some extent against sheets, chair restraints, or other devices; maintains relatively good position in chair or bed most of the time but occasionally slides down |

| | | Date of Assessment | | | | |
|---|---|---|---|---|---|---|

| | | | | | | |
|---|---|---|---|---|---|---|
| **3 Slightly limited:** Responds to verbal commands but can't always communicate discomfort or need to be turned<br>**OR**<br>Has some sensory impairment that limits ability to feel pain or discomfort in one or two extremities | **4 No impairment:** Responds to verbal commands; has no sensory deficit that would limit ability to feel or voice pain or discomfort | | | | | |
| **3 Occasionally moist:** Skin is occasionally moist; linens require an extra change approximately once per day | **4 Rarely moist:** Skin is usually dry; linens require changing only at routine intervals | | | | | |
| **3 Walks occasionally:** Walks occasionally during day, but for very short distances, with or without assistance; spends majority of each shift in bed or chair | **4 Walks frequently:** Walks outside room at least twice per day and inside room at least once every 2 hours during waking hours | | | | | |
| **3 Slightly limited:** Makes frequent though slight changes in body or extremity position independently | **4 No limitations:** Makes major and frequent changes in body or extremity position without assistance | | | | | |
| **3 Adequate:** Eats more than half of most meals; eats four servings of protein (meat and dairy products) per day; occasionally refuses a meal but will usually take a supplement if offered<br>**OR**<br>Is on a tube feeding or total parenteral nutrition regimen that probably meets most nutritional needs | **4 Excellent:** Eats most of every meal and never refuses a meal; usually eats four or more servings of meat and dairy products per day; occasionally eats between meals; doesn't require supplementation | | | | | |
| **3 No apparent problem:** Moves in bed and in chair independently and has sufficient muscle strength to lift up completely during move; maintains good position in bed or chair at all times | | | | | | |
| | **Total score: 6 to 23** | | | | | |

# Guide to topical agents for pressure ulcers

| Topical agents | Nursing considerations |
| --- | --- |
| **Antibiotics** <br> silver sulfadiazine, triple antibiotics | ▶ Consider a 2-week trial of topical antibiotics for clean or exudated pressure ulcers that aren't responding to moist-wound healing therapy. |
| **Circulatory stimulants** <br> (Granulex, Proderm) | ▶ Use these agents to promote blood flow. Both contain balsam of Peru and castor oil, but Granulex also contains trypsin, an enzyme that facilitates debridement. |
| **Enzymes** <br> collagenase (Santyl), sutilains (Travase) | ▶ Apply collagenase in thin layers after cleaning the wound with normal saline solution. <br> ▶ Avoid concurrent use of collagenase with agents that decrease enzymatic activity, including detergents, hexachlorophene, antiseptics with heavy-metal ions, iodine, and such acid solutions as Burow's solution. <br> ▶ Use collagenase cautiously near the patient's eyes. If contact occurs, flush the eyes repeatedly with normal saline solution or sterile water. <br> ▶ If using sutilains and topical antibacterials, apply sutilains ointment first. <br> ▶ Avoid applying sutilains to ulcers in major body cavities, areas with exposed nerve tissue, or fungating neoplastic lesions. Don't use sutilains in women of childbearing age or in the patient with limited cardiopulmonary reserve. <br> ▶ Store sutilains at a cool temperature: 35.6° to 50° F (2° to 10° C). <br> ▶ Use sutilains cautiously near the patient's eyes. If contact occurs, flush the eyes repeatedly with normal saline solution or sterile water. |
| **Exudate absorbers** <br> dextranomer beads (Debrisan) | ▶ Use dextranomer beads on secreting ulcers. Discontinue use when secretions stop. <br> ▶ Clean, but don't dry, the ulcer before applying dextranomer beads. Don't use in tunneling ulcers. <br> ▶ Remove gray-yellow beads (which indicate saturation) by irrigating with sterile water or normal saline solution. <br> ▶ Use cautiously near the eyes. If contact occurs, flush the eyes repeatedly with normal saline solution or sterile water. |
| **Isotonic solutions** <br> normal saline solution | ▶ This agent moisturizes tissue without injuring cells. |

or serous drainage, accelerating debridement and promoting wound healing.

Nurses usually perform or coordinate treatments according to facility policy. The procedures detailed below address cleaning and dressing the pressure ulcer. Always follow the standard precautions guidelines of the Centers for Disease Control and Prevention.

## Equipment

Hypoallergenic tape or elastic netting ● overbed table ● piston-type irrigating system ● two pairs of gloves ● normal saline solution as ordered ● sterile 4"x 4" gauze pads ● sterile cotton swabs ● selected topical dressing ● linen-saver pads ● disposable wound-measuring device ● impervious plastic trash bag

### Preparation of equipment

Assemble equipment at the patient's bedside. Cut tape into strips for securing dressings. Loosen lids on cleaning solutions and medications for easy removal. Loosen existing dressing edges and tapes before putting on gloves. Attach an impervious plastic trash bag to the overbed table to hold used dressings and refuse.

## Implementation

▶ Before any dressing change, wash your hands and review the principles of standard precautions.

### Cleaning the pressure ulcer

▶ Provide privacy, and explain the procedure to the patient to allay his fears and promote cooperation.

▶ Position the patient in a way that maximizes his comfort while allowing easy access to the pressure ulcer site.

▶ Cover bed linens with a linen-saver pad to prevent soiling.

▶ Open the normal saline solution container and the piston syringe. Carefully pour normal saline solution into an irrigation container to avoid splashing. (The container may be clean or sterile, depending on facility policy.) Put the piston syringe into the opening provided in the irrigation container.

▶ Open the packages of supplies.

▶ Put on gloves to remove the old dressing and expose the pressure ulcer. Discard the soiled dressing in the impervious plastic trash bag to avoid contaminating the sterile field and spreading infection.

▶ Inspect the wound. Note the color, amount, and odor of drainage and necrotic debris. Measure the wound perimeter with the disposable wound-measuring device (a square, transparent card with concentric circles arranged in bull's-eye fashion and bordered with a straight-edge ruler).

▶ Using the piston syringe, apply full force to irrigate the pressure ulcer to remove necrotic debris and help decrease bacteria in the wound. In non-necrotic wounds, gentle pressure is used so new tissue is not harmed.

▶ Remove and discard your soiled gloves, and put on a fresh pair.

▶ Insert a gloved finger or sterile cotton swab into the wound to assess wound tunneling or undermining. Tunneling usually signals wound extension along fascial planes. Gauge tunnel depth by determining how far you can insert your finger or the cotton swab.

▶ Next, reassess the condition of the skin and the ulcer. Note the character of the clean wound bed and the surrounding skin.

▶ If you observe adherent necrotic material, notify a wound care specialist or a doctor to ensure appropriate debridement.

▶ Prepare to apply the appropriate topical dressing. Directions for typical moist saline gauze, hydrocolloid, transparent, alginate, foam, and hydrogel dressings follow. For other dressings or topical agents, follow your facility's protocol or the supplier's instructions.

### Applying a moist saline gauze dressing

▶ Irrigate the pressure ulcer with normal saline solution. Blot the surrounding skin dry.

▶ Moisten the gauze dressing with normal saline solution.

▶ Gently place the dressing over the surface of the ulcer. To separate surfaces within the wound, gently place a dressing between opposing wound surfaces. To avoid damage to tissues, don't pack the gauze tightly.

▶ Change the dressing often enough to keep the wound moist. (See *Choosing a pressure ulcer dressing,* page 612.)

### Applying a hydrocolloid dressing

▶ Irrigate the pressure ulcer with normal saline solution. Blot the surrounding skin dry.

▶ Choose a clean, dry, presized dressing, or cut one to overlap the pressure ulcer by about 1″ (2.5 cm). Remove the dressing from its package, pull the release paper from the adherent side of the dressing, and apply the dressing to the wound. To minimize irritation, carefully smooth out wrinkles as you apply the dressing.

▶ If the dressing's edges need to be secured with tape, apply a skin sealant to the intact skin around the ulcer. After the area dries, tape the dressing to the skin. The sealant protects the skin and promotes tape adherence. Avoid using tension or pressure when applying the tape.

▶ Remove your gloves and discard them in the impervious plastic trash bag. Dispose of refuse according to facility policy, and wash your hands.

▶ Change a hydrocolloid dressing every 2 to 3 days or as necessary—for example, if the patient complains of pain, the dressing no longer adheres, or leakage occurs. Discoloration of the dressing is a sign that infection is present.

# Choosing a pressure ulcer dressing

The patient's needs and the ulcer's characteristics determine which type of dressing to use on a pressure ulcer.

### Gauze dressings

Made of absorptive cotton or synthetic fabric, these dressings are permeable to water, water vapor, and oxygen and may be impregnated with petroleum jelly or another agent. When uncertain about which dressing to use, you may apply a gauze dressing moistened in saline solution until a wound specialist recommends definitive treatment.

Be sure not to get moist dressing on skin areas surrounding the wound because it will cause maceration and further skin breakdown.

### Hydrocolloid dressings

These adhesive, moldable wafers are made of a carbohydrate-based material and usually have waterproof backings. They are impermeable to oxygen, water, and water vapor, and most have some absorptive properties.

### Transparent film dressings

Clear, adherent, and nonabsorptive, these polymer-based dressings are permeable to oxygen and water vapor, but not to water. Their transparency allows visual inspection. Because they can't absorb drainage, transparent film dressings are used on partial-thickness wounds with minimal exudate.

### Alginate dressings

Made from seaweed, these nonwoven, absorptive dressings are available as soft, white, sterile pads or ropes. They absorb excessive exudate and may be used on infected wounds. As these dressings absorb exudate, they turn into a gel that keeps the wound bed moist and promotes healing. When exudate is no longer excessive, switch to another type of dressing.

### Foam dressings

These spongelike polymer dressings may be impregnated or coated with other materials. Somewhat absorptive, they may be adherent. Foam dressings promote moist wound healing and are useful when a nonadherent surface is desired.

### Hydrogel dressings

Water-based and nonadherent, these polymer-based dressings have some absorptive properties. They're available as a gel in a tube, as flexible sheets, and as saturated gauze packing strips. They may have a cooling effect, which eases pain.

---

## Applying a transparent dressing

▶ Irrigate the pressure ulcer with normal saline solution. Blot the surrounding skin dry.
▶ Clean and dry the wound as described above.
▶ Select a dressing to overlap the ulcer by 2″ (5 cm).
▶ Gently lay the dressing over the ulcer. To prevent shearing force, don't stretch the dressing. Press firmly on the edges of the dressing to promote adherence. Although this type of dressing is self-adhesive, you may have to tape the edges to prevent them from curling.
▶ If necessary, aspirate accumulated fluid with a 21G needle and syringe. After aspirating the pocket of fluid, clean the aspiration site with an alcohol pad and cover it with another strip of transparent dressing.
▶ Change the dressing every 2 to 3 days, depending on the amount of drainage.

## Applying an alginate dressing

▶ Irrigate the pressure ulcer with normal saline solution. Blot the surrounding skin dry.
▶ Apply the alginate dressing to the ulcer surface. Cover the area with a secondary dressing (such as gauze pads) as ordered. Secure the dressing with tape or elastic netting.
▶ If the wound is draining heavily, change the dressing once or twice daily for the first 3 to 5 days. As drainage decreases, change the dressing less frequently—every 2 to 4 days or as ordered. When the drainage

stops or the wound bed looks dry, stop using alginate dressing.

### Applying a foam dressing

▶ Irrigate the pressure ulcer with normal saline solution. Blot the surrounding skin dry.

▶ Gently lay the foam dressing over the ulcer.

▶ Use tape, elastic netting, or gauze to hold the dressing in place.

▶ Change the dressing when the foam no longer absorbs the exudate.

### Applying a hydrogel dressing

▶ Irrigate the pressure ulcer with normal saline solution. Blot the surrounding skin dry.

▶ Apply gel to the wound bed.

▶ Cover the area with a secondary dressing.

▶ Change the dressing daily or as needed to keep the wound bed moist.

▶ If the dressing you select comes in sheet form, cut the dressing to match the wound base; otherwise, the intact surrounding skin can become macerated.

▶ Hydrogel dressings also come in a prepackaged, saturated gauze for wounds that require "dead space" to be filled. Follow the manufacturer's directions for usage.

### Preventing pressure ulcers

▶ Turn and reposition the patient every 1 to 2 hours unless contraindicated. For a patient who can't turn himself or who is turned on a schedule, use a pressure-reducing device, such as air, gel, or a 4″ foam mattress overlay. Low- or high-air-loss therapy may be indicated to reduce excessive pressure and promote evaporation of excess moisture. As appropriate, implement active or passive range-of-motion exercises to relieve pressure and promote circulation. To save time, combine these exercises with bathing if applicable.

▶ When turning the patient, lift him rather than slide him because sliding increases friction and shear. Use a turning sheet and get help from coworkers if necessary.

▶ Use pillows to position your patient and increase his comfort. Be sure to eliminate sheet wrinkles that could increase pressure and cause discomfort.

▶ Post a turning schedule at the patient's bedside. Adapt position changes to his situation. Emphasize the importance of regular position changes to the patient and his family, and encourage their participation in treatment and prevention of pressure ulcers by having them perform a position change correctly after you have demonstrated how.

▶ Avoid placing the patient directly on the trochanter. Instead, place him on his side, at about a 30-degree angle.

▶ Except for brief periods, avoid raising the head of the bed more than 30 degrees to prevent shearing force.

▶ Direct the patient confined to a chair or wheelchair to shift his weight every 15 minutes to promote blood flow to compressed tissues. Show a paraplegic patient how to shift his weight by doing push-ups in the wheelchair. If the patient needs your help, sit next to him and help him shift his weight to one buttock for 60 seconds; then repeat the procedure on the other side. Provide him with pressure-relieving cushions as appropriate. However, avoid seating the patient on a rubber or plastic doughnut, which can increase localized pressure at vulnerable points.

▶ Adjust or pad appliances, casts, or splints as needed to ensure proper fit and avoid increased pressure and impaired circulation.

▶ Tell the patient to avoid heat lamps and harsh soaps because they dry the skin. Applying lotion after bathing will help keep his skin moist. Also tell him to avoid vigorous massage because it can damage capillaries.

▶ If the patient's condition permits, recommend a diet that includes adequate calories, protein, and vitamins. Dietary therapy may involve nutritional consultation, food supplements, enteral feeding, or total parenteral nutrition.

▶ If diarrhea develops or if the patient is incontinent, clean and dry soiled skin. Then apply a protective moisture barrier to prevent skin maceration.

▶ Make sure the patient, family members, and caregivers learn pressure ulcer prevention and treatment strategies so that they understand the importance of care, the choices that are available, the rationales for treatments, and their own role in selecting goals and shaping the plan of care.

### Special considerations

▶ Avoid using elbow and heel protectors that fasten with a single narrow strap. The strap may impair neurovascular function in the involved hand or foot.

▶ Avoid using too-tight leg straps for urinary catheters.

▶ Avoid using artificial sheepskin. It doesn't reduce pressure, and it may create a false sense of security.

▶ Repair of stage 3 and stage 4 ulcers may require surgical intervention, such as direct closure, skin grafting, and flaps, depending on the patient's needs.

### Complications

Infection may cause foul-smelling drainage, persistent pain, severe erythema, induration, and elevated skin and body temperatures. Advancing infection or cellulitis can lead to septicemia. Severe erythema may signal worsening cellulitis, which indicates that the offending organisms have invaded the tissue and are no longer localized.

### Documentation

▶ Record the date and time of initial and subsequent treatments. Note the specific treatment given. Detail preventive strategies performed.

▶ Document the pressure ulcer's location and size (length, width, and depth); color and appearance of the wound bed; amount, odor, color, and consistency of drainage; and condition of the surrounding skin.

▶ Update the plan of care as required. Note any change in the condition or size of the pressure ulcer and any elevation of skin temperature on the clinical record.

▶ Document when the doctor was notified of any pertinent abnormal observations.

▶ Record the patient's temperature daily on the graphic sheet to allow easy assessment of body temperature patterns.

**REFERENCES**

Chua, P.C., et al. "Vacuum-Assisted Wound Closure," *AJN* 100(12):45-48, December 2000.

Greer, S., et al. "Technologies for Applying Subatmospheric Pressure Dressing to Wounds in Difficult Regions of the Anatomy," *Journal of Wound, Ostomy, and Continence Nursing* 26(5):250-53, September 1999.

Ovington, L.G. "Hanging Wet-to-Dry Dressing Out to Dry," *Home Healthcare Nurse* 19(8): 477-83, August 2001.

Ovington, L.G. "Wound Care Protocols: How to Choose," *Home Healthcare Nurse* 19(4):224-31, April 2001.

Thomas, D.R. "Prevention and Treatment of Pressure Ulcers: What Works? What Doesn't?" *Cleveland Clinic Journal of Medicine* 68(8):704-22, August 2001.

Wound, Ostomy and Continence Nurses Society. *Position Statement: Conservative Sharp Wound Debridement for Registered Nurses.* Costa Mesa, Calif.: WOCN, 1996. *www.wocn.org/publications/posstate/ debride.htm*

Wound, Ostomy and Continence Nurses Society. *Position Statement: Staging of Pressure Ulcers.* Costa Mesa, Calif.: WOCN, 1996. *www.wocn.org/publications/posstate/ staging.htm*

## Skin biopsy

Skin biopsy is a diagnostic test in which a small piece of tissue is removed, under local anesthesia, from a lesion that is suspected of being malignant or from another dermatosis.

One of three techniques may be used: shave biopsy, punch biopsy, or excisional biopsy. Shave biopsy cuts the lesion above the skin line, which allows further biopsy of the site. Punch biopsy removes an oval core from the center of the lesion. Excisional biopsy removes the entire lesion and is indicated for rapidly expanding lesions; for sclerotic, bullous, or atrophic lesions; and for examination of the border of a lesion surrounding normal skin.

Lesions suspected of being malignant usually have changed color, size, or appearance or have failed to heal properly after injury. Fully developed lesions should be selected for biopsy whenever possible because they provide more diagnostic information than lesions that are resolving or in early stages of development. For example, if the skin shows blisters, the biopsy should include the most mature ones.

Normal skin consists of squamous epithelium (epidermis) and fibrous connective tissue (dermis). Histologic examination of the tissue specimen obtained during biopsy may reveal a benign or malignant lesion. Benign growths include cysts, seborrheic keratoses, warts, pigmented nevi (moles), keloids, dermatofibromas, and neurofibromas. Malignant tumors include basal cell carcinoma, squamous cell carcinoma, and malignant melanoma.

## Equipment

Gloves ● #15 scalpel for shave or excisional biopsy ● local anesthetic ● specimen bottle containing 10% formaldehyde solution ● 4-0 sutures for punch or excisional biopsy ● adhesive bandage ● forceps ● adhesive strips

## Implementation

▶ Explain to the patient that the biopsy provides a skin specimen for microscopic study. Describe the procedure and tell him who will perform it. Answer any questions he may have to ease anxiety and ensure cooperation.

▶ Inform the patient that he need not restrict food or fluids.

▶ Tell him that he'll receive a local anesthetic for pain.

▶ Inform him that the biopsy will take about 15 minutes and that the test results are usually available in 1 day.

▶ Have the patient or an appropriate family member sign a consent form.

▶ Check the patient's history for hypersensitivity to the local anesthetic.

▶ Position the patient comfortably and clean the biopsy site before the local anesthetic is given.

▶ For a shave biopsy, the protruding growth is cut off at the skin line with a #15 scalpel. The tissue is placed immediately in a properly labeled specimen bottle containing 10% formaldehyde solution. Apply pressure to the area to stop the bleeding. Apply an adhesive bandage.

▶ For a punch biopsy, the skin surrounding the lesion is pulled taut, and the punch is firmly introduced into the lesion and rotated to obtain a tissue specimen. The plug is lifted with forceps or a needle and is severed as deeply into the fat layer as possible. The specimen is placed in a properly labeled specimen bottle containing 10% formaldehyde solution or in a sterile container, if indicated. Closing the wound depends on the size of the punch: A 3-mm punch requires only an adhesive bandage, a 4-mm punch requires one suture, and a 6-mm punch requires two sutures.

▶ For an excisional biopsy, a #15 scalpel is used to excise the lesion; the incision is made as wide and as deep as necessary. The tissue specimen is removed and placed immediately in a properly labeled specimen bottle containing 10% formaldehyde solution. Apply pressure to the site to stop the bleeding. The wound is closed using a 4-0 suture. If the incision is large, a skin graft may be required. If the incision is small, adhesive strips may be applied.

▶ Check the biopsy site for bleeding.

▶ Send the specimen to the laboratory immediately.

▶ If the patient experiences pain, give analgesics.

## Special considerations

▶ Advise the patient going home with sutures to keep the area clean and as dry as possible. Tell him that facial sutures will be removed in 3 to 5 days and trunk sutures, in 7 to 14 days.

▶ Instruct the patient with adhesive strips to leave them in place for 14 to 21 days.

## Complications

Possible complications include bleeding and infection of the surrounding tissue.

## Documentation

▶ Document the time and location where the specimen was obtained, the appearance of the specimen and site, and whether bleeding occurred at the biopsy site.

## REFERENCES

Chiller, K., et al. "Efficacy of Curettage Before Excision in Clearing Surgical Margins of Nonmelanoma Skin Cancer," *Archives of Dermatology* 136(11):1327-32, November 2000.

Edward, D., et al. *Bedside Critical Care Manual.* Philadelphia: Lippincott Williams & Wilkins, 2001.

# Skin graft care

A skin graft consists of healthy skin taken either from the patient (autograft) or a donor (allograft) and applied to a part of the patient's body. There the graft resurfaces an area damaged by burns, traumatic injury, or surgery. Care procedures for an autograft or an allograft are essentially the same. How-

# Understanding types of grafts

A burn patient may receive one or more of the graft types described below.

### Split-thickness

The type used most commonly for covering open burns, a split-thickness graft includes the epidermis and part of the dermis. It may be applied as a sheet (usually on the face or neck to preserve the cosmetic result) or as a mesh. A mesh graft has tiny slits cut in it, which allow the graft to expand up to nine times its original size. Mesh grafts prevent fluid from collecting under the graft and typically are used over extensive full-thickness burns.

### Full-thickness

This graft type includes the epidermis and the entire dermis. Consequently, the graft contains hair follicles, sweat glands, and sebaceous glands, which typically aren't included in split-thickness grafts. Full-thickness grafts usually are used for small burns that cause deep wounds.

### Pedicle-flap

This full-thickness graft includes not only skin and subcutaneous tissue but also subcutaneous blood vessels to ensure a continued blood supply to the graft. Pedicle-flap grafts may be used during reconstructive surgery to cover previous defects.

ever, an autograft requires care for two sites: the graft site and the donor site.

The graft itself may be one of several types: split-thickness, full-thickness, or pedicle-flap. (See *Understanding types of grafts*.) Successful grafting depends on various factors, including clean wound granulation with adequate vascularization, complete contact of the graft with the wound bed, aseptic technique to prevent infection, adequate graft immobilization, and skilled care.

The size and depth of the patient's burns determine whether the burns will require grafting. Grafting usually occurs at the completion of wound debridement. The goal is to cover all wounds with an autograft or allograft within 2 weeks. With enzymatic debridement, grafting may be per-

formed 5 to 7 days after debridement is complete; with surgical debridement, grafting can occur the same day as the surgery.

Depending on your facility's policy, a doctor or a specially trained nurse may change graft dressings. The dressings usually stay in place for 3 to 5 days after surgery to avoid disturbing the graft site. Meanwhile, the donor graft site needs diligent care. (See *How to care for a donor graft site*.)

## Equipment

Ordered analgesic • clean and sterile gloves • sterile gown • cap • mask • sterile forceps • sterile scissors • sterile scalpel • sterile 4"x 4" gauze pads • Xeroflo gauze • elastic gauze dressing • warm normal saline solution • moisturizing cream • topical medication (such as micronized silver sulfadiazine cream) • optional: sterile cotton-tipped applicators

### Preparation of equipment

Assemble the equipment on the dressing cart.

## Implementation

▶ Explain the procedure to the patient and provide privacy.
▶ Give an analgesic as ordered 20 to 30 minutes before beginning the procedure. Alternatively, give an I.V. analgesic immediately before the procedure.
▶ Wash your hands.
▶ Put on the sterile gown, sterile gloves, mask, and cap.
▶ Gently lift off all outer dressings. Soak the middle dressings with warm saline solution. Remove these carefully and slowly to avoid disturbing the graft site. Leave the Xeroflo intact to avoid dislodging the graft.
▶ Remove and discard the gloves, wash your hands, and put on the sterile gloves.
▶ Assess the condition of the graft. If you see purulent drainage, notify the doctor.
▶ Remove the Xeroflo with sterile forceps and clean the area gently. If necessary, soak the Xeroflo with warm saline solution to facilitate removal.
▶ Inspect an allograft for signs of rejection, such as infection and delayed healing. Inspect a sheet graft frequently for blebs. If ordered, evacuate them carefully with a sterile scalpel. (See *Evacuating fluid from a sheet graft*.)

# How to care for a donor graft site

Autografts are usually taken from another area of the patient's body with a dermatome, an instrument that cuts uniform, split-thickness skin portions—typically about 0.013 to 0.05 cm thick. Autografting makes the donor site a partial-thickness wound, which may bleed, drain, and cause pain.

This site needs scrupulous care to prevent infection, which could convert the site to a full-thickness wound. Depending on the graft's thickness, tissue may be obtained from the donor site again in as few as 10 days.

Usually, Xeroflo gauze is applied postoperatively. The outer gauze dressing can be taken off on the first postoperative day; the Xeroflo will protect the new epithelial proliferation.

### Dressing the wound

Care for the donor site as you care for the autograft, using dressing changes at the initial stages to prevent infection and promote healing. Use the following guidelines:

▶ Wash your hands and put on sterile gloves.
▶ Remove the outer gauze dressings within 24 hours. Inspect the Xeroflo for signs of infection; then leave it open to the air to speed drying and healing.
▶ Leave small amounts of fluid accumulation alone. Using aseptic technique, aspirate larger amounts through the dressing with a small-gauge needle and syringe.
▶ Apply a lanolin-based cream daily to completely healed donor sites to keep skin tissue pliable and to remove crusts.

---

▶ Apply topical medication, if ordered.
▶ Place a fresh Xeroflo over the site to promote wound healing and prevent infection. Use sterile scissors to cut it to the appropriate size. Cover this with 4″ × 4″ gauze and elastic gauze dressing.
▶ Clean any completely healed areas and apply a moisturizing cream to them to keep the skin pliable and to retard scarring.

## Special considerations

▶ To avoid dislodging the graft, hydrotherapy is usually discontinued as ordered for 3

# Evacuating fluid from a sheet graft

When small pockets of fluid (called blebs) accumulate beneath a sheet graft, you'll need to evacuate the fluid using a sterile scalpel and sterile cotton-tipped applicators. First, carefully perforate the center of the bleb with the scalpel.

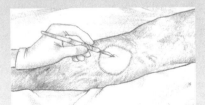

Gently express the fluid with the cotton-tipped applicators.

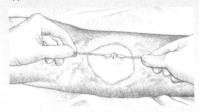

Never express fluid by rolling the bleb to the edge of the graft. This disturbs healing in other areas.

---

to 4 days after grafting. Avoid using a blood pressure cuff over the graft. Don't tug or pull dressings during dressing changes. Keep the patient from lying on the graft.
▶ If the graft dislodges, apply sterile skin compresses to keep the area moist until the surgeon reapplies the graft. If the graft affects an arm or a leg, elevate the affected extremity to reduce postoperative edema. Check for bleeding and signs or symptoms of neurovascular impairment, such as increasing pain, numbness or tingling, coolness, and pallor.

## Home care

Teach the patient how to apply moisturizing cream. Stress the importance of using a sunscreen containing titanium dioxide or oxybenzone that has a sun protection factor of 20 or higher on all grafted areas to avoid sunburn and discoloration.

## Complications
Graft failure may result from traumatic injury, hematoma or seroma formation, infection, an inadequate graft bed, rejection, or compromised nutritional status.

## Documentation
▶ Record the time and date of all dressing changes.
▶ Document all medications used, and note the patient's response to the medications.
▶ Describe the condition of the graft and note any signs of infection or rejection.
▶ Record any additional treatment and note the patient's reaction to the graft.

### REFERENCES
Donato, M., et al. "Skin Grafting: Historical and Practical Approaches," *Clinics in Podiatric Medicine and Surgery* 17(4):561-98, October 2000.
Francis, A. "Nursing Management of Skin Graft Sites," *Nursing Standard* 12(33): 41-44, May 1998.

# Skin staple and clip removal

Skin staples or clips may be used instead of standard sutures to close lacerations or surgical wounds. Because they can secure a wound more quickly than sutures, they may substitute for surface sutures when cosmetic results aren't a prime consideration such as in abdominal closure. When properly placed, staples and clips distribute tension evenly along the suture line with minimal tissue trauma and compression, facilitating healing and minimizing scarring. Because staples and clips are made from surgical stainless steel, tissue reaction to them is minimal. Usually, doctors remove skin staples and clips, but some facilities permit qualified nurses to perform this procedure.

Skin staples and clips are contraindicated when wound location requires cosmetically superior results or when the incision site makes it impossible to maintain at least a 5-mm distance between the staple and underlying bone, vessels, or internal organs.

## Equipment
Waterproof trash bag ● adjustable light ● clean gloves, if needed ● sterile gloves ● sterile gauze pads ● sterile staple or clip extractor ● povidone-iodine solution or other antiseptic cleaning agent ● sterile cotton-tipped applicators ● optional: butterfly adhesive strips or Steri-Strips and compound benzoin tincture or other skin protectant
Prepackaged, sterile, disposable staple or clip extractors are available.

### Preparation of equipment
Assemble all equipment in the patient's room. Check the expiration date on each sterile package and inspect for tears. Open the waterproof trash bag and place it near the patient's bed. Position the bag properly to avoid reaching across the sterile field or the wound when disposing of soiled articles. Form a cuff by turning down the top of the bag to provide a wide opening and prevent contamination of instruments or gloves by touching the bag's edge.

## Implementation
▶ If your facility allows you to remove skin staples and clips, check the doctor's order to confirm the exact timing and details for this procedure.
▶ Check for patient allergies, especially to adhesive tape and povidone-iodine or other topical solutions or medications.
▶ Explain the procedure to the patient. Tell him that he may feel a slight pulling or tickling sensation but little discomfort during staple removal. Reassure him that because his incision is healing properly, removing the supporting staples or clips won't weaken the incision line.
▶ Provide privacy and place the patient in a comfortable position that doesn't place undue tension on the incision. Because some patients experience nausea or dizziness during the procedure, have the patient recline, if possible. Adjust the light to shine directly on the incision.
▶ Wash your hands thoroughly.
▶ If the patient's wound has a dressing, put on clean gloves and carefully remove it. Discard the dressing and the gloves in the waterproof trash bag.
▶ Assess the patient's incision. Notify the doctor of gaping, drainage, inflammation, and other signs of infection.
▶ Establish a sterile work area with all the equipment and supplies you'll need for re-

moving staples or clips and for cleaning and dressing the incision. Open the package containing the sterile staple or clip extractor, maintaining asepsis. Put on sterile gloves.

▶ Wipe the incision gently with sterile gauze pads soaked in an antiseptic cleaning agent or with sterile cotton-tipped applicators to remove surface encrustations.

▶ Pick up the sterile staple or clip extractor. Then, starting at one end of the incision, remove the staple or clip. (See *Removing a staple.*) Hold the extractor over the trash bag and release the handle to discard the staple or clip.

▶ Repeat the procedure for each staple or clip until all are removed.

▶ Apply a sterile gauze dressing, if needed, to prevent infection and irritation from clothing. Then discard your gloves.

▶ Make sure the patient is comfortable. According to the doctor's preference, inform the patient that he may shower in 1 or 2 days if the incision is dry and healing well.

▶ Properly dispose of solutions and the trash bag and clean or dispose of soiled equipment and supplies according to facility policy.

### Special considerations

▶ Carefully check the doctor's order for the time and extent of staple or clip removal. The doctor may want you to remove only alternate staples or clips initially and to leave the others in place for an additional day or two to support the incision.

▶ When removing a staple or clip, place the extractor's jaws carefully between the patient's skin and the staple or clip to avoid patient discomfort. If extraction is difficult, notify the doctor; staples or clips placed too deeply within the skin or left in place too long may resist removal.

▶ If the wound dehisces after staples or clips are removed, apply butterfly adhesive strips or Steri-Strips to approximate and support the edges and call the doctor immediately to repair the wound. (See *Types of adhesive skin closures,* page 620.)

▶ You may also apply butterfly adhesive strips or Steri-Strips after removing staples or clips even if the wound is healing normally to give added support to the incision and prevent lateral tension from forming a wide scar. Use a small amount of compound benzoin tincture or other skin pro-

## Removing a staple

Position the extractor's lower jaws beneath the span of the first staple (as shown below).

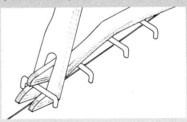

Squeeze the handles until they're completely closed; then lift the staple away from the skin (as shown below). The extractor changes the shape of the staple and pulls the prongs out of the intradermal tissue.

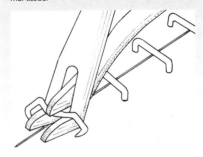

tectant to ensure adherence. Leave the strips in place for 3 to 5 days.

### Home care

If the patient is being discharged, teach him how to remove the dressing and care for the wound. Instruct him to call the doctor immediately if he observes wound discharge or any other abnormal change. Tell him that the redness surrounding the incision should gradually disappear and that, after a few weeks, only a thin line should be visible.

### Documentation

▶ Record the date and time of staple or clip removal, number of staples or clips removed, appearance of the incision, dressings or butterfly strips applied, signs of wound complications, and patient's tolerance of the procedure.

# Types of adhesive skin closures

Steri-Strips are used as a primary means of keeping a wound closed after suture removal. They're made of thin strips of sterile, nonwoven, porous fabric tape.

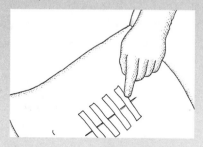

Butterfly closures consist of sterile, waterproof adhesive strips. A narrow, nonadhesive "bridge" connects the two expanded adhesive portions. These strips are used to close small wounds and assist healing after suture removal.

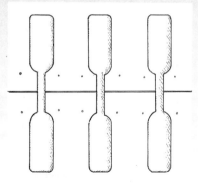

## REFERENCES

Edward, D., et al. *Bedside Critical Care Manual.* Philadelphia: Lippincott Williams & Wilkins, 2001.

Kanegaye, J.T., and McCaslin, R.I. "Pediatric Scalp Laceration Repair Complicated by Skin Staple Migration," *The American Journal of Emergency Medicine* 17(2): 157-59, March 1999.

# Surgical wound management

When caring for a surgical wound, you carry out procedures that help prevent infection by stopping pathogens from entering the wound. In addition to promoting patient comfort, such procedures protect the skin surface from maceration and excoriation caused by contact with irritating drainage. They also allow you to measure wound drainage to monitor healing and fluid and electrolyte balance.

The two primary methods used to manage a draining surgical wound are dressing and pouching. Dressing is preferred unless caustic or excessive drainage is compromising your patient's skin integrity. Usually, lightly seeping wounds with drains and wounds with minimal purulent drainage can be managed with packing and gauze dressings. Some wounds, such as those that become chronic, may require an occlusive dressing.

A wound with copious, excoriating drainage calls for pouching to protect the surrounding skin. If your patient has a surgical wound, you must monitor him and choose the appropriate dressing.

Dressing a wound calls for sterile technique and sterile supplies to prevent contamination. You may use the color of the wound to help determine which type of dressing to apply. (See *Tailoring wound care to wound color.*)

Change the dressing often enough to keep the skin dry. Always follow standard precautions set by the Centers for Disease Control and Prevention (CDC).

## Equipment

Waterproof trash bag ● clean gloves ● sterile gloves ● gown and face shield or goggles, if indicated ● sterile 4"x 4" gauze pads ● large absorbent dressings, if indicated ● povidone-iodine swabs ● sterile cotton-tipped applicators ● sterile dressing set ● topical medication, if ordered ● adhesive or other tape ● soap and water ● optional: forceps; skin protectant; nonadherent pads; collodion spray or acetone-free adhesive remover; sterile normal saline solution; graduated biohazard container; and fishnet tube elasticized dressing support, Montgomery straps, or T-binder

# Tailoring wound care to wound color

Promote healing by keeping the wound moist, clean, and free from debris. For open wounds, use the wound color to guide the specific management approach and to assess how well the wound is healing.

### Red wounds

Red, the color of healthy granulation tissue, indicates normal healing. When a wound begins to heal, a layer of pale pink granulation tissue covers the wound bed. As this layer thickens, it becomes beefy red. Cover a red wound, keep it moist and clean, and protect it from trauma. Use a transparent dressing (such as Tegaderm or Op-site), a hydrocolloidal dressing (such as DuoDerm), or a gauze dressing moistened with sterile normal saline solution or impregnated with petroleum jelly or an antibiotic. Red shouldn't surround the wound itself. This could indicate the presence of infection.

### Yellow wounds

Yellow is the color of exudate produced by microorganisms in an open wound. When a wound heals without complications, the immune system removes microorganisms. However, if there are too many microorganisms to remove, exudate accumulates and becomes visible. Exudate usually appears whitish yellow, creamy yellow, yellowish green, or beige. Dry exudate appears darker.

If the patient has a yellow wound, clean it and remove exudate, using high-pressure irrigation; then cover it with a moist dressing. Use absorptive products (for example, Debrisan beads and paste) or a moist gauze dressing with or without an antibiotic. You may also use hydrotherapy with whirlpool or high-pressure irrigation.

### Black wounds

Black, the least healthy color, signals necrosis. Dead, avascular tissue slows healing and provides a site for microorganisms to proliferate.

You should debride a black wound. After removing dead tissue, apply a dressing to keep the wound moist and guard against external contamination. As ordered, use enzyme products (such as Elase or Travase), surgical debridement, hydrotherapy with whirlpool or high-pressure irrigation, or a moist gauze dressing.

### Multicolored wounds

You may note two or even all three colors in a wound. In this case, you would classify the wound according to the least healthy color present. For example, if the patient's wound is both red and yellow, classify it as a yellow wound.

---

*For a wound with a drain*
Sterile scissors ● sterile 4″ × 4″ gauze pads without cotton lining ● sump drain ● ostomy pouch or another collection bag ● sterile precut tracheostomy pads or drain dressings ● adhesive tape (paper or silk tape if the patient is hypersensitive) ● surgical mask

*For pouching a wound*
Collection pouch with drainage port ● sterile gloves ● skin protectant ● sterile gauze pads

## Preparation of equipment
Ask the patient about allergies to tapes and dressings. Assemble all equipment in the patient's room. Check the expiration date on each sterile package and inspect for tears.

Open the waterproof trash bag and place it near the patient's bed. Position the bag properly to avoid reaching across the sterile field or the wound when disposing of soiled articles. Form a cuff by turning down the top of the trash bag to provide a wide opening and prevent contamination of instruments or gloves by touching the bag's edge.

## Implementation
❱ Explain the procedure to the patient to allay his fears and ensure his cooperation.

## Removing the old dressing
❱ Check the doctor's order for specific wound care and medication instructions. Note the location of surgical drains to avoid dislodging them during the procedure.

## How to put on sterile gloves

Using your nondominant hand, pick up the opposite glove by grasping the exposed inside of the cuff.

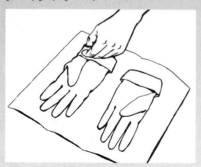

Slip the gloved fingers of your dominant hand under the glove of the loose glove to pick it up.

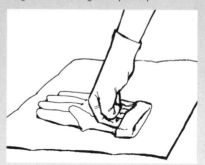

Pull the glove onto your dominant hand. Keep your thumb folded inward to avoid touching the sterile part of the glove. Allow the glove to come uncuffed as you finish inserting your hand, but don't touch the outside of the glove.

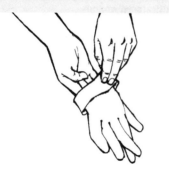

Slide your nondominant hand into the glove, holding your dominant thumb as far away as possible to avoid brushing against your arm. Allow the glove to come uncuffed as you finish putting it on, but don't touch the skin side of the cuff with your other gloved hand.

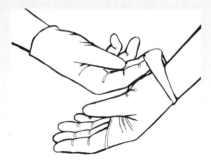

▶ Assess the patient's condition.
▶ Identify the patient's allergies, especially to adhesive tape, povidone-iodine or other topical solutions, or medications.
▶ Provide privacy and position the patient as necessary. To avoid chilling him, expose only the wound site.
▶ Wash your hands thoroughly. Put on a gown and a face shield, if necessary. Then put on clean gloves.
▶ Loosen the soiled dressing by holding the patient's skin and pulling the tape or dressing toward the wound. This protects the newly formed tissue and prevents stress on the incision. Moisten the tape with acetone-free adhesive remover, if necessary, to make the tape removal less painful (particularly if the skin is hairy). Don't apply solvents to the incision because they could contaminate the wound.
▶ Slowly remove the soiled dressing. If the gauze adheres to the wound, loosen the gauze by moistening it with sterile normal saline solution.
▶ Observe the dressing for the amount, type, color, and odor of drainage.
▶ Discard the dressing and gloves in the waterproof trash bag.

## Caring for the wound

▶ Wash your hands. Establish a sterile field with all the equipment and supplies you'll need for suture-line care and the dressing change, including a sterile dressing set and povidone-iodine swabs. If the doctor has ordered ointment, squeeze the needed amount onto the sterile field. If you're using an antiseptic from a nonsterile bottle, pour the antiseptic cleaning agent into a sterile container so you won't contaminate your gloves. Then put on sterile gloves. (See *How to put on sterile gloves.*)

▶ Saturate the sterile gauze pads with the prescribed cleaning agent. Avoid using cotton balls because they may shed fibers in the wound, causing irritation, infection, or adhesion.

▶ If ordered, obtain a wound culture; then proceed to clean the wound.

▶ Pick up the moistened gauze pad or swab and squeeze out the excess solution.

▶ Working from the top of the incision, wipe once to the bottom and then discard the gauze pad. With a second moistened pad, wipe from top to bottom in a vertical path next to the incision (as shown below).

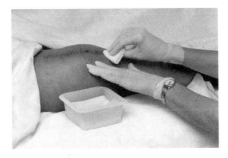

▶ Continue to work outward from the incision in lines running parallel to it. Always wipe from the clean area toward the less clean area (usually from top to bottom). Use each gauze pad or swab for only one stroke to avoid tracking wound exudate and normal body flora from surrounding skin to the clean areas. Remember that the suture line is cleaner than the adjacent skin and the top of the suture line is usually cleaner than the bottom because more drainage collects at the bottom of the wound.

▶ Use sterile, cotton-tipped applicators for efficient cleaning of tight-fitting wire sutures, deep and narrow wounds, and wounds with pockets. Because the cotton on the swab is tightly wrapped, it's less likely than a cotton ball to leave fibers in the wound. Remember to wipe only once with each applicator.

▶ If the patient has a surgical drain, clean the drain's surface last. Because moist drainage promotes bacterial growth, the drain is considered the most contaminated area. Clean the skin around the drain by wiping in half or full circles from the drain site outward.

▶ Clean all areas of the wound to wash away debris, pus, blood, and necrotic material. Try not to disturb sutures or irritate the incision. Clean to at least 1″ (2.5 cm) beyond the end of the new dressing. If you aren't applying a new dressing, clean to at least 2″ (5 cm) beyond the incision.

▶ Check to make sure that the edges of the incision are lined up properly and check for signs of infection (such as heat, redness, swelling, induration, and odor), dehiscence, and evisceration. If you observe such signs or if the patient reports pain at the wound site, notify the doctor.

▶ Irrigate the wound as ordered.

▶ Wash skin surrounding the wound with soap and water and pat dry using a sterile 4″x 4″ gauze pad. Avoid oil-based soap because it may interfere with pouch adherence. Apply any prescribed topical medication.

▶ Apply a skin protectant, if needed.

▶ If ordered, pack the wound with gauze pads or strips folded to fit, using a sterile forceps. Avoid using cotton-lined gauze pads because cotton fibers can adhere to the wound surface and cause complications. Pack the wound, using the wet-to-damp method. Soaking the packing material in solution and wringing it out so that it's slightly moist provides a moist wound environment that absorbs debris and drainage. However, removing the packing won't disrupt new tissue. Don't pack the wound tightly; doing so will exert pressure and may damage the wound.

## Applying a fresh gauze dressing

▶ Gently place sterile 4″x 4″ gauze pads at the center of the wound and move progressively outward to the edges of the wound site. Extend the gauze at least 1″ (2.5 cm) beyond the incision in each direction and cover the wound evenly with enough ster-

ile dressings (usually two or three layers) to absorb all drainage until the next dressing change. Use large absorbent dressings to form outer layers, if needed, to provide greater absorbency.
▶ Secure the dressing's edges to the patient's skin with strips of tape to maintain the sterility of the wound site (as shown below). Or secure the dressing with a T-binder or Montgomery straps to prevent skin excoriation, which may occur with repeated tape removal necessitated by frequent dressing changes. (See *How to make Montgomery straps.*) If the wound is on a limb, secure the dressing with a fishnet tube elasticized dressing support.

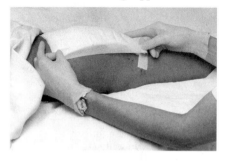

▶ Make sure that the patient is comfortable.
▶ Properly dispose of the solutions and trash bag and clean or discard soiled equipment and supplies according to your facility's policy. If your patient's wound has purulent drainage, don't return unopened sterile supplies to the sterile supply cabinet because this could cause cross-contamination of other equipment.

### Dressing a wound with a drain
▶ Prepare a drain dressing by using sterile scissors to cut a slit in a sterile 4"x 4" gauze pad. Fold the pad in half; then cut inward from the center of the folded edge. Don't use a cotton-lined gauze pad because cutting the gauze opens the lining and releases cotton fibers into the wound. Prepare a second pad the same way, or use commercially precut gauze.
▶ Gently press one folded pad close to the skin around the drain so that the tubing fits into the slit. Press the second folded pad around the drain from the opposite direction so that the two pads encircle the tubing.
▶ Layer as many uncut sterile 4"x 4" gauze pads or large absorbent dressings around

the tubing as needed to absorb expected drainage. Tape the dressing in place, or use a T-binder or Montgomery straps.

### Pouching a wound
▶ If your patient's wound is draining heavily or if drainage may damage surrounding skin, you'll need to apply a pouch.
▶ Measure the wound. Cut an opening ⅜" (1 cm) larger than the wound in the facing of the collection pouch (as shown below).

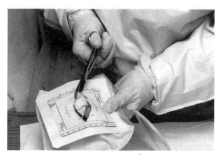

▶ Apply a skin protectant as needed. (Some protectants are incorporated within the collection pouch and also provide adhesion.)
▶ Before you apply the pouch, keep in mind the patient's usual position. Then plan to position the pouch's drainage port so that gravity facilitates drainage.
▶ Make sure that the drainage port at the bottom of the pouch is closed firmly to prevent leaks. Then gently press the contoured pouch opening around the wound, starting at its lower edge to catch any drainage (as shown below).

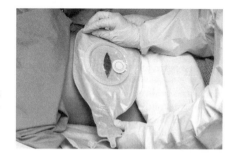

▶ To empty the pouch, put on clean gloves and a face shield or mask and goggles to avoid any splashing. Then insert the pouch's bottom half into a graduated biohazard container and open the drainage

# How to make Montgomery straps

An abdominal dressing requiring frequent changes can be secured with Montgomery straps to promote the patient's comfort. If ready-made straps aren't available, take the following steps to make your own:

▶ Cut four to six strips of 2"- or 3"-wide hypoallergenic tape of sufficient length to allow the tape to extend about 6" (15 cm) beyond the wound on each side. (The length of the tape varies, depending on the patient's size and the type and amount of dressing.)

▶ Fold one of each strip 2" to 3" (5 to 7.5 cm) back on itself (sticky sides together) to form a nonadhesive tab. Then cut a small hole in the folded tab's center, close to its top edge. Make as many pairs of straps as you'll need to snugly secure the dressing.

▶ Clean the patient's skin to prevent irritation. After the skin dries, apply a skin protectant. Then apply the sticky side of each tape to a skin barrier sheet composed of opaque hydrocolloidal or nonhydrocolloidal materials and apply the sheet directly to the skin near the dressing. Next, thread a separate piece of gauze tie, umbilical tape, or twill tape (about 12" [30.5 cm])

through each pair of holes in the straps and fasten each tie as you would a shoelace. Don't stress the surrounding skin by securing the ties too tightly.

▶ Repeat this procedure according to the number of Montgomery straps needed.

▶ Replace Montgomery straps whenever they become soiled (every 2 to 3 days). If skin maceration occurs, place new tapes about 1" (2.5 cm) away from any irritation.

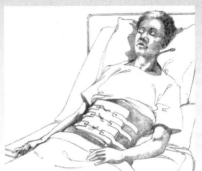

port (as shown below). Note the color, consistency, odor, and amount of fluid. If ordered, obtain a culture specimen and send it to the laboratory immediately. Remember to follow the CDC's standard precautions when handling infectious drainage.

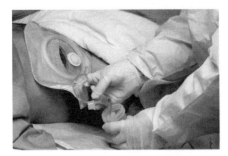

▶ Wipe the bottom of the pouch and the drainage port with a sterile gauze pad to remove any drainage that could irritate the patient's skin or cause an odor. Then reseal the port. Change the pouch only if it leaks or fails to adhere. More frequent changes are unnecessary and only irritate the patient's skin.

## Special considerations

▶ If the patient has two wounds in the same area, cover each wound separately with layers of sterile 4"x 4" gauze pads. Then cover each site with a large absorbent dressing secured to the patient's skin with tape. Don't use a single large absorbent dressing to cover both sites because drainage quickly saturates a pad, promoting cross-contamination.

▶ When packing a wound, don't pack it too tightly because this compresses adjacent capillaries and may prevent the wound edges from contracting. Avoid overlapping damp packing onto surrounding skin because it macerates the intact tissue.

▶ To save time when dressing a wound with a drain, use sterile precut tracheostomy pads or drain dressings instead of custom-cutting gauze pads to fit around the drain. If your patient is sensitive to adhesive tape, use paper or silk tape because it's less likely to cause a skin reaction and peels off more easily than adhesive tape. Use a surgical mask to cradle a chin or jawline dressing; this provides a secure dressing and avoids the need to shave the patient's hair.

▶ If ordered, use a collodion spray or similar topical protectant instead of a gauze dressing. Moisture- and contaminant-proof, this covering dries in a clear, impermeable film that leaves the wound visible for observation and avoids the friction caused by a dressing.

▶ If a sump drain isn't adequately collecting wound secretions, reinforce it with an ostomy pouch or another collection bag. Use waterproof tape to strengthen a spot on the front of the pouch near the adhesive opening; then cut a small "X" in the tape. Feed the drain catheter into the pouch through the "X" cut. Seal the cut around the tubing with more waterproof tape; then connect the tubing to the suction pump. This method frees the drainage port at the bottom of the pouch so you don't have to remove the tubing to empty the pouch. If you use more than one collection pouch for a wound or wounds, record drainage volume separately for each pouch. Avoid using waterproof material over the dressing because it reduces air circulation and promotes infection from accumulated heat and moisture.

▶ Because many doctors prefer to change the first postoperative dressing themselves to check the incision, don't change the first dressing unless you have specific instructions to do so. If you have no such order and drainage comes through the dressings, reinforce the dressing with fresh sterile gauze. Request an order to change the dressing, or ask the doctor to change it as soon as possible. A reinforced dressing shouldn't remain in place longer than 24 hours because it's an excellent medium for bacterial growth.

▶ For the recent postoperative patient or a patient with complications, check the dressing every 15 to 30 minutes or as ordered. For the patient with a properly healing wound, check the dressing at least once every 8 hours.

▶ If the dressing becomes wet from the outside (for example, from spilled drinking water), replace it as soon as possible to prevent wound contamination.

▶ If your patient will need wound care after discharge, provide appropriate teaching. If he'll be caring for the wound himself, stress the importance of using aseptic technique and teach him how to examine the wound for signs of infection and other complications. Also, show him how to change dressings and give him written instructions for all procedures to be performed at home.

▶ In elderly patients, adhesive tape may cause skin tears. Extra care should be taken when removing old tape.

## Complications

A major complication of a dressing change is an allergic reaction to an antiseptic cleaning agent, a prescribed topical medication, or an adhesive tape. This reaction may lead to skin redness, rash, excoriation, or infection.

## Documentation

▶ Document the date, time, and type of wound management procedure; amount of soiled dressing and packing removed; wound appearance (size, condition of margins, presence of necrotic tissue) and odor (if present); type, color, consistency, and amount of drainage (for each wound); presence and location of drains; additional procedures, such as irrigation, packing, or application of a topical medication; type and amount of new dressing or pouch applied; and patient's tolerance of the procedure.

▶ Document special or detailed wound care instructions and pain management steps on the plan of care. Record the color and amount of drainage on the intake and output sheet.

## REFERENCES

Edward, D., et al. *Bedside Critical Care Manual.* Philadelphia: Lippincott Williams & Wilkins, 2001.

Sams, H.H., et al. "Graftskin Treatment of Difficult to Heal Diabetic Foot Ulcers: One Center's Experience," *Dermatologic Surgery* 28(8):698-703, August 2002.

# Suture removal

The goal of suture removal is to remove skin sutures from a healed wound without damaging newly formed tissue. The timing of suture removal depends on the shape, size, and location of the sutured incision; the absence of inflammation, drainage, and infection; and the patient's general condition. Usually, for a sufficiently healed wound, sutures are removed 7 to 10 days after insertion. Techniques for removal depend on the method of suturing, but all require sterile procedure to prevent contamination. Although sutures usually are removed by a doctor, in many facilities, a nurse may remove them on the doctor's order.

## Equipment

Waterproof trash bag ● adjustable light ● clean gloves, if the wound is dressed ● sterile gloves ● sterile forceps or sterile hemostat ● normal saline solution ● sterile gauze pads ● antiseptic cleaning agent ● sterile curve-tipped suture scissors ● povidone-iodine pads ● optional: adhesive butterfly strips or Steri-Strips and compound benzoin tincture or other skin protectant

Prepackaged, sterile suture-removal trays are available.

### Preparation of equipment

Assemble all equipment in the patient's room. Check the expiration date on each sterile package and inspect for tears. Open the waterproof trash bag and place it near the patient's bed. Position the bag properly to avoid reaching across the sterile field or the suture line when disposing of soiled articles. Form a cuff by turning down the top of the trash bag to provide a wide opening and prevent contamination of instruments or gloves by touching the bag's edge.

## Implementation

▶ If your facility allows you to remove sutures, check the doctor's order to confirm the details for this procedure.
▶ Check for patient allergies, especially to adhesive tape and povidone-iodine or another topical solution or medication.
▶ Tell the patient that you're going to remove the stitches from his wound. Assure him that this procedure typically is painless but that he may feel a tickling sensation as the stitches come out. Reassure him that because his wound is healing properly, removing the stitches won't weaken the incision.
▶ Provide privacy and position the patient so he's comfortable without placing undue tension on the suture line. Because some patients experience nausea or dizziness during the procedure, have the patient recline, if possible. Adjust the light to have it shine directly on the suture line.

▶ Wash your hands thoroughly. If the patient's wound has a dressing, put on clean gloves and carefully remove the dressing. Discard the dressing and the gloves in the waterproof trash bag.
▶ Observe the patient's wound for possible gaping, drainage, inflammation, signs of infection, and embedded sutures. Notify the doctor if the wound has failed to heal properly. The absence of a healing ridge under the suture line 5 to 7 days after insertion indicates that the line needs continued support and protection during the healing process.
▶ Establish a sterile work area with all the equipment and supplies you'll need for suture removal and wound care. Put on sterile gloves and open the sterile suture-removal tray if you're using one.
▶ Using sterile technique, clean the suture line to decrease the number of microorganisms present and reduce the risk of infection. The cleaning process should also moisten the sutures sufficiently to ease removal. Soften them further, if needed, with normal saline solution.
▶ Then proceed according to the type of suture you're removing. (See *Methods for removing sutures,* page 628.) Because the visible part of a suture is exposed to skin bacteria and considered contaminated, cut sutures at the skin surface on one side of the visible part of the suture. Remove the suture by lifting and pulling the visible end off the skin to avoid drawing this contaminated portion back through subcutaneous tissue.
▶ If ordered, remove every other suture to maintain some support for the incision. Then go back and remove the remaining sutures.
▶ After removing sutures, wipe the incision gently with sterile gauze pads soaked in an antiseptic cleaning agent or with a povidone-iodine pad. Apply a light sterile gauze dressing, if needed, to prevent infection and irritation from clothing. Then discard your gloves.
▶ Make sure the patient is comfortable. According to the doctor's preference, inform the patient that he may shower in 1 or 2 days if the incision is dry and heals well.
▶ Properly dispose of the solutions and trash bag and clean or dispose of soiled equipment and supplies according to your facility's policy.

# Methods for removing sutures

Removal techniques depend in large part on the type of sutures to be removed. The illustrations here show removal steps for four common suture types. Keep in mind that for all suture types, it's important to grasp and cut sutures in the correct place to avoid pulling the exposed (thus contaminated) suture material through subcutaneous tissue.

### Plain interrupted sutures

Using sterile forceps, grasp the knot of the first suture and raise it off the skin. This will expose a small portion of the suture that was below skin level. Place the rounded tip of sterile curved-tip suture scissors against the skin and cut through the exposed portion of the suture. Then, still holding the knot with the forceps, pull the cut suture up and out of the skin in a smooth continuous motion to avoid causing the patient pain. Discard the suture. Repeat the process for every other suture initially; if the wound doesn't gape, you can then remove the remaining sutures as ordered.

### Mattress interrupted sutures

If possible, remove the small, visible portion of the suture opposite the knot by cutting it at each visible end and lifting the small piece away from the skin to prevent pulling it through and contaminating subcutaneous tissue. Then remove the rest of the suture by pulling it out in the direction of the knot. If the visible portion is too small to cut twice, cut it once and pull the entire suture out in the opposite direction. Repeat these steps for the remaining sutures and monitor the incision carefully for infection.

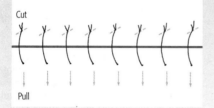

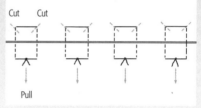

### Plain continuous sutures

Cut the first suture on the side opposite the knot. Next, cut the same side of the next suture in line. Then lift the first suture out in the direction of the knot. Proceed along the suture line, grasping each suture where you grasped the knot on the first one.

### Mattress continuous sutures

Follow the procedure for removing mattress interrupted sutures, first removing the small visible portion of the suture, if possible, to prevent pulling it through and contaminating subcutaneous tissue. Then extract the rest of the suture in the direction of the knot.

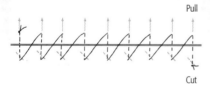

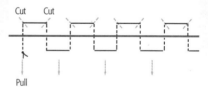

## Special considerations

▶ Check the doctor's order for the time of suture removal. Usually, you'll remove sutures on the head and neck 3 to 5 days after insertion; on the chest and abdomen, 5 to 7 days after insertion; and on the lower extremities, 7 to 10 days after insertion.

▶ If the patient has interrupted sutures or an incompletely healed suture line, remove only those sutures specified by the doctor.

He may want to leave some sutures in place for an additional day or two to support the suture line.

▶ If the patient has both retention and regular sutures in place, check the doctor's order for the sequence in which they're to be removed. Because retention sutures link underlying fat and muscle tissue and give added support to the obese or slow-healing patient, they usually remain in place for 14 to 21 days.

▶ Be particularly careful to clean the suture line before attempting to remove mattress sutures. This decreases the risk of infection when the visible, contaminated part of the stitch is too small to cut twice for sterile removal and must be pulled through tissue. After you have removed mattress sutures this way, monitor the suture line carefully for subsequent infection.

▶ If the wound dehisces during suture removal, apply butterfly adhesive strips or Steri-Strips to support and approximate the edges and call the doctor immediately to repair the wound.

▶ Apply butterfly adhesive strips or Steri-Strips after any suture removal, if desired, to give added support to the incision line and prevent lateral tension on the wound from forming a wide scar. Use a small amount of compound benzoin tincture or other skin protectant to ensure adherence. Leave the strips in place for 3 to 5 days.

## Home care

If the patient is being discharged, teach him how to remove the dressing and care for the wound. Instruct him to call the doctor immediately if he observes wound discharge or any other abnormal change. Tell him that the redness surrounding the incision should gradually disappear and only a thin line should show after a few weeks.

## Complications

Wound dehiscence and evisceration may occur if sutures are removed too soon or if the patient's healing is decreased because of diabetes or an immunocompromised condition.

## Documentation

▶ Record the date and time of suture removal, type and number of sutures, appearance of the suture line, signs of wound complications, dressings or butterfly strips applied, and patient's tolerance of the procedure.

## REFERENCES

Edward, D., et al. *Bedside Critical Care Manual*. Philadelphia: Lippincott Williams & Wilkins, 2001.

Kettle, C., et al. "Continuous Versus Interrupted Perineal Repair with Standard or Rapidly Absorbed Sutures after Spontaneous Vaginal Birth: A Randomised Controlled Trial," *Lancet* 359(9325):2217-23, June 2002.

# Traumatic wound care

Traumatic wounds include abrasions, lacerations, puncture wounds, and amputations. In an abrasion, the skin is scraped, with partial loss of the skin surface. In a laceration, the skin is torn, causing jagged, irregular edges; the severity of a laceration depends on its size, depth, and location. A puncture wound occurs when a pointed object, such as a knife or glass fragment, penetrates the skin. Traumatic amputation refers to removal of part of the body, a limb, or part of a limb.

Initial care concentrates on controlling bleeding, usually by applying firm, direct pressure and elevating the extremity. If bleeding continues, you may need to compress a pressure point. Assess the condition of the wound. Management and cleaning techniques usually depend on the specific type of wound and degree of contamination.

## Equipment

Sterile basin ● normal saline solution ● sterile 4″ × 4″ gauze pads ● sterile gloves ● clean gloves ● dry sterile dressing, nonadherent pad, or petroleum gauze ● linen-saver pad ● optional: scissors, towel, goggles, mask, gown, 50-ml catheter-tip syringe, surgical scrub brush, antibacterial ointment, porous tape, sterile forceps, sutures and suture set, hydrogen peroxide

### Preparation of equipment

Place a linen-saver pad under the area to be cleaned. Remove any clothing covering the wound. If necessary, cut hair around the wound with scissors to promote cleaning and treatment.

Assemble needed equipment at the patient's bedside. Fill a sterile basin with normal saline solution. Make sure the treatment area has enough light to allow close observation of the wound. Depending on the nature and location of the wound, wear sterile or clean gloves to avoid spreading infection.

## Implementation

▶ Check the patient's medical history for previous tetanus immunization and, if needed and ordered, arrange for immunization.
▶ Give pain medication, if ordered.
▶ Wash your hands.
▶ Use appropriate protective equipment, such as a gown, mask, and goggles, if spraying or splashing of body fluids is possible.

### For an abrasion

▶ Flush the scraped skin with normal saline solution.
▶ Remove dirt or gravel with a sterile 4″ × 4″ gauze pad moistened with normal saline solution. Rub in the opposite direction from which the dirt or gravel became embedded.
▶ If the wound is extremely dirty, you may use a surgical brush to scrub it.
▶ With a small wound, allow it to dry and form a scab. With a larger wound, you may need to cover it with a nonadherent pad or petroleum gauze and a light dressing. Apply antibacterial ointment if ordered.

### For a laceration

▶ Moisten a sterile 4″ × 4″ gauze pad with normal saline solution. Clean the wound gently, working outward from its center to about 2″ (5 cm) beyond its edges. Discard the soiled gauze pad and use a fresh one as necessary. Continue until the wound appears clean.
▶ If the wound is dirty, you may irrigate it with a 50-ml catheter-tip syringe and normal saline solution.
▶ Assist the doctor in suturing the wound edges using the suture kit, or apply sterile strips of porous tape.
▶ Apply the prescribed antibacterial ointment to help prevent infection.
▶ Apply a dry sterile dressing over the wound to absorb drainage and help prevent bacterial contamination.

### For a puncture wound

▶ If the wound is minor, allow it to bleed for a few minutes before cleaning it.
▶ For a larger puncture wound, you may need to irrigate it before applying a dry dressing.
▶ Stabilize any embedded foreign object until the doctor can remove it. After he removes the object and bleeding is stabilized, clean the wound as you'd clean a laceration or deep puncture wound.

### For an amputation

▶ Apply a gauze pad moistened with normal saline solution to the amputation site. Elevate the affected part and immobilize it for surgery.
▶ Recover the amputated part and prepare it for transport to a facility where microvascular surgery is performed.

## Special considerations

▶ When irrigating a traumatic wound, avoid using more than 8 psi of pressure. High-pressure irrigation can seriously interfere with healing, kill cells, and allow bacteria to infiltrate the tissue.
▶ To clean the wound, you may use hydrogen peroxide; its foaming action facilitates debris removal. However, peroxide should never be instilled into a deep wound because of the risk of embolism from the evolving gases. Be sure to rinse your hands well after using hydrogen peroxide.
▶ After a wound has been cleaned, the doctor may want to debride it to remove dead tissue and reduce the risk of infection and scarring. If this is necessary, pack the wound with gauze pads soaked in normal saline solution until debridement.
▶ Observe for signs and symptoms of infection, such as warm red skin at the site or purulent discharge. Infection of a traumatic wound can delay healing, increase scar formation, and trigger systemic infection such as septicemia.
▶ Observe all dressings. If edema is present, adjust the dressing to avoid impairing circulation to the area.

## Complications

Cleaning and care of traumatic wounds may temporarily increase the patient's pain. Excessive, vigorous cleaning may further disrupt tissue integrity.

## Documentation
▶ Document the date and time of the procedure, wound size and condition, medication administration, specific wound care measures, and patient teaching.

### REFERENCES
Dickerson, P., et al. "Traumatic Wound Care," *Dermatology Nursing* 11(1):53-56, 60-63, 80, February 1999. (Review.)
Kehoe, A., and Elmore, M.F. "Woundoscopy: A New Technique for Examining Deep, Nonhealing Wounds," *Ostomy Wound Management* 48(4):30-33, April 2002.

# Unna's boot therapy

Named for dermatologist Paul Gerson Unna, this boot can be used to treat uninfected, nonnecrotic leg and foot ulcers that result from such conditions as venous insufficiency and stasis dermatitis. A commercially prepared, medicated gauze compression dressing, Unna's boot wraps around the affected foot and leg. Alternatively, a preparation known as Unna's paste (gelatin, zinc oxide, calamine lotion, and glycerin) may be applied to the ulcer and covered with lightweight gauze. The boot's effectiveness results from compression applied by the bandage combined with moisture supplied by the paste.

Unna's boot is contraindicated in patients allergic to any ingredient used in the paste and in patients with arterial ulcers, weeping eczema, or cellulitis.

## Equipment
Scrub sponge with ordered cleaning agent • normal saline solution • commercially prepared gauze bandage saturated with Unna's paste (or Unna's paste and lightweight gauze) • bandage • scissors • gloves • elastic bandage to cover Unna's boot • optional: extra gauze for excessive drainage

## Implementation
▶ Explain the procedure to the patient and provide privacy.
▶ Wash your hands and put on gloves.
▶ Assess the ulcer and the surrounding skin. Evaluate ulcer size, drainage, and appearance. Perform a neurovascular assessment of the affected foot to ensure adequate circulation. If you don't detect a pulse in the foot, check with the ordering doctor before applying Unna's boot.
▶ Clean the affected area gently with the sponge and cleaning agent to retard bacterial growth and to remove dirt and wound debris, which may create pressure points after you apply the bandage. Rinse with normal saline solution.
▶ If a commercially prepared gauze bandage isn't ordered, spread Unna's paste evenly on the leg and foot. Then cover the leg and foot with the lightweight gauze. Apply three or four layers of paste interspersed with layers of gauze. In a prepared bandage, the bandage is impregnated with the paste.
▶ Apply gauze or the prepared bandage in a spiral motion, from just above the toes to the knee. Be sure to cover the heel. The wrap should be snug but not tight. To cover the area completely, make sure each turn overlaps the previous one by half the bandage width. (See *How to wrap Unna's boot,* page 632.)
▶ Continue wrapping the patient's leg up to the knee, using firm, even pressure. Stop the dressing 1″ (2.5 cm) below the popliteal fossa to prevent irritation when the knee is bent. Mold the boot with your free hand as you apply the bandage to make it smooth and even.
▶ Cover the boot with an elastic bandage to provide external compression.
▶ Instruct the patient to remain in bed with his leg outstretched and elevated on a pillow until the paste dries (approximately 30 minutes). Observe the patient's foot for signs of impairment, such as cyanosis, loss of feeling, and swelling. These signs indicate that the bandage is too tight and must be removed.
▶ Leave the boot on for 5 to 7 days or as ordered. Instruct the patient to walk on and handle the wrap carefully to avoid damaging it. Tell him the boot will stiffen but won't be as hard as a cast.
▶ Change the boot weekly, or as ordered, to assess the underlying skin and ulcer healing. Remove the boot by unwrapping the bandage from the knee back to the foot.

## Special considerations
▶ If the boot is applied over a swollen leg, it must be changed as the edema subsides—if necessary, more frequently than every 5 days.

# How to wrap Unna's boot

After cleaning the patient's skin thoroughly, flex his knee. Then, starting with the foot positioned at a right angle to the leg, wrap the medicated gauze bandage firmly, but not tightly, around the patient's foot. Make sure the dressing covers the heel. Continue wrapping upward, overlapping the dressing slightly with each turn. Smooth the boot with your free hand as you go, as shown below.

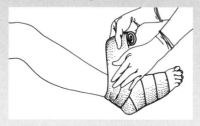

Stop wrapping about 1" (2.5 cm) below the knee. If necessary, make a 2" (5 cm) slit in the boot just below the knee to relieve constriction that may develop as the dressing hardens.

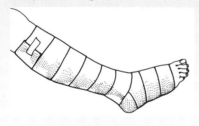

If drainage is excessive, you may wrap a roller gauze dressing over the Unna's boot. As the final layer, wrap an elastic bandage in a figure-eight pattern.

---

▶ Don't make reverse turns while wrapping the bandage. This could create excessive pressure areas that may cause discomfort as the bandage hardens.
▶ For bathing, instruct the patient to cover the boot with a plastic kitchen trash bag sealed at the knee with an elastic bandage to avoid wetting the boot. A wet boot softens and loses it effectiveness. If the patient's safety is a concern, instruct him to take a sponge bath.

## Complications

Contact dermatitis may result from hypersensitivity to Unna's paste.

## Documentation

▶ Record the date and time of application and the presence of a pulse in the affected foot.
▶ Specify which leg you bandaged.
▶ Describe the appearance of the patient's skin before and after boot application.
▶ Name the equipment used (a commercially prepared bandage or Unna's paste and lightweight gauze).
▶ Describe any allergic reaction.

### REFERENCES

Burdette-Taylor, S.R., and Kass, J. "Heel Ulcers in Critical Care Units: A Major Pressure Problem," *Critical Care Nursing Quarterly* 25(2):41-53, August 2002. (Review.)

Edward, D., et al. *Bedside Critical Care Manual.* Philadelphia: Lippincott Williams & Wilkins, 2001.

# Wound dehiscence and evisceration care

Although surgical wounds typically heal without incident, occasionally the edges of a wound may fail to join or may separate after they seem to be healing normally. This development, called wound dehiscence, may lead to an even more serious complication: evisceration, in which a portion of the viscera (usually a bowel loop) protrudes through the incision. Evisceration, in turn, can lead to peritonitis and septic shock. (See *Recognizing dehiscence and evisceration.*)

## Equipment

Two sterile towels ● 1 L of sterile normal saline solution ● sterile irrigation set, including a basin, solution container, and 50-ml catheter-tip syringe ● several large abdominal dressings ● sterile, waterproof drape ● linen-saver pads ● sterile gloves

If the patient will return to the operating room, also gather the following equipment: I.V. administration set and I.V. fluids ● equipment for nasogastric intubation ● preoperative medications as ordered ● suction apparatus.

## Implementation

▶ Provide reassurance and support to ease the patient's anxiety. Tell him to stay in bed. If possible, stay with him while someone else notifies the doctor and collects the necessary equipment.

▶ Place a linen-saver pad under the patient to keep the sheets dry when you moisten the exposed viscera.

▶ Using sterile technique, unfold a sterile towel to create a sterile field. Open the package containing the irrigation set and place the basin, solution container, and 50-ml syringe on the sterile field.

▶ Open the bottle of normal saline solution and pour about 400 ml into the solution container. Also pour about 200 ml into the sterile basin.

▶ Open several large abdominal dressings and place them on the sterile field.

▶ Put on the sterile gloves and place one or two of the large abdominal dressings into the basin to saturate them with saline solution.

▶ Place the moistened dressings over the exposed viscera. Then place a sterile, waterproof drape over the dressings to prevent the sheets from getting wet.

▶ Moisten the dressings every hour by withdrawing saline solution from the container through the syringe and then gently squirting the solution on the dressings.

▶ When you moisten the dressings, inspect the color of the viscera. If it appears dusky or black, notify the doctor immediately. With its blood supply interrupted, a protruding organ may become ischemic and necrotic.

▶ Keep the patient on absolute bed rest in low Fowler's position (elevated no more than 20 degrees) with his knees flexed. This prevents injury and reduces stress on an abdominal incision.

▶ Don't allow the patient to have anything by mouth to decrease the risk of aspiration during surgery.

▶ Monitor the patient's pulse, respirations, blood pressure, and temperature every 15 minutes to detect shock.

▶ If necessary, prepare the patient to return to the operating room.

▶ Continue to reassure the patient while you prepare him for surgery. Make sure that he has signed a consent form and that the operating room staff has been informed about the procedure.

## Recognizing dehiscence and evisceration

In wound dehiscence (top), the layers of the surgical wound separate. In evisceration (bottom), the viscera (in this case, a bowel loop) protrude through the surgical incision.

**WOUND DEHISCENCE**

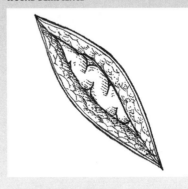

**EVISCERATION OF BOWEL LOOP**

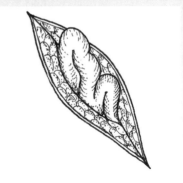

## Special considerations

▶ The best treatment is prevention. If you're caring for a postoperative patient who's at risk for poor healing, make sure he gets an adequate supply of protein, vitamins, and calories. Monitor his dietary deficiencies and discuss any problems with the doctor and the dietitian.

▶ When changing wound dressings, always use sterile technique. Inspect the incision with each dressing change and, if you recognize the early signs of infection, start treatment before dehiscence or evisceration can occur.

## Complications

Infection, which can lead to peritonitis and, possibly, septic shock, is the most severe and most common complication of wound dehiscence and evisceration. Caused by bacterial contamination or by drying of normally moist abdominal contents, infection can impair circulation and lead to necrosis of the affected organ.

## Documentation

▶ Note when the problem occurred, the patient's activity preceding the problem, his condition, and the time the doctor was notified.

▶ Describe the appearance of the wound or eviscerated organ; amount, color, consistency, and odor of any drainage; and nursing actions taken.

▶ Record the patient's vital signs, his response to the incident, and the doctor's actions.

### REFERENCES

Waldhausen, J.H., and Davies, L. "Pediatric Postoperative Abdominal Wound Dehiscence: Transverse Versus Vertical Incisions," *Journal of the American College of Surgeons* 190(6):688-91, June 2000.

Schessel, E.S., et al. "The Management of the Postoperative Disrupted Abdominal Wall," *American Journal of Surgery* 184(3):263-68, September 2002.

# Wound irrigation

Irrigation cleans tissues and flushes cell debris and drainage from an open wound. Irrigation with a commercial wound cleaner helps the wound heal properly from the inside tissue layers outward to the skin surface; it also helps prevent premature surface healing over an abscess pocket or infected tract. Performed properly, wound irrigation requires strict sterile technique. After irrigation, open wounds usually are packed to absorb additional drainage. Always follow the standard precaution guidelines of the Centers for Disease Control and Prevention (CDC).

## Equipment

Waterproof trash bag • linen-saver pad • emesis basin • clean gloves • sterile gloves • goggles • gown, if indicated • prescribed irrigant such as sterile normal saline solution • sterile water or normal saline solution • soft rubber or plastic catheter • sterile container • materials as needed for wound care • sterile irrigation and dressing set • commercial wound cleaner • 35-ml piston syringe with 19G needle or catheter • skin protectant wipe

### Preparation of equipment

Assemble all equipment in the patient's room. Check the expiration date on each sterile package and inspect for tears. Check the sterilization date and the date that each bottle of irrigating solution was opened; don't use any solution that has been open longer than 24 hours.

Using sterile technique, dilute the prescribed irrigant to the correct proportions with sterile water or normal saline solution, if necessary. Let the solution stand until it reaches room temperature, or warm it to 90° to 95° F (32.2° to 35° C).

Open the waterproof trash bag and place it near the patient's bed. Position the bag to avoid reaching across the sterile field or the wound when disposing of soiled articles. Form a cuff by turning down the top of the trash bag to provide a wide opening, which will keep instruments or gloves from touching the bag's edge, thus preventing contamination.

## Implementation

▶ Check the doctor's order and assess the patient's condition. Identify the patient's allergies, especially to povidone-iodine or other topical solutions or medications.

▶ Explain the procedure to the patient, provide privacy, and position the patient correctly for the procedure. Place the linen-saver pad under the patient to catch any spills and avoid linen changes. Place the emesis basin below the wound so that the irrigating solution flows from the wound into the basin.

▶ Wash your hands thoroughly. If necessary, put on a gown to protect your clothing from wound drainage and contamination. Put on clean gloves.

▶ Remove the soiled dressing; then discard the dressing and gloves in the trash bag.

▶ Establish a sterile field with all the equipment and supplies you'll need for irrigation and wound care. Pour the prescribed amount of irrigating solution into a sterile container so you won't contaminate your sterile gloves later by picking up unsterile containers. Put on sterile gloves, gown, and goggles, if indicated.

▶ Fill the syringe with the irrigating solution; then connect the catheter to the syringe. Gently instill a slow, steady stream of irrigating solution into the wound until the syringe empties. (See *Irrigating a deep wound*.) Make sure the solution flows from the clean to the dirty area of the wound to prevent contamination of clean tissue by exudate. Also make sure the solution reaches all areas of the wound.

▶ Refill the syringe, reconnect it to the catheter, and repeat the irrigation.

▶ Continue to irrigate the wound until you've given the prescribed amount of solution or until the solution returns clear. Note the amount of solution given. Then remove and discard the catheter and syringe in the waterproof trash bag.

▶ Keep the patient positioned to allow further wound drainage into the basin.

▶ Clean the area around the wound with normal saline solution; wipe intact skin with a skin protectant wipe and allow it to dry well to help prevent skin breakdown and infection.

▶ Pack the wound, if ordered, and apply a sterile dressing. Remove and discard your gloves and gown.

▶ Make sure the patient is comfortable.

▶ Properly dispose of drainage, solutions, and trash bag and clean or dispose of soiled equipment and supplies according to facility policy and CDC guidelines. To prevent contamination of other equipment, don't return unopened sterile supplies to the sterile supply cabinet.

## Special considerations

▶ Try to coordinate wound irrigation with the doctor's visit so that he can inspect the wound.

▶ Use only the irrigant specified by the doctor because others may be erosive or otherwise harmful. When using an irritating irrigant, such as Dakin's solution, spread sterile petroleum jelly around the wound site to protect the patient's skin.

▶ Remember to follow your facility's policy and CDC guidelines concerning wound and skin precautions.

▶ Irrigate with a bulb syringe if the wound is small or not particularly deep or if a piston syringe is unavailable. However, use a bulb syringe cautiously because this type of syringe doesn't deliver enough pressure to adequately clean the wound.

# Irrigating a deep wound

When preparing to irrigate a wound, attach a 19G needle or catheter to a 35-ml piston syringe. This setup delivers an irrigation pressure of 8 pounds per square inch, which is effective in cleaning the wound and reducing the risk of trauma and wound infection. To prevent tissue damage or, in an abdominal wound, intestinal perforation, avoid forcing the needle or catheter into the wound.

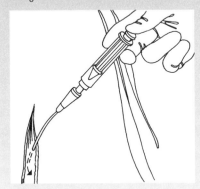

Irrigate the wound with gentle pressure until the solution returns clean. Then position the emesis basin under the wound to collect any remaining drainage.

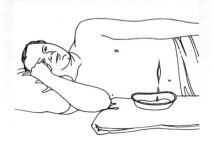

## Home care

If the wound must be irrigated at home, teach the patient or a family member how to perform this procedure using strict aseptic technique. Ask for a return demonstration of the proper technique. Provide written instructions. Arrange for home health supplies and nursing visits, as appropriate. Urge the patient to call the doctor if he detects signs of infection.

## Complications

Wound irrigation increases the risk of infection and may cause excoriation and increased pain. Pressure over 15 psi causes trauma to the wound and directs bacteria back into the tissue.

## Documentation

▶ Record the date and time of irrigation, amount and type of irrigant, appearance of the wound, sloughing tissue or exudate, amount of solution returned, skin care performed around the wound, dressings applied, and patient's tolerance of the treatment.

### REFERENCES

Bansal, B.C., et al. "Tap Water for Irrigation of Lacerations," *American Journal of Emergency Medicine* 20(5):469-72, September 2002.

Marberry, K.M., et al. "Surfactant Wound Irrigation for the Treatment of Staphylococcal Clinical Isolates," *Clinical Orthopaedics* 403:73-79, October 2002.

# 12

# Endocrine and hematologic care

C OLLECTING SPECIMENS PROMPTLY AND CORRECTLY CAN DIRECTLY AFFECT A PATIENT'S DIAG-
nosis, treatment, and recovery. In many cases, the nurse alone is responsible for collecting appropriate specimens. The nurse may have to teach the patient how to perform some procedures at home, for example, blood glucose and fecal occult blood tests.
This chapter contains protocols for managing patients with diabetes mellitus and hypoglycemia, as well as those receiving radioactive iodine therapy. It also describes procedures for bedside glucose and hemoglobin tests, urine glucose and ketone tests, and radioactive iodine therapy.

# Protocols

## Managing the patient receiving radioactive iodine treatment

### Purpose
To provide safe, economical treatment for the patient who must receive radioactive iodine treatment

### Collaborative level
Dependent

### Expected patient outcomes
▶ The patient will display a serum thyroid level within normal limits.
▶ The patient will comply with require-ments to increase treatment effectiveness, especially if therapy is administered on an outpatient basis.

### Definition of terms
▶ *Hyperthyroidism:* A disorder character-ized by overproduction of thyroid hor-mones, which accelerates the body's meta-bolic processes.
▶ *Hypothyroidism:* A disorder character-ized by underproduction of thyroid hor-mones, which slows the body's metabolic processes.
▶ *Myxedema:* A severe form of hypothy-roidism characterized by swelling of the face, hands, and feet.
▶ *Thyroxine:* The major hormone pro-duced by the thyroid gland; it primarily controls the metabolic rate.
▶ *Triiodothyronine:* A thyroid hormone ex-creted in smaller amounts than thyroxine;

among other actions, it helps control the metabolic rate.

### Indications
Treatment
▶ Hyperthyroidism
▶ Thyroid cancer

Prevention
▶ Thyroid crisis
▶ Heart failure

### Assessment guidance
Signs and symptoms
▶ Nervousness
▶ Tremors
▶ Mood swings
▶ Exophthalmos
▶ Goiter
▶ Tachycardia and palpitations
▶ Loose bowel movements
▶ Diaphoresis
▶ Poor coordination
▶ Heat intolerance
▶ Soft, thin hair

Diagnostic studies
*Laboratory tests*
▶ Serum thyroxine test
▶ Serum triiodothyronine test
▶ Triiodothyronine resin uptake test
▶ Thyrotropin-releasing hormone test

*Imaging tests*
▶ Radioactive iodine uptake test

## Nursing interventions
### Outpatient care
▶ Make sure the patient discontinues levothyroxine (Synthroid) 6 weeks before treatment and begins taking liothyronine (Cytomel). Liothyronine has a shorter half-life, which allows it to be discontinued for less time before radioactive iodine therapy.

▶ Stop liothyronine administration 2 weeks before radioactive iodine therapy. This produces a hypothyroid state, which increases iodine uptake.

▶ Ask the female patient if she's pregnant or breast-feeding. Perform a pregnancy test. Instruct her to avoid sexual intercourse until therapy is complete.

▶ Prepare the patient for testing by telling him to consume a low-iodine diet 1 week before treatment. Such a diet eliminates iodized salt, fish, shellfish, dairy products, canned foods, cured meats, white bread, teas, citrus, salty foods, and red dyes.

▶ Perform laboratory tests 2 days before treatment to confirm that the patient is now hypothyroid. Repeat the pregnancy test to confirm that the female patient isn't pregnant.

▶ Prepare the patient for a whole-body radioactive iodine scan, which takes 4 to 6 hours, before radioactive iodine therapy begins.

▶ Refer the patient to a home health program, if needed, to encourage compliance.

### Inpatient care
▶ For inpatient care (usually for those with cancerous thyroid glands), expect the patient to be hospitalized for the first 3 days of therapy.

▶ Place the patient in isolation to protect facility personnel and visitors. Allow only brief visits.

▶ Because all personal items brought to the facility will be destroyed after discharge, encourage the use of puzzles, paperback books, and television. Warn the patient that craft items, stuffed animals, and pillows from home will absorb radiation and can't be allowed in the room.

## Patient teaching
▶ Emphasize the importance of complying with all instructions and precautions. Absolute compliance is necessary for the success of radioactive iodine treatment.

▶ To encourage compliance, provide verbal and written instructions in the patient's language.

▶ Advise the patient to return in 3 days for laboratory tests and a whole-body scan and to return in 6 days for final laboratory tests and a second whole-body scan.

▶ Instruct the patient to drink plenty of water to flush the radioactive isotope out of his system, when appropriate.

▶ Instruct the patient to avoid exposing family members and others to radiation. To do this, advise him to wash his clothing and linens separately from family items. Tell him to wash the sink, toilet, and bathtub or shower after each use. Instruct him to wash his hands with soap and water after toileting, using tissues, or eating, and to dry his hands on a towel only he uses. Encourage him to use disposable dishes and utensils and not taste foods while cooking. Tell the patient to sleep alone and avoid sexual contact. Instruct him to avoid contact with children and pregnant women.

▶ Inform the patient who received outpatient therapy that he should continue radiation precautions until 3 days after the final results of laboratory tests and scans have been received.

▶ Inform the patient who received inpatient therapy that he should continue radiation precautions for 1 month—rather than 3 days—after the final test and scan results are known. The longer precaution period is necessary because inpatient dosages of radioactive iodine are much higher.

## Precautions
▶ Expect to reserve radioactive iodine therapy for middle-aged and elderly patients. Thyroid surgery or antithyroid medications, such as propylthiouracil or methimazole (Tapazole), are more desirable for younger patients.

▶ During radioactive iodine therapy, radiation exposure is a risk for family members or health care workers. Ensure that everyone who comes in contact with the patient or his environment follows radiation precautions.

## Contraindications
Patients who are hypersensitive to iodine or shellfish shouldn't receive iodine therapy because of the possibility of anaphylaxis. Pregnant or breast-feeding patients

shouldn't receive this therapy because the radioactive isotope will damage or destroy the developing thyroid gland of the fetus or child.

## Documentation
▶ Document the results of all baseline and follow-up diagnostic studies.
▶ Record all patient teaching.

## Related procedures
▶ Cardiac monitoring
▶ Electrocardiography
▶ Endotracheal intubation
▶ Indwelling catheter care and removal
▶ Indwelling catheter insertion
▶ Mechanical ventilation
▶ Oral drugs
▶ Peripheral I.V. line insertion
▶ Peripheral I.V. line maintenance
▶ Physical assessment
▶ Radioactive iodine therapy
▶ Standard precautions
▶ Use of isolation equipment
▶ Venipuncture

**REFERENCES**
Apgar, B. "Radioiodine Therapy for Multinodular Goiter," *American Family Physician* 60(9):2680, December 1999.
Christensen, B. *Adult Health Nursing*, 4th ed. Philadelphia: W.B. Saunders Co., 2003.
Nygard, B., et al. "Radioiodine Therapy Multinodular Toxic Goiter," *Archives of Internal Medicine* 159(12):1364, June 1999.

**ORGANIZATIONS**
The Thyroid Society for Education and Research: *www.the-thyroid-society.org*

# Managing the patient with diabetes mellitus

## Purpose
To maintain the patient's blood glucose level within normal limits by balancing food intake with medication and activity

## Collaborative level
Interdependent

## Expected patient outcomes
▶ The patient will maintain a normal blood glucose level by balancing diet, exercise, and medication.
▶ The patient will avoid cardiovascular, renal, and neurologic complications.

## Definition of terms
▶ *Diabetes mellitus:* A complex endocrine disorder characterized by the complete or relative lack of insulin production or by defective insulin receptors.
▶ *Diabetic ketoacidosis* (DKA): An acute complication of type 1 diabetes that occurs when the patient fails to inject sufficient insulin. The body begins breaking down body tissues to try to nourish cells; this produces ketones as a byproduct and leads to acidosis.
▶ *Gestational diabetes:* A form of diabetes that occurs when the body attempts to keep the blood glucose level high to nourish the fetus during pregnancy. It usually subsides after delivery, but may return as type 2 diabetes later.
▶ *Hyperglycemic hyperosmolar nonketotic coma* (HHNC): An acute complication of type 2 diabetes that develops gradually from inadequate treatment. It can cause the blood glucose level to exceed 1,000 mg/dl.
▶ *Hyperlipidemia:* A common complication of diabetes. It produces excessive circulating fats and cholesterol, which lead to vascular lesions that result in sensory deficits (blindness and neuropathy); vascular degeneration that results in nephropathy, peripheral vascular disease, stroke, and myocardial infarction (MI); and retarded healing related to poor tissue perfusion.
▶ *Type 1 diabetes:* A form of diabetes mellitus that requires daily insulin injections and is caused by destruction of beta cells in the pancreas. This destruction may result from a viral infection or trauma. The onset of type 1 diabetes is commonly near puberty.
▶ *Type 2 diabetes:* A form of diabetes mellitus associated with insulin resistance or excessive insulin demand related to excessive calorie intake or stress. Previously thought to be a disease of middle age, type 2 diabetes is known to affect preteens who have a sedentary lifestyle and consume a high-fat, high-carbohydrate diet.

## Indications
Treatment
▶ Blood glucose level above 200 mg/dl

### Prevention
▶ DKA
▶ HHNC
▶ Nephropathy
▶ Renal failure
▶ Stroke
▶ MI
▶ Delayed or incomplete wound healing
▶ Amputation
▶ Blindness
▶ Neuropathy
▶ Peripheral vascular disease

## Assessment guidance
### Signs and symptoms
▶ Recent weight gain or loss
▶ Sluggishness, weakness, and apathy
▶ Cuts or sores that don't heal
▶ Polyphagia (extreme hunger)
▶ Polydipsia (extreme thirst)
▶ Polyuria (frequent urination of large amounts)
▶ Nausea and vomiting or dry heaves
▶ Blurred vision
▶ Signs of dehydration, such as hypotension and dry oral mucosa despite consumption of large quantities of water
▶ Fruity or acetone breath odor
▶ Rapid, deep respirations
▶ Warm, very dry skin
▶ Decreased bowel sounds

### Diagnostic studies
*Laboratory tests*
▶ Blood glucose level
▶ Glycosylated hemoglobin test
▶ Arterial blood gas (ABG) analysis
▶ Fluid and electrolyte levels
▶ Blood osmolality
▶ Urine ketone test
▶ Urinalysis

*Imaging tests*
▶ Electrocardiography (ECG)

## Nursing interventions
### Care related to DKA or HHNC
▶ Notify the patient's doctor.
▶ Administer normal saline solution I.V. until the blood glucose level falls to 200 mg/dl or less; then change I.V. solution to dextrose 5% in water.
▶ Give the patient insulin by I.V. drip. Titrate the flow rate based on the results of hourly bedside glucose monitoring.
▶ Replace electrolytes based on laboratory test results monitored every 2 to 4 hours.

▶ Maintain airway patency and ensure adequate ventilation.
▶ Provide continuous ECG monitoring.
▶ Establish baseline ABG levels and treat imbalances.
▶ Assess the patient's vital signs and urine output hourly.
▶ Observe for signs and symptoms of more serious complications, such as GI bleeding, infection, apnea, and cardiac arrest.
▶ Protect the patient from harming himself—for example, by climbing over the side rails or falling.

### Care related to diabetes mellitus
▶ If the patient isn't in a state of emergency, perform bedside glucose monitoring before each meal and at bedtime; intervene as appropriate based on the glucose level.
▶ If the patient's blood glucose level is elevated at bedtime or if he reports symptoms at night, monitor him and provide treatment during the night also.
▶ Administer all medications based on blood glucose and electrolyte levels.
▶ Treat the disorder that brought the patient to the hospital, such as an infection or cardiac or renal problem.
▶ Provide an appropriate diet such as the one approved by the American Diabetes Association (ADA).
▶ Encourage the patient to provide self-care while you observe as much as possible.
▶ Assess the patient for recent changes in diet, lifestyle, activity, and medications.

## Patient teaching
▶ Teach the patient and his family how the exchange diet works. If needed, refer the patient to a dietitian or other resource who can reinforce dietary teaching. Provide written dietary guidelines for independent use. If the diet seems restrictive, review the wide variety of minimally processed foods the patient can enjoy. Discuss portion control to help the patient control his weight and blood glucose level.
▶ Encourage the patient to follow a regular exercise program to control weight, preserve cardiovascular status, and allow greater food intake. By eating the same and getting the same amount of activity daily, the patient will maintain a more steady blood glucose level.
▶ Instruct the patient with diabetes to wear well-fitting shoes with socks most of the

time. Explain that reduced sensation and poor wound healing can pose risks because the patient may be unaware when he steps on a sharp object. Suggest regular trips to the podiatrist or weekly trips to a reputable salon for a pedicure, which will help protect against foot problems that can lead to amputation.

▶ Have the patient demonstrate his expertise in administering insulin or other antihyperglycemic medications. Give him a sliding scale and ensure that he knows how to use it to adjust his medication according to his daily needs.

▶ Observe the patient performing a needle stick to obtain a blood sample and using the blood glucose monitor that he'll use at home. Reinforce the concept that insulin, other medications, and changes in activity level and stress can cause his blood glucose level to change.

▶ Urge the patient to have his eyes examined by an ophthalmologist annually to help preserve his eyesight. Inform him that prescription lenses may need to be changed more frequently if diabetes is poorly controlled.

▶ Give the patient a doctor-approved protocol for managing sick days. Most doctors encourage the patient to continue routine insulin or medication doses, but to monitor the blood glucose level every 2 hours, to check the urine for ketones, and to notify the doctor if ketones are present or if the glucose level exceeds a certain level.

▶ Suggest that the patient join a support group. The ADA and many facilities have established programs for patients to share information and enhance their compliance with the diabetic regimen.

▶ Teach the patient how to dispose of needles safely to protect his family and sanitation workers.

## Documentation

▶ Record the patient's blood glucose levels and medication administration regularly.

▶ Document the patient's electrolyte levels, fluid intake and output, daily weight, level of consciousness, and cardiac rhythm. If changes occur in these parameters, also note their treatment.

▶ Note all symptoms that the patient reports and all signs detected by physical assessment.

▶ Record the patient's statements about his compliance and noncompliance.

▶ Document your notification of the doctor regarding laboratory test results and subsequent interventions.

▶ Record all patient teaching.

▶ Note the patient's reaction to your teaching to help determine the level of outpatient and home health resources he may need.

## Related procedures

▶ Arterial pressure monitoring
▶ Bedside blood glucose and hemoglobin testing
▶ Blood glucose tests
▶ Cardiac monitoring
▶ Electrocardiography
▶ Endotracheal intubation
▶ I.M. injection
▶ Mechanical ventilation
▶ Oxygen administration
▶ Peripheral I.V. line insertion
▶ Peripheral I.V. line maintenance
▶ Physical assessment
▶ Pulse and ear oximetry
▶ Subcutaneous injection
▶ Urine collection
▶ Urine glucose and ketone tests
▶ Venipuncture

## REFERENCES

Beckman, J., et al. "Diabetes and Atherosclerosis," *JAMA* 287(19):2570, May 2002.

Hoeger, T., et al. "Cost Effectiveness of Interventions for Type 2 Diabetes," *JAMA* 287(19):2542, May 2002.

Rewers, A., et al. "Predictors of Acute Complications in Children with Type 1 Diabetes," *JAMA* 287(19):2511, May 2002.

## ORGANIZATIONS

American Association of Diabetes Educators: *www.aadenet.org*
American Diabetes Association: *www.diabetes.org*
Diabetes Watch: www.*diabeteswatch.com*

# Managing the patient with hypoglycemia

## Purpose
To provide rapid, effective treatment for hypoglycemia; to minimize complications of hypoglycemia and assist in diagnosing its cause

## Collaborative level
Interdependent

## Expected patient outcomes
▶ The patient will maintain airway patency and adequate circulation.
▶ The patient will display no change in neurologic status.
▶ The patient will demonstrate a blood glucose level between 60 and 150 mg/dl.

## Definition of terms
▶ *Hypoglycemia:* A blood glucose level below 60 mg/dl. It may result from uncontrolled diet, inappropriate medication or insulin dosage, cancer, hormonal changes, organ failure, or alcohol or recreational drug use.

## Indications
Treatment
▶ Symptoms of hypoglycemia

Prevention
▶ Seizure
▶ Cardiovascular collapse
▶ Respiratory failure

## Assessment guidance
Signs and symptoms
▶ Irritability
▶ Confusion
▶ Anxiety
▶ Hunger
▶ Tachycardia and palpitations
▶ Blurred vision
▶ Seizures or loss of consciousness
▶ Tremors
▶ Cool, clammy skin
▶ Hypotension

Diagnostic studies
*Laboratory data*
▶ Blood glucose level
▶ Electrolyte levels

## Nursing interventions
▶ Ensure a patent airway.
▶ Administer liquids that contain glucose.
▶ If the patient is alert, give him juice with sugar added, followed by protein and complex carbohydrates to prevent hypoglycemia from recurring in the next hour.
▶ If the patient has a decreased level of conciousness, establish a large-bore I.V. line and administer 50 ml of 50% dextrose as a bolus. If he doesn't regain consciousness in 15 minutes, repeat the bolus of dextrose.
▶ If I.V. access can't be established, administer glucose gel under the patient's tongue or give glucose-rich liquids by nasogastric tube instead of providing the I.V. dextrose solution.
▶ If none of the above interventions is possible, administer glucagon or epinephrine I.M.
▶ Repeat the measurement of the blood glucose level in 1 hour.
▶ Monitor the patient's heart rate, cardiac rhythm, and blood pressure.
▶ Administer a normal saline bolus if hypotension occurs.
▶ Replace electrolytes based on laboratory test results.
▶ Help determine the cause of hypoglycemia by interviewing the patient and reviewing his history. Be sure to inquire about such common causes as poor food intake, medication changes, alcohol or other recreational drug use, hepatic or renal impairment that prevents gluconeogenesis, pancreatic tumor, or an endocrine disorder, including impaired pituitary, thyroid, parathyroid, or adrenal glands.
▶ Be aware that postprandial hypoglycemia may occur with many conditions, but especially after gastric bypass surgery.

## Patient teaching
▶ After determining which factors contributed to this incident of hypoglycemia, help the patient understand how to prevent its recurrence.
▶ Teach the patient to recognize early signs and symptoms of hypoglycemia.
▶ Teach the patient how to use a glucometer at home if a chronic condition may cause hypoglycemia to recur.
▶ Emphasize the importance of having glucose tablets, hard candy, or other food containing simple sugars readily available.

▶ Encourage the patient to wear a medical identification bracelet or necklace or similar identification.

## Documentation

▶ Record the patient's blood glucose level before treatment.
▶ Document the route used to administer glucose.
▶ Note interventions to maintain the patient's airway and circulation.
▶ Document your notification of the doctor.
▶ Record the patient's response to each treatment.
▶ Document all patient teaching.

## Related procedures

▶ Arterial pressure monitoring
▶ Arterial puncture for blood gas analysis
▶ Bedside blood glucose and hemoglobin testing
▶ Blood glucose testing
▶ Buccal, sublingual, and translingual drugs
▶ Cardiac monitoring
▶ Electrocardiography
▶ Endotracheal intubation
▶ I.M. injection
▶ I.V. bolus injection
▶ Indwelling catheter insertion
▶ Mechanical ventilation
▶ Nasogastric tubes
▶ Oxygen administration
▶ Peripheral I.V. line insertion
▶ Peripheral I.V. line maintenance
▶ Physical assessment
▶ Pulse and ear oximetry
▶ Standard precautions
▶ Urine collection
▶ Urine glucose and ketone tests
▶ Venipuncture

## REFERENCES

Coker, R.H., et al. "Prevention of Overt Hypoglycemia During Exercise: Stimulation of Endogenous Glucose Production Independent of Hepatic Catecholamine Action and Changes in Pancreatic Hormone Concentration." *Diabetes* 51(5):1310, May 2002.
Essig, M. "Splitting Evening Doses Reduces Nocturnal Hypoglycemia," *Diabetes Week* 2, June 2002.
Tkacs, N. "Hypoglycemia Awareness: Your Patients with Diabetes Won't Always Know Their Blood Sugar Is Low," *AJN* 102(20):34, February 2002.

## ORGANIZATIONS

The Mayo Clinic: *www.mayoclinic.com*

# Procedures

# Bedside blood glucose and hemoglobin testing

Increasingly, nurses are monitoring blood glucose and hemoglobin (Hb) levels at the patient's bedside. The fast, accurate results obtained this way allow immediate intervention, if necessary. By contrast, blood samples obtained from traditional monitoring methods must be sent to the laboratory for interpretation. A blood sample that sits at room temperature for an hour may undergo glycolysis, which reduces glucose concentration by 3% to 30%, leading to inaccurate test results.

Numerous testing systems are available for bedside monitoring. Bedside systems are also convenient for the patient's home use.

Normal glucose values range from 70 to 100 mg/dl. An above-normal glucose level (hyperglycemia) may indicate diabetes mellitus or the use of steroid drugs. A below-normal glucose level may indicate overly rapid glucose use, which may occur with strenuous exercise or infection, resulting in tissues receiving insufficient glucose.

Normal Hb values range from 12.5 to 15 g/dl. A below-normal Hb value may indicate anemia, recent hemorrhage, or fluid retention, causing hemodilution. An elevated Hb value suggests hemoconcentration from polycythemia or dehydration.

## Equipment

Lancet • microcuvette • photometer • gloves • alcohol pad • gauze pads

## Implementation

▶ Take the equipment to the patient's bedside and explain the test's purpose to him. Tell the patient he'll feel a pinprick in his finger during blood sampling.
▶ Turn the photometer on. If it hasn't been used recently, insert the control cuvette to make sure that the photometer is working properly.
▶ Prepare the photometer according to the manufacturer's directions.
▶ Wash your hands and put on gloves.
▶ Select an appropriate puncture site. You'll usually use a fingertip or an earlobe for an adult. The middle and fourth fingers are the best choices. The second finger is usually the most sensitive, and the thumb may have thickened skin or calluses. Blood should circulate freely in the finger from which you're collecting blood, so avoid using a ring-bearing finger.

◆ **ALERT!** For an infant, use the heel or great toe.

▶ Keep the patient's finger straight and ask him to relax it. Holding his finger between the thumb and index finger of your nondominant hand, gently rock the patient's finger as you move your fingers from his top knuckle to his fingertip. This causes blood to flow to the sampling point.
▶ Use an alcohol pad to clean the puncture site, wiping in a circular motion from the center of the site outward. Dry the site thoroughly with a gauze pad.
▶ Pierce the skin quickly and sharply with the lancet and apply the microcuvette, which automatically collects about 5 µl of blood.
▶ Place the microcuvette into the photometer. Results will appear on the photometer screen in from 40 seconds to 4 minutes.
▶ Place a gauze pad over the puncture site until the bleeding stops.

▶ Dispose of the lancet and microcuvette according to your facility's policy. Take off your gloves and wash your hands. Notify the doctor if the test result is outside the expected parameters.

## Special considerations

▶ Before using a microcuvette, note its expiration date. After the microcuvette vial is opened, the shelf life is 90 days.
▶ Before collecting a blood sample, operate the photometer with the control cuvette to check for proper function. To ensure an adequate blood sample, don't use a cold, cyanotic, or swollen area as the puncture site.

## Documentation

▶ Document the values obtained from the photometer as well as the date and time of the test and any interventions performed.

### REFERENCES

Edward, D., et al. *Bedside Critical Care Manual.* Philadelphia: Lippincott Williams & Wilkins, 2001.
Salardi, S., et al. "The Glucose Area Under the Profiles Obtained with Continuous Glucose Monitoring System Relationships With HbA$_{1c}$ in Pediatric Type 1 Diabetic Patients," *Diabetes Care* 25(10):1840-44, October 2002.

# Blood glucose tests

Rapid, easy-to-perform reagent strip tests (such as Glucostix, Chemstrip bG, and Multistix) use a drop of capillary blood obtained by fingerstick, heelstick, or earlobe puncture as a sample. Newer machines (Free Style and One Touch Ultra) require smaller amounts of blood, so the puncture may be done on the patient's arm. These tests can detect or monitor elevated blood glucose levels in patients with diabetes, screen for diabetes mellitus and neonatal hypoglycemia, and help distinguish diabetic coma from nondiabetic coma. They can be performed in the facility, the doctor's office, or the patient's home.

In blood glucose tests, a reagent patch on the tip of a handheld plastic strip changes color in response to the amount of glucose in the blood sample. Comparing the color change with a standardized color chart provides a semiquantitative measurement of blood glucose levels; inserting the strip in a portable blood glucose meter (such as Accu-Chek Easy and One Touch) provides quantitative measurements that compare in accuracy with other laboratory tests. Some meters store successive test results electronically to help determine glucose patterns.

### Equipment

Reagent strips ● gloves ● portable blood glucose meter, if available ● alcohol pads ● gauze pads ● disposable lancets or mechanical blood-letting device ● small adhesive bandage ● watch or clock with a second hand

### Implementation

▶ Explain the procedure to the patient or the child's parents.
▶ Next, select the puncture site, usually the fingertip or earlobe for an adult or a child.

◆ **ALERT!** Select the heel or great toe for an infant.

▶ Wash your hands and put on gloves.
▶ If necessary, dilate the capillaries by applying warm, moist compresses to the area for about 10 minutes.
▶ Wipe the puncture site with an alcohol pad and dry it thoroughly with a gauze pad.
▶ To collect a sample from the fingertip with a disposable lancet (smaller than 2 mm), position the lancet on the side of the patient's fingertip, perpendicular to the lines of the fingerprints. Pierce the skin sharply and quickly to minimize the patient's anxiety and pain and to increase blood flow. Alternatively, you can use a mechanical blood-letting device such as an Autolet, which uses a spring-loaded lancet.
▶ After puncturing the fingertip, don't squeeze the puncture site to avoid diluting the sample with tissue fluid.
▶ Touch a drop of blood to the reagent patch on the strip; make sure you cover the entire patch.
▶ After collecting the blood sample, briefly apply pressure to the puncture site to prevent painful extravasation of blood into subcutaneous tissues. Ask the adult patient to hold a gauze pad firmly over the puncture site until bleeding stops.

▶ Make sure you leave the blood on the strip for the amount of time required by the glucometer.
▶ If you're using a blood glucose meter, follow the manufacturer's instructions. Meter designs vary, but they all analyze a drop of blood placed on a reagent strip that comes with the unit and provide a digital display of the resulting glucose level.
▶ After bleeding has stopped, you may apply a small adhesive bandage to the puncture site.
▶ In patients experiencing a shock state, consider using blood from an arterial line, because capillary blood may be diluted with interstitial fluid.

### Special considerations

▶ To help detect abnormal glucose metabolism and diagnose diabetes mellitus, the doctor may order other blood glucose tests. (See *Oral and I.V. glucose tolerance tests.*)
▶ Before using reagent strips, check the expiration date on the package and replace outdated strips. Check for special instructions related to the specific reagent. The reagent area of a fresh strip should match the color of the "0" block on the color chart. Protect the strips from light, heat, and moisture.
▶ Before using a blood glucose meter, calibrate it and run it with a control sample to ensure accurate test results. Follow the manufacturer's instructions for calibration.
▶ Avoid selecting cold, cyanotic, or swollen puncture sites to ensure an adequate blood sample. If you can't obtain a capillary sample, perform venipuncture and place a large drop of venous blood on the reagent strip. If you want to test blood from a refrigerated sample, allow the blood to return to room temperature before testing it.

### Home care

If the patient will be using the reagent strip system at home, teach him the proper use of the lancet or Autolet, reagent strips and color chart, and portable blood glucose meter as necessary. Also provide written guidelines.

### Documentation

▶ Record the reading from the reagent strip (using a portable blood glucose meter or a

# Oral and I.V. glucose tolerance tests

For monitoring trends in glucose metabolism, these two tests may offer benefits over blood testing with reagent strips.

## Oral glucose tolerance test

The most sensitive test for detecting borderline diabetes mellitus, the oral glucose tolerance test (OGTT) measures carbohydrate metabolism after ingestion of a challenge dose of glucose. The body absorbs this dose rapidly, causing plasma glucose levels to rise and peak within 30 minutes to 1 hour. The pancreas responds by secreting insulin, causing glucose levels to return to normal within 2 to 3 hours. During this period, plasma and urine glucose levels are monitored to assess insulin secretion and the body's ability to metabolize glucose.

Although you may not collect the blood and urine specimens (usually five of each) required for this test, you are responsible for preparing the patient for the test and monitoring his physical condition during the test.

Begin by explaining the OGTT to the patient. Then tell him to maintain a high-carbohydrate diet for 3 days and to fast for 10 to 16 hours before the test, as ordered. The patient must not smoke, drink coffee or alcohol, or exercise strenuously for 8 hours before the test or during the test. Inform him that he'll then receive a challenge dose of 100 g of carbohydrate (usually a sweetened carbonated beverage or gelatin).

Tell the patient who will perform the venipunctures and when and that he may feel slight discomfort from the needle punctures and the pressure of the tourniquet. Reassure him that collecting each blood sample usually takes less than 3 minutes. As ordered, withhold drugs that may affect test results. Remind him not to discard the first urine specimen voided after waking.

During the test period, watch for signs and symptoms of hypoglycemia — weakness, restlessness, nervousness, hunger, and sweating — and report them to the doctor immediately. Encourage the patient to drink plenty of water to promote adequate urine excretion. Provide a bedpan, urinal, or specimen container when necessary.

## I.V. glucose tolerance test

The I.V. glucose tolerance test may be chosen for patients who can't absorb an oral dose of glucose — for example, those with malabsorption disorders and short-bowel syndrome or those who have had a gastrectomy. This test measures blood glucose after an I.V. infusion of 50% glucose over 3 to 4 minutes. Blood samples are then collected after 30 minutes, 1 hour, 2 hours, and 3 hours. After an immediate glucose peak of 300 to 400 mg/dl (accompanied by glycosuria), the normal glucose curve falls steadily, reaching fasting levels within 1 to 1¼ hours. Failure to achieve fasting glucose levels within 2 to 3 hours typically confirms diabetes.

---

color chart) in your notes or on a special flowchart, if available.
▶ Record the time and date of the test.

## REFERENCES

Hempe, J., et al. "High and Low Hemoglobin Glycation Phenotypes in Type 1 Diabetes. A Challenge for Interpretation of Glycemic Control," *Journal of Diabetes and its Complications* 16(5):313, September-October 2002.

Salardi, S., et al. "The Glucose Area Under the Profiles Obtained with Continuous Glucose Monitoring System Relationships With HbA$_{1c}$ in Pediatric Type 1 Diabetic Patients," *Diabetes Care* 25(10):1840-44, October 2002.

# Radioactive iodine therapy

Because the thyroid gland concentrates iodine, radioactive iodine 131 ($^{131}$I) can be used to treat thyroid cancer. Usually administered orally, this isotope is used to treat postoperative residual cancer, recurrent disease, inoperable primary thyroid tumors, invasion of the thyroid capsule, and thyroid ablation as well as cancers that have metastasized to cervical or mediastinal lymph nodes or other distant sites.

Because $^{131}$I is absorbed systemically, all body secretions, especially urine, must be considered radioactive. For $^{131}$I treatments, the patient usually is placed in a private room (with its own bathroom) located as

## What to do after $^{131}$I treatment

▶ Instruct the patient to report long-term adverse reactions. In particular, review signs and symptoms of hypothyroidism and hyperthyroidism. Also ask him to report signs and symptoms of thyroid cancer, such as enlarged lymph nodes, dyspnea, bone pain, nausea, vomiting, and abdominal discomfort.

▶ Although the patient's radiation level at discharge will be safe, suggest that he take extra precautions during the 1st week, such as using separate eating utensils, sleeping in a separate bedroom, and avoiding bodily contact, especially with infants and children.

▶ Sexual intercourse may be resumed 1 week after iodine 131 ($^{131}$I) treatment. However, urge a female patient to avoid pregnancy for 6 months after treatment and tell a male patient to avoid impregnating his partner for 3 months after treatment.

---

far away from high-traffic areas as practical. Adjacent rooms and hallways may also need to be restricted. Consult your facility's radiation safety policy for specific guidelines.

In lower doses, $^{131}$I also may be used to treat hyperthyroidism. Most patients receive this treatment on an outpatient basis and are sent home with appropriate home care instructions.

### Equipment
Film badges, pocket dosimeters, or ring badges ● RADIATION PRECAUTION sign for door ● RADIATION PRECAUTION warning labels ● waterproof gowns ● clear and red plastic bags for contaminated articles ● plastic wrap ● absorbent plastic-lined pads ● masking tape ● radioresistant gloves ● trash cans ● emergency tracheotomy tray ● optional: portable lead shield

### Preparation of equipment
Assemble all necessary equipment in the patient's room. Keep an emergency tracheotomy tray just outside the room or in a handy place at the nurses' station. Place the RADIATION PRECAUTION sign on the door. Affix warning labels to the patient's chart and Kardex to ensure staff awareness of the patient's radioactive status.

Place an absorbent plastic-lined pad on the bathroom floor and under the sink; if the patient's room is carpeted, cover it with such a pad as well. Place an additional pad over the bedside table. Secure plastic wrap over the telephone, television controls, bed controls, mattress, call button, and toilet. These measures prevent radioactive contamination of working surfaces.

Keep large trash cans in the room lined with plastic bags (two clear bags inserted inside an outer red bag). Monitor all objects before they leave the room.

Notify the dietitian to supply foods and beverages only in disposable containers and with disposable utensils.

### Implementation
▶ Explain the procedure and review treatment goals with the patient and his family. Before treatment begins, review the facility's radiation safety procedures and visitation policies, potential adverse effects, interventions, and home care procedures. (See *What to do after $^{131}$I treatment*.)

▶ Verify that the doctor has obtained informed consent.

▶ Check for allergies to iodine-containing substances, such as contrast media and shellfish. Review the medication history for thyroid-containing or thyroid-altering drugs and for lithium carbonate, which may increase $^{131}$I uptake.

▶ Review the patient's health history for vomiting, diarrhea, productive cough, and sinus drainage, which could increase the risk of radioactive secretions.

▶ If necessary, remove the patient's dentures to avoid contaminating them and to reduce radioactive secretions. Tell him that they'll be replaced 48 hours after treatment.

▶ Affix a RADIATION PRECAUTION warning label to the patient's identification wristband.

▶ Encourage the patient to use the toilet rather than a bedpan or urinal and to flush it three times after each use to reduce radiation levels.

▶ Tell the patient to remain in his room except for tests or procedures. Allow him to ambulate.

▶ Unless contraindicated, instruct the patient to increase his daily fluid intake to 3 qt (2.8 L).

▶ Encourage the patient to chew or suck on hard candy to keep salivary glands stimulated and prevent them from becoming inflamed (which may develop in the first 24 hours).

▶ Ensure that all laboratory tests are performed before beginning treatment. If laboratory work is required, the badged laboratory technician obtains the specimen, labels the collection tube with a RADIATION PRECAUTION warning label, and alerts the laboratory personnel before transporting it. If urine tests are needed, ask the radiation oncology department or laboratory technician how to transport the specimens safely.

▶ Wear a film badge or dosimeter at waist level during the entire shift. Turn in the radiation badge monthly or according to your facility's protocol and record your exposures accurately. Pocket dosimeters measure immediate exposures. These measurements may not be part of the permanent exposure record but help to ensure that nurses receive the lowest possible exposure.

▶ Each nurse must have a personal, nontransferable film badge or ring badge. Badges document each person's cumulative lifetime radiation exposure. Only primary caregivers are badged and allowed into the patient's room.

▶ Wear gloves to touch the patient or objects in his room.

▶ Wear a waterproof gown and gloves when handling the patient's body secretions (for example, when moving his emesis basin).

▶ Allow visitors to stay no longer than 30 minutes every 24 hours with the patient. Stress that no visitors will be allowed who are pregnant or trying to conceive or father a child.

**ALERT!** Visitors younger than age 18 aren't allowed.

▶ Restrict direct contact to no longer than 30 minutes or 20 millirems per day. If the patient is receiving 200 millicuries of $^{131}I$, remain with him only 2 to 4 minutes and stand no closer than 18″ (30.5 cm) away. If standing 38″ (0.9 m) away, the time limit is 20 minutes; if standing 58″ (1.5 m) away, the limit is 30 minutes.

▶ Give essential nursing care only; omit bed baths. If ordered, provide perineal care, making sure that wipes, sanitary pads, and similar items are bagged correctly.

▶ If the patient vomits or urinates on the floor, notify the nuclear medicine depart-

ment and use nondisposable radioresistant gloves when cleaning the floor. After cleanup, wash your gloved hands, remove the gloves and leave them in the room, and then rewash your hands.

▶ If the patient must be moved from his room, notify the appropriate department of his status so that receiving personnel can make appropriate arrangements to receive him. When moving the patient, ensure that the route is clear of equipment and other people and that the elevator, if there is one, is keyed and ready to receive the patient. Move the patient in a bed or wheelchair, accompanied by two badged caregivers. If delayed, stand as far away from him as possible until you can continue.

▶ The patient's room must be cleaned by the radiation oncology department, not by housekeeping. The room must be monitored daily, and disposables must be monitored and removed according to facility guidelines.

▶ At discharge, schedule the patient for a follow-up examination. Also, arrange for a whole-body scan about 7 to 10 days after $^{131}I$ treatment.

▶ Inform the patient and his family of community support services for cancer patients.

## Special considerations

▶ Nurses and visitors who are pregnant or trying to conceive or father a child must not attend or visit patients receiving $^{131}I$ therapy because the gonads and developing embryo and fetus are highly susceptible to the damaging effects of ionizing radiation.

▶ If a code is called on a patient undergoing $^{131}I$ therapy, follow your facility's code procedures as well as the following steps: Notify the code team of the patient's radioactive status to exclude any team member who is pregnant or trying to conceive or father a child. Also, notify the radiation oncology department. Don't allow anything out of the patient's room until it's monitored. The primary care nurse must remain in the room (as far as possible from the patient) to act as a resource person and to provide film badges or dosimeters to code team members.

▶ If the patient dies on the unit, notify the radiology safety officer, who will determine which precautions to follow before postmortem care is provided and before the body can be removed to the morgue.

## Complications

Myelosuppression is common in patients who undergo repeated $^{131}$I treatments. Radiation pulmonary fibrosis may develop if extensive lung metastasis was present when $^{131}$I was administered.

Other complications may include nausea, vomiting, headache, radiation thyroiditis, fever, sialadenitis, and pain and swelling at metastatic sites.

## Documentation

▶ Record radiation precautions taken during treatment, any teaching given to the patient and his family, the patient's tolerance of (and the family's compliance with) isolation procedures, and referrals to local cancer counseling services.

### REFERENCES

Stocker, D.J., et al. "Bilateral External Laryngoceles Following Radioiodine Ablation for Graves Disease," *Archives of Internal Medicine* 162(17):2007-09, September 2002.

Wang, W., et al. "Resistance of [18f]-Fluorodeoxyglucose-avid Metastatic Thyroid Cancer Lesions to Treatment with High-dose Radioactive Iodine," *Thyroid* 11(12): 1169-75, December 2001.

# Urine glucose and ketone tests

Reagent tablet and strip tests are used to monitor urine glucose and ketone levels and to screen for diabetes. Urine glucose tests are less accurate than blood glucose tests and are used less frequently because of the increasing convenience of blood self-testing. Urine ketone tests monitor fat metabolism, help diagnose carbohydrate deprivation and diabetic ketoacidosis, and help distinguish between diabetic and nondiabetic coma.

Glucose oxidase tests (such as Diastix, Tes-Tape, and Clinistix strips) produce color changes when patches of reagents implanted in handheld plastic strips react with glucose in the patient's urine; urine ketone strip tests (such as Keto-Diastix and Ketostix) are similar. All test results are read by comparing color changes with a standardized reference chart.

## Equipment

*For reagent strip test*

Specimen container ● gloves ● glucose or ketone test strip ● reference color chart

## Implementation

▶ Explain the test to the patient and, if he's a newly diagnosed diabetic, teach him how to perform the test himself. Check his history for medications that may interfere with test results.

▶ Before each test, instruct the patient not to contaminate the urine specimen with stool or toilet tissue.

▶ Test the urine specimen immediately after the patient voids.

### Glucose oxidase strip tests

▶ Explain the test to the patient and, if he's diagnosed as diabetic, teach him to perform it himself. Check his history for medications that may interfere with test results. Put on gloves before collecting a specimen for the test and remove them to record test results.

▶ Instruct the patient to void. Ask him to drink a glass of water, if possible, and collect a second-voided specimen after 30 to 45 minutes.

▶ If you're using a *Clinistix* strip, dip the reagent end of the strip into the urine for 2 seconds. Remove excess urine by tapping the strip against the specimen container's rim, wait for exactly 10 seconds, and then compare its color with the color chart on the test strip container. Ignore color changes that occur after 10 seconds. Record the result.

▶ If you're using a *Diastix* strip, dip the reagent end of the strip into the urine for 2 seconds. Tap off excess urine from the strip, wait for exactly 30 seconds, and then compare the strip's color with the color chart on the test strip container. Ignore color changes that occur after 30 seconds. Record the result.

▶ If you're using a *Tes-Tape* strip, pull about 1½" (4 cm) of the reagent strip from the dispenser and dip one end about ¼" (0.5 cm) into the specimen for 2 seconds. Tap off excess urine from the strip, wait exactly 60 seconds, and then compare the darkest part of the tape with the color chart on the dispenser. If the test result exceeds 0.5%, wait an additional 60 seconds and make a final comparison. Record the result.

## Ketone strip tests

▶ Explain the test to the patient and, if he's diagnosed as diabetic, teach him to perform it himself. Check his medication history.

▶ Put on gloves and collect a second-voided midstream specimen.

▶ If you're using a *Ketostix* strip, dip the reagent end of the strip into the specimen and remove it immediately. Wait exactly 15 seconds and then compare the color of the strip with the color chart on the test strip container. Ignore color changes that occur after 15 seconds. Remove and discard your gloves and record the test result.

▶ If you're using a *Keto-Diastix* strip, dip the reagent end of the strip into the specimen and remove it immediately. Tap off excess urine from the strip and hold the strip horizontally to prevent mixing of chemicals between the two reagent squares. Wait exactly 15 seconds and then compare the color of the ketone part of the strip with the color chart on the test strip container. After 30 seconds, compare the color of the glucose part of the strip with the color chart. Remove and discard gloves and record the test results.

## Special considerations

Keep reagent tablets and strips in a cool, dry place at a temperature below 86° F (30° C), but don't refrigerate them. Keep the container tightly closed. Don't use discolored or outdated tablets or strips.

Wear gloves as barrier protection when performing all urine tests.

## Documentation

▶ Record test results according to the information on the reagent containers, or use a flowchart designed to record this information. Indicate whether the doctor was notified of the test results. If you're teaching a patient how to perform the test, keep a record of his progress.

▶ Record any treatment given as a result of the testing.

### REFERENCES

Edward, D., et al. *Bedside Critical Care Manual.* Philadelphia: Lippincott Williams & Wilkins, 2001.

Parikh, C.R., et al. "Screening for Microalbuminuria Simplified by Urine Specific Gravity," *American Journal of Nephrology* 22(4):315-19, July-August 2002.

# Index

*i* refers to an illustration; *t* refers to a table.

*i* refers to an illustration; *t* refers to a table.

*i* refers to an illustration; *t* refers to a table.

*i* refers to an illustration; *t* refers to a table.

*i* refers to an illustration; *t* refers to a table.

*i* refers to an illustration; *t* refers to a table.

*i* refers to an illustration; *t* refers to a table.

*i* refers to an illustration; *t* refers to a table.